T0234599

More information about this series at http://www.springer.com/series/7412

Lecture Notes in Computer Science 9007

Daniel Cremers · Ian Reid
Hideo Saito · Ming-Hsuan Yang (Eds.)

Computer Vision – ACCV 2014

12th Asian Conference on Computer Vision
Singapore, Singapore, November 1–5, 2014
Revised Selected Papers, Part V

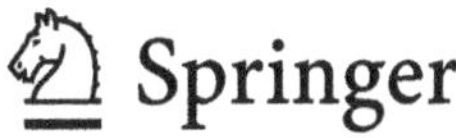

Editors
Daniel Cremers
Technische Universität München
Garching
Germany

Hideo Saito
Keio University
Yokohama, Kanagawa
Japan

Ian Reid
University of Adelaide
Adelaide, SA
Australia

Ming-Hsuan Yang
University of California at Merced
Merced, CA
USA

Videos to this book can be accessed at
http://www.springerimages.com/videos/978-3-319-16813-5

ISSN 0302-9743 ISSN 1611-3349 (electronic)
Lecture Notes in Computer Science
ISBN 978-3-319-16813-5 ISBN 978-3-319-16814-2 (eBook)
DOI 10.1007/978-3-319-16814-2

Library of Congress Control Number: 2015934895

LNCS Sublibrary: SL6 – Image Processing, Computer Vision, Pattern Recognition, and Graphics

Springer Cham Heidelberg New York Dordrecht London

Printed on acid-free paper

Springer International Publishing AG Switzerland is part of Springer Science+Business Media
(www.springer.com)

Preface

ACCV 2014 received a total of 814 submissions, a reflection of the growing strength of Computer Vision in Asia. We note, particularly, that a number of Area Chairs commented very positively on the overall quality of the submissions. The conference had submissions from all continents (except Antarctica, a challenge for the 2016 organizers perhaps) with 64 % from Asia, 20 % from Europe, and 10 % from North America.

The Program Chairs assembled a geographically diverse team of 36 Area Chairs who handled between 20 and 30 papers each. Area Chairs recommended reviewers for papers, and each paper received at least three reviews from the 638 reviewers who participated in the process. Paper decisions were finalized at an Area Chair meeting held in Singapore in September 2014. At this meeting, Area Chairs worked in triples to reach collective decisions about acceptance, and in panels of 12 to decide on the oral/poster distinction. The total number of papers accepted was 227, an overall acceptance rate of 28 %. Of these, 32 were selected for oral presentation.

We extend our immense gratitude to the Area Chairs and Reviewers for their generous participation in the process – the conference would not be possible if it were not for this huge voluntary investment of time and effort. We acknowledge particularly the contribution of 35 reviewers designated as "Outstanding Reviewers" (see page 14 in this booklet for a full list) who were nominated by Area Chairs and Program Chairs for having provided a large number of helpful, high-quality reviews.

The Program Chairs are also extremely grateful for the support, sage advice, and occasional good-natured prompting provided by the General Chairs. Each of them helped with matters that in other circumstances might have been left to the Program Chairs, so that it regularly felt as if we had a team of seven, not four Program Chairs. The PCs are very grateful for this.

Finally, we wish to thank the authors and delegates. Without their participation there would be no conference. The conference was graced with a uniformly high quality of presentations and posters, and we offer particular thanks to the three eminent keynote speakers, Stephane Mallat, Minoru Etoh, and Dieter Fox, who delivered outstanding talks.

Computer Vision in Asia is growing, and the quality of ACCV steadily climbing so that it is now, rightly, considered as one of the top conferences in the field. We look forward to future editions.

November 2014

Daniel Cremers
Ian Reid
Hideo Saito
Ming-Hsuan Yang

Preface

[illegible]

Organization

Organizing Committee

General Chairs

Michael S. Brown	National University of Singapore, Singapore
Tat-Jen Cham	Nanyang Technological University, Singapore
Yasuyuki Matsushita	Microsoft Research Asia, China

Program Chairs

Daniel Cremers	Technische Universität München, Germany
Ian Reid	University of Adelaide, Australia
Hideo Saito	Keio University, Japan
Ming-Hsuan Yang	University of California at Merced, USA

Organizing Chair

Teck Khim Ng	National University of Singapore, Singapore
Junsong Yuan	Nanyang Technological University, Singapore

Workshop Chairs

C.V. Jawahar	IIIT Hyderabad, India
Shiguang Shan	Institute of Computing Technology, Chinese Academy of Sciences, China

Demo Chairs

Bohyung Han	POSTECH, Korea
Koichi Kise	Osaka Prefecture University, Japan

Tutorial Chairs

Chu-Song Chen	Academia Sinica, Tawain
Brendan McCane	University of Otago, New Zealand

Publication Chairs

Terence Sim	National University of Singapore, Singapore
Jianxin Wu	Nanjing University, China

Industry Chairs

Hongcheng Wang	United Technologies Corporation, USA
Brian Price	Adobe, USA
Antonio Robles-Kelly	NITCA, Australia

Steering Committee

In-So Kweon KAIST, Korea
Yasushi Yagi Osaka University, Japan
Hongbin Zha Peking University, China

Honorary Chair

Katsushi Ikeuchi University of Tokyo, Japan

Area Chairs

Lourdes Agapito Queen Mary University of London/University College London, UK
Thomas Brox University of Freiburg, Germany
Tat-Jun Chin University of Adelaide, Australia
Yung-Yu Chuang National Taiwan University, Taiwan
Larry Davis University of Maryland, USA
Yasutaka Furukawa Washington University in St. Louis, USA
Bastian Goldluecke University of Konstanz, Germany
Bohyung Han POSTECH, Korea
Hiroshi Ishikawa Waseda University, Japan
C.V. Jawahar IIIT Hyderabad, India
Jana Kosecka George Mason University, USA
David Kriegman University of California, San Diego, USA
Shang-Hong Lai National Tsing-Hua University, Taiwan
Ivan Laptev Inria Rocquencourt, France
Kyoung Mu Lee Seoul National University, Korea
Vincent Lepetit École Polytechnique Fédérale de Lausanne, Switzerland
Jongwoo Lim Hanyang University, Korea
Simon Lucey CSIRO/University of Queensland, Australia
Ajmal Mian University of Western Australia, Australia
Hajime Nagahara Kyushu University, Japan
Ko Nishino Drexel University, USA
Shmuel Peleg The Hebrew University of Jerusalem, Israel
Imari Sato National Institute of Informatics, Japan
Shin'ichi Satoh National Institute of Informatics, Japan
Stefano Soatto University of California, Los Angeles, USA
Jamie Shotton Microsoft Research, UK
Ping Tan Simon Fraser University, Canada
Lorenzo Torresani Dartmouth College, USA
Manik Varma Microsoft Research, India
Xiaogang Wang Chinese University of Hong Kong, China
Shuicheng Yan National University of Singapore, Singapore
Qing-Xiong Yang City University of Hong Kong, Hong Kong
Jingyi Yu University of Delaware, USA

Junsong Yuan	Nanyang Technological University, Singapore
Hongbin Zha	Peking University, China
Lei Zhang	Hong Kong Polytechnic University, Hong Kong, China

Program Committee Members

Catherine Achard
Hanno Ackermann
Haizhou Ai
Emre Akbas
Naveed Akhtar
Karteek Alahari
Mitsuru Ambai
Dragomir Anguelov
Yasuo Ariki
Chetan Arora
Shai Avidan
Alper Ayvaci
Venkatesh Babu
Xiang Bai
Vineeth Balasubramanian
Jonathan Balzer
Atsuhiko Banno
Yufang Bao
Adrian Barbu
Nick Barnes
John Bastian
Abdessamad Ben Hamza
Chiraz BenAbdelkader
Moshe Ben-Ezra
AndrewTeoh Beng-Jin
Benjamin Berkels
Jinbo Bi
Alberto Del Bimbo
Horst Bischof
Konstantinos Blekas
Adrian Bors
Nizar Bouguila
Edmond Boyer
Steve Branson
Hilton Bristow
Asad Butt
Ricardo Cabral
Cesar Cadena
Francesco Camastra
Xun Cao
Gustavo Carneiro
Joao Carreira
Umberto Castellani
Carlos Castillo
Turgay Celik
Antoni Chan
Kap Luk Chan
Kwok-Ping Chan
Bhabatosh Chanda
Manmohan Chandraker
Sharat Chandran
Hong Chang
Kuang-Yu Chang
Che-Han Chang
Vincent Charvillat
Santanu Chaudhury
Yi-Ling Chen
Yi-Lei Chen
Jieying Chen
Yen-Lin Chen
Kuan-Wen Chen
Chia-Ping Chen
Yi-Ting Chen
Tsuhan Chen
Xiangyu Chen
Xiaowu Chen
Haifeng Chen
Hwann-Tzong Chen
Bing-Yu Chen
Chu-Song Chen
Qiang Chen
Jie Chen
Jiun-Hung Chen
MingMing Cheng
Hong Cheng
Shyi-Chyi Cheng
Yuan Cheng
Wen-Huang Cheng
Jen-Hui Cheng
Liang-Tien Chia
Chen-Kuo Chiang
Shao-Yi Chien
Minsu Cho
Nam Ik Cho
Jonghyun Choi
Wongun Choi
Mario Christoudias
Wen-Sheng Chu
Albert C.S. Chung
Pan Chunhong
Arridhana Ciptadi
Javier Civera
Carlo Colombo
Yang Cong
Sanderson Conrad
Olliver Cossairt
Marco Cristani
Beleznai Csaba
Jinshi Cui
Fabio Cuzzolin
Jeremiah D. Deng
Alessio Del Bue
Fatih Demirci
Xiaoming Deng
Joachim Denzler
Anthony Dick
Julia Diebold
Thomas Diego
Csaba Domokos
Qiulei Dong
Gianfranco Doretto
Ralf Dragon
Bruce Draper
Tran Du
Lixin Duan
Kun Duan
Fuqing Duan

Zoran Duric
Michael Eckmann
Hazim Ekenel
Naoko Enami
Jakob Engel
Anders Eriksson
Francisco Escolano
Virginia Estellers
Wen-Pinn Fang
Micha Feigin
Jiashi Feng
Francesc Ferri
Katerina Fragkiadaki
Chi-Wing Fu
Yun Fu
Chiou-Shann Fuh
Hironobu Fujiyoshi
Giorgio Fumera
Takuya Funatomi
Juergen Gall
Yongsheng Gao
Ravi Garg
Arkadiusz Gertych
Bernard Ghanem
Guy Godin
Roland Goecke
Vladimir Golkov
Yunchao Gong
Stephen Gould
Josechu Guerrero
Richard Guest
Yanwen Guo
Dong Guo
Huimin Guo
Vu Hai
Lin Hai-Ting
Peter Hall
Onur Hamsici
Tony Han
Hu Han
Zhou Hao
Kenji Hara
Tatsuya Harada
Mehrtash Harandi
Jean-Bernard Hayet
Ran He
Shengfeng He
Shinsaku Hiura
Jeffrey Ho
Christopher Hollitt
Hyunki Hong
Ki Sang Hong
Seunghoon Hong
Takahiro Horiuchi
Timothy Hospedales
Kazuhiro Hotta
Chiou-Ting Candy Hsu
Min-Chun Hu
Zhe Hu
Kai-Lung Hua
Gang Hua
Chunsheng Hua
Chun-Rong Huang
Fay Huang
Kaiqi Huang
Peter Huang
Jia-Bin Huang
Xinyu Huang
Yi-Ping Hung
Mohamed Hussein
Cong Phuoc Huynh
Du Huynh
Sung Ju Hwang
Naoyuki Ichimura
Ichiro Ide
Yoshihisa Ijiri
Sei Ikeda
Nazli Ikizler-Cinbis
Atsushi Imiya
Kohei Inoue
Yani Ioannou
Catalin Ionescu
Go Irie
Rui Ishiyama
Yoshio Iwai
Yumi Iwashita
Arpit Jain
Hueihan Jhuang
Yangqing Jia
Yunde Jia
Kui Jia
Yu-Gang Jiang
Shuqiang Jiang
Xiaoyi Jiang
Jun Jiang
Kang-Hyun Jo
Matjaz Jogan
Manjunath Joshi
Frederic Jurie
Ioannis Kakadiaris
Amit Kale
Prem Kalra
George Kamberov
Kenichi Kanatani
Atul Kanaujla
Mohan Kankanhalli
Abou-Moustafa Karim
Zoltan Kato
Harish Katti
Hiroshi Kawasaki
Christian Kerl
Sang Keun Lee
Aditya Khosla
Hansung Kim
Kyungnam Kim
Seon Joo Kim
Byungsoo Kim
Akisato Kimura
Koichi Kise
Yasuyo Kita
Itaru Kitahara
Reinhard Klette
Georges Koepfler
Iasonas Kokkinos
Kazuaki Kondo
Xiangfei Kong
Sotiris Kotsiantis
Junghyun Kown
Arjan Kuijper
Shiro Kumano
Kashino Kunio
Yoshinori Kuno
Cheng-hao Kuo
Suha Kwak
Iljung Kwak
Junseok Kwon
Alexander Ladikos
Hamid Laga

Antony Lam
Francois Lauze
Duy-Dinh Le
Guee Sang Lee
Jae-Ho Lee
Chan-Su Lee
Yong Jae Lee
Bocchi Leonardo
Marius Leordeanu
Matt Leotta
Wee-Kheng Leow
Bruno Lepri
Frederic Lerasle
Fuxin Li
Hongdong Li
Rui Li
Jia Li
Yufeng Li
Yongmin Li
Yung-Hui Li
Cheng Li
Xin Li
Peihua Li
Xirong Li
Annan Li
Xi Li
Chia-Kai Liang
Shu Liao
T. Warren Liao
Jenn-Jier Lien
Joseph Lim
Ser-Nam Lim
Huei-Yung Lin
Haiting Lin
Weiyao Lin
Wen-Chieh (Steve) Lin
Yen-Yu Lin
RueiSung Lin
Yuanqing Lin
Yen-Liang Lin
Haibin Ling
Hairong Liu
Cheng-Lin Liu
Qingzhong Liu
Miaomiao Liu
Jingchen Liu
Ligang Liu
Haowei Liu
Guangcan Liu
Feng Liu
Shuang Liu
Shuaicheng Liu
Xiaobai Liu
Si Liu
Lingqiao Liu
Chen Change Loy
Feng Lu
Tong Lu
Zhaojin Lu
Le Lu
Huchuan Lu
Ping Luo
Lui Luoqi
Ludovic Macaire
Arif Mahmood
Robert Maier
Yasushi Makihara
Koji Makita
Yoshitsugu Manabe
Rok Mandeljc
Al Mansur
Gian-Luca Marcialis
Stephen Marsland
Takeshi Masuda
Thomas Mauthner
Stephen Maybank
Chris McCool
Xing Mei
Jason Meltzer
David Michael
Anton Milan
Gregor Miller
Dongbo Min
Ikuhisa Mitsugami
Anurag Mittal
Daisuke Miyazaki
Henning Müller
Thomas Moellenhoff
Pascal Monasse
Greg Mori
Bryan Morse
Yadong Mu
Yasuhiro Mukaigawa
Jayanta Mukhopadhyay
Vittorio Murino
Atsushi Nakazawa
Myra Nam
Anoop Namboodiri
Liangliang Nan
Loris Nanni
P.J. Narayanan
Shawn Newsam
Thanh Ngo
Bingbing Ni
Jifeng Ning
Masashi Nishiyama
Mark Nixon
Shohei Nobuhara
Vincent Nozick
Tom O'Donnell
Takeshi Oishi
Takahiro Okabe
Ryuzo Okada
Takayuki Okatani
Gustavo Olague
Martin Oswald
Wanli Ouyang
Yuji Oyamada
Paul Sakrapee Paisitkriangkrai
Kalman Palagyi
Hailang Pan
Gang Pan
Sharath Pankanti
Hsing-Kuo Pao
Hyun Soo Park
Jong-Il Park
Ioannis Patras
Nick Pears
Helio Pedrini
Pieter Peers
Yigang Peng
Bo Peng
David Penman
Janez Pers
Wong Ya Ping
Hamed Pirsiavash
Robert Pless
Dilip Prasad
Dipti Prasad Mukherjee
Andrea Prati

Vittal Premachandran
Brian Price
Oriol Pujol Pujol
Pulak Purkait
Zhen Qian
Xueyin Qin
Bogdan Raducanu
Luis Rafael Canali
Visvanathan Ramesh
Ananth Ranganathan
Nalini Ratha
Edel Garcia Reyes
Hamid Rezatofighi
Christian Riess
Antonio Robles-Kelly
Mikel Rodriguez
Olaf Ronneberger
Guy Rosman
Arun Ross
Amit Roy Chowdhury
Xiang Ruan
Raif Rustamov
Fereshteh Sadeghi
Satoshi Saga
Ryusuke Sagawa
Fumihiko Sakaue
Mathieu Salzmann
Jorge Sanchez
Nong Sang
Pramod Sankar
Angel Sappa
Michel Sarkis
Tomokazu Sato
Yoichi Sato
Jun Sato
Harpreet Sawhney
Walter Scheirer
Bernt Schiele
Frank Schmidt
Dirk Schnieders
William Schwartz
McCloskey Scott
Faisal Shafait
Shishir Shah
Shiguang Shan
Li Shen
Chunhua Shen
Xiaohui Shen
Shuhan Shen
Sanketh Shetty
Boxin Shi
YiChang Shih
Huang-Chia Shih
Atsushi Shimada
Nobutaka Shimada
Ilan Shimshoni
Koichi Shinoda
Abhinav Shrivastava
Xianbiao Shu
Gautam Singh
Sudipta Sinha
Eric Sommerlade
Andy Song
Li Song
Yibing Song
Mohamed Souiai
Richard Souvenir
Frank Steinbruecker
Ramanathan Subramanian
Yusuke Sugano
Akihiro Sugimoto
Yasushi Sumi
Yajie Sun
Weidong Sun
Xiaolu Sun
Deqing Sun
Min Sun
Ju Sun
Jian Sun
Ganesh Sundaramoorthi
Jinli Suo
Rahul Swaminathan
Yuichi Taguchi
Yu-Wing Tai
Taketomi Takafumi
Jun Takamatsu
Hugues Talbot
Toru Tamaki
Xiaoyang Tan
Robby Tan
Masayuki Tanaka
Jinhui Tang
Ming Tang
Kevin Tang
João Manuel R.S. Tavares
Mutsuhiro Terauchi
Ali Thabet
Eno Toeppe
Matt Toews
Yan Tong
Akihiko Torii
Yu-Po Tsai
Yi-Hsuan Tsai
Matt Turek
Seiichi Uchida
Hideaki Uchiyama
Toshio Ueshiba
Norimichi Ukita
Julien Valentin
Pascal Vasseur
Ashok Veeraraphavan
Matthias Vestner
Xiaoyu Wang
Dong Wang
Ruiping Wang
Sheng-Jyh Wang
Shenlong Wang
Lei Wang
Song Wang
Xianwang Wang
Yang Wang
Yunhong Wang
Yu-Chiang Frank Wang
Hanzi Wang
Hongcheng Wang
Chaohui Wang
Chen Wang
Cheng Wang
Changhu Wang
Li-Yi Wei
Longyin Wen
Gordon Wetzstein
Paul Wohlhart
Chee Sun Won
Kwan-Yee Kenneth Wong
John Wright
Jianxin Wu

Xiao Wu
Yi Wu
Xiaomeng Wu
Rolf Wurtz
Tao Xiang
Yu Xiang
Yang Xiao
Ning Xu
Li Xu
Changsheng Xu
Jianru Xue
Mei Xue
Yasushi Yagi
Koichiro Yamaguchi
Kota Yamaguchi
Osamu Yamaguchi
Toshihiko Yamasaki
Takayoshi Yamashita
Pingkun Yan
Keiji Yanai
Jie Yang
Ruigang Yang
Ming Yang
Hao Yang
Meng Yang
Xiaokang Yang
Yi Yang
Yongliang Yang
Jimei Yang
Chih-Yuan Yang
Bangpeng Yao
Jong Chul Ye
Mao Ye
Sai Kit Yeung
Kwang Moo Yi
Alper Yilmaz
Zhaozheng Yin
Xianghua Ying
Ryo Yonetani
Ju Hong Yoon
Kuk-Jin Yoon
Lap Fai Yu
Gang Yu
Xenophon Zabulis
John Zelek
Zheng-Jun Zha
De-Chuan Zhan
Kaihua Zhang
Tianzhu Zhang
Yu Zhang
Zhong Zhang
Yinda Zhang
Xiaoqin Zhang
Liqing Zhang
Xiaobo Zhang
Changshui Zhang
Cha Zhang
Hong Hui Zhang
Hui Zhang
Guofeng Zhang
Xiao-Wei Zhao
Rui Zhao
Gangqiang Zhao
Shuai Zheng
Yinqiang Zheng
Zhonglong Zheng
Weishi Zheng
Wenming Zheng
Lu Zheng
Baojiang Zhong
Lin Zhong
Bolei Zhou
Jun Zhou
Feng Zhou
Feng Zhu
Ning Zhu
Pengfei Zhu
Cai-Zhi Zhu
Zhigang Zhu
Andrew Ziegler
Danping Zou
Wangmeng Zuo

Best Paper Award Committee

James Rehg	Georgia Institute of Technology, USA
Horst Bischof	Graz University of Technology, Austria
Kyoung Mu Lee	Seoul National University, South Korea

Best Paper Awards

1. Saburo Tsuji Best Paper Award

A Message Passing Algorithm for MRF inference with Unknown Graphs and Its Applications
Zhenhua Wang (University of Adelaide), Zhiyi Zhang (Northwest A&F University), Geng Nan (Northwest A&F University)

2. Sang Uk Lee Best Student Paper Award [Sponsored by Nvidia]

Separation of Reflection Components by Sparse Non-negative Matrix Factorization
Yasuhiro Akashi (Tohoku University), Takayuki Okatani (Tohoku University)

3. Songde Ma Best Application Paper Award [Sponsored by NICTA]

Stereo Fusion using a Refractive Medium on a Binocular Base
Seung-Hwan Baek (KAIST), Min H. Kim (KAIST)

4. Best Paper Honorable Mention

Singly-Bordered Block-Diagonal Form for Minimal Problem Solvers
Zuzana Kukelova (Czech Technical University, Microsoft Research Cambridge), Martin Bujnak (Capturing Reality), Jan Heller (Czech Technical University), Tomas Pajdla (Czech Technical University)

5. Best Student Paper Honorable Mention [Sponsored by Nvidia]

On Multiple Image Group Cosegmentation
Fanman Meng (University of Electronic Science and Technology of China), Jianfei Cai (Nanyang Technological University), Hongliang Li (University of Electronic Science and Technology of China)

6. Best Application Paper Honorable Mention [Sponsored by NICTA]

Massive City-scale Surface Condition Analysis using Ground and Aerial Imagery
Ken Sakurada (Tohoku University), Takayuki Okatani (Tohoku Univervisty), Kris Kitani (Carnegie Mellon University)

ACCV 2014 – Outstanding Reviewers

Emre Akbas
Jonathan Balzer
Steve Branson
Sanderson Conrad
Marco Cristani
Alessio Del Bue
Anthony Dick
Bruce Draper
Katerina Fragkiadaki
Tatsuya Harada
Mehrtash Harandi
Nazli Ikizler-Cinbis
Catalin Ionescu
Suha Kwak
Junseok Kwon
Fuxin Li
Chen-Change Loy
Scott McCloskey
Xing Mei
Yasushi Makihara
Guy Rosman
Mathieu Salzmann
Pramod Sankar
Walter Scheirer
Bernt Schiele
Chunhua Shen
Sudipta Sinha
Deqing Sun
Yuichi Taguchi
Toru Tamaki
Dong Wang
Yu-Chiang Frank Wang
Paul Wohlhart
John Wright
Bangpeng Yao

ACCV 2014 Sponsors

Platnium	Singapore Tourism Board
Gold	Omron Nvidia Garena Samsung
Silver	Adobe ViSenze
Bronze	Lee Foundation Morpx Microsoft Research NICTA

Contents – Part V

Poster Session 3

Improving Human Action Recognition Using Score Distribution and Ranking

Minh Hoai[1,2(✉)] and Andrew Zisserman[1]

[1] Visual Geometry Group, Department of Engineering Science, University of Oxford, Oxford, UK
minhhoai@cs.stonybrook.edu

[2] Department of Computer Science, Stony Brook University, Stony Brook, NY, USA

Abstract. We propose two complementary techniques to improve the performance of action recognition systems. The first technique addresses the temporal interval ambiguity of actions by learning a classifier score distribution over video subsequences. A classifier based on this score distribution is shown to be more effective than using the maximum or average scores. The second technique learns a classifier for the relative values of action scores, capturing the correlation and exclusion between action classes. Both techniques are simple and have efficient implementations using a Least-Squares SVM. We demonstrate that taken together the techniques exceed the state-of-the-art performance by a wide margin on challenging benchmarks for human actions.

1 Introduction

Action recognition is an active research area. Recent research focuses on realistic datasets collected from TV shows [1], movies [2,3], and web videos [3]. However, there exists an inherent ambiguity for actions in realistic data: when does an action begin and end? Consider the action "handshake." When is the precise moment that two people begin to shake hands? When they start extending their hands or when the two hands are in contact? Moreover, when does the action end? For TV shows and movies, this is even more difficult to determine due to the existence of shot boundaries. Should we consider the action has ended when the camera cuts to a different shot? What if the action extends over multiple shots? Many works in action recognition ignore this temporal ambiguity problem, and simply classify the entire video clip, e.g., [1–4]. However, as shown in [5,6], refining the temporal extent of actions can improve the recognition performance.

So, how should we handle this ambiguity? A possible approach is to treat the temporal extent of an action as a latent variable (e.g., [7–11]) and embed the problem in a Multiple Instance Learning (MIL) framework such as [12,13]. MIL [14] is a generalization of supervised classification in which class labels are associated with sets of samples (called bags) instead of individual samples (called instances). For action recognition, a bag is a video clip, and the instances in each bag can be generated by varying the temporal extent of sequences within the clip (e.g., all subsequences of a video).

D. Cremers et al. (Eds.): ACCV 2014, Part V, LNCS 9007, pp. 3–20, 2015.
DOI: 10.1007/978-3-319-16814-2_1

However, the efficacy of MIL for solving the temporal ambiguity of action in video is unproven. Moreover, the underlying assumptions and design principles of MIL are often violated. For example, the MIL algorithms of [15,16] implicitly assume that instances are drawn i.i.d. (independently and identically distributed) from some distribution and randomly placed into bags. This is not valid for action recognition where there exist temporal correlation between subsequences of a video. Another basic assumption of MIL is that a bag is positive if at least one of its instances is positive. This leads to a practical procedure adopted by most MIL algorithms (e.g., MI-SVM [12]): an instance classifier is learned (or iteratively learned) and the maximum classifier score is used to find the positive instance of a bag (for prediction during testing or for iterative update during training). In practice using only the maximum score is not robust, especially in action recognition where the state-of-the-art classifiers are far from perfect [4].

Empirical evidence also suggests the inadequacy of using the maximum subsequence score for video classification. In many test cases of our experiments, which will be seen in Sect. 5, we observe that using the average score of video subsequences is better than using the maximum score. In another context of MIL beyond action recognition, this observation has also been reported [17]. For example, [18] observed that MIL algorithms could be outperformed by a simple approach that used supervised learning together with label inheritance, which simply assigned the bag label to its instances.

On the other hand, the mean is not always better than the max. The mean works well when the influence of negative instances in positive bags is low. This does not hold if the percentage of positive instances in a positive bag is small. In that situation, the mean score is inferior to the maximum score, which will be empirically confirmed in Sects. 3.2 and 5. Note, if we consider the instances of a bag as the output of a generative process with a latent variable, the comparison between the max and the mean is equivalent to the comparison between the maximum and marginal likelihoods. Others have used measures between the mean and the max, or defined set kernels for bags of multiple instances [19–27].

In this paper, we propose to use the *distribution* of classifier scores, rather than just the max or mean, to improve action recognition. We first train a base classifier and then use the scores of *all* subsequences of a video clip to predict its label (Fig. 1(a)). The scores of video subsequences are ordered and combined using a weight vector, which can be learned from the same set of training data that is used to train the base classifier. We will show that the ordered score distribution preserves more information than both extreme (i.e., max) and summary (i.e., mean) statistics, and it is more effective in practice.

Complementary to using the score distribution, this paper addresses another fundamental drawback of many current action recognition systems that action classes are recognized independently. In the second part of the paper, we propose an approach to learn the correlation and exclusion between action classes. In particular, we learn a classifier that reweights the action score based on the ordered scores of other classes, as illustrated in Fig. 1(b).

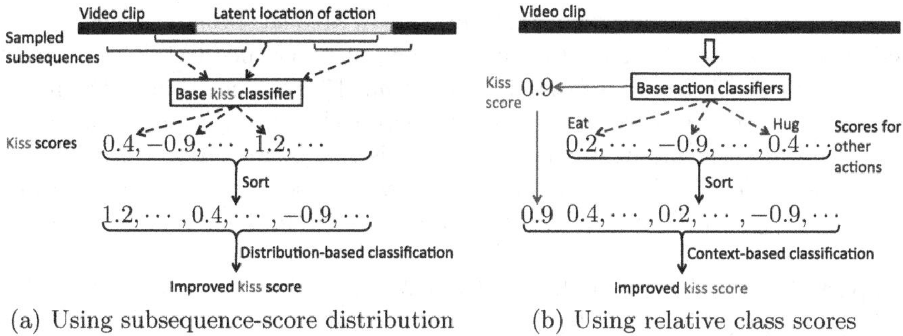

(a) Using subsequence-score distribution (b) Using relative class scores

Fig. 1. Complementary techniques to improve recognition performance. (a): improved action score is computed based on the score distribution of video subsequences. (b): an improved action score is computed based on the relative action scores

The rest of this paper is structured as follows. Section 2 reviews related prior work. Section 3 shows that using the score distribution is more effective than using the maximum and average scores (and shed some light on the poor performance of using maximum score for action recognition and MIL in general). Section 4 presents a learning formulation to capture the correlation and exclusion of the actions to improve the performance of action classifiers. Section 5.1 details the experimental setup on Hollywood2, TVHI, and HMDB51, which are among the most challenging datasets for human action recognition. Section 5.1 also describes another technical contribution of our work, which is the use of data augmentation to obtain stronger performance. Since a video and its left-right mirrored video depict the same action, we propose to learn a classifier that is invariant to flipping by data augmentation. This is related to several works that use virtual samples [28,29]. Section 5.2 demonstrates that our proposed techniques significantly improve the state-of-the-art performance. This is achieved using standard, publicly available, features and encodings.

2 Reviews of Related Work and Least-Squares SVM

The need for considering the temporal extent of actions in training or testing has been studied before. Duchenne *et al.* [6] and Satkin & Hebert [5] observed that temporal boundaries of actions in training videos are not precisely defined in practice. They proposed methods to crop training videos using discriminative clustering and cross-validation performance. Nowozin *et al.* [30] and Nguyen *et al.* [31] presented algorithms that sought discriminative subsequences in video. Yuan *et al.* [32] proposed a branch-and-bound algorithm for 3D bounding-box cropping, by maximizing the mutual information of features and actions. Hoai *et al.* [33] performed joint segmentation and classification. Gaidon *et al.* [34] learned actoms for modeling and localizing actions. Accurate temporal localization, however, is not a focus of this paper. Instead, our effort is to improve the classifier performance based on the distribution of classification scores.

The inadequacy of using the maximum score in MIL has been observed before. Cheung & Kwok [35] suggested combining bag and instance feature vectors to improve the classification performance. Hu *et al.* [17] considered both the maximum and the average scores, and reported better classification performance for the average score in many experiments. In this paper, we propose to consider the classifier scores of all instances instead. It will be seen that the distribution-based decision is more effective than both the extreme (max) and summary (mean) statistics.

A part of this work is related to Ordered Weighted Averaging (OWA) [36,37], which is an aggregation operator for multiple criteria. Our work is also based on ranking and aggregation, but it considers a single criterion of multiple instances instead. There are also some multiple instance learning formulations that use OWA or a similar fusion operator [38,39].

High-level representation from the outputs of multiple classifiers have been shown to help object detection and image classification. Aytar *et al.* [40] combined the outputs of multiple concept detectors to improve retrieval results. Rabinovich *et al.* [41] incorporated semantic object context to improve a categorization model. Torresani *et al.* [42], Li *et al.* [43], and Sadanand & Corso [44] proposed classemes, object bank, and action bank, respectively, which are generic classifiers for generating high-level feature vectors. Bourdev *et al.* [45] obtained attribute classifiers from poselet outputs. Song *et al.* [46] proposed Context-SVM that provided mutual benefits for object detection and image classification. Felzenszwalb *et al.* [13] re-scored a detector based on the scores and locations of multiple detectors. Unlike the aforementioned approaches that consider a fixed order of classifiers, our methods ground the decisions on the distribution and ordering of action scores. As will be seen, this is crucial for action recognition.

Least-Squares SVM. We propose to use Least-Squares Support Vector Machines (LSSVM) [47]. LSSVM, also known as kernel Ridge regression [48], has been shown to perform equally well as SVM in many classification benchmarks [49]. LSSVM has a closed-form solution, which is a computational advantage over SVM. Furthermore, once the solution of LSSVM has been computed, the solution for a reduced training set obtaining by removing any training data point can found efficiently. This enables reusing training data for further calibration (e.g., used in [50,51]). This section reviews LSSVM and the leave-one-sample-out formula.

Given a set of n data points $\{\mathbf{x}_i | \mathbf{x}_i \in \Re^d\}_{i=1}^n$ and associated labels $\{y_i | y_i \in \{1, -1\}\}_{i=1}^n$, LSSVM optimizes the following:

$$\underset{\mathbf{w},b}{\text{minimize}} \ \lambda ||\mathbf{w}||^2 + \sum_{i=1}^{n} (\mathbf{w}^T \mathbf{x}_i + b - y_i)^2. \tag{1}$$

For high dimensional data ($d \gg n$), it is more efficient to obtain the solution for $(\mathbf{w}, b)$ via the representer theorem, which states that $\mathbf{w}$ can be expressed as a linear combination of training data, i.e., $\mathbf{w} = \sum_{i=1}^n \alpha_i \mathbf{x}_i$. Let $\mathbf{K}$ be the kernel matrix, $k_{ij} = \mathbf{x}_i^T \mathbf{x}_j$. The optimal coefficients $\{\alpha_i\}$ and the bias term b can be found using closed-form formula: $[\boldsymbol{\alpha}^T, b]^T = \mathbf{M}\mathbf{y}$. Where $\mathbf{M}$ and other auxiliary variables are defined as:

$$\mathbf{R} = \begin{bmatrix} \lambda\mathbf{K} & \mathbf{0}_n \\ \mathbf{0}_n^T & 0 \end{bmatrix}, \mathbf{Z} = \begin{bmatrix} \mathbf{K} \\ \mathbf{1}_n^T \end{bmatrix}, \mathbf{C} = \mathbf{R} + \mathbf{Z}\mathbf{Z}^T, \mathbf{M} = \mathbf{C}^{-1}\mathbf{Z}, \mathbf{H} = \mathbf{Z}^T\mathbf{M}. \quad (2)$$

If $\mathbf{x}_i$ is removed from the training data, the optimal coefficients can be computed:

$$\begin{bmatrix} \boldsymbol{\alpha}_{(i)} \\ b_{(i)} \end{bmatrix} = \begin{bmatrix} \boldsymbol{\alpha} \\ b \end{bmatrix} + \left(\frac{[\boldsymbol{\alpha}^T \ b]\mathbf{z}_i - y_i}{1 - h_{ii}} \right) \mathbf{m}_i. \quad (3)$$

Here, $\mathbf{z}_i$ is the ith column vector of $\mathbf{Z}$ and h_{ii} is the ith element in the diagonal of $\mathbf{H}$. Note that $\mathbf{R}, \mathbf{Z}, \mathbf{C}, \mathbf{M}$, and $\mathbf{H}$ are independent of the label vector $\mathbf{y}$. Thus, training LSSVMs for multiple classes is efficient as these matrices need to be computed once. A more gentle derivation of the above formula is given in [52].

3 Subsequence-Score Distribution (SSD)

To handle the ambiguity of the temporal extent of an action in a video clip, we sample subsequences of the video clip at multiple locations and scales. We compute the improved action score for the video clip based on the score distribution of the subsequences.

3.1 Formulation

Assume we have learned a base classifier for a particular action. Given a video clip $\mathbf{x}$, we sample l subsequences $\mathbf{x}^1 \cdots \mathbf{x}^l$ of $\mathbf{x}$ with replacement, compute their action scores, and sort the scores in descending order to obtain a vector $\mathbf{d}$, i.e., $\mathbf{d} = [sort(f(\mathbf{x}^1), \cdots, f(\mathbf{x}^l))]^T$. Here, *sort* is the function that reorders the inputs in descending order. With a sufficiently large l, $\mathbf{d}$ represents the score distribution of subsequences from $\mathbf{x}$. In practice, for computational efficiency, it is unnecessary to sample from the set of all video subsequences because of strong temporal correlation between nearby frames. We therefore restrict our consideration to a subset of video subsequences. In particular, we divide a video clip into several intervals, and only consider the subsequences that can be obtained by concatenating a set of adjacent intervals. For example, if a video is divided into 10 intervals, then there are $l = 55$ possible subsequences. Details of how a video is divided into intervals and the number of subsequences are given in Sect. 5.1.

Given n video clips $\{\mathbf{x}_i\}_{i=1}^n$, each represented by the distribution feature vector $\mathbf{d}_i$, we learn an SSD classifier by optimizing the following objective:

$$\underset{\mathbf{s}, b}{\text{minimize}} \sum_{i=1}^{n} \max(1 - y_i(\mathbf{s}^T \mathbf{d}_i + b), 0) \quad (4)$$

$$\text{s.t.} \sum_{j=1}^{l} s_j = 1, \text{and } s_1 \geq s_2 \geq \cdots \geq s_l \geq 0. \quad (5)$$

The above optimization problem seeks a weight vector $\mathbf{s}$ and the bias term b for separating between score distribution vectors of positive and negative data. The objective in Eq. (4) is the sum of Hinge losses, as used in the standard SVM objective. Constraint (5) requires the weights to be non-negative, monotonic, and have unit sum. Recall that $\mathbf{d}_i$ are classification scores sorted in descending order. The weights should be non-negative and monotonic to emphasize the relative importance of higher classification scores. The weights should have unit sum because we are learning the weights for score distributions. The feasible set of $\mathbf{s}$ subsumes two special cases:

1. $s_1 = 1, s_2 = \cdots = s_l = 0$. This corresponds to using the maximum score.
2. $s_1 = s_2 \cdots = s_l = \frac{1}{l}$. This corresponds to using the average score.

The optimization problem (4) is linear. It can be efficiently solved by any linear programming tool, e.g., Cplex[1]. Once $\mathbf{s}, b$ have been learned, we compute the improved recognition score for a test video $\mathbf{x}$ as follows. First, sample l subsequences $\mathbf{x}^1, \cdots, \mathbf{x}^l$ of $\mathbf{x}$. The improved classifier is defined as: $f^*(\mathbf{x}) = \mathbf{s}^T[sort(f(\mathbf{x}^1), \cdots, f(\mathbf{x}^l))]^T + b$. This technique is illustrated in Fig. 1(a).

The same set of training data can be used to learn the base classifier f and the improved classifier f^*. To avoid overfitting, we compute $\mathbf{d}_i$ using the leave-one-out versions of f. Let f' be the base classifier by removing $\mathbf{x}_i$ from the training data, $\mathbf{d}_i = [sort(f'(\mathbf{x}_i^1), \cdots, f'(\mathbf{x}_i^l))]^T$. If LSSVM is used, the leave-one-out classifiers can be computed efficiently with closed form formula, as shown in Sect. 2. Nevertheless, the technique proposed here can be applied to any type of classifiers.

3.2 Controlled Experiments on Synthetic Data

When would it be beneficial to use SSD and how much improvement should we expect? To answer this question, we perform a set of controlled experiments on synthetic data. We vary two important factors that affect the difficulty of action recognition: (i) the separation between positive and negative descriptors; and (ii) the proportion of the target action in each video clip.

We generate 200 positive and 2000 negative video clips, half of them are used for training and half for testing. Each positive video contains the action of interest, however, only a portion of the video depicts the action. The percentage of the video that corresponds to the action is a controlled parameter of the experiment, which will be referred as the *action percentage*. For simplicity, we assume the action part is contiguous, and its location is randomly distributed. Each video is represented by a sequence of 1000 synthetic descriptors; these descriptors are analogous to dense trajectory descriptors for real videos [4] (explained in Sect. 5.1). Negative descriptors (for negative videos or outside the non-action parts of positive videos) are generated from a 10-dimensional Normal distribution. Positive descriptors (for the action parts of positive videos) are also generated from a 10-dimensional Normal distribution, except for the

[1] http://www-01.ibm.com/software/commerce/optimization/cplex-optimizer/.

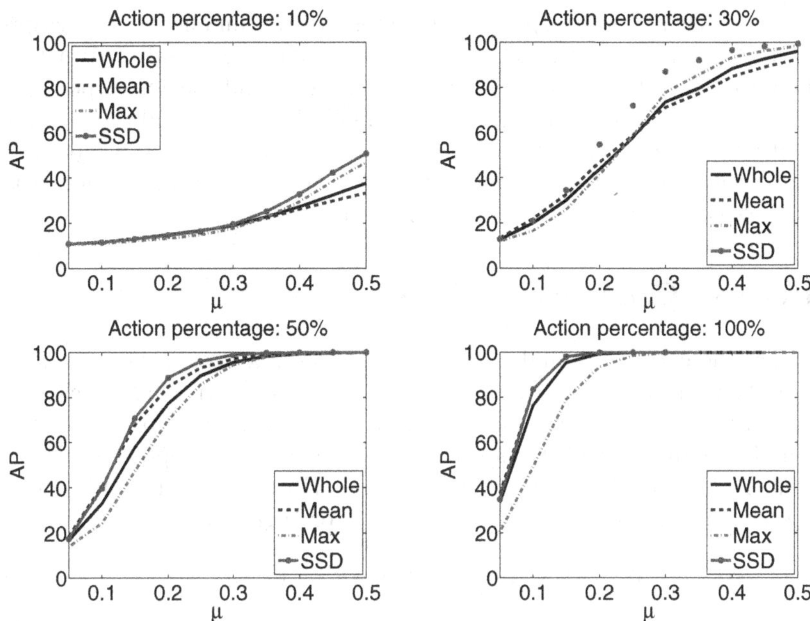

Fig. 2. Average precision as a function of: (i) the action percentage, which is the percentage in each positive video that depicts the action; and (ii) the separation between positive and negative descriptors. SSD (red solid curves) outperforms competing approaches, but the relative advantage depends on these two factors (Colour figure online)

first dimension which is shifted by a value μ. μ is a controlled parameter of this experiment, and it inversely correlates with the difficulty of separating between positive and negative descriptors. We use Fisher vector [53] with two Gaussians to encode descriptors. Each video is divided into 10 intervals, and 55 possible video subsequences are considered, each is represented by a Fisher vector. As will be seen in Sect. 5, except for using synthetic data, the experiment setup here is the same as the setup for real data.

For each setting of the controlled parameters, we repeat the experiment 50 times and average the results. We compare SSD with *Whole*, *Max*, and *Mean*. Whole is the method that is trained on the whole video clips and tested on the whole video clips. Whole is the base classifier for Max, Mean, and SSD. Max is the method that uses the maximum subsequence score, while Mean uses the average score. SSD is the method that is based on the entire score distribution.

Figure 2 plots the Average Precision (AP) for action recognition as a function of: (i) the action percentage; and (ii) the offset between positive and negative descriptors. The four subplots correspond to four different action percentages, which are 10 %, 30 %, 50 %, 100 %. The black solid lines are the performance curves of Whole, which correlate with the action percentage and μ. In general, using the maximum score of video subsequences (Max) is better than using the average score when the the separation between positive and negative descriptors is easy (high μ) and when the action percentage is low. Conversely, it is better to use the mean when the base classifier is less accurate and the action percentage is higher. The proposed approach outperforms both the max and the mean, but the relative advantage depends on the action percentage and the separability between positive and negative descriptors. For more experiments and further analysis, please see the supplementary material.

4 Relative Class Scores (RCS)

To capture the correlation and exclusion among action classes, we learn a classifier for the ranked list of action scores. This section describes this technique.

Consider a particular action and suppose we have learned a base classifier f. Given a video clip $\mathbf{x}$, $f(\mathbf{x})$ is the score for the given action. Suppose we also have m classifiers $f_1 \cdots f_m$ for m other action classes. For each training video clip $\mathbf{x}_i$, we construct a Relative Class Score (RCS) vector (Fig. 1(b)) as follows:

$$\mathbf{a}_i = [f(\mathbf{x}_i), sort(f_1(\mathbf{x}_i), \cdots, f_m(\mathbf{x}_i))]^T. \tag{6}$$

We train a linear SVM to separate between RCS vectors of positive data from RCS vectors of negative data, obtaining a weight vector $\mathbf{v}$ and bias term b. The improved classifier for the target action is defined as:

$$f^*(\mathbf{x}) = \mathbf{v}^T[f(\mathbf{x}), sort(f_1(\mathbf{x}), \cdots, f_m(\mathbf{x}))]^T + b. \tag{7}$$

The same set of training data can be used to learn the base classifiers $f, f_1, \cdots, f_m$ and the improved classifier f^*. To avoid overfitting, we compute $\mathbf{a}_i$ using the leave-one-out classifiers $f', f'_1, \cdots, f'_m$, obtained by removing $\mathbf{x}_i$ from the training data. This technique is applicable to any type of classifiers. However, if LSSVM is used, the leave-one-out classifiers can be computed efficiently using closed form formula, as shown in Sect. 2.

An alternative to the above is to calculate the RCS vector keeping the order of classes: $\mathbf{a}_i = [f(\mathbf{x}_i), f_1(\mathbf{x}_i), \cdots, f_m(\mathbf{x}_i)]^T$ (without sorting), as is often done. However, this performs poorly for action recognition, as will be seen in Sect. 5.2.

5 Experiments on Real Data

5.1 Experimental Setup

Datasets. This section describes Hollywood2, HMDB51, TVHI, which are three datasets used in our experiments. These challenging datasets are widely used for benchmarking human action recognition methods.

The Hollywood2 dataset [2] has 12 action classes and contains 1707 video clips collected from 69 different Hollywood movies. The videos are split into a training set of 823 videos and a testing set of 884 videos. The training and testing videos come from different movies.

The TVHI dataset [1] consists of 300 video clips compiled from 23 different TV shows. There are four classes, corresponding to four types of human interaction: Handshake, Highfive, Hug, and Kiss. Each of these interactions has 50 videos. There are 100 negative examples, which do not contain any of the above interactions. We keep the training/testing split of the dataset [1].

The HMDB51 dataset [3] contains 6766 video sequences for 51 action categories. The videos are collected from various sources including digitized movies and YouTube videos. We follow the suggested protocol for three train-test splits [3]. For every class and split, there are 70 videos for training and 30 videos for testing. We report the mean performance over the three splits as the overall performance. Note that we use the original videos and not the stabilized ones.

We measure performance using Average Precision (AP), which is an accepted standard for action recognition [1,2,54–58]. We only compute Accuracy (ACC) for HMDB51 to compare with published results [3,4,59]. In this paper, the default reporting performance is in AP, if not stated otherwise.

Trajectory Features. The feature representation is based on improved Dense-Trajectory Descriptors (DTDs) [4]. DTD extracts dense trajectories and encodes gradient and motion cues along trajectories. Each trajectory leads to four feature vectors: Trajectory, HOG, HOF, and MBH, which have dimensions of 30, 96, 108, and 192 respectively. We refer the reader to [4] for more details.

The procedure for extracting DTDs is the same as [4] with two subtle modifications: (i) videos are normalized to have the height of 360 pixels, and (ii) frames are extracted at 25 fps. These modifications are added to standardize the feature extraction procedure across videos and datasets. They do not significantly alter the performance of the action recognition system, as verified in our experiments.

Fisher Vector Encoding. To encode features, we use Fisher vector [53]. Fisher vector encodes both first and second order statistics between the feature descriptors and a Gaussian Mixture Model (GMM). In [4], Fisher vector shows an improved performance over bag of features for action classification. Following [4,53], we first reduce the dimension of DTDs by a factor of two using Principal Component Analysis (PCA). We set the number of Gaussians to $k = 256$ and randomly sample a subset of 1,000,000 features from the training sets of TVHI and Hollywood2 to learn the GMM. There is one GMM for each feature type. A video sequence is represented by a $2dk$ dimensional Fisher vector for each descriptor type, where d is the descriptor dimension after performing PCA. As in [4,53], we apply power ($\alpha = 0.5$) and L_2 normalization to the Fisher vectors. We combine all descriptor types by concatenating their normalized Fisher vectors, leading to a single feature vector of 109,056 dimensions.

Video Subsequences. We divide each video clip into roughly 10 intervals and only consider video subsequences that can be composed by concatenating adjacent intervals. The division into intervals is based on shot boundaries and shot lengths.

We first run a shot boundary detection algorithm (explained below) to obtain all shot boundaries. We divide the video clip into intervals such that intervals either include or do not include shot boundaries. The video clip is divided into a sequence of intervals that alternate between those straddling shot boundaries (which are restricted to about 0.6 s in duration) and those in between. This division is unique and can be constructed deterministically. If the number of intervals is more than or equal 10, we terminate the interval division procedure. If the number of intervals is less than 10, we partition the longest intervals (those within shots) to create a total of 10 intervals. Thus, a video clip is normally divided into 10 intervals except when the video clip has many shot boundaries. The number of intervals can be smaller than 10 if the clip length is less than 25 frames (1 s). If a video clip is divided into k intervals, the total number of different subsequences is $k(k+1)/2$. Regardless of k, we sample a fixed l number of subsequences with replacement. We found $l = 1100$ sufficiently large for the sample set to represent the true distribution of subsequences. Note that if k was constant, it would be sufficient to use $l = k(k+1)/2$, i.e., to use all subsequences. But since k varies around 10, we use $l = 1100$ ($\gg k(k+1)/2$) for the sample set for the sample set to be a stable fixed length vector (i.e., not too sensitive to randomness in the sampling process).

For shot boundary detection, we develop an algorithm based on normalized color histograms, HOG, and SIFT. Based on normalized color histograms and HOG, the algorithm produces a set of candidate shot boundaries by thresholding the difference between pairs of consecutive frames. Subsequently, SIFT matching is used to remove false candidates. Evaluated on the TVHI dataset, this shot boundary detection algorithm has 0 false positive and 1 false negative.

5.2 Experimental Results

SVM, LSSVM, and the Validity of Feature Extraction. To validate our video processing and feature extraction procedure, we compare the baseline performance with published results [4]. We evaluate LSSVM and SVM on the Fisher vectors computed for the entire video clips of the Hollywood2 dataset. These classifiers achieve APs of 64.63 % and 64.71 %, respectively. These numbers are comparable to the AP of 64.30 % published by [4]. On HMDB51, LSSVM and SVM achieve ACCs of 56.3 and 57.0, which are comparable to ACC of 57.2 published by [4]. On the TVHI dataset, LSSVM and SVM yield APs of 61.94 % and 61.92 %, respectively. From this experiment, we conclude that: (i) the features are properly extracted and consistent with [4], and (ii) LSSVM and SVM perform similarly. In subsequent experiments, we choose LSSVM because of its computational advantage.

Data Augmentation. Based on the observation that a video and its left-right mirrored video depict the same concept, we propose data augmentation to improve the performance. We double the amount of training data by adding videos obtained by left-right flipping. In testing, we average the classification scores of a test video and its mirrored version. This leads to a few percent improvement in AP. Specifically, on Hollywood2, TVHI, and HMDB51 datasets, the APs increase from 64.63 %, 61.94 %, 57.53 % to 66.68 %, 66.6 %, 59.70 %, respectively. These improved results will serve as the new baselines in subsequent experiments.

Discussion of Results. Table 1 displays the APs of various methods on three datasets. Overall, the proposed methods (SSD, RCS, SSD+RCS) significantly outperform the improved baseline (Whole+). On the HMDB51 dataset, RCS and SSD+RCS outperform Whole+, but SSD does not. On this dataset, Mean and Max also yield lower performance than Whole+. This is due to the idiosyncrasy of HMDB51 as it consists of very short video clips (2–3 s), which are well clipped to the target actions.

For a more detailed analysis, Table 1 also reports the APs for individual action classes of Hollywood2. This reveals some notable facts. Max generally performs poorly, leading to inferior results than Whole+ and Mean. This is perhaps because human action recognition is a hard problem, so the base classifier is far from perfect and the maximum subsequence score is unreliable. However, Max can sometimes outperforms both Whole+ and Mean, e.g., for HandShake. Among Whole+, Mean, Max, and SSD, the proposed method SSD performs

Table 1. Average Precisions on three datasets. Whole: the classifier is trained on the whole video clips and tested on the whole video clips. Whole+: same as Whole, but with data augmentation. Other methods in the table use Whole+ as the base classifier. Mean, Max: using either the mean or maximum score. SSD: learned classifier for the score distribution of video subsequences. RCS: improved classifier based on scores of multiple action classes. SSD+RCS: combined method

			With proposed data augmentation					
		Baseline	New baseline			Proposed		
	Class/Mean	Whole	Whole+	Mean	Max	SSD	RCS	SSD+RCS
	Hollywood2-Mean	64.6	66.7	68.1	64.8	69.1	69.9	**72.7**
	TVHI-Mean	61.9	66.6	69.1	65.0	69.5	67.0	**70.6**
	HMDB51-Mean	57.5	59.7	58.4	55.9	58.3	**63.1**	62.2
Hollywood2	AnswerPhone	29.0	33.9	34.0	23.8	32.7	44.6	**45.4**
	DriveCar	94.7	94.5	94.9	92.4	94.7	95.1	**96.0**
	Eat	65.2	65.8	69.3	66.4	**69.6**	63.9	68.6
	FightPerson	84.8	86.1	85.7	86.0	87.4	88.4	**89.1**
	GetOutCar	62.4	67.6	70.7	63.1	70.9	72.4	**74.3**
	HandShake	44.7	48.0	50.3	57.1	57.1	56.9	**65.0**
	HugPerson	51.5	53.4	51.0	48.7	52.8	57.8	**58.6**
	Kiss	65.5	66.2	67.8	61.4	66.3	67.0	**68.7**
	Run	86.1	87.4	87.7	86.2	88.6	88.7	**90.4**
	SitDown	78.3	79.0	81.4	75.6	80.8	82.9	**84.6**
	SitUp	35.4	38.6	41.1	38.0	44.2	39.2	**46.4**
	StandUp	77.8	79.8	82.8	79.2	84.0	81.6	**85.4**

the best or close to the best in all cases. The combination of SSD and RCS is consistently outstanding.

The results provided in Table 1 are obtained with the base classifiers trained on the whole video clips. We consider an alternative way of training the base classifiers as follows. We represent a training video clip by the average of Fisher vectors computed for its subsequences. We train the base classifiers for this feature representation. These base classifiers improve the performance of all methods on Hollywood2 and TVHI datasets, but yield lower results on HMDB51. On the Hollywood2 dataset, the APs for Whole+ (tested on the whole video clips), Mean, Max, SSD, RCS, SSD+RCS are 67.6, 68.9, 66.0, 70.0, 72.4, **73.6**, respectively. On TVHI dataset, the APs for Whole+, Mean, Max, SSD, RCS, SSD+RCS are 66.5, 68.6, 65.8, 69.9, 70.0, **71.1**, respectively.

Table 2 compares the performances from SSD+RCS to previously published results. It is evident that the performance exceeds the previous state of the art results by a wide margin. Very recently, after the completion of this work, the state-of-the-art accuracy on HMDB51 was reestablished to be 66.8 [60]. However, [60] used different feature representation and encoding, which may also gain benefit from SSD and RCS.

A complementary technique to the proposed methods is to use temporal pyramid. Following this direction, we develop a method with a 2-layer pyramid: (i) divide a video clip into two halves, (ii) compute the Fisher vectors for both halves and the whole video clip, and (iii) represent the video clip by concatenating the three Fisher vectors. We will refer to this method as TempoPyra. TempoPyra (with data augmentation) outperforms Whole+ on Hollywood2 and HMDB51, but not on TVHI. Specifically, the APs of TempoPyra on Hollywood2, TVHI, and HMDB51, are 68.7, 66.0, and 62.4, respectively. These results are lower than the performance of the proposed methods. Furthermore, it is important to emphasize that TempoPyra and the proposed methods are complementary, as video clips and video subsequences can be represented using a temporal pyramid. For example,

Table 2. Comparison with previously published results. The proposed methods (last row) outperform state-of-the-art approaches on Hollywood2 and TVHI datasets. The second last row is our reproduction results for Wang *et al* [4]. These methods and ours use exactly the same features

Hollywood2	AP	TVHI	AP	HMDB51	ACC	AP
Vig *et al.* [54]	59.4	Marin *et al.* [55]	39.2	Kliper *et al.* [59]	29.2	–
Jiang *et al.* [56]	59.5	Patron *et al.* [1]	42.4	Jiang *et al.* [56]	40.7	–
Mathe *et al.* [57]	61.0	Gaidon *et al.* [58]	55.6	Jain *et al.* [61]	52.1	–
Jain *et al.* [61]	62.5	Yu *et al.* [62]	55.9	Wang *et al.* [4]	57.2	–
Wang *et al.* [4]	64.3	Hoai *et al.* [63]	56.3	Peng *et al.* [60]	**66.8**	–
DTD-SVM [4]	64.7	DTD-SVM [4]	61.9	DTD-SVM [4]	57.0	57.8
SSD+RCS	**73.6**	SSD+RCS	**71.1**	TempoPyra+RCS	60.8	**65.9**

the combination of TempoPyra and RCS yields an AP of **65.9** on HMDB51, which outperforms the state-of-the-art results, as shown in Table 2.

Analysis of SSD Classifiers. Figure 3 shows the weight distribution of SSD classifiers for several actions of the Hollywood2 dataset. Recall that the scores are sorted in descending order and the weights decrease monotonically. For AnswerPhone, our algorithm suggests to aggregate the scores from the top 80 percentile. Meanwhile, for HandShake, the algorithm suggests to consider the top 35 percentile only. These results are intuitively consistent with the analysis in Sect. 3.2. For a handshake in Hollywood movies, the temporal extent of the actual handshake is usually brief, and it could possibly interrupted when the camera switches to showing other people watching the handshake. In contrast, a video clip for AnswerPhone often shows one or two actors talking on the phone for a period time, as long as the length of the phone conversation. Empirical evidence in Table 1 also confirms this intuition. Mean outperforms Max for AnswerPhone, and Max outperforms Mean for HandShake. SSD learns from data, and it performs close to the best of Max and Mean in both cases. For some other actions such as FightPerson and SitUp, SSD outperforms both Max and Mean.

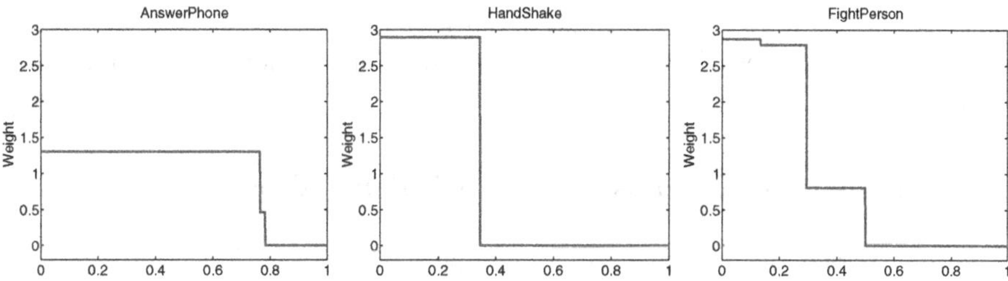

Fig. 3. Weights for SSD classifiers for Hollywood2 dataset. Each subplot depicts the weights for the score distribution. Weights decrease monotonically, and the area under the curve is always 1. AnswerPhone aggregates scores from 80 % of video subsequences, while HandShake only uses the top 35 percentile

Analysis of RCS Classifiers. Figure 4 shows the RCS weights for the combined SSD+RCS classifiers on the Hollywood2 dataset. For all actions, the RCS classifier emphasizes the score of the target class by using a high positive weight, and it penalizes the highest scores of the other classes (negative weights). The spread of the penalty weights depends on the action, which is learned from the data. The use of RCS drastically improves AP (e.g., from 32.7 to 45.4 for AnswerPhone, and from 57.1 to 65.0 for HandShake).

It is crucial to sort the scores of other action classes when constructing the feature vectors to train the RCS classifier. If not, the RCS classifier brings no benefit. Specifically, if the scores are kept based on the order of the classes, the APs for SSD+RCS on Hollywood2 and TVHI are 69.3 and 69.4. These APs are similar to the APs of not using RCS; SSD alone achieves APs of 69.1 and 69.5

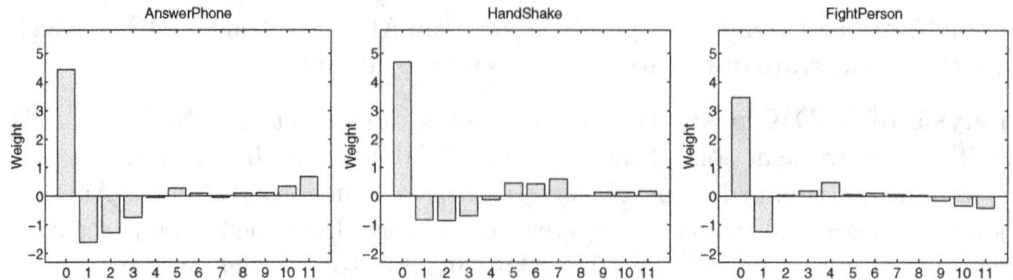

Fig. 4. RCS weights for actions of Hollywood2 dataset. In each subplot, the first bar is the weight for the base classifier of the target action. The remaining bars show the weights for the sorted scores of other classes. All RCS classifiers penalize the top-rank score of other classifiers (negative weights)

on these two datasets. We also experimented with applying the sigmoid function on the raw SVM scores before learning the RCS classifier with unsorted scores, but this also performs poorly.

Parameter Setting. The proposed methods require tuning few parameters. LSSVM has only a single parameter (λ in Eq. (1)), and its classification performance is not too sensitive to λ. In all of our experiments, we set $\lambda = 10^{-3} \times n$, where n is the number of training examples. The formulation for learning SSD classifiers has no parameter.

6 Conclusions, Discussions, and Future Work

We have proposed several techniques for human action recognition, improving the state-of-the-art performance on three challenging benchmark datasets. First, we used data augmentation to learn a flipping invariant classifier. Second, we replaced SVMs by Least-Squares SVMs, which performed equally well and are more computationally efficient. Moreover, Least-Squares SVM enabled reusing training data for further tuning and calibration. Third, we proposed distribution-based classifiers to address the temporal ambiguity of actions, proving its advantage over using maximum and average scores. Fourth, we showed action recognition can benefit from exploiting the correlation and exclusion between action classes, by learning a classifier for the relative action scores.

We have applied the aforementioned techniques to improve the performance of base classifiers. In this paper, we simply obtained the base classifiers by training them on the whole video clips. We have not considered updating the base classifiers after improvement. A direction for future work is to investigate an iterative scheme for updating and improving the base classifiers, as in MI-SVM [12].

Empirical evidence in this paper suggests that using the maximum score leads to poor performance in many cases. On the one hand, this is consistent with empirical observation reported earlier [17,35]. On the other hand, it seems to conflict with the success of several weakly-supervised learning systems such as the Deformable Part Model (DPM) [13] for object detection. There are several possible reasons for the good performance of DPM. First, it is trained on supervised data, where the object location is given. Second, the location of a part of a DPM is heavily regularized by a quadratic function enforcing the part to remain close to an anchor point. This prevents the model selecting the part location using the maximum score alone. If this is indeed a reason for the success of the DPM, we could possibly adapt it for action recognition by putting regularization on the location of the action. This is another direction for future investigation.

Acknowledgements. This work was supported by the EPSRC grant EP/I012001/1 and a Royal Society Wolfson Research Merit Award.

References

1. Patron-Perez, A., Marszalek, M., Reid, I., Zisserman, A.: Structured learning of human interactions in tv shows. IEEE Trans. Pattern Anal. Mach. Intell. **34**, 2441–2453 (2012)
2. Marszalek, M., Laptev, I., Schmid, C.: Actions in context. In: Proceedings of the IEEE Conference on Computer Vision and Pattern Recognition (2009)
3. Kuehne, H., Jhuang, H., Garrote, E., Poggio, T., Serre, T.: HMDB: a large video database for human motion recognition. In: Proceedings of the International Conference on Computer Vision (2011)
4. Wang, H., Schmid, C.: Action recognition with improved trajectories. In: Proceedings of the International Conference on Computer Vision (2013)
5. Satkin, S., Hebert, M.: Modeling the temporal extent of actions. In: Daniilidis, K., Maragos, P., Paragios, N. (eds.) ECCV 2010. LNCS, vol. 6311, pp. 536–548. Springer, Heidelberg (2010)
6. Duchenne, O., Laptev, I., Sivic, J., Bach, F.R., Ponce, J.: Automatic annotation of human actions in video. In: Proceedings of the International Conference on Computer Vision (2009)
7. Buehler, P., Everingham, M., Zisserman, A.: Learning sign language by watching TV (using weakly aligned subtitles). In: Proceedings of the IEEE Conference on Computer Vision and Pattern Recognition (2009)
8. Niebles, J.C., Chen, C.-W., Fei-Fei, L.: Modeling temporal structure of decomposable motion segments for activity classification. In: Daniilidis, K., Maragos, P., Paragios, N. (eds.) ECCV 2010. LNCS, vol. 6312, pp. 392–405. Springer, Heidelberg (2010)
9. Lan, T., Wang, Y., Mori, G.: Discriminative figure-centric models for joint action localization and recognition. In: Proceedings of the International Conference on Computer Vision (2011)
10. Shapovalova, N., Vahdat, A., Cannons, K., Lan, T., Mori, G.: Similarity constrained latent support vector machine: an application to weakly supervised action classification. In: Fitzgibbon, A., Lazebnik, S., Perona, P., Sato, Y., Schmid, C. (eds.) ECCV 2012. LNCS, pp. 55–68. Springer, Heidelberg (2012)
11. Prest, A., Schmid, C., Ferrari, V.: Weakly supervised learning of interactions between humans and objects. IEEE Trans. Pattern Anal. Mach. Intell. **34**, 601–614 (2012)
12. Andrews, S., Tsochantaridis, I., Hofmann, T.: Support vector machines for multiple-instance learning. In: Advances in Neural Information Processing Systems (2003)

13. Felzenszwalb, P.F., Girshick, R.B., McAllester, D., Ramanan, D.: Object detection with discriminatively trained part based models. IEEE Trans. Pattern Anal. Mach. Intell. **32**, 1627–1645 (2010)
14. Dietterich, T., Lathrop, R., Lozano-Pérez, T.: Solving the multiple-instance problem with axis-parallel rectangles. Artif. Intell. **89**, 31–71 (1997)
15. Maron, O., Lozano-Pérez, T.: A framework for multiple-instance learning. In: Advances in Neural Information Processing Systems (1998)
16. Zhang, Q., Goldman, S.A.: EM-DD: an improved multiple-instance learning technique. In: Advances in Neural Information Processing Systems (2002)
17. Hu, Y., Li, M., Yu, N.: Multiple-instance ranking: learning to rank images for image retrieval. In: Proceedings of the IEEE Conference on Computer Vision and Pattern Recognition (2008)
18. Ray, S., Craven, M.: Supervised versus multiple instance learning: an empirical comparison. In: Proceedings of the International Conference on Machine Learning (2005)
19. Wohlhart, P., Köstinger, M., Roth, P.M., Bischof, H.: Multiple instance boosting for face recognition in videos. In: Proceedings of the International Conference on Pattern Recognition (2011)
20. Gartner, T., Flach, P.A., Kowalczyk, A., Smola, A.J.: Multi-instance kernels. In: Proceedings of the International Conference on Machine Learning (2002)
21. Chen, Y., Bi, J., Wang, J.Z.: Miles: multiple-instance learning via embedded instance selection. IEEE Trans. Pattern Anal. Mach. Intell. **28**, 1931–1947 (2006)
22. Kwok, J.T., Cheung, P.M.: Marginalized multi-instance kernels. In: International Joint Conference on Artificial Intelligence (2007)
23. Ping, W., Xu, Y., Wang, J., Hua, X.S.: FAMER: making multi-instance learning better and faster. In: International Conference on Data Mining (2011)
24. Zhou, Z.H., Sun, Y.Y., Li, Y.F.: Multi-instance learning by treating instances as non-i.i.d. samples. In: Proceedings of the International Conference on Machine Learning (2009)
25. Ping, W., Xu, Y., Ren, K., Chi, C.H., Shen, F.: Non-I.I.D. multi-instance dimensionality reduction by learning a maximum bag margin subspace. In: AAAI Conference on Artificial Intelligence (2010)
26. Li, W., Duan, L., Xu, D., Tsang, I.W.H.: Text-based image retrieval using progressive multi-instance learning. In: Proceedings of the International Conference on Computer Vision (2011)
27. Hajimirsadeghi, H., Li, J., Mori, G., Sayed, T., Zaki, M.: Multiple instance learning by discriminative training of markov networks. In: Proceedings of the Conference on Uncertainty in Artificial Intelligence (2013)
28. Poggio, T., Vetter, T.: Recognition and structure from one 2D model view: observations on prototypes, object classes and symmetries. Technical report AIM-1347, MIT (1992)
29. Vedaldi, A., Blaschko, M., Zisserman, A.: Learning equivariant structured output svm regressors. In: Proceedings of the International Conference on Computer Vision (2011)
30. Nowozin, S., Bakir, G., Tsuda, K.: Discriminative subsequence mining for action classification. In: Proceedings of the International Conference on Computer Vision (2007)
31. Nguyen, M.H., Torresani, L., De la Torre, F., Rother, C.: Weakly supervised discriminative localization and classification: a joint learning process. In: Proceedings of the International Conference on Computer Vision (2009)

32. Yuan, J., Liu, Z., Yu, Y.: Discriminative subvolume search for efficient action detection. In: Proceedings of the IEEE Conference on Computer Vision and Pattern Recognition (2009)
33. Hoai, M., Lan, Z.Z., De la Torre, F.: Joint segmentation and classification of human actions in video. In: Proceedings of the IEEE Conference on Computer Vision and Pattern Recognition (2011)
34. Gaidon, A., Harchaoui, Z., Schmid, C.: Actom sequence models for efficient action detection. In: Proceedings of the IEEE Conference on Computer Vision and Pattern Recognition (2011)
35. Cheung, P.M., Kwok, J.T.: A regularization framework for multiple-instance learning. In: Proceedings of the International Conference on Machine Learning (2006)
36. Yager, R.R.: On ordered weighted averaging aggregation operators in multicriteria decisionmaking. IEEE Trans. Syst. Man Cybern. **18**, 183–190 (1988)
37. Yager, R.R., Filev, D.P.: Induced ordered weighted averaging operators. IEEE Trans. Syst. Man Cybern. **29**, 141–150 (1999)
38. Hajimirsadeghi, H., Mori, G.: Multiple instance real boosting with aggregation functions. In: Proceedings of the International Conference on Pattern Recognition (2012)
39. Li, F., Sminchisescu, C.: Convex multiple-instance learning by estimating likelihood ratio. In: Advances in Neural Information Processing Systems (2010)
40. Aytar, Y., Orhan, O.B., Shah, M.: Improving semantic concept detection and retrieval using contextual estimates. In: ICME (2007)
41. Rabinovich, A., Vedaldi, A., Galleguillos, C., Wiewiora, E., Belongie, S.: Objects in context. In: Proceedings of the International Conference on Computer Vision (2007)
42. Torresani, L., Szummer, M., Fitzgibbon, A.: Efficient object category recognition using classemes. In: Daniilidis, K., Maragos, P., Paragios, N. (eds.) ECCV 2010. LNCS, vol. 6311, pp. 776–789. Springer, Heidelberg (2010)
43. Li, L.J., Su, H., Xing, E.P., Fei-Fei, L.: Object bank: a high-level image representation for scene classification and semantic feature sparsification. In: Advances in Neural Information Processing Systems (2010)
44. Sadanand, S., Corso, J.J.: Action bank: a high-level representation of activity in video. In: Proceedings of the IEEE Conference on Computer Vision and Pattern Recognition (2012)
45. Bourdev, L., Maji, S., Malik, J.: Describing people: a poselet-based approach to attribute classification. In: Proceedings of the International Conference on Computer Vision, pp. 1543–1550 (2011)
46. Song, Z., Chen, Q., Huang, Z., Hua, Y., Yan, S.: Contextualizing object detection and classification. In: Proceedings of the IEEE Conference on Computer Vision and Pattern Recognition (2010)
47. Suykens, J.A.K., Vandewalle, J.: Least squares support vector machine classifiers. Neural Process. Lett. **9**, 293–300 (1999)
48. Saunders, C., Gammerman, A., Vovk, V.: Ridge regression learning algorithm in dual variables. In: Proceedings of the International Conference on Machine Learning (1998)
49. Suykens, J.A.K., Gestel, T.V., Brabanter, J.D., DeMoor, B., Vandewalle, J.: Least Squares Support Vector Machines. World Scientific, Singapore (2002)
50. Tommasi, T., Caputo, B.: The more you know, the less you learn: from knowledge transfer to one-shot learning of object categories. In: Proceedings of the British Machine Vision Conference (2009)

51. Hoai, M.: Regularized max pooling for image categorization. In: Proceedings of the British Machine Vision Conference (2014)
52. Cawley, G.C., Talbot, N.L.: Fast exact leave-one-out cross-validation of sparse least-squares support vector machines. Neural Netw. **17**, 1467–1475 (2004)
53. Perronnin, F., Sánchez, J., Mensink, T.: Improving the fisher kernel for large-scale image classification. In: Daniilidis, K., Maragos, P., Paragios, N. (eds.) ECCV 2010. LNCS, vol. 6314, pp. 143–156. Springer, Heidelberg (2010)
54. Vig, E., Dorr, M., Cox, D.: Space-variant descriptor sampling for action recognition based on saliency and eye movements. In: Fitzgibbon, A., Lazebnik, S., Perona, P., Sato, Y., Schmid, C. (eds.) ECCV 2012. Lecture Notes in Computer Science, vol. 7578, pp. 84–97. Springer, Heidelberg (2012)
55. Marin-Jimenez, M.J., Yeguas, E., de la Blanca, N.P.: Exploring stip-based models for recognizing human interactions in tv videos. PRL **34**, 1819–1828 (2013)
56. Jiang, Y.-G., Dai, Q., Xue, X., Liu, W., Ngo, C.-W.: Trajectory-based modeling of human actions with motion reference points. In: Fitzgibbon, A., Lazebnik, S., Perona, P., Sato, Y., Schmid, C. (eds.) ECCV 2012. LNCS, vol. 7576, pp. 425–438. Springer, Heidelberg (2012)
57. Mathe, S., Sminchisescu, C.: Dynamic eye movement datasets and learnt saliency models for visual action recognition. In: Fitzgibbon, A., Lazebnik, S., Perona, P., Sato, Y., Schmid, C. (eds.) ECCV 2012. LNCS, vol. 7573, pp. 842–856. Springer, Heidelberg (2012)
58. Gaidon, A., Harchaoui, Z., Schmid, C.: Recognizing activities with cluster-trees of tracklets. In: Proceedings of the British Machine Vision Conference (2012)
59. Kliper-Gross, O., Gurovich, Y., Hassner, T., Wolf, L.: Motion interchange patterns for action recognition in unconstrained videos. In: Fitzgibbon, A., Lazebnik, S., Perona, P., Sato, Y., Schmid, C. (eds.) ECCV 2012. LNCS, vol. 7577, pp. 256–269. Springer, Heidelberg (2012)
60. Peng, X., Zou, C., Qiao, Y., Peng, Q.: Action recognition with stacked fisher vectors. In: Fleet, D., Pajdla, T., Schiele, B., Tuytelaars, T. (eds.) ECCV 2014. LNCS, vol. 8693, pp. 581–595. Springer, Heidelberg (2014)
61. Jain, M., Jégou, H., Bouthemy, P.: Better exploiting motion for better action recognition. In: Proceedings of the IEEE Conference on Computer Vision and Pattern Recognition (2013)
62. Yu, G., Yuan, J., Liu, Z.: Propagative hough voting for human activity recognition. In: Fitzgibbon, A., Lazebnik, S., Perona, P., Perona, P., Sato, Y., Schmid, C. (eds.) ECCV 2012. lncs, vol. 7574, pp. 693–706. Springer, Heidelberg (2012)
63. Hoai, M., Zisserman, A.: Talking heads: detecting humans and recognizing their interactions. In: Proceedings of the IEEE Conference on Computer Vision and Pattern Recognition (2014)

Context-Aware Activity Forecasting

Anirban Chakraborty and Amit K. Roy-Chowdhury(✉)

Electrical and Computer Engineering, University of California,
Riverside, CA, USA
amitrc@ece.ucr.edu

Abstract. In this paper, we investigate the problem of forecasting future activities in continuous videos. Ability to successfully forecast activities that are yet to be observed is a very important video understanding problem, and is starting to receive attention in the computer vision literature. We propose an activity forecasting strategy that models the simultaneous and/or sequential nature of human activities on a graph and combines that with the interrelationship between static scene cues and dynamic target trajectories, termed together as the 'activity and scene context'. The forecasting problem is then posed as an inference problem on a MRF model defined on the graph. We perform experiments on the publicly available challenging VIRAT ground dataset and obtain high forecasting accuracy for most of the activities, as evidenced by the results.

1 Introduction

In computer vision literature, one major topic of interest is to automatically detect and recognize human activities in a video. The methods developed in the literature on activity recognition range from analyzing simple individual actions such as those discussed in [1,2] to more natural and complex human activities involving one or more actors in the scene [3–5]. However, these methods provide 'after-the-fact' recognition once the activity of interest is complete. Forecasting activities into the future much before they are observed is an important problem for many application scenarios and can be useful in designing anomalous event detection schemes. However, it hasn't yet received much attention in the computer vision community.

We have seen some recent developments in the field of activity prediction or forecasting and two classes of such problems have been introduced in the literature. The first class of problems looks into early recognition of ongoing activities [6–8] and is defined in the literature as an inference of the ongoing activity given temporally incomplete observations. In this problem, the first few frames of the video sequence containing an activity are observed and an early classification of the ongoing activity needs to be achieved. The second class of the problems seeks to forecast future activities in continuous videos [9] well

---

Electronic supplementary material The online version of this chapter (doi:10.1007/978-3-319-16814-2_2) contains supplementary material, which is available to authorized users.

D. Cremers et al. (Eds.): ACCV 2014, Part V, LNCS 9007, pp. 21–36, 2015.
DOI: 10.1007/978-3-319-16814-2_2

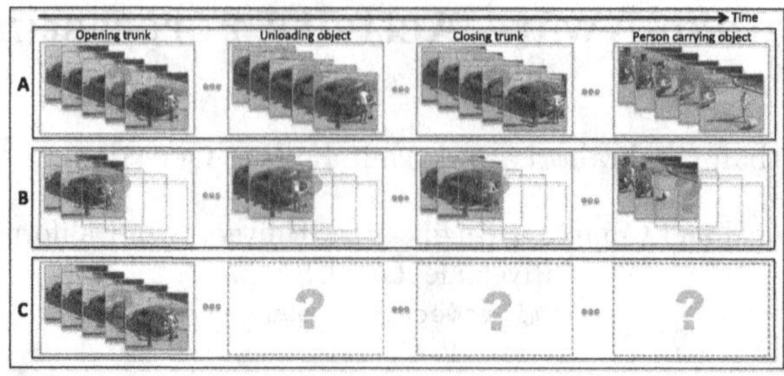

Fig. 1. Different types of problems in human activity analysis. The figure shows four consecutive activity sequences for an actor - opening the trunk of a vehicle, unloading an object from the vehicle, closing the trunk, and the actor carrying the unloaded object, performed in that order. Three categories of activity analysis problems are presented on these sequences. (A) The classic activity recognition problem: each of the activity sequences is fully observed before the activity labels are predicted. (B) Early prediction of ongoing activity: only a few initial frames per activity sequence is observed and the goal is an early prediction of the activity classes from these incomplete observation sets. (C) Forecasting of future activities in absence of observation: at any point of time in a continuous video all activities occurring upto that time point are observed and the goal is to forecast the labels for future activities without the availability of observation for any of them.

before they are observed. This problem can be generally stated as an anticipation about future activity classes in a continuous video, where no observation of any future activity is available and all past activities are observed. The differences between these two problems and how each of them are principally different from a standard activity recognition problem are described through Fig. 1.

In this paper, we propose a method that not only attempts to solve the problem of forecasting unseen future activities (the second class of problem) but also jointly recognizes the activities that have already taken place and were observed. In most cases, it can be observed that activities performed by an actor occur following fixed temporal sequences. For example, if a person carries a bag and walks towards the trunk of a parked car, s/he is most likely to open the trunk, load the bag into it and then close the trunk. Also, for collective activities it can often be seen that actions of the actors involved are strongly synchronized with each other within a spatio-temporal window. All of these are collectively termed in this paper as 'activity and scene context' and we leverage upon these contextual information for successful recognition of observed activities and forecasting of unobserved future activities.

We formulate the joint recognition and forecasting problem probabilistically. The past, present and future activities in a video are modeled as the nodes of a graph and the activity and scene context are modeled as a Markov Random Field on the proposed graph structure. Then a suitable inference strategy is adapted for recognition and forecasting of the activity classes. We show experiments on a challenging and realistic activity dataset - the VIRAT ground dataset release 2 [10]. This dataset comprises of long duration video clips, each containing multiple activities that take place either simultaneously or sequentially, thereby making these datasets both challenging and suitable for testing the proposed spatio-temporal context based activity forecasting method.

2 Relation to Existing Work

In computer vision research, majority of the works related to human activity in video has focused on the task of recognition of simple to more complex activities [11]. Many existing works exploring context focus on spati-temporal relationship of features [3,12], interactions of objects and actions/activities [5,13,14], AND-OR graph based scene representation [15,16]. Methods such as [17–22] studied spatio-temporal relationship between activities in a scene.

There have been some recent works on the emerging topic of early recognition of ongoing activities. The method in [6] approached this problem by representing an activity as an integral histogram of spatio-temporal features and subsequently used a novel dynamic bag-of-words approach to model how these feature distributions change over time. Authors in [7] developed a 'spatial-temporal implicit shape model' which characterizes the space time structure of the sparse activity features extracted from a video and the early recognition is done using a random forest structure. The authors in [8] proposed a max-margin framework based on structured SVM to recognize partially observed events. However, these methods rely on the availability of a partial set of information for the ongoing activity where a typical activity forecasting problem should be able to forecast probable future activities well before the start of the activity segments.

Very recently, the activity forecasting problem was introduced in [9]. The authors combined semantic scene labeling with inverse optimal control to forecast probable actor trajectories, which in turn help predict destinations and future actions. However, there are a number of differences between our method and [9]. Kitani et al. [9] investigates the effect of the static scene environment on future activities, whereas we use both static cues from the scene and dynamic cues from target trajectories and model their interrelationships for forecasting future activities. Unlike a pure trajectory based approach in [9], we combine the target trajectory information with the motion based activity recognition methods in a dynamical model. Finally, we show results on the recent release of VIRAT dataset containing 11 diverse activities where [9] tested their forecasting method on a dataset of three activities.

3 Overview of the Proposed Method

In this work, we propose a strategy to jointly recognize and forecast activities in long duration continuous videos. The method attempts to recognize activities that have already been observed in a video while forecasting the most probable categories of future activities, yet to be observed in that video sequence.

A typical surveillance video contains multiple activities occurring simultaneously or in succession at different portions of the scene. In such videos, it can be

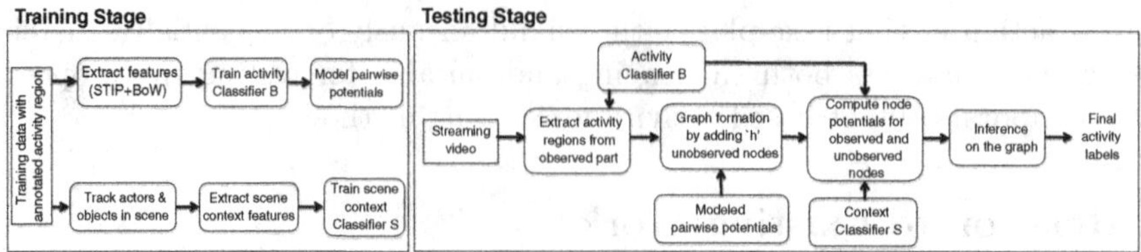

Fig. 2. The overall pipeline: training and testing.

observed that a specific activity by an actor is often followed by another activity by the same actor and this pattern repeats itself through and across the videos given the similarity in scenes. Therefore, an actor's future activities can often be inferred from one or more of its previous activities. Moreover, in group activities where multiple actors are involved, one actor's observed activity pattern can help us forecast another's future actions. We call this 'activity context' and it can be modeled on the edges of an *activity graph* to aid recognition and prediction. As the number of observed activities can increase with time, the graph formation strategy is dynamic with an aim to keeping the size of the graph constant. This is discussed in Sect. 4.1.

After graph formation, a 'Markov Random Field' (MRF) (see Sect. 4.2) is defined on the graph. The edge potentials defined on each of the edges of the graph are modeled using the frequencies of occurrence of pairs of activities in a tight spatio-temporal proximity (Sect. 4.3) and are directly learned from a set of annotated training videos. The node potentials for the observed nodes (observed activities) are obtained using the likelihood of the activities, given by a set of activity classifiers when applied on the features (STIP+BoW) extracted from the observed activity regions (Fig. 2). The node potentials for all the unobserved nodes (unobserved future activities) are initially set as uniform distributions in absence of any other specific information. However, as in most cases, the activity can be characterized by the proximity and motion of the actor relative to a number of key points and detected secondary objects in the scene. These scene specific information, termed as the *scene context*, help modifying the observation/node potential of the first unobserved activity node in immediate future for every actor (Fig. 3). Please note that these scene contexts and the previously introduced spatio-temporal activity context are collectively termed as 'activity and scene context'.

An object detector and a person tracker are employed to extract and estimate various scene context features (see Sect. 4.4) for each actor in the scene at each time point. A trained classifier, when applied on the scene context features extracted from the observed video, provides us with the observation potentials of the aforementioned nodes. The edge potentials remain fixed for the graph across all time points. Finally, the joint activity recognition and forecasting problem can be posed as an inference problem on the MRF just described, which is solved using an iterative 'message passing' algorithm.

4 Activity Forecasting Framework

Let a complete continuous video clip be V, v_t being the portion of V that is observed upto time t and let $v_t^{'}$ be the portion that is yet to be observed. Therefore, $v_t \cup v_t^{'} = V$. v_t contains a number of activity regions and the set of K most recent observations from these activity regions is given as $Y = \{y_1, y_2, \cdots y_K\}$. More clearly, the observation y_k denotes the image observation of an activity, i.e., the features computed from the kth activity region amongst the most recent K activity observations. A subset of these observations is the set of observed activities by one individual actor. If there are n^o actors $O = \{o_1, o_2, \cdots o_{n^o}\}$ in the scene at time t, the set of activities by actor $o_i \in O$, observed so far would be $Y^i = \{y_1^i, y_2^i, \cdots y_{N^i}^i\}$. Further, we define a forecasting horizon h over which we intend to do activity forecasting. Note that h is not a time window, rather it denotes the number of future activities per actor we would be predicting ahead of the current time instant. Therefore, we can define a total of $(K + n^o.h)$ variables representing the hidden activity labels, which we estimate. Let the set of these labels be $X_t = \{x_1, x_2, \cdots x_K, x_{K+1}, \cdots x_{K+n^o.h}\}$. The two subsets of this label set are the one containing the labels with associated observations, $X_t^{obs} = \{x_1, x_2, \cdots x_K\}$ and another containing the labels for which no observation is available, $X_t^{unobs} = \{x_{K+1}, x_{K+2}, \cdots x_{K+n^o.h}\}$. Let the hidden variable/label for k^{th} activity by actor o_i be represented as $x_k^i \in X_t$.

In the next subsections we introduce the structure of an ‘activity graph’, the potential functions associated with an MRF defined on it and how to do recognition and prediction as inference on this MRF to obtain the labels of the hidden states X_t.

4.1 Activity Graph Formation

A graph is built with the atomic activities (both observed and unobserved) as nodes and the activity contexts are modeled on the edges of the graph. The characteristics and definitions of various components of the graph are, as follows,

Each node in the graph is an atomic activity. Let the set of all the nodes in the graph at any given time instant t be $\mathcal{N}_t$. Let a node corresponding to an activity by actor o_i be n_k^i. Then, $n_k^i \in \mathcal{N}_t$. The hidden variable corresponding to the node n_k^i is x_k^i (the activity label), the value of which is to be estimated. An edge between two activity nodes represents the spatio-temporal context between them. Let the set of all the edges in the graph be $\mathcal{E}_t$. The nodes corresponding to the already observed activities in the video are called observed nodes ($\mathcal{N}_t^{obs}$, blue nodes in Fig. 3). The unobserved activities are represented by the unobserved nodes ($\mathcal{N}_t^{unobs}$, white nodes in Fig. 3). Observed edges are those which connect two observed nodes ($\mathcal{E}_t^{obs}$, blue lines in Fig. 3). If both the terminal nodes of an edge are unobserved, it is called an unobserved edge ($\mathcal{E}_t^{unobs}$, red lines in Fig. 3). If an edge connects two nodes one of which is observed and the other unobserved, it is called a semi-observed edge ($\mathcal{E}_t^{semi-obs}$, black lines in Fig. 3).

Two observed nodes are connected by an edge if the corresponding activities occur in a predefined spatio-temporal proximity. But for the unobserved

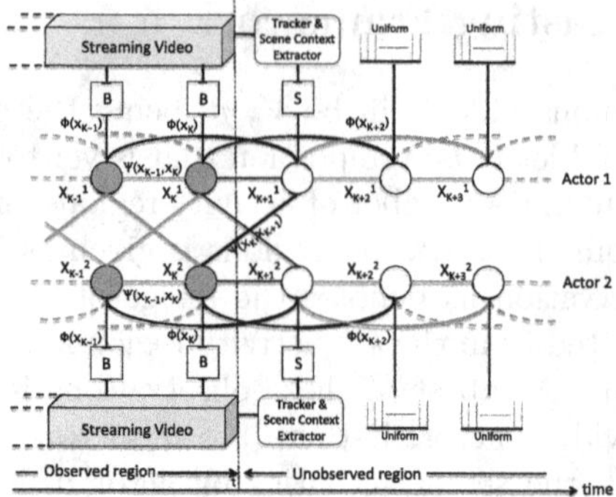

Fig. 3. A snapshot of the graph structure for activity forecasting for two actors in the scene at any time instant 't'. 'B' denotes a trained activity classifier for observed activity recognition and 'S' denotes a scene-context classifier.

nodes and edges, this strategy cannot be adapted as we are unaware of both the spatial location and time of any future activity. Even the exact number of future activities in a video clip at any observational time point is also unknown. Therefore, whenever an activity is observed, we add one more unobserved node (corresponding to the actor of that activity) in the graph and drop the node corresponding to the oldest observed activity. Thus the total number of observed (K) and unobserved ($n^o.h$) nodes remains constant through the video. Please note that an actor might exit the scene, or the video sequence might end before all the future activity nodes are observed. The unobserved nodes are time ordered and two consecutive unobserved nodes pertaining to the activities to be performed by the same actor are connected using an *unobserved edge.* Second order connections are also made for two unobserved nodes. Finally, the *semi-observed edges* are used to connect the last two observed nodes per actor and the two unobserved nodes in the immediate future.

4.2 Markov Random Field Modeling

The set of random variables associated with nodes $\mathcal{N}_t$ is $X_t = \{x_1, x_2, \cdots x_K, x_{K+1}, \cdots x_{K+n^o.h}\}$, which are to be estimated given all observations Y_t. These random variables correspond to the state of each node in the graph and the support for each of these variables is the candidate set of activities (C).

Then the overall MRF is expressed as

$$P(X_t; Y_t) = \frac{1}{Z} \prod_{k=1}^{K+n^o.h} \phi(x_k, y_k) \prod_{\substack{(k,l) \\ :\ (n_k, n_l) \in \mathcal{E}_t}} \psi(x_k, x_l) \tag{1}$$

Here $\phi(x_k, y_k)$ represents the node potential of any node $n_k \in \mathcal{N}_t$, and $\psi(x_k, x_l)$ is the edge potential from node n_k to node n_l. To estimate the optimal state for every node, we have to maximize $P(X_t; Y_t)$. Towards that objective, we first estimate the approximate marginal distributions $P(x_k; Y_t)$ at each node using a belief propagation scheme as described later. The optimal states that maximize the posterior distribution could be then estimated by maximizing the marginals independently.

4.3 Edge/Activity Context Potential

The activity context potential is defined on the edges of the graph, in each of $\mathcal{E}_t^{obs}$, $\mathcal{E}_t^{unobs}$, $\mathcal{E}_t^{semi-obs}$. This potential function models the association between any two activities occurring immediately one after the other or in close spatio-temporal succession. For any two nodes n_k^i and n_l^j (the corresponding labels being x_k^i and x_l^j respectively) such that $\left(n_k^i, n_l^j\right) \in \mathcal{E}_t$, the inter-activity potential is given as,

$$
\begin{aligned}
\psi\left(x_k^i = c_m, x_l^j = c_n\right) &= f_{mn,1}^s \text{ if } i = j, |l-k| = 1 \\
&= f_{mn,2}^s \text{ if } i = j, |l-k| = 2 \\
&= f_{mn}^d \text{ if } i \neq j
\end{aligned} \tag{2}
$$

All these values $f_{mn,1}^s$, $f_{mn,2}^s$ and f_{mn}^d are computed from the annotated training data. $f_{mn,1}^s$ is computed as the ratio of the number of times the same actor performs the activities c_m and c_n immediately one after another to the total number of times the activity c_m is performed in the training data. $f_{mn,2}^s$ is computed as the number of times the same actor performs activities c_m and c_n with the gap of exactly one activity in between them, and it is expressed as a ratio to the total number of times the activity c_m is performed. Finally, f_{mn}^d is obtained as the ratio of the number of times activities c_m and c_n are performed in a close spatio-temporal vicinity by two different actors to the number of times c_m is observed in the video. The same spatio-temporal proximity thresholds are also used in forming the graph, as discussed in Sect. 4.1.

For computing the activity context, only close spatio-temporal neighbors (1st and 2nd order connections) are considered, as we have observed that sub-sequences of relatively smaller length show stronger trends in repeating themselves than the longer activity sequences. Thus in the training videos, we examine all such 2 and 3-tuples of activity sub-sequences and model their pairwise relationships. This also helps us in correcting for any false positives and missing activities.

4.4 Node Potentials

The node potential is the likelihood of occurrence of a particular type of activity as observed in the video data. As there are specifically two types of nodes in our graph (observed and unobserved), we devise separate strategies for computing node potentials for these two categories of nodes.

Observed Nodes: From the annotated training data, we identify the activity regions and we train one activity classifier, the output of which is the probability of a given activity belonging to a particular category. Features at these activity regions are the observation variables and if any of the observation variables is associated with the kth observed activity by actor o_i, it is denoted as y_k^i. A classifier can be employed to estimate the probability of an observation y_k^i resulting from an activity belonging to a particular category $c_p \in C$. Thus, if the set of trained baseline classifiers is B, then the observation/node potentials of the node n_k^i is given as

$$\phi\left(x_k^i, y_k^i\right) = p\left(x_k^i | y_k^i, B\right), \text{ if } n_k^i \in \mathcal{N}_t^{obs} \tag{3}$$

Although we have mentioned a particular feature and type of baseline classifier in the experiments section, any other discriminative classifier and low level motion features could be used for this purpose.

Unobserved Nodes: The node potentials, thus obtained above, are potentials for the observed nodes. However, for an unobserved node n_k^i, observation y_k^i is yet to be obtained (i.e., $y_k^i = \emptyset$) and hence a future activity is equally likely to belong to any category out of the M possible activity types in the dataset, i.e.,

$$\phi\left(x_k^i, y_k^i = \emptyset\right) = (1/M)\mathbf{1}^T, \text{ if } n_k^i \in \mathcal{N}_t^{unobs} \tag{4}$$

Although no low level motion feature is available for a future activity, its likelihood of being categorized as a specific activity can sometimes be substantially improved over $1/M$ with the help of some secondary observations from the scene, termed as the 'scene context' through this paper.

Scene Context Classifier: Often times, an activity is characterized by its interaction with other objects in the scene. For example, in [10], 'opening trunk'/ 'closing trunk', 'loading a vehicle'/'unloading a vehicle', 'getting into a vehicle'/'getting out of a vehicle' - all these activities have at least one thing in common, i.e. the actor interacts with a parked car in all of them. Similarly, 'entering a facility'/'exiting a facility' are both associated with a detectable entry-exit point of a facility in the scene, probably the doorway of a building. Therefore, knowledge about the locations of these objects, key scene elements and whether an actor is going to interact with either of them in near future could help us ascertain that the future activity belongs to a much smaller subset of all possible activities. These information, as a whole, is termed as the 'scene context'. It is represented by a set of variables comprising of the locations/bounding boxes of all the secondary objects, and key points in the scene that are related to one or more types of activities, location and motion information of the actor relative to these objects/key points. Please note that the scene context is computed individually for every actor in the scene and the values of them naturally change with time. Details on such context features in relation to experiments on VIRAT data is given in Sect. 5.

The computed scene context features are averaged over a predefined time window to generate a smoothed scene context feature vector per actor at each time point. Let, at time point t, the scene context feature computed for actor o_i be $f_t^{o_i} = \left\langle f_{t,1}^{o_i}, f_{t,2}^{o_i}, \cdots f_{t,N^f}^{o_i} \right\rangle$. As these features are computed in between two successive activities, the pair $(f_t^{o_i}, a_{k+1})$ completes the representation of the scene context, where $f_t^{o_i}$ is computed at a time t, after which the next activity o_i is going to perform is a_{k+1}. Such features for all the actors over the entire training dataset are combined and a scene-context classifier S is trained. Given a test video, at each time point, whenever we want to run the recognition and prediction, we compute the scene context features. If an actor o_i has already performed k activities and its computed scene context features at time t is $f_t^{o_i}$, then the classifier S provides us with the likelihood of the next activity (X_{k+1}^i) that o_i is going to perform, which is also the node potential for the first unobserved activity node for o_i at time t. Therefore,

$$\phi\left(x_{k+1}^i, y_{k+1}^i = \emptyset\right) = p\left(x_{k+1}^i \mid f_t^{o_i},\ S\right), \tag{5}$$

where $n_k^i \in \mathcal{N}_t^{obs}$, $n_{k+1}^i \in \mathcal{N}_t^{unobs}$. For all other future unobserved nodes for actor o_i, the node potentials remain uniform (see Eq. 4) until the next observation is obtained. It can be noted that as $f_t^{o_i}$ is time varying, the estimated node potential also changes from frame to frame and needs to be re-estimated.

4.5 Inference: Loopy Belief Propagation

The next step is to do the inference on the MRF, which involves the computation of the marginal probability distributions for the states x_k of each node $n_k \in \mathcal{N}_t$, given the observations Y_t. For computation of the marginals at each node, we choose to use *Loopy Belief Propagation* (LBP) based on the *Sum-Product* algorithm [23]. If LBP converges at iteration L, the estimated marginals at each node would be $P^{(L)}(x_k; Y_t)$ and the MAP estimates for the most likely states is computed as $\hat{x_k} = \arg_{x_k} \max P^{(L)}(x_k; Y_t)$. This optimum state corresponds either to the recognized or the predicted label of activity node n_k depending on the type of the node.

5 Experimental Results

To assess the effectiveness of our proposed method in activity forecasting, we perform experiments on the publicly available state-of-the-art VIRAT ground dataset [10] that contains 11 activities in different scenes (see supplementary for the list of activities). We perform two similar sets of experiments corresponding to two recognition schemes used for labeling observed activities, viz. 1. An automated classifier (BOW+SVM), 2. Ground truth activity labels. For experiment set 1, we use half of the data for each scene for training our model and the rest is used for testing. For experiment set 2, however, training is only needed for the scene context based future activity classifier and only a fifth of the data in each scene is used for training and we test our method on the rest of the data.

5.1 Preprocessing

Given a test video sequence, the first task is to obtain the observed activity regions. As activity regions overlap with the motion regions in a video, a background subtraction method [24] can be used to locate the motion regions. Moving persons and vehicles are identified by using an available software [25]. Doors, bags, boxes etc. are detected by using a detector similar to [26] on the entire scene. A tracking method [27], when applied on the detected actors' bounding boxes, provides us with the trajectories of the actors.

5.2 Extraction of Scene Context Features

For our experiments on VIRAT dataset, the set of scene context features computed are - 1. Are cars parked in the scene? (1-Y, 0-N), 2. Distance from the closest parked vehicle normalized by length of diagonal of the car bounding box, 3. Heading towards the closest parked vehicle, 4. Largest overlap of the actor bounding box with the bounding box of a parked vehicle normalized by area of the actor bounding box, 5. Is there one or more entry/exit points to facilities in the scene? (1-Y, 0-N), 6. Distance from the closest entry/exit point normalized by the length of the diagonal of the actor bounding box, 7. Heading towards the closest entry/exit point, 8. Is an object seen on the actor? (1-Y, 0-N), 9. Average velocity of the actor, 10. Time elapsed since last observed activity. For other datasets, the objects of interest will be recognized from the segmented training videos and the generalized scene context features can be estimated by keeping the same relationship between actor and objects. The features are estimated at every frame for every actor using the actor track and locations of detected objects in the scene. The features extracted from the training videos are further used to train a *bag of decision trees* containing 200 fully grown trees. At every frame, the next activity class is used as label. In training videos, given a scene context feature vector extracted at any frame, the trees individually vote and the normalized votes are used as the likelihood for probable future activity class labels.

5.3 Motion Feature Extraction for Observed Activities

In experimental setup 1 (automated classifier based labels for observed activities), we have used a 'Bag-of-Features' approach over 'Space Time Interest Points' (STIP) [28] due to its popularity in the literature for recognition of atomic activities. The STIPs based on Harris and Förstner operators are computed for every activity region in the training data. Feature vectors computed at each point are clustered and quantized to generate a codebook during the training phase and each activity category is modeled as a distribution over this codebook. A multiclass SVM classifier is trained with these features and the corresponding activity labels obtained from the annotated training data. Similarly, for test video inputs, the STIPs are computed and probable activity regions are identified where a significant number of points from the trained vocabulary is observed.

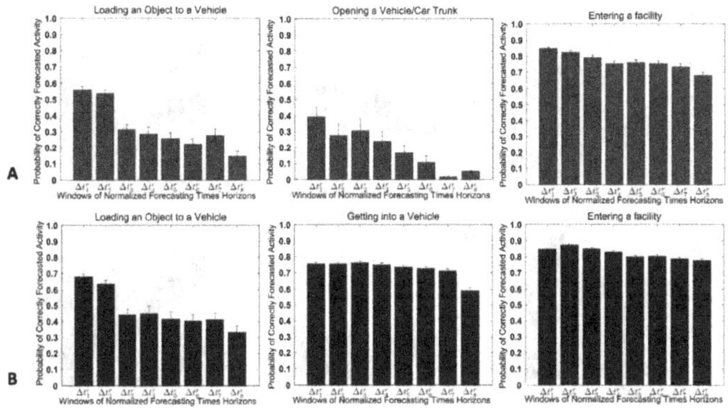

Fig. 4. Increasing trend of forecasting probabilities for different classes of activity (observed in the test set) with time. The positive direction of the time axis indicates increasing time gap from the instant at which the activity to be forecast happens. (A) Probability with which the ground truth activity is forecast as the next activity in exp. setup 1, (B) Similar increasing trend as observed in exp. setup 2.

5.4 Experiment Set 1

In this section, we present the experimental results when a classifier (BOW + SVM) is used to generate node potentials corresponding to already observed activities. At every fifth frame between two activities in a continuous video, we forecast the next activities that an actor is going to perform using the previously observed activities in the video as well as estimated scene context at that frame. At any given time before an activity is performed, the proposed method estimates the probabilities of various candidate future activity labels and these forecasting probabilities can vary with time as the actor moves and the scene context changes. In Figs. 4(A) and 5(A), we examine this variation in forecasting probabilities with time for the next activity that an actor may perform.

Let us assume that an actor has already performed an activity A_{last} upto time t_{last} (or just entered the scene) and is going to perform A_{next} at time t_{next}. At every time point t between t_{last} and t_{next}, we estimate the probability with which A_{next} is forecast as the next unobserved activity label, and thus $t^r = (t - t_{next})$ is the forecasting horizon. The average probability of forecasting the ground truth activity(A_{next}) over all instances of A_{last} in the dataset is computed and its time evolution is observed. Please note that for the same future activity performed, the time gap $[t_{last}, t_{next}]$ varies for different instances and hence is normalized between $[-1, 0]$ (-1 denotes the end time of last observed activity or the time of actor's first appearance and 0 is the time when the next activity is going to occur in future). This time gap is split into 8 equal ranges ($\Delta t_i^r, i = 1, \cdots 8$) and the average probabilities (with standard errors) of the next ground truth activities are plotted.

Figure 4(A) shows the time evolution of probabilities of three activity types (loading obj. to vehicle, opening trunk, entering facility) as the next activity in

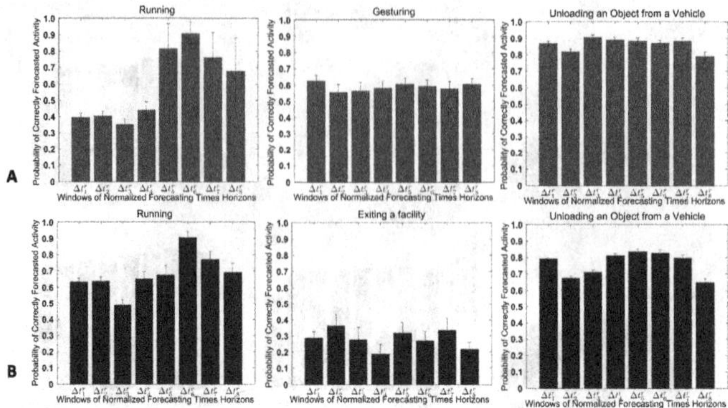

Fig. 5. Time evolution of forecasting probabilities for different classes of activity (in the test set), where no apparent trend is observed. The positive direction of the time axis indicates increasing time gap from the instant at which the activity to be forecast happens. (A) Probability with which the ground truth activity is forecast as the next activity in exp. setup 1, (B) Similar absence of trend, as observed in exp. setup 2.

exp. setup 1. It can be observed that for these activities, the probabilities rapidly increase as the forecasting horizon closes to zero (t closes to t_{next}), especially for the first two car related activities. This is because, during this time range an actor typically walks upto the vehicle and as the actor gets closer to the vehicle (t closes to t_{next}), the model gets more confident that the person is going to interact with the car and hence one of these activities is going to be performed. The last observed activity label and the spatio-temporal context further refines the forecasting probabilities to put preference to a particular activity label.

However, this increasing trend in forecasting probability is largely activity specific as for some of the activities in the dataset, there may not be any tightly associated scene context variable. Thus, even large changes in computed scene context variables minimally affect the forecasting probabilities when these activities would occur in immediate future. For VIRAT, some examples of such activities are Running, Gesturing etc. As seen in Fig. 5(A), there is no visible trend in the time evolution of forecasting probabilities for these activities. Again, for activities such as 'unloading object from a vehicle', the relevant scene context variables (e.g. distance from a car, overlap with a car bounding box etc.) remain largely constant, thereby resulting in uniform average probabilities through the forecasting time range (Fig. 5(A)).

5.5 Experiment Set 2

The probabilities and accuracies for forecasting future activities are affected by the accuracy of the recognition module used for already observed activities. Therefore, to factor out the effect of the errors in the observed activity recognition module on the forecasting results, we repeat the same experiments as in exp. set 1 with only the classifier replaced by a perfect recognition scheme. As we

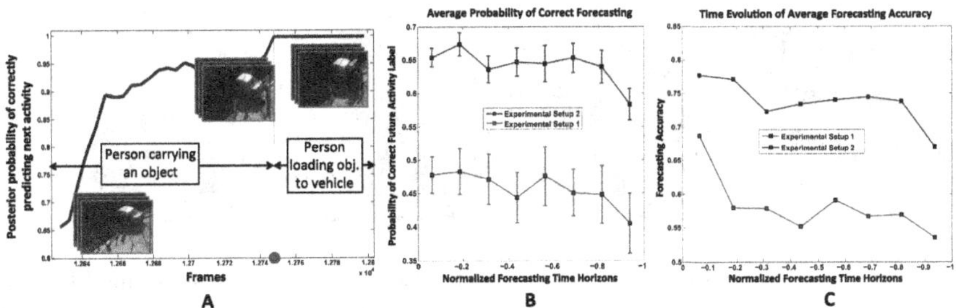

Fig. 6. (A) An example showing how the posterior probability of forecasting increases with time and stabilizes once the next observation is obtained. (B) Time evolution of forecasting probability averaged over all activity classes in exp. setups 1 and 2. (C) Average accuracy of forecasting correct labels for the immediately next unobserved activities in both the experimental setups.

observe an activity, we retrieve its ground truth label and set the activity recognition probability for that particular activity at a very high value, and close to zero for the rest. The evolution of forecasting probabilities with normalized time horizon is shown in Fig. 4(B) for the activities that show an increasing trend in forecasting probabilities and Fig. 5(B) for the activities without any apparent trend in the time evolution of probabilities. The figures are visually similar to those for the same activities in exp. setup 1. However, the average forecasting probabilities for most of the activities are typically higher than that in the classifier based recognition case (set 1).

An example showing the increasing forecasting probability for the next unobserved activity is presented in Fig. 6(A) (in exp. setup 2). In a video segment, an actor in observed to 'carry an object' and the *unobserved* future activity would be 'person loading object to a vehicle'. A parked car is detected in the scene and the posterior probability of the next activity being labeled as 'person loading obj.' rapidly increases as the person walks straight towards the car and gets closer to it. Fluctuation in the probability is seen due to occlusion of the detected object on person. The posterior probability gets close to 1 just before the start of the next activity. Once the next observation is obtained, the posterior represents recognition probability and remains constant for the rest of the video. The time evolutions of forecasting probability averaged over all activity classes for both exp. setup 1 and 2 are shown in Fig. 6(B) and in both the cases they show an overall increasing trend. As expected, the average probabilities in exp. setup 2 is higher than that in exp. setup 1. Similar trends are also observed in Fig. 6(C), which shows the time evolution of average forecasting accuracies. An increasing trend very similar to that of forecasting probabilities is observed.

As the proposed method is capable of forecasting activities deeper into the future beyond the immediately next activity, we also compute the time evolution of forecasting probabilities and accuracies for activities one step ahead (the 'next-to-next' activities). Time evolution of forecasting probabilities for the next-to-next activities are given in the supplementary. The overall forecasting accuracies

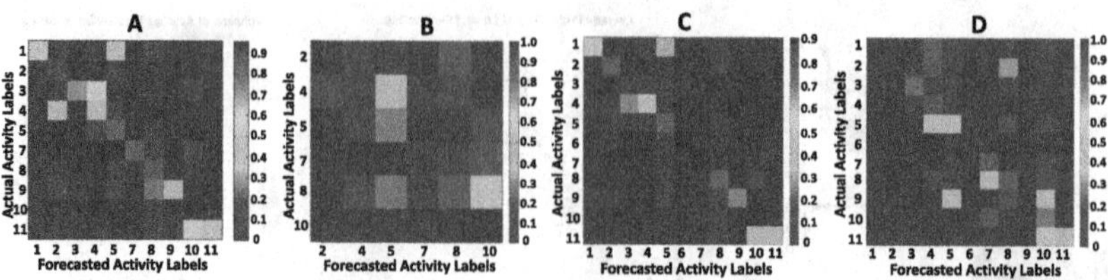

Fig. 7. Confusion matrices showing the overall forecasting accuracies obtained for each class of activity. (A–B) Accuracies for forecasting activities in immediate future and one step ahead (next-to-next) in experimental setup 1, (C–D) Accuracies for next and next-to-next activities respectively in experimental setup 2.

of all next and next-to-next activities in exp. setup 1 are shown in Fig. 7(A–B). The accuracies for most activities happening in immediate future is high. As we predict activities deeper into future, the accuracies tend to go down, as evidenced by Fig. 7(B). Similar trends are seen for activities in exp. setup 2 (Fig. 7(C–D)). Please note that, as there is no baseline activity classifier to train in exp. setup 2 and we need only 20 % of the data for training the scene context classifier, we have the entire remaining dataset for testing and that is why results for all 11 activities could be investigated. With an ideal activity recognition scheme (setup 2), the expected improvements in forecasting accuracy can immediately be evidenced by the confusion matrices shown in Fig. 7(C–D).

The effect and importance of individual components of the proposed model can be understood by analyzing the results above. Figures 4 and 6 show improvement in forecasting probability and accuracy as the scene context based node potential changes from uniform (no scene context) to a more definitive distribution. Figures 6(B,C) and 7 also show how scene context improves forecasting over simple temporal activity context as the next unobserved activity nodes benefit from scene context, but the next-to-next activities do not.

6 Conclusion

In this paper, we have presented a novel approach towards the problem of forecasting future activities in long duration continuous videos. We have shown that the forecasting problem can be posed as a graph inference problem on a MRF where individual activities in a sequence are nodes on the graph. The method combines the spatio-temporal inter activity context and inter-relationship between actors' tracks and detected key points and objects in the scene with a standard activity recognition classifier to forecast activities that are yet to be observed. We show detailed experimental results on the challenging VIRAT [10] dataset and achieve meaningful and encouraging results. Future work would include anomalous activity detection using the method proposed in this paper.

Acknowledgement. This work is partially supported by the National Science Foundation grant IIS-1316934.

References

1. Schuldt, C., Laptev, I., Caputo, B.: Recognizing human actions: a local svm approach. In: International Conference on Pattern Recognition, vol. 3, pp. 32–36 (2004)
2. Dollar, P., Rabaud, V., Cottrell, G., Belongie, S.: Behavior recognition via sparse spatio-temporal features. In: Visual Surveillance and Performance Evaluation of Tracking and Surveillance, pp. 65–72 (2005)
3. Ryoo, M.S., Aggarwal, J.K.: Spatio-temporal relationship match: video structure comparison for recognition of complex human activities. In: International Conference on Computer Vision (2009)
4. Nayak, N.M., Zhu, Y., Roy-Chowdhury, A.K.: Exploiting spatio-temporal scene structure for wide-area activity analysis in unconstrained environments. IEEE Trans. Inf. Forensics Secur. **8**, 1610–1619 (2013)
5. Choi, W., Shahid, K., Savarese, S.: Learning context for collective activity recognition. In: Computer Vision and Pattern Recognition (2011)
6. Ryoo, M.S.: Human activity prediction: early recognition of ongoing activities from streaming videos. In: International Conference on Computer Vision, pp. 1036–1043 (2011)
7. Yu, G., Yuan, J., Liu, Z.: Predicting human activities using spatio-temporal structure of interest points. In: ACM Multimedia, pp. 1049–1052. ACM (2012)
8. Hoai, M., De la Torre, F.: Max-margin early event detectors. Comput. Vis. Pattern Recogn. **107**, 191–202 (2014)
9. Kitani, K.M., Ziebart, B.D., Bagnell, J.A., Hebert, M.: Activity forecasting. In: Fitzgibbon, A., Lazebnik, S., Perona, P., Sato, Y., Schmid, C. (eds.) ECCV 2012, Part IV. LNCS, vol. 7575, pp. 201–214. Springer, Heidelberg (2012)
10. Oh, S., Hoogs, A., Perera, A.G.A., Cuntoor, N.P., Chen, C.C., Lee, J.T., Mukherjee, S., Aggarwal, J.K., Lee, H., Davis, L.S., Swears, E., Wang, X., Ji, Q., Reddy, K.K., Shah, M., Vondrick, C., Pirsiavash, H., Ramanan, D., Yuen, J., Torralba, A., Song, B., Fong, A., Chowdhury, A.K.R., Desai, M.: A large-scale benchmark dataset for event recognition in surveillance video. In: CVPR, pp. 3153–3160. IEEE (2011)
11. Poppe, R.: A survey on vision-based human action recognition. Image Vis. Comput. **28**, 976–990 (2010)
12. Gaur, U., Zhu, Y., Song, B., Roy-Chowdhury, A.K.: A "string of feature graphs" model for recognition of complex activities in natural videos. In: International Conference on Computer Vision (2011)
13. Yao, B., Feifei, L.: Modeling mutual context of object and human pose in human object interaction activities. In: Computer Vision and Pattern Recognition (2010)
14. Lan, T., Wang, Y., Robinovitch, S.N., Mori, G.: Discriminative latent models for recognizing contextual group activities. IEEE Trans. Pattern Anal. Mach. Intell. **34**, 1549–1562 (2012)
15. Gupta, A., Srinivasan, P., Shi, J., Davis, L.S.: Understanding videos, constructing plots learning a visually grounded storyline model from annotated videos. In: Computer Vision and Pattern Recognition (2009)
16. Si, Z., Pei, M., Yao, B., Zhu, S.: Unsupervised learning of event and-or grammar and semantics from video. In: International Conference on Computer Vision (2011)
17. Zhu, Y., Nayak, N.M., Roy-Chowdhury, A.K.: Context-aware modeling and recognition of activities in video. In: Computer Vision and Pattern Recognition (2013)
18. Zhu, Y., Nanyak, N.M., Roy-Chowdhury, A.K.: Vector field analysis for multi-object behavior modeling. IEEE J. Sel. Top. Sign. Proces. (J-STSP) **7**, 91–101 (2013)

19. Nayak, N., Zhu, Y., Roy-Chowdhury, A.K.: Exploiting spatio-temporal scene structure for wide-area activity analysis in unconstrained environments. IEEE Trans. Inf. Forensics Secur. **8**, 1610–1619 (2013)
20. Benmokhtar, R., Laptev, I.: INRIA-WILLOW at TRECVid2010: Surveillance Event Detection. In: TRECVID (2010)
21. Morariu, V.I., Davis, L.S.: Multi-agent event recognition in structured scenarios. In: Computer Vision and Pattern Recognition (2011)
22. Tang, K., Fei-Fei, L., Koller, D.: Learning latent temporal structure for complex event detection. In: Computer Vision and Pattern Recognition (2012)
23. Kschischang, F.R., Frey, B.J., Loeliger, H.A.: Factor graphs and the sum-product algorithm. IEEE Trans. Inf. Theory **47**, 498–519 (1998)
24. Zivkovic, Z.: Improved adaptive gaussian mixture model for background subtraction. In: International Conference on Pattern Recognition, pp. 28–31 (2004)
25. Felzenszwalb, P.F., Girshick, R.B., McAllester, D., Ramanan, D.: Object detection with discriminatively trained part based models. IEEE Trans. Pattern Anal. Mach. Intell. **32**, 1627–1645 (2010)
26. Dalal, N., Triggs, B.: Histograms of oriented gradients for human detection. In: Computer Vision and Pattern Recognition, pp. 886–893 (2005)
27. Song, B., Jeng, T.Y., Staudt, E., Roy-Chowdhury, A.K.: A stochastic graph evolution framework for robust multi-target tracking. In: Daniilidis, K., Maragos, P., Paragios, N. (eds.) ECCV 2010, Part I. LNCS, vol. 6311, pp. 605–619. Springer, Heidelberg (2010)
28. Gorelick, L., Blank, M., Shechtman, E., Irani, M., Basri, R.: Actions as space-time shapes. In: International Conference on Computer Vision, pp. 1395–1402 (2005)

DMM-Pyramid Based Deep Architectures for Action Recognition with Depth Cameras

Rui Yang[1,2] and Ruoyu Yang[1,2](✉)

[1] State Key Laboratory for Novel Software Technology, Nanjing University, Nanjing, China
ryang@smail.nju.edu.cn

[2] Department of Computer Science and Technology, Nanjing University, Nanjing, China
yangry@nju.edu.cn

Abstract. We propose a method for training deep convolutional neural networks (CNNs) to recognize the human actions captured by depth cameras. The depth maps and 3D positions of skeleton joints tracked by depth camera like Kinect sensors open up new possibilities of dealing with recognition task. Current methods mostly build classifiers based on complex features computed from the depth data. As a deep model, convolutional neural networks usually utilize the raw inputs (occasionally with simple preprocessing) to achieve classification results. In this paper, we train both traditional 2D CNN and novel 3D CNN for our recognition task. On the basis of Depth Motion Map (DMM), we propose the DMM-Pyramid architecture, which can partially keep the temporal ordinal information lost in DMM, to preprocess the depth sequences so that the video inputs can be accepted by both 2D and 3D CNN models. The combination of networks with different depth is used to improve the training efficiency and all the convolutional operations and parameters updating are based on the efficient GPU implementation. The experimental results applied to some widely used benchmark outperform the state of the art methods.

1 Introduction

Human action recognition is an important topic in computer vision. As a key step in an overall human action understanding system, action recognition is applied for many applications including human computer interaction, video surveillance, game control system and etc. [1,2]. Based on the traditional video sequences captured by RGB cameras, spatio-temporal features are widely used for the recognition task [3]. With the recent development of high-speed depth cameras, we can capture depth information of body's 3D position and motion in real-time [4]. Compared with the 2D information, the depth information has obvious advantages because it can distinguish the human actions from more than one view because the z-index displacement information which is lost in 2D frames is valued here. The new data format has motivated researchers to propose more innovative methods which are able to make full use of the depth information.

D. Cremers et al. (Eds.): ACCV 2014, Part V, LNCS 9007, pp. 37–49, 2015.
DOI: 10.1007/978-3-319-16814-2_3

Convolutional neural network [5,6] is an efficient recognition algorithm which is widely used in pattern recognition, image processing and other fields. The weight sharing network structure is of significance to reduce the complexity of network model and more similar to the biological neural network. As a special design of a multi-layer perceptron for the recognition of 2D shapes, this network structure has high invariance to translation, scaling, inclination and some other anamorphosis. [6–9] have shown CNNs' powerful ability in visual object recognition on the premise of appropriate training and parameter adjustment. In the field of human action recognition, [10] treats video frames as still images and apply CNNs to recognize actions at the individual frame level. [11–13] successfully extract spatial and the temporal features by performing 3D convolutions. But, impressive as these successes are, few research has been done on action recognition with the depth inputs.

In this paper, we firstly propose a 2D-CNN based deep model for human action recognition using depth maps captured by Kinect. The challenging datasets in this field usually provide us a lot of video clips and each clip only perform one complete action. Since traditional CNN is good at dealing with 2D inputs (usually the natural images), we need to engrave the frame sequences along the time axis into a static image before building the neural network model. The overall shape and position after superposition are used to indicate the action performed by the clip. Motion History Image (MHI) [14,15] and the Motion Energy Image (MEI) [15] are two great engraving methods due to their simplicity and good performance. Here we use Depth Motion Maps (DMM) [16] which looks like MHI to a certain extent. DMM can accumulate global activities through entire video sequences to represent the motion intensity but the temporal ordinal relationship is lost. So we extend the DMM to DMM-Pyramid in order to avoid losing too much temporal features. We regard all the DMMs in a DMM-Pyramid as different channels of an image and the image is the final input for our architecture. With the steps of DMM-Pyramid calculation done, a modified CNN model is built to achieve the recognition result.

Secondly we propose a 3D-CNN based deep model in order to learn spatio-temporal features automatically. Compared with the preprocessing work in 2D-CNN model, the most difference is that here we divide the depth sequence in a clip evenly into N parts and apply DMM calculation to these parts respectively (In fact, it can be seen as the bottom layer of DMM-Pyramid). Then we stack multiple contiguous DMMs together to form a DMM cube (with size $Width \times Height \times N$) rather than a group of individual DMMs in 2D architecture. After that we convolute a 3D kernel to the cube. The remanning work is quite similar to the previous model. Both of the 2D/3D models are evaluated on two benchmark datasets: MSR Action3D dataset [1] and MSR Gesture3D dataset [17] which are captured with depth cameras.

The key contributions of this work can be summarized as follows:

- We propose to apply 2D/3D convolutional networks to recognize the human actions captured by depth cameras. We use convolution operation to extract spatial and temporal features from low-level video data automatically.

- We extend DMM to DMM-Pyramid and then we can organize the raw depth sequence into formats which can be accepted by both 2D and 3D convolutional networks. The preprocessing work is simple enough and will keep the raw information as much as possible.
- We propose to combine deep CNN models with different depth to further boost the performance. We train multiple models at the same time and apply a linear weighted combination to their outputs. Experimental result has proved the operation's effectiveness.
- We evaluate our models on the MSR Action3D dataset and MSR Gesture3D dataset in comparison with the state-of-the-art methods. Experimental results show that the proposed models significantly outperforms other ones.

The rest of the paper is organized as follows. Section 2 reviews the recent research work on human action recognition using the advantages of depth data. Sections 3 and 4 describe the 2D/3D-CNN architectures we proposed in detail. The experimental results and comparisons are given in Sect. 5. Section 6 concludes the paper with future work.

2 Related Works

Li et al. [1] model the dynamics of the action by building an action graph and describe the salient postures by a bag-of-points (BOPs). It's an effective method which is similar to some traditional 2D silhouette-based action recognition methods. The method does not perform well in the cross subject test due to some significant variations in different subjects from MSR Action3D dataset.

Wu et al. [18] extract features from depth maps based on Extended-Motion-History-Image (Extended-MHI) and use the Multi-view Spectral Embedding (MSE) algorithm. They try to find the frames that are similar to the beginning and ending frame in the unsegmented testing video sequence for temporal segmentation.

Yang et al. [16] are motivated by the success of Histograms of Oriented Gradients (HOG) in human detection. They extract Multi-perspective HOG descriptors from DMM as representations of human actions. They also illustrate how many frames are sufficient to build DMM-HOG representation and give satisfactory experimental results on MSR Action3D dataset. Before that, they have proposed an EigenJoints-based action recognition system by using a NBNN classifier [19] with the same goal.

In order to deal with the problems of noise and occlusion in depth maps, Jiang et al. extracts semi-local features called random occupancy pattern (ROP) [20]. They propose a weighted sampling algorithm to reduce the computational cost and claim that their method performs better in accuracy and computationally efficiency than SVM trained by raw data. After that they further propose Local Occupancy Patterns (LOP) features [21] which are similar to ROP in some case and improve their results to some extent.

Oreifej et al. [22] propose to capture the observed changing structure using a histogram of oriented 4D surface normals (HON4D). They demonstrate that their method captures the complex and articulated structure and motion within the sequence using a richer and more discriminative descriptor than other ones.

Different from all above approaches, our methods do not try to extract any complex or so-called "rich" features from the depth sequences. We just leave the task of building high-level features from low-level ones to the deep CNN models. The preprocessing work on the raw inputs is quite simple.

3 A 2D-CNN Architecture

This section describes the 2D-CNN based deep model in detail. It shows how we stack contiguous frames together into still images and convert action recognition to a task which looks like traditional image classification based on CNN.

3.1 Depth Motion Map

Yang et al. [16] details the framework to compute action representation of DMM-HOG. In this subsection, the HOG descriptor is no longer needed. The only thing we care about is using DMM to stack depth sequences into the inputs which can be accepted by CNN model.

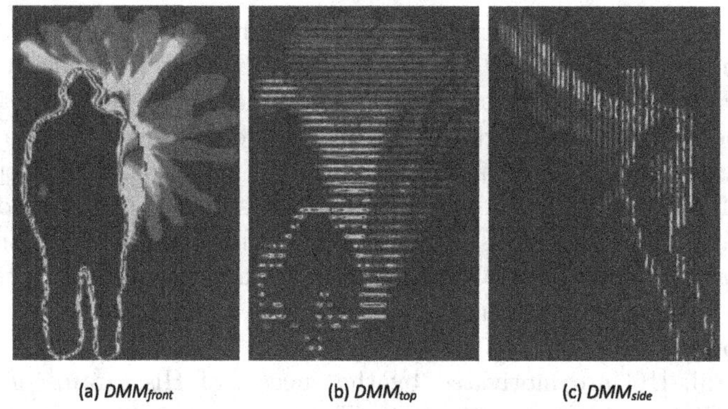

Fig. 1. Three DMMs represent the action "high arm wave". They summarize the body motion in the depth sequence from three orthogonal views.

To put it simply, DMMs are used to summarize the difference between each two consecutive depth maps in a clip. Each 3D depth frame generates three 2D binary maps including front views map map_f, side views map map_s, and top views map map_t. Then DMM is denoted as:

$$DMM_v = \sum_{i=1}^{N-1} |map_v^i - map_v^{i+1}|, \tag{1}$$

where $v \in \{front, side, top\}$ and N is the number of frames in a given clip. Figure 1 shows an example of three DMM maps generated by the depth maps sequence which performs the action "high arm wave".

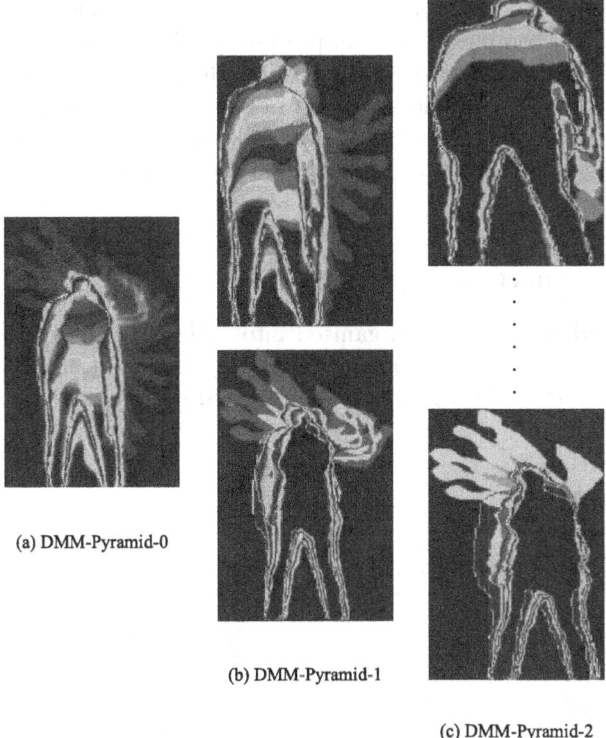

Fig. 2. A DMM-Pyramid architecture represents the action "pick up & throw" in different levels.

3.2 DMM-Pyramid

While we utilize DMM to summarize each whole video clip, we can not avoid losing some temporal information. For an example, there is a complex action called "pick up & throw" in the benchmark. This action contains two consecutive sub-actions: "bend to pick up" and "high throw". If we only use one "general" DMM (even from three perspectives) to do the representation work, the confusion may occur between "pick up & throw" and "high throw" or "high arm wave" because their total depth motions are similar to each others'.

In order to capture some temporal features of the DMM, we propose a simple temporal-pyramid method to extend DMM. We recursively segment the action into several parts along the time axis and then apply the DMM calculation to each part respectively, i.e., if we use the dichotomy to segment the depth sequence, the number of DMMs from top to bottom in the pyramid will be $1, 2, 4, \cdots, 2^{h-1}$ where h is the hierarchy label. Figure 2 shows a DMM-Pyramid architecture which describes the action "pick up & throw" more closely. In this case, we can see that sub-actions in the complex action can be observed clearly with the pyramid growing. So we believe that using DMM-Pyramid as input will improve the classification performance.

On the other hand, the "not-too-deep-hierarchy" pyramid will not increase the computational complexity. In the process of DMM generation, calculating the motions between each two consecutive depth maps and stacking them are most time-consuming. But the work will not be repeated during the pyramid generation because we can directly get high-level DMMs by overlapping low-level DMMs together (e.g. overlapping two images in Fig. 2(b) can get the image in Fig. 2(a)).

3.3 CNN Architecture

Since all the videos have been organized into DMM-Pyramids, we can simply apply the model similar to the one introduced by LeCun et al. [23] to the classification task. The final architecture is illustrated in Fig. 3.

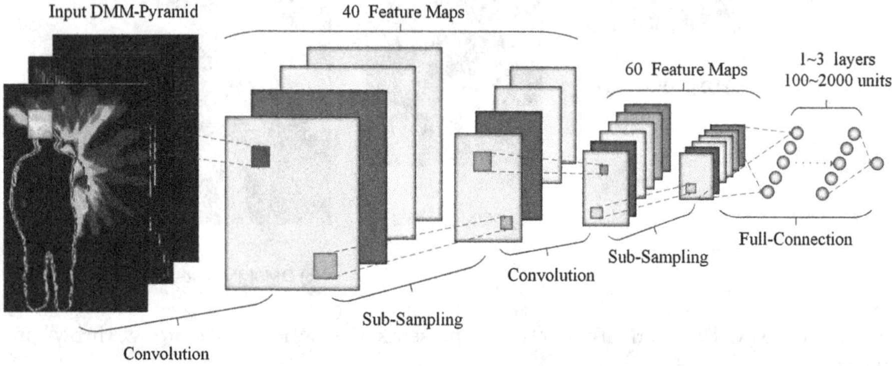

Fig. 3. Our 2D-CNN architecture for human action recognition with DMM-Pyramid as input. The architecture consists of two convolution layers, two sub-sampling layers, and one full connection part consisting of 1–3 layers.

Including the input layer, the architecture consists of 7–9 layers. We can observe the performance when the full connected multi-layer perceptron part varies. The shape of the filters in two convolution layers is alternative and the poolsize of sub-sampling layers is fixed to 2×2. The size of DMMs is rescaled to 100×100. The first convolution layer consists of 40 feature maps of size 88×88 pixels with the 13×13 filter shape. After max-pooling, the layer connected to the first convolution layer is composed of 40 feature maps of size 44×44. Following the same principle, the second convolution layer has 60 feature maps of size 34×34 and the filter shape is 11×11. Then the following sub-sampling layer has 60 feature maps of size 17×17. The layers of the multilayer perceptron part is not fixed. Finally, we can instantiate the network by using a logistic regression layer in the end of the whole architecture.

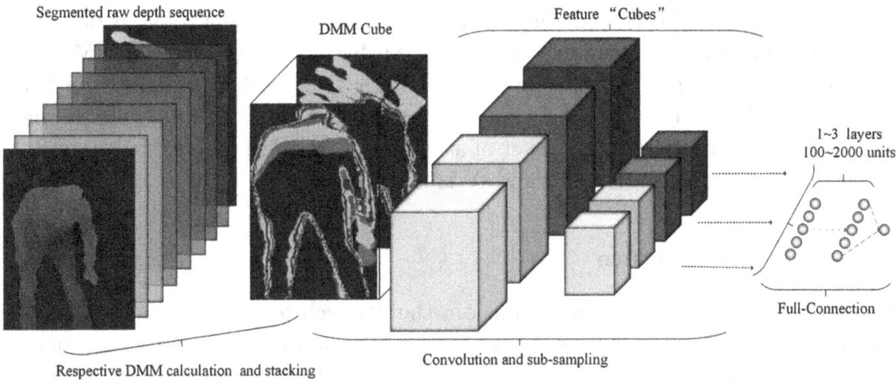

Fig. 4. Our 3D-CNN architecture for human action recognition with DMM cube as input. The architecture consists of two convolution layers, two sub-sampling layers, and one full connection part consisting of 1–3 layers.

3.4 Strategies for Performance Improvement

Since the benchmarks for human action recognition with depth cameras are usually not large-scale, our architecture's size seems to be much larger than some famous ones. The implementation of the convolution and parameters updating is based on Theano [24] so that we can use fast GPUs to accelerate our experiments. We employ the regularization here to overcome the overffting. L1-norm and L2-sqrt are added in the cost function. More anecdotally, we find that the output probability distribution for each action class changes with the depth of the architecture. So it is plausible that combining the results of single architectures with different depth will improve the performance. Our final strategy is that training three models with different depth (7–9 in this paper) and combining their outputs after each N iterations. The inverse of validation errors of each model are set as weights. In fact, our experiment in Sect. 5 has proved that the combination can both improve the precision and reduce training time.

4 A 3D-CNN Architecture

Compared with 2D CNN, 3D convolution is more straightforward to handle video inputs (depth maps sequence in this paper). The extended convolution in time dimension help us to learn spatio-temporal features automatically. The architecture is shown in Fig. 4.

4.1 DMM Segmentation and Stacking

Unlike 2D model, the inputs for 3D model need to keep information for the convolution operation on the temporal axis. Single images are no longer applicable here. Our preprocessing method is dividing the depth sequence in a clip evenly into N parts and applying DMM calculation to these parts respectively. So we get N segmented DMMs and they have temporal ordinal relationship between each other. Then we stack these contiguous DMMs together to form a DMM cube (with size $Width \times Height \times N$) and convolute a 3D kernel to it. An example is shown in the left part of Fig. 4. From another perspective, the final cube is just composed of stacking a bottom layer of a DMM-Pyramid (The DMM-Pyramid-2 in Fig. 2 can form a usable cube and N is 4 in this case).

4.2 CNN Architecture

Regardless of the difference in dimension, the 3D architecture is almost same as the 2D one. The 3D kernel we used is same as the one in [11]. In our experiment, the input layer gets cubes with size $50 \times 50 \times 8$, then the 3D filter shape is $7 \times 7 \times 3$ so that the 40 "feature cubes" in the first convolution have the size $44 \times 44 \times 6$. We apply 2×2 max-pooling (in the spatial dimension) on each of the feature cubes in the sub-sampling layer and the cubes' size is reduced to $22 \times 22 \times 6$. The next 3D filter shape is $8 \times 8 \times 4$ and sub-sampling size is 3×3. So the size of final input for the full connected multi-layer perceptron part is $60 \times 5 \times 5 \times 3$ (60 filters). The last part is exactly the same as the full connection part in 2D-CNN architecture.

5 Experimental Results and Discussion

In this section, we show our experimental results produced by applying our method to the public domain MSR Action3D/Gesture3D datasets and compare them with the existing methods.

5.1 Action Recognition on MSR Action3D Dataset

There are 20 action types in the MSR Action3D dataset. Each action type contains 10 subjects and they performed the same action 2–3 times for each subject. 567 depth map sequences are provided in total and 10 of them are abandoned because the skeletons are either missing or too erroneous. The resolution is 320×240. Each depth map sequence we used is regarded as a clip. We compare our method with the state-of-the-art methods on the cross-subject test setting [1], where half subjects are used for training and the rest ones are used for testing.

The performances of our method are shown in Table 1. Intuitively, we see that our work has shown a significant improvement comparing to other methods. The two results of our methods in this table are achieved under the optimal parameters and the combination strategy which is described in Sect. 3.4. Using 2D-CNN with DMM-Pyramid as inputs we obtain the accuracy 91.21 %. It shows that the DMM-Pyramid is able to retain enough original information of the video clip and the CNN successfully learns high-level features from it. On the other hand, the 3D-CNN's performance (86.08 %) is not as good as expected. We believe that the resolution 50×50 for the entire human motion is too small. It will lose much details of body shape and the temporal features in the dataset may not be as important as spatial features.

Table 1. Recognition accuracies (%) comparison based on MSR Action3D dataset

Method	Accuracy %
2D-CNN with DMM-Pyramid	**91.21**
3D-CNN with DMM-Cube	86.08
HON4D + D_{disc} [22]	88.89
Jiang et al. [21]	88.20
Jiang et al. [20]	86.50
Yang et al. [16]	85.52

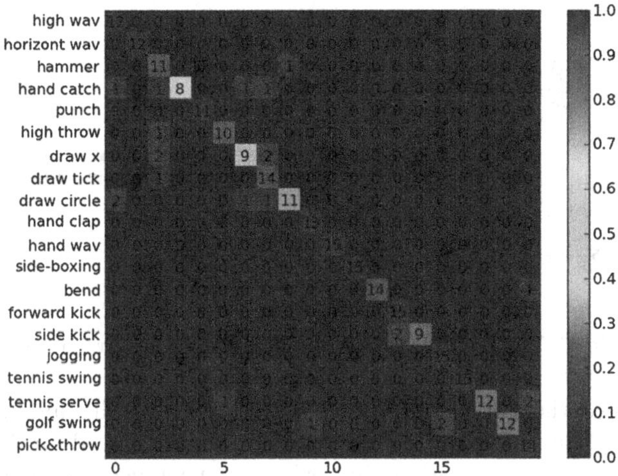

Fig. 5. The overall confusion matrix for the fixed cross subject test.

Figure 5 shows the confusion matrix of the 2D-CNN (91.21 %). The error distribution made by our architecture seems to be more uniform than [21,22]. Many classification errors occur if two actions are too similar to each other, such as "hand catch" and "high throw" in [21] (25.00 %) or "draw X" and "draw circle" in [22] (46.7 %). By contrast, the lowest recognition accuracy for single action class in our experiment is 66.67 % ("hand catch"). In fact, our method works very well for almost all of the actions.

Figure 6 shows the pace of decline of different models' error rate. The depth of these models ranges from 7 to 9. The error rate decreases fast in the first 10 to 15 iterations and then becomes very stable. For a single model, the one with depth of 9 performs best and takes only 30 iterations to achieve a better result (89.02 %) than HON4D [22] and Actionlet Ensemble [21]. On the contrary, the most shallow model reaches 88.28 % at iteration 49 and will take another 150 iterations to reach 88.65 %. At the same time you may see that the combination of three models touches the 90 % line at amazing iteration 13 and the best result showed in Table 1 is achieved at iteration 33. It take no more than 30 min to learn parameters while the single model cannot reach the accuracy by using

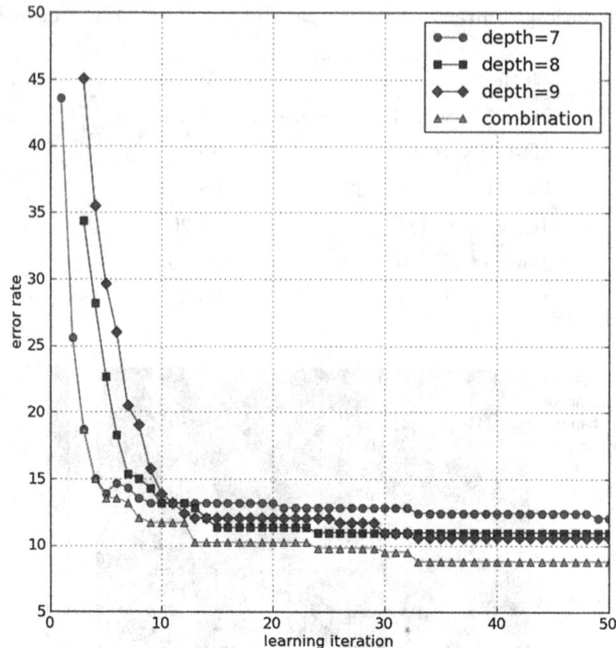

Fig. 6. The pace of decline of different models' error rate.

days of time. Another interesting thing is that increasing the number of hidden units in the multilayer perceptron part can also slightly speed up the error rate decreasing but a single iteration time will be longer because there are more parameters to train.

5.2 Gesture Recognition on MSR Gesture3D Dataset

There are 12 dynamic American Sign Language (ASL) gestures in MSR Gesture3D dataset: "bathroom", "blue", "finish", "green", "hungry", "milk", "past", "pig", "store", "where", "j", "z". All of the gestures were captured by a Kinect device. There are 336 files in total, each corresponding to a depth sequence just like MSR Action3D dataset. We follow the experiment setup in [17]. Table 2

Table 2. Recognition accuracies (%) comparison based on MSR Gesture3D dataset

Method	Accuracy %
2D-CNN with DMM-Pyramid	**94.35**
3D-CNN with DMM-Cube	92.25
HON4D + D_{disc} [22]	92.45
Jiang et al. [21]	88.50
Yang et al. [16]	89.20

shows that our architecture outperforms the state of the art methods. We also notice that the 3D-CNN architecture performs much better here than in Action3D dataset. We believe that low resolution will not cause too much impact on the recognition of local motion like gestures.

6 Conclusion

In this paper, we presented two deep architectures based on convolutional neural networks for human action recognition from depth sequences. In 2D-CNN based architecture, we proposed a DMM-Pyramid method to stack contiguous frames together into still images and convert action recognition to "image classification" work. In 3D-CNN based architecture, we use the DMM Cube as the inputs for the networks and expect to learn more temporal features. Both of the architectures aim to learn spatial and temporal features automatically from the raw inputs without complex preprocessing. We also find that applying a linear weighted combination to CNN models with different depth can significantly improve the precision and reduce learning time. Our experiments on some widely-used and challenging datasets show that the proposed architectures give competitive results, among the best of related work, both on MSR Action3D (91.21 %) and MSR Gesture3D (94.35 %). Our methods are easy to implement based on the open-source python library Theano and anyone can reproduce the experiment to achieve the good (or even better) results following the setup described in Sect. 5.

Furthermore, although the MSR Action3D dataset remains to be the most widely used dataset for human action recognition with depth inputs, there are some other challenging datasets (especially more realistic) for us to verify our architectures' genericity, e.g. MSR DailyActivity3D dataset [21] and Subtle Walking From CMU Mocap Dataset [25]. We also plan to do a large-scale experiment to confirm our CNN models' performance in practice.

Acknowledgement. This work was supported in part by the National Natural Science Foundation of China under Grant Nos. 61321491 and 61272218.

References

1. Li, W., Zhang, Z., Liu, Z.: Action recognition based on a bag of 3d points. In: 2010 IEEE Computer Society Conference on Computer Vision and Pattern Recognition Workshops (CVPRW), pp. 9–14. IEEE (2010)
2. Shotton, J., Sharp, T., Kipman, A., Fitzgibbon, A., Finocchio, M., Blake, A., Cook, M., Moore, R.: Real-time human pose recognition in parts from single depth images. Commun. ACM **56**, 116–124 (2013)
3. Li, W., Zhang, Z., Liu, Z.: Expandable data-driven graphical modeling of human actions based on salient postures. IEEE Trans. Circuits Syst. Video Technol. **18**, 1499–1510 (2008)
4. Zhang, S.: Recent progresses on real-time 3d shape measurement using digital fringe projection techniques. Opt. Lasers Eng. **48**, 149–158 (2010)

5. Lawrence, S., Giles, C.L., Tsoi, A.C., Back, A.D.: Face recognition: a convolutional neural-network approach. IEEE Trans. Neural Netw. **8**, 98–113 (1997)
6. Krizhevsky, A., Sutskever, I., Hinton, G.E.: Imagenet classification with deep convolutional neural networks. In: Advances in Neural Information Processing Systems, pp. 1097–1105 (2012)
7. Farabet, C., Couprie, C., Najman, L., LeCun, Y.: Learning hierarchical features for scene labeling. IEEE Trans. Pattern Anal. Mach. Intell. **35**, 1915–1929 (2013)
8. Kavukcuoglu, K., Sermanet, P., Boureau, Y.L., Gregor, K., Mathieu, M., Cun, Y.L.: Learning convolutional feature hierarchies for visual recognition. In: Advances in Neural Information Processing Systems, pp. 1090–1098 (2010)
9. Ciresan, D., Meier, U., Schmidhuber, J.: Multi-column deep neural networks for image classification. In: 2012 IEEE Conference on Computer Vision and Pattern Recognition (CVPR), pp. 3642–3649. IEEE (2012)
10. Ning, F., Delhomme, D., LeCun, Y., Piano, F., Bottou, L., Barbano, P.E.: Toward automatic phenotyping of developing embryos from videos. IEEE Trans. Image Process. **14**, 1360–1371 (2005)
11. Ji, S., Xu, W., Yang, M., Yu, K.: 3d convolutional neural networks for human action recognition. IEEE Trans. Pattern Anal. Mach. Intell. **35**, 221–231 (2013)
12. Baccouche, M., Mamalet, F., Wolf, C., Garcia, C., Baskurt, A.: Sequential deep learning for human action recognition. In: Salah, A.A., Lepri, B. (eds.) HBU 2011. LNCS, vol. 7065, pp. 29–39. Springer, Heidelberg (2011)
13. Karpathy, A., Toderici, G., Shetty, S., Leung, T., Sukthankar, R., Fei-Fei, L.: Large-scale video classification with convolutional neural networks. In: IEEE Conference on Computer Vision and Pattern Recognition (CVPR) (2014)
14. Ahad, M.A.R., Tan, J.K., Kim, H., Ishikawa, S.: Motion history image: its variants and applications. Mach. Vis. Appl. **23**, 255–281 (2012)
15. Han, J., Bhanu, B.: Individual recognition using gait energy image. IEEE Trans. Pattern Anal. Mach. Intell. **28**, 316–322 (2006)
16. Yang, X., Zhang, C., Tian, Y.: Recognizing actions using depth motion maps-based histograms of oriented gradients. In: Proceedings of the 20th ACM International Conference on Multimedia, pp. 1057–1060. ACM (2012)
17. Kurakin, A., Zhang, Z., Liu, Z.: A real time system for dynamic hand gesture recognition with a depth sensor. In: 2012 Proceedings of the 20th European Signal Processing Conference (EUSIPCO), pp. 1975–1979. IEEE (2012)
18. Wu, D., Zhu, F., Shao, L.: One shot learning gesture recognition from rgbd images. In: 2012 IEEE Computer Society Conference on Computer Vision and Pattern Recognition Workshops (CVPRW), pp. 7–12. IEEE (2012)
19. Yang, X., Tian, Y.: Eigenjoints-based action recognition using naive-bayes-nearest-neighbor. In: 2012 IEEE Computer Society Conference on Computer Vision and Pattern Recognition Workshops (CVPRW), pp. 14–19. IEEE (2012)
20. Wang, J., Liu, Z., Chorowski, J., Chen, Z., Wu, Y.: Robust 3d action recognition with random occupancy patterns. In: Fitzgibbon, A., Lazebnik, S., Perona, P., Sato, Y., Schmid, C. (eds.) ECCV 2012, Part II. LNCS, vol. 7573, pp. 872–885. Springer, Heidelberg (2012)
21. Wang, J., Liu, Z., Wu, Y., Yuan, J.: Mining actionlet ensemble for action recognition with depth cameras. In: 2012 IEEE Conference on Computer Vision and Pattern Recognition (CVPR), pp. 1290–1297. IEEE (2012)
22. Oreifej, O., Liu, Z.: Hon4d: histogram of oriented 4d normals for activity recognition from depth sequences. In: 2013 IEEE Conference on Computer Vision and Pattern Recognition (CVPR), pp. 716–723. IEEE (2013)

23. LeCun, Y., Bengio, Y.: Convolutional networks for images, speech, and time series. In: Leung, T., Malik, J. (eds.) The Handbook of Brain Theory and Neural Networks. MIT press, Cambridge (1995)
24. Bergstra, J., Breuleux, O., Bastien, F., Lamblin, P., Pascanu, R., Desjardins, G., Turian, J., Warde-Farley, D., Bengio, Y.: Theano: a CPU and GPU math expression compiler. In: Proceedings of the Python for Scientific Computing Conference (SciPy), vol. 4, p. 3 (2010)
25. Han, L., Wu, X., Liang, W., Hou, G., Jia, Y.: Discriminative human action recognition in the learned hierarchical manifold space. Image Vis. Comput. **28**, 836–849 (2010)

Discriminative Orderlet Mining for Real-Time Recognition of Human-Object Interaction

Gang Yu[1](✉), Zicheng Liu[2], and Junsong Yuan[1]

[1] School of Electrical and Electronic Engineering, Nanyang Technological University, Singapore, Singapore
gyu1@e.ntu.edu.sg, jsyuan@ntu.edu.sg
[2] Microsoft Research, Redmond, WA, USA
zliu@microsoft.com

Abstract. This paper presents a novel visual representation, called orderlets, for real-time human action recognition with depth sensors. An orderlet is a middle level feature that captures the ordinal pattern among a group of low level features. For skeletons, an orderlet captures specific spatial relationship among a group of joints. For a depth map, an orderlet characterizes a comparative relationship of the shape information among a group of subregions. The orderlet representation has two nice properties. First, it is insensitive to small noise since an orderlet only depends on the comparative relationship among individual features. Second, it is a frame-level representation thus suitable for real-time online action recognition. Experimental results demonstrate its superior performance on online action recognition and cross-environment action recognition.

1 Introduction

Human movement exhibits strong coordination patterns among the skeleton joints. Each type of action typically involves a subset of joints, and the spatial configurations of these joints are strong characteristics of the action. For example, when people talk over phone, the hand that holds the phone is usually close to the ear no matter whether the person is sitting, bending, standing, or walking. This particular spatial configuration between the hand and the ear is thus a characteristic of the talking-over-phone action. We believe that if we can model such action-dependent inter-joint coordination patterns, it will provide us with an effective tool for action recognition. This paper is one step along this direction.

We propose to use an ordinal representation, called orderlets, to encode the spatial configuration of a group of skeleton joints. Generally speaking, an orderlet captures the ordinal information among a group of primitive feature values. For example, if we use the X-coordinate as the primitive feature, then the ordinal information represents which joint is the leftmost and which joint is the rightmost.

G. Yu—The work was done when Gang Yu was an intern at Microsoft Research. This work is supported in part by Singapore MoE Tier-1 grant.

D. Cremers et al. (Eds.): ACCV 2014, Part V, LNCS 9007, pp. 50–65, 2015.
DOI: 10.1007/978-3-319-16814-2_4

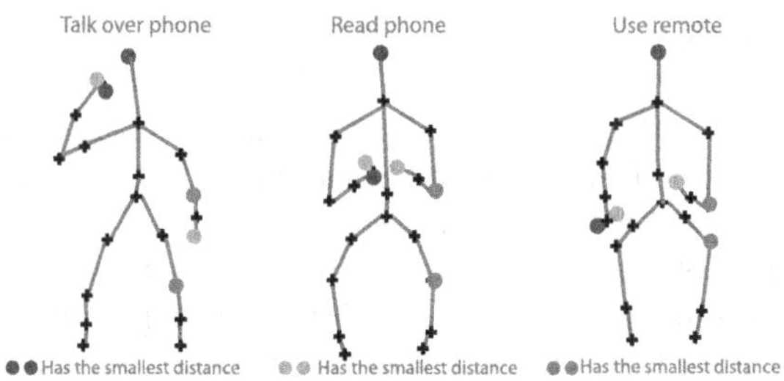

Fig. 1. An illustration of our orderlet representation.

If we use the pairwise Euclidean distances between the joints as the primitive features, then the ordinal information represents which joint pair is the closest and which joint pair is the farthest apart. Again consider the talking-over-phone action. Instead of requiring the distance between the ear and the hand to be a small value, we can require the hand-ear distance to be smaller than the distance between left hand and right hand. One example can be found in Fig. 1.

Such ordinal representation is also applicable to shape features to describe object shape information. Given a hypothesized object patch, we can divide the patch into multiple subregions. The comparative relationship between the shape features in the subregions can be captured by orderlets. In this way, both the skeleton information and the object shape information can be represented by orderlets and combined to recognize human-object interactions.

The orderlet representation has the following two properties. First, it is insensitive to small noise. An orderlet only depends on the comparative relationship among the primitive feature values. Such information is less sensitive to noise than the numerical values. Also, it is capable of handling missing or incorrect joints caused by occlusions or skeleton tracking module. Many orderlets only depend on a small group of skeleton joints. They can be correctly detected as long as the joints that they depend on are not missing. Second, the orderlet representation is well suited for real-time online action recognition from unsegmented streams since an orderlet is a frame-level representation. We have developed a real-time online action recognition system from a commodity depth sensor. The system does not require temporal segmentation, and it can handle natural transitions between two consecutive actions. Our contributions can be summarized as follows:

- We propose a novel middle level representation, called orderlets, for action recognition. It is robust to noises and missing joints, and is flexible to handle large intra-class variations.
- An orderlet mining algorithm is presented to effectively discover the discriminative orderlets from a large pool of candidates.
- We build a real time system that continuously recognizes human-object interactions using a RGB-D camera. To evaluate the performance, we collect a new dataset that contains both segmented video sequences for offline action recognition and unsegmented video sequences for online action recognition.

2 Related Work

In the past decade, there has been tremendous amount of work on human action recognition and detection from static images and 2D video sequences. It is impossible to list them all, and we only mention a few [10,11,25,26,28–32]. Recently, with the development of the commodity depth sensors like Kinect, there has been a lot of interests in human action recognition from depth data [4,12,24]. Like other visual recognition tasks, the performance of action recognition depends on the visual representation. In [13], spatial-temporal interest points are proposed to represent an action where histogram of gradients and histogram of optical flows are used to describe the extracted interest points [9]. Different from sparse interest points as in [13], a dense cuboid feature is presented in [14] for action recognition. Recently, dense trajectory [15,16] based algorithm achieved promising results on the challenging datasets like HMDB and Hollywood2.

For depth data, [1,19,21,27] utilize skeleton information as features for action recognition. In [4], it proposed the actionlet ensemble framework. Our work differs from [4] in two key aspects. First, an actionlet does not encode the spatial relationship between its joints. Second, the actionlet ensemble is a sequence-level representation that requires a segmented sequence for feature extraction and recognition. It is not suitable for online action recognition from unsegmented streams.

Instead of relying on skeleton information, many researchers have developed features based on depth maps. Wang et al. [5] proposed to randomly sample a large number of occupancy features in the 4D space of a depth sequence. Encouraged by the work of using 3D normal vectors for object recognition [7,12] proposed the histogram of oriented 4D normal features. Xia and Aggarwal [17] extended the spacetime interest point features to the depth sequences, and developed a filtering technique to suppress the noises in the depth maps thus improving the quality of the interest point detection. Other interesting action representations based on depth streams include [20,22].

Order representation has been widely used in image indexing and search. In [2], min-hash is employed for near-duplicate image search. Winner-take-all hash is presented in [3] for image search. A set of random patterns are generated and the element with the minimum value is encoded. However, there are two main differences between our work and the previous order representations. First, the previous order representations fix the group size of the primitive features, which is the number of items in an orderlet. This is not suitable for action recognition because different actions may involve different number of joints. In contrast, we allow arbitrary group size in the orderlets. Second, the order features are usually randomly generated in the previous work [3] while we use a data mining process to select the discriminative orderlets.

The orderlet representation is related to the attribute representation [8,33] in that both are higher level representations compared to the basic low-level features. There are two main differences between the orderlets and attributes. First, attribute is a sequence-level representation while orderlet is a frame-level representation. Thus orderlets are more suitable for online action recognition.

Second, attributes can be designed manually as demonstrated by [8] where manually designed attributes are important for action recognition performance. In contrast, all the orderlets are discovered automatically by a data-driven process.

3 Orderlet

Suppose we have a training dataset with N_R videos: $\mathcal{R} = \{(\mathcal{V}_i, y_i), i = 1, 2, \cdots, N_R\}$, where $y_i \in \{0, 1\}$ refers to the label of the video. $\mathcal{V} = [I_1, I_2, \cdots, I_T]$ refers to a video sequence from a RGB-D camera, where $I_t, t = 1, 2, \cdots, T$, is a video frame.

3.1 Primitive Skeleton Feature

The pose of human skeleton provides strong cues to recognize human-object interaction, as illustrated in Fig. 1. Thanks to [1], skeleton feature now can be extracted from a RGB-D video sequence. For frame I_t, the skeleton information is denoted as $\mathbf{S}^t = \{\mathbf{s}_1^t, \mathbf{s}_2^t, \cdots, \mathbf{s}_{N_S}^t\}$, where $\mathbf{s}_i^t = (x_i^t, y_i^t, z_i^t)$ refers to the coordinate position of joint i on the t-th frame and $N_S = 20$ is the total number of joints.

We propose three types of primitive features extracted from human skeleton:

- Pairwise joint distance:
$$\lambda^{(1)} = ||\mathbf{s}_i^t - \mathbf{s}_j^t||. \tag{1}$$
- Spatial coordinate of a joint:
$$\lambda^{(2)} = x_i^t \ \ or \ \ y_i^t \ \ or \ \ z_i^t. \tag{2}$$
- Temporal variation of a joint location:
$$\lambda^{(3)} = ||\mathbf{s}_i^t - \mathbf{s}_i^{t-\Delta}||, \tag{3}$$

where Δ denotes a time duration.

Pairwise joint distance feature (Eq. 1) can be used to describe the distance between joint pair in one frame. One example can be found in Fig. 1 where the distance between each pair of dots can be considered as one primitive feature. Spatial coordinate feature (Eq. 2), on the other hand, is to describe the joint's coordinate position. For example, $\lambda^{(2)} = z_i$ can be used to indicate which joint is close to the camera. Finally, temporal variation of a joint location (Eq. 3) describes the motion of one joint given a time period Δ. In general, primitive features in Eqs. 1, 2 and 3 are independent of time t.

We further denote $\Lambda^{(f)}$ as the complete primitive features of type f. Then, we have $|\Lambda^{(1)}| = N_S \times (N_S - 1)/2$, $|\Lambda^{(2)}| = N_S \times 3$, and $|\Lambda^{(3)}| = N_S \times N_\Delta$, where N_Δ refers to the number of time durations for Eq. 3.

3.2 Order Representation

There are large intra-class variations in the human actions. The same actions performed by the same person may differ a lot in terms of speed and style, not to mention the actions performed by different people in different environments. As a result, using the raw values of these primitive features is not robust.

Motivated by Fig. 1, instead of computing the raw values from the skeleton primitive features, a small set of joints with special ordinal configuration should be more meaningful for action recognition. As illustrated in Fig. 1, three joint pairs are selected with red, green and blue color, respectively. Although the raw values of the pairwise joint distance in Eq. 1 may be noisy for action classification, the ordinal configuration among the three joint pairs is actually stable for each specific human behavior. For example, for the talking-over-phone action, the red joint pair has the smallest distance among the three pairs while, for reading phone and using remote actions, the green and blue joint pairs should have the smallest distance, respectively.

Order representation has been successfully employed in image indexing and searching [2,3]. Inspired by the previous work, we propose a novel middle level representation, called orderlets. Formally, we define a size-n orderlet $\mathbf{p}$ as:

$$\mathbf{p} = (O_{\mathbf{p}}, k), \tag{4}$$

where $O_{\mathbf{p}} = [\lambda_{i_1}^{(f)}, \lambda_{i_2}^{(f)}, \cdots, \lambda_{i_n}^{(f)}]$ is a subset from $\Lambda^{(f)}$ and k is an index value for the element of $O_{\mathbf{p}}$ with the minimum value. f is denoted as the primitive feature category. The response of orderlet $\mathbf{p}$ on video frame I^t is defined as

$$\mathbf{v}_{\mathbf{p}}(I^t) = \begin{cases} 1 & \lambda_{i_k}^{(f)} \leq \lambda_{i_j}^{(f)} \text{ for all } \lambda_{i_j}^{(f)} \in O_{\mathbf{p}} \\ 0 & \text{otherwise} \end{cases} \tag{5}$$

Given a video sequence $\mathcal{V}$ with T frames, the representation of the video $\mathcal{V}$ based on orderlet $\mathbf{p}$ is:

$$\mathbf{V}_{\mathbf{p}}(\mathcal{V}) = \sum_{t=1}^{T} \mathbf{v}_{\mathbf{p}}(I^t). \tag{6}$$

3.3 Object Feature

Only using the skeleton feature is not sufficient to address the human-object interaction recognition problem. For example, it is difficult to predict the action if the actor is lifting his hand near the head position. It could be an eating action if food is held in the hand, or a picking up phone call action if the phone is in his hand. Thus, it is critical to utilize the object information for the action classification.

Different from previous work, which either extracts the object feature from the neighborhood of each joint position [4] or samples random patterns from the RGB-D space [5], we propose to focus on the potential object positions. Given the skeleton information, it is easy to model the object position relative to skeleton joints for each action class. More specifically, during the training stage, the distance between hand (both left and right) and object center is utilized for each frame and a clustering is performed to obtain several frequent hand-object shifts. Also, frequent object sizes can be obtained by a clustering process on the objects from the training data. For each testing frame, these frequent shifts and scales can be used to generate a set of potential object positions.

For each potential object position, Local Occupancy Pattern (LOP) [4] is extracted to obtain the object shape information from the depth video. Specifically, for each potential local region, it is partitioned into a grid with $N_b = N_x \times N_y \times N_z$ non-overlapping cells. The number of cloud points is computed for each cell, denoted as γ, and a sigmoid function is employed to obtain the occupancy information $l = \frac{1}{1+exp(-\beta\gamma)}$, where β is a parameter. The concatenation of all the occupancy information from each cell is the LOP feature: $\mathbf{d} = [l_1, l_2, \cdots, l_{N_b}]$.

Similar to skeleton feature in Sect. 3.2, the extracted LOP feature is further encoded by the order representation. The LOP primitive feature can be defined as:

$$\lambda^{(4)} = ||\mathbf{d}(i) - \mathbf{d}(j)|| = ||l_i - l_j||, \quad 1 \le i, j, \le N_b, \quad i \ne j. \tag{7}$$

In total, we have $|\Lambda^{(4)}| = N_b \times (N_b - 1)/2$ such features. Based on the LOP primitive feature in Eq. 7, we define LOP orderlets as in Eq. 4 of Sect. 3.2. LOP orderlets can represent the comparative relationship among the primitive shape feature of a subset of the grids, which is an important complementary feature when skeleton is ambiguous or noisy. Based on the skeleton and object orderlet representation, the next section will discuss how to obtain discriminative orderlets for action recognition.

3.4 Orderlets Discovery

We present a feature mining approach to discover a pool of discriminative orderlets, whose response $V_\mathbf{p}$ in Eq. 6 is high for the positive videos but low for the negative ones.

Initially, we have different kinds of primitive features, either from skeleton feature or object feature. Let us take the pairwise joint distance feature (Eq. 1) as an example. Suppose we have N_S joints in the skeleton, then the total number of pairwise joint distance is $|\Lambda^{(1)}| = N_S \times (N_S - 1)/2$. We start from size-2 orderlet, which can be enumerated since the total number of candidates is $|\Lambda^{(1)}| \times (|\Lambda^{(1)}| - 1)/2$.

Given a size-2 orderlet $\mathbf{p}$ and a threshold $\theta_\mathbf{p}$, we can define a classification function $\mathcal{F}_{\mathbf{p},\theta_\mathbf{p}}$ as follows:

$$\mathcal{F}_{\mathbf{p},\theta_\mathbf{p}}(\mathcal{V}) = \mathbb{1}(\mathbf{V}_\mathbf{p}(\mathcal{V}) > \theta_\mathbf{p}), \tag{8}$$

where $V_\mathbf{p}$ is the response of pattern $\mathbf{p}$ on video $\mathcal{V}$ as in Eq. 6 and $\mathbb{1}(\cdot)$ is an identity function. To handle videos with different durations, a normalization weight is added to each frame so that all the video sequences are normalized to the same duration, denoted as N_T. Thus, $\theta_\mathbf{p}$ is the response threshold on the normalized sequences. The optimal $\theta_\mathbf{p}$ can be obtained by minimizing the following classification error:

$$\epsilon_{\mathbf{p}} = \min_{\theta_{\mathbf{p}}} \frac{1}{N_R} \sum_{i=1}^{N_R} \mathbb{1}(\mathcal{F}_{\mathbf{p},\theta_{\mathbf{p}}}(\mathcal{V}) \neq y_i), \tag{9}$$

where $y_i \in \{0,1\}$ is the label of the video. For simplicity, we denote $\mathcal{F}_{\mathbf{p}}$ as the orderlet classifier with parameter $\theta_{\mathbf{p}}$ obtained from solving Eq. 9.

All the size-2 orderlets, denoted as $\mathcal{T}_2$, can be sorted based on the classification error defined in Eq. 9. To discard redundant orderlets, we remove the orderlets which have large overlapping items with previous orderlets from the sorted list. This can make our orderlet pool more diverse. Only those orderlets at the top of the list, for example, $\epsilon_{\mathbf{p}} < \mu$, are kept for further processing, where μ is an error threshold. We denote this orderlet set as $\mathcal{T}_2'$. Given the size-2 orderlets in $\mathcal{T}_2'$, they can be easily extended to size-3 orderlet set $\mathcal{T}_3$ by adding one more element from $\Lambda^{(1)}$ to the end of size-2 orderlet. Similarly, based on Eq. 9, we select a subset of them with smaller classification error. This process will continue until it reaches size-L orderlet. By generating size-$(l+1)$ orderlets from discriminative size-l orderlets, it can save us a lot of computational cost since we do not need to enumerate all the size-$(l+1)$ orderlets, but only extend those size-l orderlets with smaller classification error.

We can apply the same algorithm to the other feature types as well. Note that for spatial coordinate in Eq. 2, we require that all the items in one orderlet should use the same coordinate type (x, y, or z). Thus the total number of candidates for size-2 orderlets is: $|\Lambda^{(2)}| \times (N_S - 1)$. In general, Algorithm 1 is a description of our orderlet discovery process. After the pattern discovery process, we have an orderlet pool $\mathcal{P}^{(f)}$ for each primitive feature f.

3.5 Boosting Orderlets

As we have four types of primitive features, after mining the discriminative orderlet from each category, the combined orderlet pool is $\mathcal{P} = \mathcal{P}^{(1)} \cup \mathcal{P}^{(2)} \cup \mathcal{P}^{(3)} \cup \mathcal{P}^{(4)}$.

Algorithm 1. Orderlet Discovery

Input: Initial orderlet set $\mathcal{T}_2$, maximum orderlet size L
Output: Pattern Pool $\mathcal{P}^{(f)}$

$\mathcal{P}^{(f)} := \emptyset$
for $l := 2 \rightarrow L$ **do**
  $\mathcal{T}_l' := \{\mathbf{p}_j | \mathbf{p}_j \in \mathcal{T}_l, \epsilon_{\mathbf{p}_j} < \mu\}$
  $\mathcal{P}^{(f)} := \mathcal{P}^{(f)} \cup \mathcal{T}_l'$
  if $l < L$ **then**
    $\mathcal{T}_{l+1} := \emptyset$
    for $\lambda_{i_{l+1}}^{(f)} \in \Lambda^{(f)} - O_{\mathbf{p}_j}$ where $\mathbf{p}_j \in \mathcal{T}_l'$ **do**
      for $k := 1 \rightarrow l+1$ **do**
        $\mathbf{p}^* := ([O_{\mathbf{p}_j}, \lambda_{i_{l+1}}^{(f)}], k)$
        $\mathcal{T}_{l+1} := \mathcal{T}_{l+1} \cup \mathbf{p}^*$
      end for
    end for
  end if
end for

Now we need to further select and combine the discovered orderlets for action classification. AdaBoosting [6] is employed here due to its good performance on feature selection and combination.

Given each orderlet $\mathbf{p} \in \mathcal{P}$, we have a corresponding weak classifier $\mathcal{F}_{\mathbf{p}}(\mathcal{V})$ as defined in Eq. 8. After the boosting stage, our final classifier can be computed as:

$$g(\mathcal{V}) = \mathbb{1}(\sum_{m=1}^{M} \alpha_m \mathbb{1}(\mathcal{F}_m(\mathcal{V}) = 1) > \sum_{m=1}^{M} \alpha_m \mathbb{1}(\mathcal{F}_m(\mathcal{V}) = 0)), \tag{10}$$

where M is the number of weak learners, $\mathcal{F}_m$ is the learned orderlet weak classifier, and α_m is the weight for the m-th weak classifier $\mathcal{F}_m$.

It is easy to extend our algorithm for multi-class action recognition. Suppose we have C categories of actions, for each category, a binary one-against-rest classifier is learnt. Then the testing video $\mathcal{V}$ is labeled as the category c^* with the maximum response:

$$c^* = \arg\max_{c} \sum_{m=1}^{M} \alpha_m^c (\mathbb{1}(\mathcal{F}_m^c(\mathcal{V}) = 1) - \mathbb{1}(\mathcal{F}_m^c(\mathcal{V}) = 0)), \tag{11}$$

where $\mathcal{F}_m^c, c = 1, 2, \cdots, C$, is the m-th weak classifier and α_m^c is its corresponding weight for the category c.

4 Online Action Recognition

Online action recognition performs real-time continuous prediction for on-going testing sequence. Let us first consider two-class online action recognition. Different from the sequence-level score in Eq. 10, we define the frame-level score as:

$$h(I_t) = \sum_{m=1}^{M} \alpha_m h_m(I_t), \tag{12}$$

where $h_m(I_t)$ is the response of orderlet $\mathbf{p}_m$ (the selected orderlet for the m-th boosting stage $\mathcal{F}^m(I_t)$) on frame I_t:

$$h_m(I_t) = \frac{N_T - \theta_{\mathbf{p}_m}}{N_T} \mathbb{1}(\mathbf{v}_{\mathbf{p}_m}(I^t) = 1) - \frac{\theta_{\mathbf{p}_m}}{N_T} \mathbb{1}(\mathbf{v}_{\mathbf{p}_m}(I^t) = 0), \tag{13}$$

where $\mathbf{v}_{\mathbf{p}_m}(I^t)$ is defined in Eq. 5. $\theta_{\mathbf{p}_m}$ and N_T are defined in Sect. 3.4. The weights $\frac{N_T - \theta_{\mathbf{p}_m}}{N_T}$ and $\frac{\theta_{\mathbf{p}_m}}{N_T}$ in Eq. 13 balance the positive and negative votes based on the response threshold $\theta_{\mathbf{p}_m}$.

As it is unreliable to make a decision based on a single frame, temporal smoothness is commonly applied to bring more robust result, e.g., by using a fixed-length window. However, it is difficult to determine the optimal window size since the action speed varies and different types of actions have different durations. We thus propose to use a smoothing window with adaptive temporal length. Since each frame votes a positive score for the target class and a negative score for the other types of actions, at current frame t, we can search backward for a window with the largest accumulated score. Following the maximum subarray search [23], we present an efficient forward sub-path search algorithm which can determine the best score for the current frame without performing a backward search for every frame. The idea is to maintain a best score $\mathcal{S}(\mathcal{V}^t)$ for each frame t:

$$\mathcal{S}(\mathcal{V}^t) = \max(\ 0, \mathcal{S}(\mathcal{V}^{t-1}) + h(I_t)\ ), \quad t > 1 \tag{14}$$

where $\mathcal{S}(\mathcal{V}^1) = h(I_1)$. If the best score is smaller than 0, it will be reset as 0, indicating the start of new action. Intuitively, $\mathcal{S}(\mathcal{V}^t) > 0$ means one action is continuing and $\mathcal{S}(\mathcal{V}^t) \leq 0$ means no action is happening at current frame. This can naturally split the testing sequence based on our score response defined by Eq. 14.

For multi-class online action recognition, denote $\mathcal{S}^c(\mathcal{V}^t)$ as the score for category c, then the category with largest response $c^* = \arg\max_c \mathcal{S}^c(\mathcal{V}^t)$ is the prediction label.

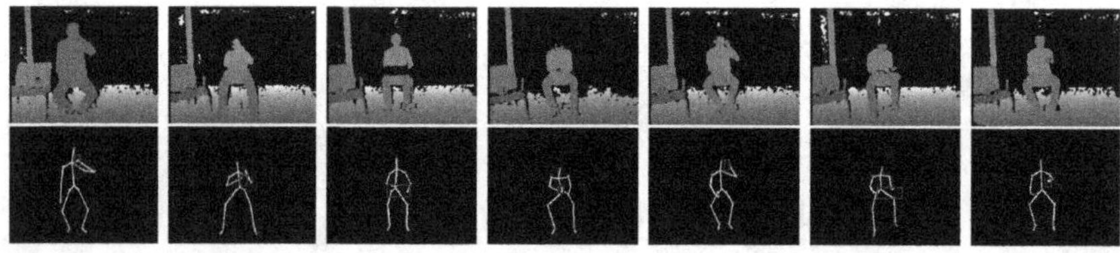

Fig. 2. Sample frames of our human-object interaction dataset. The first row is from the depth stream and the second row is from the skeleton stream with the object position marked with blue rectangle. The seven columns refer to drinking, eating, using laptop, reading phone, picking up phone, reading book, and using remote, respectively.

5 Experiments

5.1 Action Recognition on Online RGBD Action Dataset (ORGBD)

As far as we know, there does not exist a benchmark dataset for cross-environment and online action recognition with depth sensors. To that end, we collect a new dataset which simulates the living room environment: "Online RGBD Action dataset (ORGBD)"[1]. There are seven types of actions that people often do in the living room: *drinking, eating, using laptop, picking up phone, reading phone (sending SMS), reading book*, and *using remote*. All these actions are human-object interactions. The bounding box of the object in each frame is manually labelled. The object location labels are used only for training. Figure 2 gives an illustration of the seven action categories.

[1] The dataset can be downloaded from http://research.microsoft.com/en-us/um/people/zliu/ActionRecoRsrc/default.htm.

Three sets of depth sequences are collected by using a Kinect device. The first set, which is designed for action recognition in the same environment, contains 16 subjects and each subject performs every action two times. The second set contains 8 new subjects which are recorded in different environments from the first one. This set is used for cross-environment action recognition. In the third set, each sequence consists of multiple unsegmented actions. This set is for real-time online action recognition.

Same-Environment Action Recognition. We first evaluate our algorithm based on video sequences in the same environment: half-of the subjects in the first set are used for the training and the other half subjects are used for testing. 2-fold cross-validation is used and the mean value is reported in Table 1. It shows the significant improvement if multiple features are combined together compared with using a single feature. This verifies that our skeleton and object features are complementary. In addition to using boosting to select the discriminative orderlets, we also perform the experiment with linear SVM to learn the weights for each orderlet. Table 1 shows that boosting works better than linear SVM. Compared with the state-of-art algorithms [4,17,19,27], our algorithm has obvious performance advantage.

Table 1. Comparison of recognition results on human-object interaction dataset.

Method	Accuracy
Pairwise joint distance only (Eq. 1)	0.633
Spatial coordinate only (Eq. 2)	0.544
Temporal variation only (Eq. 3)	0.455
Object feature only (Eq. 7)	0.464
All the features + Boosting	**0.714**
All the features + SVM	0.687
Skeleton + LoP [4]	0.660
DSTIP + DCSF [17]	0.617
EigenJoints [19]	0.491
Moving Pose [27]	0.384
All the features & Occlusion	0.546
EigenJoints [19] & Occlusion	0.169

Figure 3 shows seven mined orderlets, one per action class, based on the pairwise joint distance. Each pair of joints is marked with the same color. The joint pair with red color refers to the minimum element index k which is defined in Eq. 4. For instance, for the drinking action, if the red color pair is of the smallest distance, then this orderlet will give a positive vote for the drinking action. The pattern statistics of our mined classifier in Eq. 10 is shown in Fig. 4. The diagram on the left shows the percentage of orderlets from each primitive feature type in the

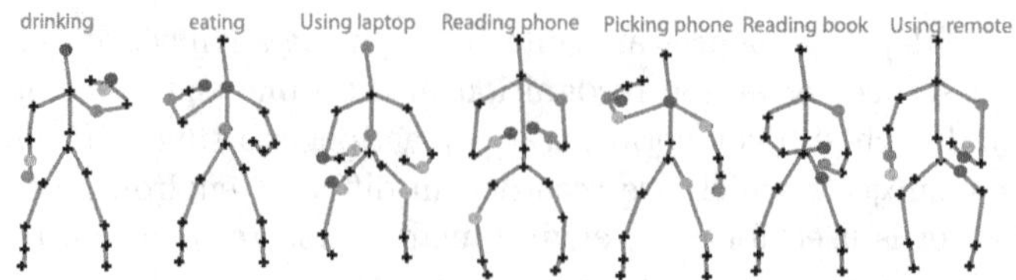

Fig. 3. Examples of mined orderlet based on pairwise joint distance. Different skeleton pairs are marked with different color (Colour figure online).

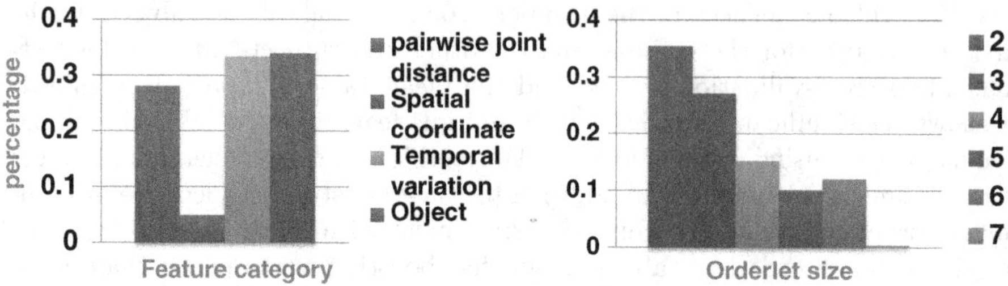

Fig. 4. Pattern statistics for our final classifier.

final classifier. The statistics of the orderlet size is shown in the right diagram of Fig. 4. We can see that both skeleton and object orderlets have a strong effect on our final classifier and most of the orderlets have size 2 or 3.

Next we test the robustness of our algorithm against missing joints caused by occlusion or skeleton tracking module. With the Kinect device, it is difficult to capture partial occlusion data because the occlusion of a subset of the joints may cause the skeleton tracking to fail on all the joints. So we simulate the occlusion scenario by randomly selecting 4 skeleton joints and consider them as being occluded (setting their coordinates to be 0). The results are shown at the bottom of Table 1. We can see that our algorithm works much better than the global skeleton feature [19]. This is because most of the orderlets involve only a small number of joints.

Cross-Environment Action Recognition. To test the robustness and generalization capability of our algorithm, we use the 8 new subjects from the second set of our human-object interaction dataset for testing. The 16 subjects in the first set are used for training. The recognition results are shown in Table 2. We can see that our algorithm is more robust than [4,17,19,27] for cross-environment action recognition.

Action Prediction on Segmented Videos. Action prediction [18] on segmented video sequences is tested to evaluate the latency of our algorithm. We follow the setting in Sect. 5.1. Figure 5 shows the result of our algorithm. Obviously, our algorithm has significant advantages over DSTIP+DCSF [17] and Moving Pose [27] especially when the observation ratio is lower than 40 %. To implement [17], 500 interest points are extracted from each depth sequence and

Table 2. Comparison of cross-environment recognition results.

Method	Accuracy
All the features	**0.661**
Skeleton + LoP [4]	0.598
DSTIP + DCSF [17]	0.215
Eigenjoints [19]	0.357
Moving Pose [27]	0.285

clustered based on a vocabulary with 1000 words. From Fig. 5, we can see that our algorithm performs very well even when only 10 % to 20 % of the frames are observed. This is an indication of the effectiveness our object feature. When more frames are observed, the skeleton feature helps to improve the prediction results.

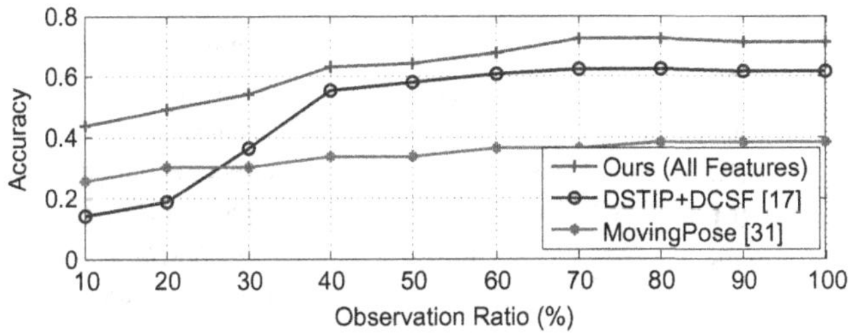

Fig. 5. Comparison of action prediction results.

Continuous Action Recognition. Different from action prediction in previous subsection, which requires to know the start frame of the action, our algorithm can also be used for online action recognition on unsegmented video. We collect 36 unsegmented action sequences from 12 new subjects. There are three unsegmented sequences for each subject. Each sequence consists of multiple actions. Seven categories of human actions as well as the background action (none of the seven actions) are recorded continuously. The duration of these video sequences lasts from 30 s to 2 min. Among the 36 continuous sequences, there are 123 actions from the seven categories and the percentage of background frames (without any of the seven actions) is around 30 %. For evaluation purpose, we manually label each frame of the video sequences but the boundary between two consecutive actions may not be very accurate since it is difficult to determine the boundary.

We train our model on the segmented data as described in Sect. 5.1 plus additional background action sequences. The 36 continuous videos are used for testing. Our algorithm can process around 25 frames per second with un-optimized code on a normal desktop PC.

Table 3 compares our algorithm with [17,19,27] based on frame-level accuracy, i.e., the percentage of frames which are correctly classified. To utilize [17]

Table 3. Comparison of online action recognition results based on frame-level accuracy.

Method	Accuracy
Our algorithm	**0.564**
DSTIP + DCSF [17]	0.321
EigenJoints [19]	0.236
Moving Pose [27]	0.50

for online action recognition, we extract 3 DSTIPs in average from each frame and make a decision based on the histogram in a sliding window of 100 frames long. Similarly, [19,27] are also modified to make a prediction based on a 100-frame sliding window. The results are shown in Table 3. We can see that our algorithm performs significantly better than the baselines [17,19,27] on the continuous action recognition.

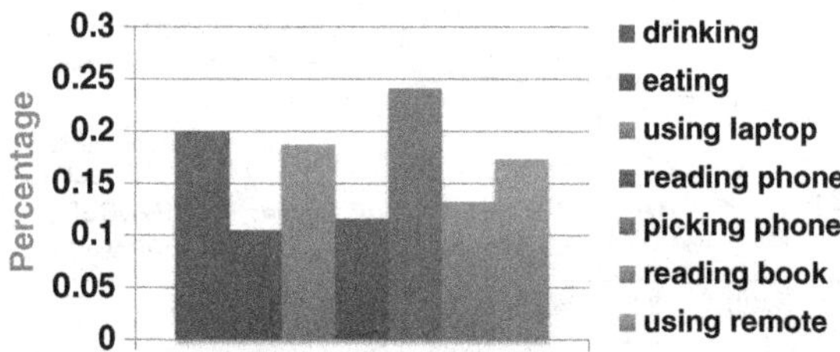

Fig. 6. Latency analysis. Y-axis refers to the percentage of frames passed until our algorithm can make the positive prediction.

Actually, there is a latency between the our prediction and the ground-truth. Figure 6 gives a latency analysis of our algorithm. 61 actions out of 123 non-background actions, which have more than 50 % overlap with ground-truth, are evaluated. Y-axis refers to the average ratio of the number of frames that have passed until our algorithm first gives a positive prediction over that action's duration. Clearly, our algorithm has a very short latency. Most of the time, it gives a correct prediction when less than 25 % of the sequence is observed.

5.2 Action Recognition on MSR Daily Activity 3D Dataset

The MSR Daily Activity 3D dataset is collected in an indoor environment with sixteen categories: *drink, eat, read book, call cellphone, write on a paper, use laptop, use vacuum cleaner, cheer up, sit still, toss paper, play game, lie down on sofa, walk, play guitar, stand up and sit down.* There are 10 subjects and each subject performs each action twice, one in sitting pose and the other in standing pose.

Continuous Action Recognition. To test continuous action recognition on MSR Daily Activity dataset, we use the videos from half of the subjects for

Table 4. Comparison of continuous action recognition results on MSR daily activity dataset. Frame-level accuracy is used for evaluating the performance.

Method	Accuracy
Our algorithm	**0.601**
DSTIP + DCSF [17]	0.246
EigenJoints [19]	0.470
Moving Pose [27]	0.452

training and the other half for testing. Similar to Sect. 5.1, frame-level accuracy is employed to evaluate the performance of action recognition based on all the frames till the current frame. As shown in Table 4, our algorithm obtains promising results compared with the baselines on the task of continuous action recognition.

Batch Action Recognition. For the batch action recognition, we follow the standard evaluation setting: half of the subjects are used for training and the other half are used for testing. Table 5 shows the action recognition results. Since many of the categories in MSR Daily Activity dataset do not contain objects interacted with human, our algorithm is only based on skeleton feature. To make it fair for comparison, we mainly compare with the algorithms on skeleton feature [4,27] (skeleton only). Although our algorithm is not as good as [4] which is based on both skeleton and depth features on batch action recognition, [4] cannot be applied for the continuous action recognition due to the batch feature representation.

Table 5. Comparison of batch action recognition results on MSR daily activity dataset.

Method	Accuracy
Our skeleton Feature	0.738
Skeleton in [4]	0.68
Both Skeleton and Depth in [4]	0.857[a]
Moving Pose [27]	0.738

[a] This result (0.857) of [4] is obtained based on both the skeleton and depth streams while the other algorithms only rely on the skeleton features.

6 Conclusion

In this paper, we proposed a novel middle level representation, called orderlets, for recognizing human-object interactions. An orderlet captures the ordinal patterns among a group of low-level features. It can be applied to skeletons to encode inter-joint coordinations as well as depth maps to encode the object's shape information. An orderlet mining algorithm is presented to discover the most representative orderlets from an extremely large pool. A boosting technique is developed to combine the discriminative orderlets for action recognition. Experiments on cross-environment action recognition, occlusion handling, and online action recognition demonstrated the effectiveness of this new representation.

References

1. Shotton, J., Fitzgibbon, A., Cook, M., Sharp, T., Finocchio, M., Moore, R., Kipman, A., Blake, A.: Real-time human pose recognition in parts from single depth images. In: CVPR (2011)
2. Chum, O., Philbin, J., Zisserman, A.: Near duplicate image detection: min-Hash and tf-idf weighting. In: BMVC (2008)
3. Yagnik, J., Strelow, D., Ross, D., Lin, R.S.: The power of comparative reasoning. In: ICCV (2011)
4. Wang, J., Liu, Z., Wu, Y., Yuan, J.: Mining actionlet ensemble for action recognition with depth cameras. In: CVPR (2012)
5. Wang, J., Liu, Z., Chorowski, J., Chen, Z., Wu, Y.: Robust 3d action recognition with random occupancy patterns. In: Fitzgibbon, A., Lazebnik, S., Perona, P., Sato, Y., Schmid, C. (eds.) ECCV 2012, Part II. LNCS, vol. 7573, pp. 872–885. Springer, Heidelberg (2012)
6. Schapire, R.: A brief introduction to boosting. In: IJCAI (1999)
7. Tang, S., Wang, X., Lv, X., Han, T.X., Keller, J., He, Z., Skubic, M., Lao, S.: Histogram of oriented normal vectors for object recognition with a depth sensor. In: Lee, K.M., Matsushita, Y., Rehg, J.M., Hu, Z. (eds.) ACCV 2012, Part II. LNCS, vol. 7725, pp. 525–538. Springer, Heidelberg (2013)
8. Liu, J., Kuipers, B., Savarese, S.: Recognizing human actions by attributes. In: CVPR (2011)
9. Schuldt, C., Laptev, I., Caputo, B.: Recognizing human actions: a local svm approach. In: ICPR (2004)
10. Yu, G., Yuan, J., Liu, Z.: Unsupervised random forest indexing for fast action search. In: IEEE Conference on Computer Vision and Pattern Recognition (2011)
11. Yu, G., Yuan, J., Liu, Z.: Propagative hough voting for human activity recognition. In: Fitzgibbon, A., Lazebnik, S., Perona, P., Sato, Y., Schmid, C. (eds.) ECCV 2012, Part III. LNCS, vol. 7574, pp. 693–706. Springer, Heidelberg (2012)
12. Oreifej, O., Liu, Z.: HON4D: histogram of oriented 4D Normals for activity recognition from depth sequences. In: CVPR (2013)
13. Laptev, I.: On space-time interest points. IJCV **64**(2–3), 107–123 (2005)
14. Dollar, P., Rabaud, V., Cottrell, G., Belongiel, S.: Behavior recognition via sparse spatio-temporal features. In: Visual Surveillance and Performance Evaluation of Tracking and Surveillance (2005)
15. Wang, H., Klaser, A., Schmid, C., Liu, C.L.: Action recognition by dense trajectories. In: CVPR (2011)
16. Jiang, Y.-G., Dai, Q., Xue, X., Liu, W., Ngo, C.-W.: Trajectory-based modeling of human actions with motion reference points. In: Fitzgibbon, A., Lazebnik, S., Perona, P., Sato, Y., Schmid, C. (eds.) ECCV 2012, Part V. LNCS, vol. 7576, pp. 425–438. Springer, Heidelberg (2012)
17. Xia, L., Aggarwal, J.K.: Spatio-temporal depth cuboid similarity feature for activity recognition using depth camera. In: CVPR (2013)

18. Ryoo, M.S.: Human activity prediction: early recognition of ongoing activities from streaming videos. In: ICCV (2011)
19. Yang, X., Tian, Y.: EigenJoints-based action recognition using Naive-Bayes-Nearest-Neighbor. In: CVPRW (2012)
20. Yang, X., Zhang, C., Tian, Y.: Recognizing actions using depth motion maps-based histograms of oriented gradients. In: ACM Multimedia (2012)
21. Chen, H.S., Chen, H.T., Chen, Y.W., Lee, S.Y.: Human action recognition using star skeleton. In: ACM International Workshop on Video Surveillance and Sensor Networks (2006)
22. Li, W., Zhang, Z., Liu, Z.: Action recognition based on a bag of 3d points. In: CVPRW (2010)
23. Bentley, J.: Programming pearls: algorithm design techniques. Commun. ACM **27**(9), 865–873 (1984)
24. Zhu, Y., Chen, W., Guo, G.D.: Fusing spatiotemporal features and joints for 3D action recognition. In: CVPRW (2013)
25. Hoai, M., DelaTorre, F.: Max-margin early event detectors. In: CVPR (2012)
26. Zhou, B., Wang, X., Tang, X.: Understanding collective crowd behaviors: learning a mixture model of dynamic pedestrian-agents. In: CVPR (2012)
27. Zanfir, M., Leordeanu, M., Sminchisescu, C.: The moving pose: an efficient 3d kinematics descriptor for low-latency action recognition and detection. In: ICCV (2013)
28. Yu, G., Norberto, A., Yuan, J., Liu, Z.: Fast action detection via discriminative random forest voting and top-K subvolume search. IEEE Trans. Multimedia **13**(3), 507–517 (2011)
29. Sadanand, S., Corso, J.J.: Action bank: a high-level representation of activity in video. In: CVPR (2012)
30. Chen, C.Y., Grauman, K.: Efficient activity detection with max-subgraph search. In: CVPR (2012)
31. Gupta, A., Davis, L.S.: Objects in action: an approach for combining action understanding and object perception. In: CVPR (2007)
32. Jain, A., Gupta, A., Rodriguez, M., Davis, L.S.: Representing videos using mid-level discriminative patches. In: CVPR (2013)
33. Parikh, D., Grauman, K.: Relative attributes. In: ICCV (2011)

Anomaly Detection via Local Coordinate Factorization and Spatio-Temporal Pyramid

Tan Xiao[1,2(✉)], Chao Zhang[1], Hongbin Zha[1], and Fangyun Wei[1]

[1] Key Laboratory of Machine Perception, Peking University, Beijing, P.R. China
pkuxiaotan@pku.edu.cn, {chzhang,zha}@cis.pku.edu.cn, wei494300527@163.com
[2] CRSC Communication & Information Corporation, Beijing, P.R. China

Abstract. Anomaly detection, which aims to discover anomalous events, defined as having a low likelihood of occurrence, from surveillance videos, has attracted increasing interest and is still a challenge in computer vision community. In this paper, we propose an efficient anomaly detection approach which can perform both real-time and multi-scale detection. Our approach can handle the change of background. Specifically, Local Coordinate Factorization is utilized to tell whether a spatio-temporal video volume (STV) belongs to an anomaly, which can effectively detect spatial, temporal and spatio-temporal anomalies. And we employ Spatio-temporal Pyramid (STP) to capture the spatial and temporal continuity of an anomalous event, enabling our approach to handle multi-scale and complicated events. We also propose an online method to update the local coordinates, which makes our approach self-adaptive to background change which typically occurs in real-world setting. We conduct extensive experiments on several publicly available datasets for anomaly detection, and the results show that our approach can outperform state-of-the-art approaches, which verifies the effectiveness of our approach.

1 Introduction

Recent years, surveillance system has been applied to almost everywhere in a city. However, current systems require human operators to watch a large number of screens [1] showing the content captured by differen cameras. One of the main tasks of human operators is to detect or discover suspicious and unusual individuals or events [2], or anomalies. However, with more cameras in city, more human efforts are required, and it's becoming more difficult for human operators and their performance may degrades significantly [3]. To address this problem, automatic anomaly detection approaches attract increasing interests in recent years. These techniques can automatically analyze video streams to warn, possibly in real-time, the human operators that an anomalous event is taking place.

This research was supported by National Key Basic Research Project of China (973 Program) 2011CB302400 and National Nature Science Foundation of China (NSFC Grant No. 61071156 and 61131003).

D. Cremers et al. (Eds.): ACCV 2014, Part V, LNCS 9007, pp. 66–82, 2015.
DOI: 10.1007/978-3-319-16814-2_5

In computer vision community, anomaly detection is defined as discovering events with low likelihood of occurrence. Recent works can be summarized into three categories based on how they construct their models: supervised [4–8], semi-supervised [9,10] and unsupervised [11–17]. Actually, considering that anomalies are always rare and they can be quite different from each other with unpredictable variations, recent works [16,17] concentrate more on unsupervised scenarios. Furthermore, since it's almost impossible to define all the anomalous events in advance, unsupervised approaches are more practical.

Several unsupervised approaches have been proposed. Trajectories based approaches [18–21] aim to track motions of objects and persons by their spatial location. But these methods only consider spatial deviations, thus abnormal appearance or motion of a target following a "normal" track is not detected. And they are difficult to cope with crowd scenes where precise segmentation of a target is nearly impossible. Optical flow has also been used to model typical motion patterns [11–13]. However, these methods perform unreliably in crowded scenes, as mentioned in [18]. Furthermore, two kinds of approaches above mainly focus on the motion of objects, i.e., they only considers anomalous motion while ignoring anomalous appearance. Instead, [16] and [17] propose to use densely sampled local spatio-temporal descriptor which represents both motion and appearance and possesses some degree of robustness to unimportant variations in data. A non-parametric statistic model is utilized in [16] to measure the degree of anomaly. And [17] proposes to organize spatio-temporal video volumes into large contextual graphs and decompose spatio-temporal contextual information into unique spatial and temporal contexts. Both methods achieve promising results for real-time anomaly detection on several publicly available datasets.

An effective real-time anomaly detection approach should have the following properties. (1) It should be unsupervised because it's almost impossible to define all anomalous events in advance and it's burdensome for human operators to do so. (2) It can detect both spatial and temporal anomalies. (3) It can detect multi-scale events. Actually, it's also hard to know in advance the range of an anomaly, e.g. how large the abnormal object is, how fast the abnormal object moves, or how long the abnormal event lasts. (4) It should be self-adaptive to scene change, both in appearance and motion, which has also emphasized in [16] and [17]. In fact, the appearance background is always changing in surveillance videos because of the lighting condition, weather, etc. (5) Of course, it should be able to effectively and efficiently detect the anomalies from surveillance videos.

In this paper, we propose a novel approach for anomaly detection in surveillance videos. Densely sampled spatio-temporal video volumes (STVs) with pixel-by-pixel analysis is utilized as the foundation of our approach. Specifically, each STV is represented by a local spatio-temporal descriptor which can capture both motion and appearance characteristic of STV. Motivated by the extensive study in employing STVs in the context of bag-of-video-words (BoVW), we propose to use Local Coordinate Factorization [22] to tell whether a STV belongs to an anomalous event. The local coordinates are updated continuously with coming surveillance videos, thus it requires no offline or supervised pre-training.

This unsupervised method enables our approach to detect anomaly which hasn't been observed before. Furthermore, the updating procedure also ensures that our approach can cope with the scene change both in appearance and motion. To detect multi-scale and complicated anomalies, we propose a Spatio-temporal Pyramid (STP), which is the temporal extension of spatial pyramid [23]. STP can describe videos by STV of different scales to detect multi-scale events. We also observe that an event is always associated with several STVs which are different in location or time or both. STP can be used to discover the relationship of different STVs associated to one event, which enables our approach to detect complicated events. Furthermore, upper level representation of STP can be easily constructed from lower level representation, which guarantees the efficiency.

The overview of our approach is summarized in Fig. 1. Given a video stream, initially it's densely sampled, i.e., sampled pixel by pixel, and a 3-D volume is constructed around a pixel. Then this volume is segmented without overlap into 8 smaller STVs. The large STV forms the upper and coarser level of STP, which can capture the overall information of an event. And the small STVs form the lower and finer level of STP, which can describe an event in detail. We can also segment any small STV into another smaller 8 STVs. But we find that a two-level STP is enough for anomaly detection. Then HOG features which can represent both motion and appearance are extracted for each STV. Interestingly,

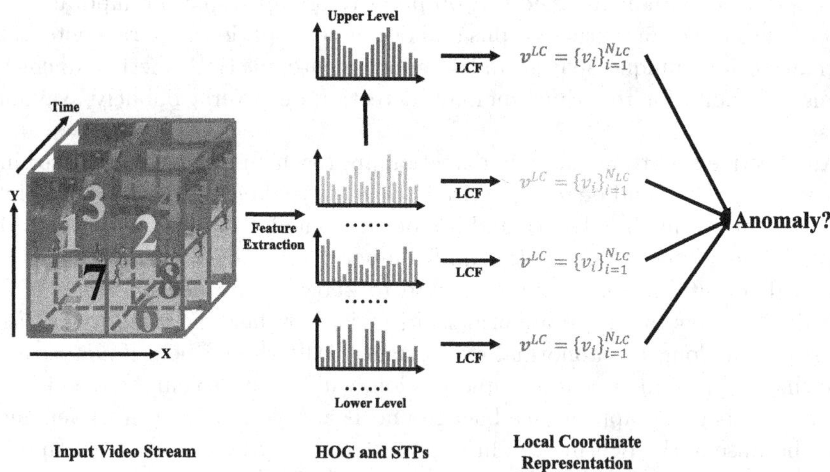

Fig. 1. Overview of our approach. This is an example of two-level spatio-temporal pyramid. The input is a video stream. Then a 3-D volume around a pixel is constructed represented by the outer red cube. Then it's segmented into 8 ($2 \times 2 \times 2$) smaller cubes denoted by different numbers in this figure. The smaller cubes form the lower but finer level of the pyramid. HOG features are extracted for each smaller cube. And the HOG features of upper level cube can be constructed efficiently from lower level cubes. Next, we apply Local Coordinate Factorization to each cube (both lower and upper level) to generate their local coordinate representation v. Finally, the anomaly judgement is given based on the combination of local coordinate representation of different levels.

we find that the HOG of upper level STV can be easily constructed from lower level STVs, implying that the pyramid doesn't require too much extra computation. So it can be quite efficient which is essential for real-time detection. Local Coordinate Factorization is then applied to the HOG features to obtain the local coordinate representation v for each STV. Furthermore, the local coordinates are updated automatically to adapt adapting themselves to scene changes. Finally, the anomaly judgement is given based on results of both levels.

The main contributions of this paper can be summarized as follows. (1) We propose a novel anomaly detection approach based on densely sampled STVs. Local Coordinate Factorization is applied to HOG features of STV to effectively judge whether this STV belongs to an anomalous event. (2) We propose to use Spatio-temporal Pyramid (STP) to capture the spatial and temporal continuity of an anomalous event. STP can also enable our approach to handle multi-scale and complicated events. (3) We propose an online method to continuously update the local coordinates so our method can adaptively learns the event patterns in the scene and thus can cope with scene changes. (4) We conduct extensive experiments on several public datasets to evaluate our approach for anomaly detection. The results show that our approach can significantly outperform several state-of-the-art approaches, which verifies the effectiveness of our approach.

2 Related Work

As mentioned above, trajectory analysis of objects are widely utilized in previous works. However, they require precise tracking methods [24,25]. Unfortunately, tracking objects is time-consuming, especially in crowded scene where a lot of objects (or persons) are moving so that precise segmentation of targets which is the foundation of tracking is nearly impossible. Optical flow is also used in several works [11–13] but they also perform unreliably in crowded scenes [16].

Recent years, approaches not requiring object detection or tracking, focusing on local spatio-temporal features are proposed and have received increasing attention [26,27]. These approaches describe the local characteristic at each pixel by low-level visual features such as color, texture and motion. Then a pixel-level background model and behavior template can be constructed [28–31]. Moreover, spatio-temporal video volumes in the context of bag-of-video-words are becoming popular [12,16,32,33]. By ignoring the order of local features, probabilistic topic models like LDA [34] can be directly applied to analysis videos [35,36]. But these methods often ignore the spatio-temporal relationship between STVs which is essential for scene understanding and event detection [37,38]. Some works have made efforts to incorporate either spatial or temporal compositions of STVs into the probabilistic topic model. But they are highly time-consuming and computationally expensive, thus they can't be applied to online and real-time tasks [39]. Furthermore, some approaches [26,29,40,41] propose to construct spatio-temporal behavior model and low-level local anomalous events can be detected by analyzing the spatio-temporal pattern of each pixel as a function of time.

However, such as in [40], they independently process each pixel but ignore the relationships between pixel in space and time, thus leading to too local detection.

In [16], Bertini *et al.* propose a multi-scale and non-parametric approach to perform real-time anomaly detection and localization. To capture both appearance and motion of objects in the scene, dense local spatio-temporal features are extracted at each pixel. And they propose to use "overlapping" features to consider the relationship between pixels. Though they achieve promising results, their approach also face challenge of efficiency to achieve accurate multi-scale detection. In fact, our Spatio-temporal Pyramid is partially motivated by their "overlapping" features. But our STP can be constructed more efficiently and can achieve much better performance. And our STP can naturally cope with multi-scale detection while their approach actually treat different scales independently.

In addition, our Local Coordinate Factorization is similar to the Sparse Reconstruction method proposed in [15]. However, their reconstruction problem is formulated as an L_1-norm regularized least squares problem which can't be solved quite efficiently, thus their method can't be applied to real-time detection. But Local Coordinate Factorization can be solved by just few simple linear matrix operations which can be highly efficient for real-time detection.

3 Local Coordinate Factorization

3.1 Spatio-Temporal Features

Firstly, we need to describe a two-level STV (we can use any-level STV, but we find two level is enough) centered at pixel (x, y, t) by meaningful spatio-temporal features. Given a STV $v \in \mathbb{R}^{n_x \times n_y \times n_t}$ with the size $n_x \times n_y \times n_t$, where $n_x \times n_y$ is the sizeof spatial window and n_t is the depth of STV in time. In this paper, we find $10 \times 10 \times 10$ is a good choice. Then we calculate the histogram of the spatio-temporal gradient of the video in polar coordinates to describe the STV [16,17,42]. Denote the spatial gradients as $G_x(x, y, t)$, $G_y(x, y, t)$, and the temporal gradient as $G_t(x, y, t)$ respectively at pixel (x, y, t). To eliminate the effect of local texture and contrast, the spatial gradient is normalized as:

$$G_s(x, y, t) = \frac{\sqrt{G_x^2(x, y, t) + G_y^2(x, y, t)}}{\sum_{x', y', t' \in v} \sqrt{G_x^2(x', y', t') + G_y^2(x', y', t')} + \epsilon} \tag{1}$$

where $G_s(x, y, t)$ is the normalized spatial gradient and ϵ is a constant to avoid numeric instabilities. In this paper, we set $\epsilon = 0.01$. Then we can construct 3D normalized gradient represented in polar coordinates as below,

$$M_{3D}(x, y, t) = \sqrt{G_s^2(x, y, t) + G_t^2(x, y, t)} \tag{2}$$

$$\theta(x, y, t) = \tan^{-1}\left(\frac{G_y(x, y, t)}{G_x(x, y, t)}\right) \tag{3}$$

$$\phi(x,y,t) = \tan^{-1}(\frac{G_t(x,y,t)}{G_s(x,y,t)}) \tag{4}$$

where $M_{3D}(x,y,t)$ is the magnitude of 3D normalized gradient, and $\phi(x,y,t) \in [-\frac{\pi}{2}, \frac{\pi}{2}]$ and $\theta(x,y,t) \in [-\pi, \pi]$ are the orientations of the gradient respectively. Now for a given STV v, we can construct a histogram of oriented gradients (HOG) by quantizing each pixel in v into $n_\phi + n_\theta$ bins by their 3D normalized gradient. In this paper, we set $n_\phi = 8$ and $n_\theta = 16$. So the HOG features for STV v, denoted as h, has 24 dimension in this paper. From the feature extraction procedure, we can see that this HOG feature can capture the characteristics of both motion and appearance in the video so that we can detect both anomalous actions and objects. Furthermore, it's also robust to unimportant variations in the data such as texture and contrast. Though it's quite simple, it shows promising performance. Moreover, we need to mention that, as a histogram feature, each element in h is non-negative. This is an essential property for the Local Coordinate Factorization, which requires non-negative input.

We can also notice that it can be efficient to calculate this HOG feature. In fact, the gradient and 3D normalized gradient for all pixels can be computed in advance. And the histogram of pixel (x,y,t), denoted as $h(x,y,t)$ can also be precomputed by quantization. Then the histogram of a STV v around pixel (x,y,t) can be computed by simply sum up all the histogram in this STV as

$$h_v(x,y,t) = \sum_{(x',y',t') \in v} h(x',y',t') \tag{5}$$

And computing the HOG of a STV can use its neighbor's HOG which has been computed to save more computations. Denote the STV around (x,y,t) and $(x+1,y,t)$ as v_1 and v_2 respectively. Then we have,

$$h_{v_2} = h_{v_1} - \sum_{(x',y',t') \in v_1 \setminus v_2} h(x',y',t') + \sum_{(x',y',t') \in v_2 \setminus v_1} h(x',y',t') \tag{6}$$

where "\" is the set minus operation. It's clear that $v_1 \setminus v_2$ is much smaller than v_1. Furthermore, the HOG feature of upper level STV can be computed by summing up the HOG features of lower level STVs in the same STP. Consider the outer red cube in Fig. 1. Given the HOG of eight lower level STVs in this cube, the HOG of the upper level, i.e., the red cube, can be computed as follow,

$$h_{v_{\text{up}}} = \sum_{(x',y',t') \in v_{\text{up}}} h(x',y',t') = \sum_{i=1}^{8} \sum_{(x',y',t') \in v_i} h(x',y',t') = \sum_{i=1}^{8} h_{v_i} \tag{7}$$

The highly efficiency of spatio-temporal feature extraction, which is guaranteed by computation tricks above, is one of the requirements for real-time detection.

3.2 Local Coordinate Selection

When statio-temporal features are extracted for STV, we can perform Local Coordinate Factorization to tell whether this STV belongs to an anomalous event.

Algorithm 1. Local Coordinate Selection

Input: $\mathbf{H}$,$\lambda = 1$, $\mathbf{S}_0$ K, c
Output: $\mathbf{S}$;
Initialize $\mathbf{Z}_0 = \mathbf{S}_0$,$a_0 = 1$
for $k = 0, 1, 2, ..., K$ **do**
  $\mathbf{S}_{k+1} = \arg\min_{\mathbf{S}} : p_{\mathbf{Z}_k,L}(\mathbf{S}) = D_{\frac{\lambda}{L}}(\mathbf{Z}_k - \frac{1}{L}\nabla f(\mathbf{Z}_k))$
  while $f_0(\mathbf{S}_{k+1}) > p_{\mathbf{Z}_k,L}(\mathbf{S}_{k+1})$ **do**
    $L = L/c$
    $\mathbf{S}_{k+1} = \arg\min_{\mathbf{S}} : p_{\mathbf{Z}_k,L}(\mathbf{S}) = D_{\frac{\lambda}{L}}(\mathbf{Z}_k - \frac{1}{L}\nabla f(\mathbf{Z}_k))$
  end while
  $a_{k+1} = (1 + \sqrt{1 + 4a_k^2})/2$
  $\mathbf{Z}_{k+1} = (\frac{a_{k+1}+a_k-1}{a_{k+1}})\mathbf{S}_{k+1} - (\frac{a_k-1}{a_{k+1}})\mathbf{S}_k$
end for

But we need to construct local coordinates first. Actually, the local coordinates for our approach can be regarded as video words for BoVW, i.e., they are some points in the feature space. Analogous to video words, local coordinates can be generated by cluster the spatio-temporal features. The obtained cluster centroids are local coordinates. However, there are some parameters for clustering algorithm, for example, we need to specify k for kmeans clustering. And we find our approach is a little sensitive to this parameter.

Instead, we propose to construct local coordinates from data. Given a set of spatio-temporal features $\mathbf{H} = [h_1, ..., h_n] \in \mathbb{R}^{d\times n}$, where $d = 24$ is the dimension of feature, and n is the size of feature set. Actually we don't need a training set. This initial feature set $\mathbf{H}$ can be constructed by using the first one or two seconds of the video. Moreover, we can also randomly select some features to reduce n so that our selection algorithm is computationally feasible. In this paper, we tune n from $10,000$ to $20,000$ based on the resolution of videos. Then we need to select some features from $\mathbf{H}$ as the local coordinates. In our method, the number of local coordinates is determined automatically by the algorithm, which is more adaptive to the test data. Following the idea in [15], we'd like to select an optimal subset of $\mathbf{H}$ as local coordinate set, such that the rest of features can be well reconstructed from it. We can formulate this criterion as follows,

$$min_{\mathbf{S}} = \frac{1}{2}\|\mathbf{H} - \mathbf{HS}\|_F^2 + \lambda\|\mathbf{S}\|_{2,1} \tag{8}$$

where $\mathbf{S} \in \mathbb{R}^{n\times n}$ is the selection matrix, $\|\mathbf{S}\|_F = \sqrt{\sum_i \sum_j \mathbf{S}_{ij}^2}$ is the Frobenius norm of $\mathbf{S}$, $\|\mathbf{S}\|_{2,1} = \sum_{i=1}^n \|\mathbf{S}_{i.}\|_2$ is the $L_{2,1}$-norm, and λ is the model parameter and we set $\lambda = 1$ in this paper. Finally, by selecting features with $\|\mathbf{S}_{i.}\| > 0$, we can obtain the local coordinates. To solve this problem, we follow the method proposed in [43]. Consider an objective function $f_0(x) = f(x) + g(x)$ where $f(x)$ is convex and smooth and $g(x)$ is convex but non-smooth. The key step is to construct $p_{Z,L}(x) = f(Z) + \langle\nabla f(Z), x - Z\rangle + \frac{L}{2}\|x - Z\|_F^2 + g(Z)$ to approximate $f_0(x)$ at point Z. Obviously, we can define $f(\mathbf{S}) = \frac{1}{2}\|\mathbf{H}-\mathbf{HS}\|_F^2$ and

$g(\mathbf{S}) = \|\mathbf{S}\|_{2,1}$. So we can construct $p_{\mathbf{Z},L}(\mathbf{S})$ as

$$p_{\mathbf{Z},L}(\mathbf{S}) = f(\mathbf{Z}) + \langle \nabla f(\mathbf{Z}), \mathbf{S} - \mathbf{Z} \rangle + \frac{L}{2}\|\mathbf{S} - \mathbf{Z}\|_F^2 + g(\mathbf{Z}) \tag{9}$$

And we can define another function $D_\tau(.) : \mathbf{M} \in \mathbb{R}^{n \times n} \mapsto \mathbf{N} \in \mathbb{R}^{n \times n}$

$$\mathbf{N}_{i.} = \begin{cases} 0, & \|\mathbf{M}_{i.}\| \leq \tau \\ (1 - \tau/\|\mathbf{M}_{i.}\|)\mathbf{M}_{i.}, & \text{otherwise} \end{cases} \tag{10}$$

Because of the limit of space, we can't show all the details to solve this problem. Instead we summarize the algorithm in Algorithm 1.

3.3 Local Coordinate Factorization

As mentioned in [15] and [16], a normal STV may be close to a cluster while an anomalous STV may be an outlier. We also observe that a normal STV is always close to some local coordinates. Denote the local coordinates obtained above as $\mathbf{U} = [u_1, u_2, ..., u_m]$, where m is the number of local coordinates. The local coordinate representation $v \in \mathbb{R}^{m \times 1}$ of a STV represented by HOG feature $h \in \mathbb{R}^{d \times 1}$ can be calculated by minimizing the following objective function,

$$\mathcal{O}_h = \|h - \mathbf{U}v\|_F^2 + \mu \sum_{i=1}^{m} |v_i| \|u_i - h\|_F^2, \quad \text{s.t.} \quad v_i \geq 0, \forall i \tag{11}$$

where μ is a model parameter and we set $\mu = 10$ in this paper. The first term in Eq. (11) aims to reconstruct h by local coordinates. The second term requires that the local coordinates selected to reconstruct h should be close to h to preserve data locality, which is motivated by [44]. Furthermore, this term also leads to sparse v, i.e., h is reconstructed just by very few local coordinates. This is important because we have $m > d$. Without it, any h can be perfectly reconstructed because $\mathbf{U}$ is over-complete in feature space. Motivated by resent study in Non-negative Matrix Factorization [45–47], we constraint that v should be non-negative, thus h is reconstructed by addition but not substraction of $\mathbf{U}$, which will lead to better performance.

Actually, when reconstructed by just few local coordinates, i.e., v is quite sparse, the normal STV can be well reconstructed with less reconstruction error, while the reconstruction error for an anomalous STV will be quite large because it's always outliers so that it's far from all local coordinates. Moreover, the local coordinate representation for normal STV is also different from representation for anomalous STV. Generally, we observe that the length of v is close to 1 for most normal STV but far from 1 for anomalous STV. This is also reasonable because normal STV is always close to some local coordinates. To incorporate both observations above for anomaly detection, we compute the degree of anomaly as

$$d_{\mathrm{a}} = \|h - \mathbf{U}v\|_F^2 + \gamma|1 - \|v\|_F^2| \tag{12}$$

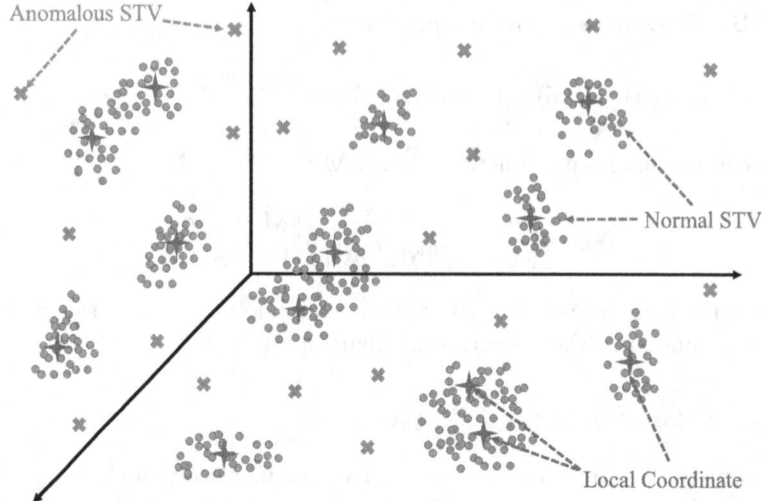

Fig. 2. Local coordinate factorization. There are a lot of local coordinates in feature space. Based on the construction method of local coordinates, normal STV can be well reconstructed by just few local coordinates, e.g., just one or two. However, there is large reconstruction error for anomalous STV. Furthermore, the local coordinate representations of normal STV and anomalous STV are also quite different.

where γ is to balance the magnitude of both terms. Then d_{a} is utilized to determine whether a STV is anomalous based on its value compared to a threshold δ. STVs with d_{a} larger than δ are determined to be anomalous. δ is determined by the anomaly probability p_a depending on the user's need. A large p_a will lead to high true positive rate and high false positive rate while a small one will lower both. Empirically, p_a can be set to 10^{-2},10^{-3},10^{-4}.... In this paper we set $p_a = 10^{-3}$. Then, as the local coordinate selection procedure, we can compute d_a for all STVs in the first one or two seconds in a test video, and set δ such that the ratio of STVs whose d_a are larger than δ is about p_a. So about p_a STVs will be treated as anomalies. We have a postprocessing step on the initial judgement to obtain better results, which will be introduced latter (Fig. 2).

Now we will show how to solve Eq. (11) to obtain v for a STV represented by h. Following some simple algebraic steps, we can rewrite Eq. (11) as follows,

$$\mathcal{O}_h = \|h - \mathbf{U}v\|_F^2 + \mu \sum_{i=1}^{m} |v_i| \|u_i - h\|_F^2 = \|h - \mathbf{U}v\|_F^2 + \mu \|(h\mathbf{1}^T - \mathbf{U})\Lambda^{\frac{1}{2}}\|_F^2 \quad (13)$$

where $\Lambda = diag(v_1, ..., v_m) \in \mathbb{R}^{m \times m}$. Noticing that $\|A\|_F^2 = tr(AA^T)$, we have

$$\mathcal{O}_h = tr(hh^T + \mathbf{U}vv^T\mathbf{U}^T - 2hv^T\mathbf{U}^T + \mu(h\mathbf{1}^T\Lambda\mathbf{1}^T h^T - 2h\mathbf{1}^T\Lambda\mathbf{U}^T + \mathbf{U}\Lambda\mathbf{U}^T)) \quad (14)$$

Now let ϕ_i be the Lagrange multiplier for constraints $v_i \geq 0$, and define $\Phi = [\phi_i]$, then the Lagrange $\mathcal{L}$ is

$$\mathcal{L} = \mathcal{O}_h + tr(\Phi v^T) \quad (15)$$

Then we can calculate the partial derivative of $\mathcal{L}$ with respect to v as follows,

$$\frac{\partial \mathcal{L}}{\partial v} = 2\mathbf{U}^T\mathbf{U}v - 2\mathbf{U}^T h + \mu(\mathbf{C} - 2\mathbf{U}^T h + \mathbf{D}) + \Phi \quad (16)$$

where column vector $\mathbf{C} = [h^T h, ..., h^T h] \in \mathbb{R}^{m\times 1}$ and $\mathbf{D} = diag(\mathbf{U}^T\mathbf{U}) \in \mathbb{R}^{m\times 1}$. Using the KKT conditions $\phi_i v_i = 0$, we obtain the following equation,

$$2(\mathbf{U}^T\mathbf{U}v)_i v_i - 2(\mathbf{U}^T h)_i v_i + \mu(\mathbf{C} - 2\mathbf{U}^T h + \mathbf{D})_i v_i = 0 \quad (17)$$

Then the equation above lead to the following update rule for v

$$v_i \leftarrow v_i \frac{2(\mu+1)(\mathbf{U}^T h)_i}{(2\mathbf{U}^T\mathbf{U}v + \mu\mathbf{C} + \mu\mathbf{D})_i} \quad (18)$$

The update rules in Eq. (18) is guaranteed to converge and the final solution will be a local optimum, and similar proof of convergency based on [46] and [48] can be found in [47].

So to solve Eq. (11), we can randomly initialize v by some non-negative values and use Eq. (18) iteratively. Equation (11) can converge in tens of iterations but we find that 5 to 10 iterations are enough to get satisfactory performance while guaranteing the efficiency, thus we set the maximum number of iterations to 5. Compared to [15] who proposes to solve a L_1-norm regularized least squares problem which can't be solved efficiently, our method just needs some simple matrix operations and few iterations which is quite efficient. Thus our approach can perform real-time detection while [15] can't.

3.4 Online Update

As discussed in [15–17], an anomaly detection system should be adaptive to the background change, both in appearance and motion. So we propose an update strategy to tune the local coordinates to capture the change in background. The basic idea is straightforward, i.e., the normal features can be well reconstructed by local coordinates, or the local coordinates should be as close as possible to normal features. Since the distribution of normal features is changing slightly all the time, we need to update the local coordinates simultaneously. Given a set of n normal features $\mathbf{H} = [h_1, ..., h_n] \in \mathbb{R}^{d\times n}$ and their local coordinate representations $\mathbf{V} = [v_1, ..., v_n] \in \mathbb{R}^{m\times n}$, the local coordinates $\mathbf{U}$ is updated by minimizing the following objective function,

$$\mathcal{O}_U = \|\mathbf{H} - \mathbf{U}\mathbf{V}\|_F^2 + \mu \sum_{i=1}^{n}\sum_{j=1}^{m} |v_{ji}| \|u_j - h_i\|_F^2 \quad \text{s.t.} \quad u_{ij} \geq 0, \forall i, j \quad (19)$$

Analogous to our strategy in Eqs. (13–15), let $\Lambda_i = diag(v_{i1}, ..., v_{im})$ $\mathbb{R}^{m\times m}$, ψ_{ij} be the Lagrange multiplier for constraints $u_{ij} \geq 0$, $\Psi = [\psi_{ij}]$, and the Lagrange $\mathcal{L}_U = \mathcal{O}_U + tr(\Psi\mathbf{U}^T)$. The partial derivatives of $\mathcal{L}_U$ to $\mathbf{U}$ is

$$\frac{\partial \mathcal{L}_U}{\partial \mathbf{U}} = 2\mathbf{U}\mathbf{V}\mathbf{V}^T - 2\mathbf{H}\mathbf{V}^T + \mu \sum_{i=1}^{n}(-2h_i\mathbf{1}^T\Lambda_i + 2\mathbf{U}\Lambda_i) + \Psi \quad (20)$$

and by using the KKT conditions $\psi_{ij}u_{ij} = 0$, we can get the update rule for $\mathbf{U}$ like Eqs. (17) and (18),

$$u_{ij} \leftarrow u_{ij} \frac{(\mathbf{H}\mathbf{V}^T + \mu \sum_{i=1}^{n} h_i \mathbf{1}^T \Lambda_i)_{ij}}{(\mathbf{U}\mathbf{V}\mathbf{V}^T + \mu \sum_{i=1}^{n} \mathbf{U}\Lambda_i)_{ij}} \tag{21}$$

Though the background may sharply change in long time, the change during a short time (e.g., two seconds) is always slight. So we just need to update $\mathbf{U}$ every two seconds. Further we can also do random sample among normal features to obtain a small n (10,000 to 20,000 based on the resolution of videos) to guarantee real-time updating. Moreover, we can use the origin $\mathbf{U}$ as the input to Eq. (19) and execute Eq. (21) just once such that the updated $\mathbf{U}$ is different but close to origin one. As a result, the local coordinates can change all the time to adapt to the background change but the change in one updating step isn't too sharp. In addition, as our feature can capture both spatial and temporal properties of videos, the update strategy proposed here can be adaptive to background change in both appearance and motion.

4 Spatio-Temporal Pyramid

In fact, there is noise in the video and our Local Coordinate Factorization method may sometimes give wrong judgement which may lower the true positive rate and lift the false positive rate. But we can observe that an anomalous event shows continuity in space and time, i.e., it's associated to a relatively large region and it lasts for a period of time. Thus considering the relationship of STVs in space and time can promote the detection performance. In this paper, we propose to use Spatio-temporal Pyramid as illustrated in Fig. 1. Specifically, we use two-level pyramid and we find that this setting can achieve satisfactory result.

As discussed in Sect. 3.1, the HOG feature of upper level STV can be constructed efficiently from lower level STVs. The upper level can capture the relationship of lower level STVs in space and time and global information of an event. And because STVs in different levels have different scales, the Spatio-temporal Pyramid can be utilized to detect multi-scale events. Given a STV in any scale (either upper level of lower level), we can tell whether it belongs to an anomalous event by Local Coordinate Factorization individually.

In our experiments, we find an interesting phenomenon. The judgement on upper level STV tends to have high precision but low recall, i.e., our approach can claim that a upper level STV is anomalous with high confidence but it may miss some anomalous STV. We think the reason is that the upper level STV can capture the global information of an event which fully considers the continuity of an event in space and time while it may ignore some important local details. On the contrary, the judgement on lower level STV tends to have high recall because it can capture the local details of anomalous event but low precision since it's too sensitive to local details and noise and ignores the relationship between STVs. So we propose to combine these two levels as Spatio-temporal Pyramid to consider both local details and global information as follows.

Firstly, when a upper STV is judged to be normal, it actually may be anomalous. So we should consider the results of (1) its six neighbors and (2) its lower STVs. In this paper, we consider an upper STV to be anomalous if (1) it's judged to be anomalous, (2) three or more of its neighbors are anomalous, and (3) five or more of its lower level STVs are anomalous. The first criterion is based on the high-precision result for upper level STV. The second criterion is based on the continuity of events. The third criterion is based on a voting scheme, because it's reasonable to assume that though one lower STV may be influenced by noise or local details, it's difficult for most STVs to generate wrong judgement.

Secondly, as a lower level STV can't capture the continuity of events, so the judgement of a STV should be incorporated with its upper level STV and neighbors. So a lower level STV is considered to be anomalous if it's judged to be anomalous and (1) two of more of its neighbors are anomalous or (2) its upper level STV is anomalous.

Based on the Spatio-temporal Pyramid and criteria above, we take into consideration the continuity of events, the relationship between STVs in space and time, and the local details simultaneously which can promote the performance significantly. Furthermore, the Spatio-temporal Pyramid allow us to perform multi-scale detection.

5 Experiments

To validate the effectiveness of the proposed approach, we test it in the following two public datasets for anomaly detection: anomaly behavior detection dataset [49][1] and UCSD pedestrian dataset [14][2]. The evaluation and comparison of different approaches are presented in precision-recall, ROC curves and EER at both frame level and pixel level. As mentioned before, we use a two-level pyramid, and the the size of lower level STV is $10 \times 10 \times 10$. To extract HOG features, we set $n_\phi = 8$ and $n_\theta = 16$. We set $\lambda = 1$ for local coordinate selection in Eq. (8), $\mu = 10$ for Local Coordinate Factorization in Eq. (11) and online update in Eq. (19), and $p_a = 10^{-3}$. In fact, our method doesn't need training procedure. It just use the first two seconds of a test video to select initial local coordinates. Furthermore, we set that the local coordinates are updated every two seconds. We compare our approach to several state-of-the-art approaches for anomaly detection: Optical Flow [11], MDT [14], Sparse Reconstruction (Cong *et al.*) [15], spatio-temporal oriented energies [49], Dominant Behavior (Roshtkhari *et al.*) [17], Saligrama *et al.* [50], Reddy *et al.* [51] and Bertini *et al.* [16].

The first dataset is *Belleview*. It's a traffic scene where the lighting conditions changes during the day gradually. Cars running from top to bottom is normal event, while cars entering or exiting from the intersection from left or right and people in the lane is the anomalous event. The second is *Boat-river* dataset. The anomalous event is a boat that passing the scene. The third is *Train* dataset

[1] http://www.cse.yorku.ca/vision/research/.

[2] http://www.svcl.ucsd.edu/projects/anomaly.

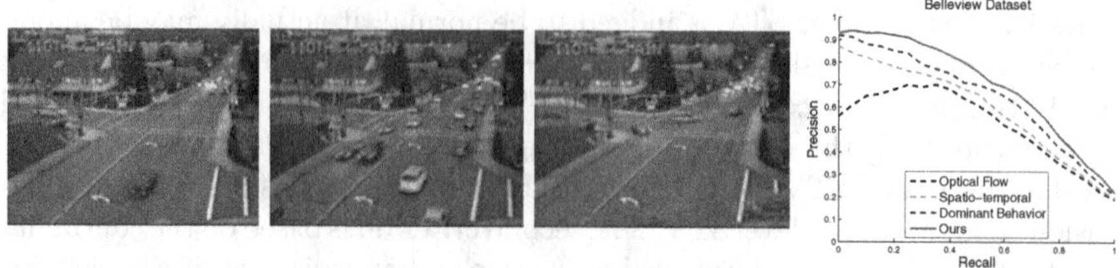

Fig. 3. Experiments on Belleview dataset

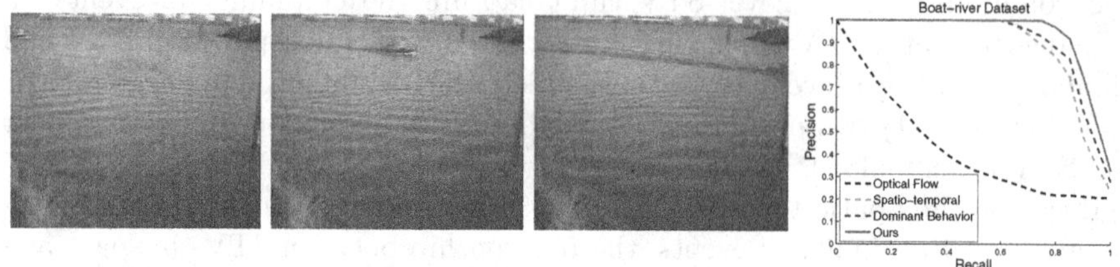

Fig. 4. Experiments on Boat-Holborn dataset

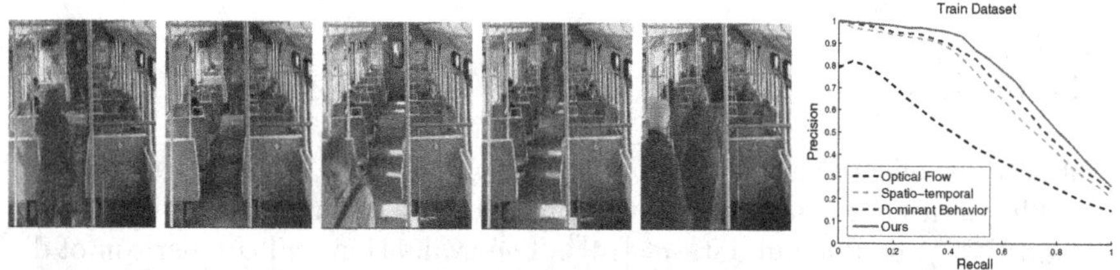

Fig. 5. Experiments on train dataset

where anomalies are moving people. The results on three datasets above, including the anomalous regions detected by our approach (highlighted in red) and the precision-recall curves of different approaches, are shown in Figs. 3, 4 and 5 respectively. We can observe that our approach is superior to state-of-the-art methods, e.g., Zaharescu *et al.* and Roshtkhari *et al.* Three main reasons are: (1) our approach can update model timely so that it's quite robust to drastic background change, (2) our approach takes a full consideration of the relationship between neighbor STVs thus it's robust to local noise, and (3) our approach considers the continuity of anomalous event in space and time.

In the UCSD datasets (Ped1 and Ped2), the anomalies are non-pedestrian entities (e.g., cyclist, skaters, small carts) and pedestrians moving in anomalous motion. We follow the evaluation utilized in [14] and [16]. In the frame level, an anomalous frame is considered correctly detected if at least one pixel is detected as anomalous. In the pixel level, an anomalous frame is considered correctly detected only if at least 40 % of the anomalous pixels are detected correctly. The anomalous regions detected and the ROC curves of other approaches for Ped1 and Ped2 datasets are shown in Figs. 6 and 7 respectively. And the Equal Error Rate (EER) for both frame level and pixel level detection of different approaches is shown in Table 1. The results show that our approach can outperform all other state-of-the-art approaches, both at frame level and pixel level. And we need to highlight that our approach is unsupervised which doesn't require any training data, and can perform real-time detection because it's quite efficient.

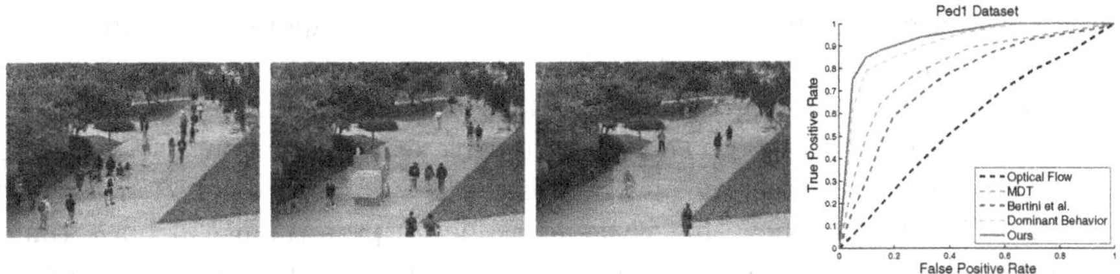

Fig. 6. Experiments on Ped1 dataset

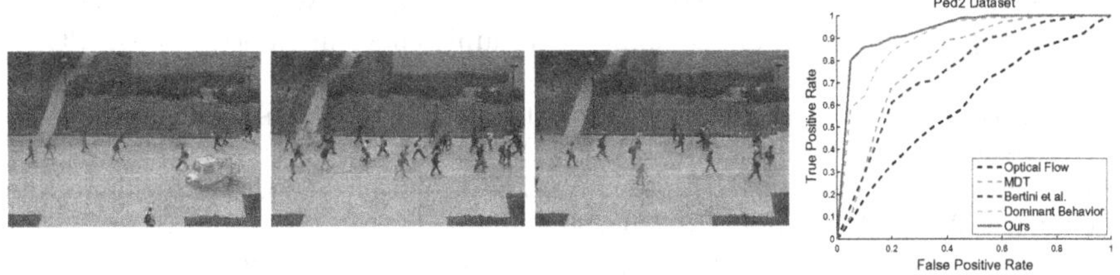

Fig. 7. Experiments on Ped2 dataset

Table 1. Comparison of the proposed approach and the state-of-the-art for anomaly detection using Ped datasets. Approaches with * can perform real-time detection.

	Ped1		Ped2	
	EER (frame)	EER (pixel)	EER (frame)	EER (pixel)
Optical Flow* [11]	38 %	76 %	42 %	80 %
Saligrama *et al.* [50]	16 %	-	19 %	-
MDT [14]	25 %	58 %	25 %	55 %
Cong *et al.* [15]	19 %	-	20 %	-
Reddy *et al.** [51]	22.5 %	32 %	21 %	31 %
Bertini *et al.** [16]	31 %	70 %	30 %	68 %
Roshtkhari *et al.** [17]	15 %	29 %	17 %	30 %
Ours*	**12** %	**25** %	**13** %	**26** %

6 Conclusions

In this paper, we propose a novel approach to perform real-time and multi-scale anomaly detection. Specifically, we use spatio-temporal features to capture the characteristics of STV in both appearance and motion in order that our approach can detect spatial, temporal, and spatio-temporal anomalies. Then we utilize Local Coordinate Factorization to efficiently tell whether a SVT belongs to an anomaly. Then to consider the relationship between STVs, and the continuity of an event in space and time, we propose to use Spatio-temporal Pyramid, which can further support multi-scale detection. We also propose an efficient online method to update local coordinates such that our approach is self-adaptive to background change. Finally, we conduct extensive experiments on several public datasets for anomaly detection and compare our approach to state-of-the-art approaches. The results show that it achieve superior performance at both frame and pixel level and our approach can outperform state-of-the-art approaches.

References

1. Troscianko, T., Holmes, A., Stillman, J., Mirmehdi, M., Wright, D., Wilson, A.: What happens next? the predictability of natural behaviour viewed through CCTV cameras. Perception **33**, 87–101 (2004)
2. Keval, H., Sasse, M.: not the usual suspects: a study of factors reducing the effectiveness of CCTV. Secur. J. **23**, 134–154 (2010)
3. Haering, N., Venetianer, P., Lipton, A.: The evolution of video surveillance: an overview. Mach. Vis. Appl. **19**, 279–290 (2008)
4. Brax, C., Niklasson, L., Smedberg, M.: Finding behavioural anomalies in public areas using video surveillance data. In: Proceedings of 11th International Conference on Information Fusion (2008)
5. Ivanov, I., Dufaux, F., Ha, T., Ebrahimi, T.: Towards generic detection of unusual events in video surveillance. In: Proceedings of IEEE International Conference on Advanced Video and Signal Based Surveillance (2009)
6. Li, J., Gong, S., Xiang, T.: Discovering multi-camera behaviour correlations for on-the-fly global activity prediction and anomaly detection. In: Proceedings of IEEE International Conference on Computer Vision Workshops (2009)
7. Liu, C., Wang, G., Ning, W., Lin, X., Li, L., Liu, Z.: Anomaly detection in surveillance video using motion direction statistics. In: Proceedings of IEEE International Conference on Image Processing (2010)
8. Loy, C., Xiang, T., Gong, S.: Detecting and discriminating behavioural anomalies. Pattern Recogn. **44**, 117–132 (2011)
9. Zhang, D., Gatica-Perez, D., Bengio, S., McCowan, I.: Semi-supervised adapted HMMs for unusual event detection. In: Proceedings of IEEE Conference on Computer Vision and Pattern Recognition (2005)
10. R. Sillito, R.F.: Semi-supervised learning for anomalous trajectory detection. In: Proceedings of British Machine Vision Conference (2008)
11. Adam, A., Rivlin, E., Shimshoni, I., Reinitz, D.: Robust real-time unusual event detection using multiple fixed-location monitors. IEEE Trans. Pattern Anal. Mach. Intell. **30**, 555–560 (2008)
12. Kim, J., Grauman, K.: Observe locally, infer globally: a spacectime MRF for detecting abnormal activities with incremental updates. In: Proceedings of IEEE Conference on Computer Vision and Pattern Recognition (2009)

13. Mehran, R., Oyama, A., Shah, M.: Abnormal crowd behavior detection using social force model. In: Proceedings of IEEE Conference on Computer Vision and Pattern Recognition (2009)
14. Mahadevan, V., Li, W., Bhalodia, V., Vasconcelos, N.: Anomaly detection in crowded scenes. In: Proceedings of IEEE Conference on Computer Vision and Pattern Recognition (2010)
15. Cong, Y., Yuan, J., Liu, J.: Sparse reconstruction cost for abnormal event detection. In: Proceedings of IEEE Conference on Computer Vision and Pattern Recognition (2011)
16. Bertini, M., Bimbo, A.D., Seidenari, L.: Multi-scale and realtime non-parametric approach for anomaly detection and localization. CVIU **116**(3), 320–329 (2012)
17. Roshtkhari, M.J., Levine, M.D.: Online dominant and anomalous behavior detection in videos. In: Proceedings of IEEE Conference on Computer Vision and Pattern Recognition (2012)
18. Kratz, L., Nishino, K.: Anomaly detection in extremely crowded scenes using spatio-temporal motion pattern models. In: Proceedings of IEEE Conference on Computer Vision and Pattern Recognition (2009)
19. Jiang, F., Wu, Y., Katsaggelos, A.: A dynamic hierarchical clustering method for trajectory-based unusual video event detection. IEEE Trans. Image Process. (TIP) **14**, 907–913 (2009)
20. Khalid, S.: Activity classification and anomaly detection using m-medoids based modelling of motion patterns. Pattern Recogn. **43**, 3636–3647 (2010)
21. Jiang, F., Yuan, J., Tsaftaris, S.A., Katsaggelos, A.K.: Anomalous video event detection using spatiotemporal context. Comput. Vis. Image Underst. **115**(3), 323–333 (2011)
22. Yu, K., Zhang, T., Gong, Y.: Nonlinear learning using local coordinate coding. In: Advances in Neural Information Processing Systems (2009)
23. Lazebnik, S., Schmid, C., Ponce, J.: Beyond bags of features: spatial pyramid matching for recognizing natural scene categories. In: Proceedings of IEEE Conference on Computer Vision and Pattern Recognition (2006)
24. Morris, B.T., Trivedi, M.M.: Trajectory learning for activity understanding: unsupervised, multilevel, and long-term adaptive approach. IEEE Trans. Pattern Anal. Mach. Intell. **33**, 2287–2301 (2011)
25. Ouivirach, K., Gharti, S., Dailey, M.N.: Incremental behavior modeling and suspicious activity detection. Pattern Recogn. **46**, 671–680 (2013)
26. Benezeth, Y., Jodoin, P.M., Saligrama, V.: Abnormality detection using low-level co-occurring events. Pattern Recogn. Lett. **32**, 423–431 (2011)
27. Hospedales, T., Gong, S., Xiang, T.: Video behaviour mining using a dynamic topic model. Int. J. Comput. Vis. **98**, 303–323 (2012)
28. Benezeth, Y., Jodoin, P.M., Saligrama, V., Rosenberger, C.: Abnormal events detection based on spatio-temporal co-occurences. In: Proceedings of IEEE Conference on Computer Vision and Pattern Recognition (2009)
29. Ermis, E.B., Saligrama, V., Jodoin, P.M., Konrad, J.: Motion segmentation and abnormal behavior detection via behavior clustering. In: Proceedings of IEEE International Conference on Image Processing (2008)
30. Kim, K., Chalidabhongse, T.H., Harwood, D., Davis, L.: Real-time foreground-background segmentation using codebook model. Real-Time Imaging **11**, 172–185 (2005)
31. Mittal, A., Monnet, A., Paragios, N.: Scene modeling and change detection in dynamic scenes: a subspace approach. CVIU **113**, 63–79 (2009)

32. Boiman, O., Irani, M.: Detecting irregularities in images and in video. Int. J. Comput. Vis. **74**, 17–31 (2007)
33. Zhu, X., Liu, Z.: Human behavior clustering for anomaly detection. Front. Comput. Sci. Chin. **5**(3), 279–289 (2011)
34. Blei, D., NG, A., Jordan, M.: Latent dirichlet allocation. J. Mach. Learn. Res. **3**, 993–1022 (2003)
35. Hospedales, T.M., Jian, L., Shaogang, G., Tao, X.: Identifying rare and subtle behaviors: a weakly supervised joint topic model. IEEE Trans. Pattern Anal. Mach. Intell. **33**(12), 2451–2464 (2011)
36. Li, J., Gong, S., Xiang, T.: Learning behavioural context. Int. J. Comput. Vis. **97**(3), 276–304 (2012)
37. Ricci, E., Zen, G., Sebe, N., Messelodi, S.: A prototype learning framework using EMD: application to complex scenes analysis. IEEE Trans. Pattern Anal. Mach. Intell. **PP**(99), 1 (2012)
38. Roshtkhari, M.J., Levine, M.D.: A multi-scale hierarchical codebook method for human action recognition in videos using a single example. In: Conference on Computer and Robot Vision (2012)
39. Hospedales, T.M., Jian, L., Shaogang, G., Tao, X.: Identifying rare and subtle behaviors: a weakly supervised joint topic model. IEEE Trans. Pattern Anal. Mach. Intell. **33**, 2451–2464 (2012)
40. P. Jodoin, J.K., Saligrama, V.: Modeling background activity for behavior subtraction. In: International Conference on Distributed Smart Cameras (2008)
41. Jodoin, P., Saligrama, V., Konrad, J.: Behavior subtraction. IEEE Trans. Image Process. (TIP) **21**(9), 4244–4255 (2012)
42. Scovanner, P., Ali, S., Shah, M.: A 3-dimensional sift descriptor and its application to action recognition. In: International Conference on Multimedia (2007)
43. Nesterov, Y.: Gradient methods for minimizing composite objective function. In: CORE (2007)
44. Wang, J., Yang, J., Yu, K., Lv, F., Huang, T., Gong, Y.: Locality-constrained linear coding for image classification. In: Proceedings of IEEE Conference on Computer Vision and Pattern Recognition (2010)
45. Lee, D.D., Seung, H.S.: Learning the parts of objects by nonnegative matrix factorization. Nature **401**(6755), 788–791 (1999)
46. Lee, D.D., Seung, H.S.: Algorithms for non-negative matrix factorization. In: Advances in Neural Information Processing Systems (2001)
47. Cai, D., He, X., Han, J., Huang, T.S.: Graph regularized nonnegative matrix factorization for data representation. IEEE Trans. Pattern Anal. Mach. Intell. **33**, 1548–1560 (2011)
48. Lin, C.J.: On the convergence of multiplicative update algorithms for non-negative matrix factorization. IEEE Trans. Neural Netw. **18**(6), 1589–1596 (2007)
49. Zaharescu, A., Wildes, R.: Anomalous behaviour detection using spatiotemporal oriented energies, subset inclusion histogram comparison and event-driven processing. In: Daniilidis, K., Maragos, P., Paragios, N. (eds.) ECCV 2010, Part I. LNCS, vol. 6311, pp. 563–576. Springer, Heidelberg (2010)
50. Saligrama, V., Zhu, C.: Video anomaly detection based on local statistical aggregates. In: Proceedings of IEEE Conference on Computer Vision and Pattern Recognition (2012)
51. Reddy, V., Sanderson, C., Lovell, B.C.: Improved anomaly detection in crowded scenes via cell-based analysis of foreground speed, size and texture. In: Proceedings of IEEE Conference on Computer Vision and Pattern Recognition Workshops (2011)

Intrinsic Image Decomposition from Pair-Wise Shading Ordering

Yuanliu Liu(✉), Zejian Yuan, and Nanning Zheng

Institute of Artificial Intelligence and Robotics,
Xi'an Jiaotong University, Xian, China
liuyuanliu88@gmail.com

Abstract. An image is composed by several intrinsic images including the reflectance and the shading. In this paper, we propose a novel approach to infer the shading image from shading orders between pairs of pixels. The pairwise shading orders are measured by two types of methods: the brightness order and the low-order fittings of local shading field. The brightness order is a non-local measure, which does not rely on local gradients, and can be applied to any pair of pixels. In contrast, the low-order fittings are effective for pixel pairs within local regions of smooth shading. These methods are complementary, and they together can capture both the local smoothness and non-local order structure of shading. Further, we evaluate the reliability of these methods by their robustness to perturbations, including the errors in reflectance clustering, the variations of reflectance and shading, and the spatial distances. We adopt a strategy of local competition and global Angular Embedding to integrate pairwise orders into a globally consistent order, taking their reliability into account. Experiments on the MIT Intrinsic Image dataset and the UIUC Shadow dataset show that our model can effectively recover the shading image including those deeply shadowed areas.

1 Introduction

An image is produced by several factors jointly, including the reflectance of the material, the shape of the surface, the positions and the colors of the illuminants and the parameters of the camera. Barrow and Tenenbaum [1] proposed to decompose a single image into intrinsic images, each of which captures a distinct aspect of the scene. The shading image captures the incident illumination at each pixel, while the reflectance image reflects the albedo of the surfaces. However it is essentially an underconstrained problem to recover the shading and reflectance from a single image. To solve this problem, additional constraints expressing the properties of the scene and the objects are needed. Most widely used properties include the local smoothness of shading [2–6], the local smoothness of reflectance [3,6–8] and the global sparsity of reflectance [4,7–9]. However, the smoothness of shading are not applicable to pixels separated by a shadow edge, while the smoothness of reflectance will be broken by the albedo change. The sparsity of global reflectance are not valid for complex scenes containing too many colors. How to add constraints to proper variables remains an open problem.

D. Cremers et al. (Eds.): ACCV 2014, Part V, LNCS 9007, pp. 83–98, 2015.
DOI: 10.1007/978-3-319-16814-2_6

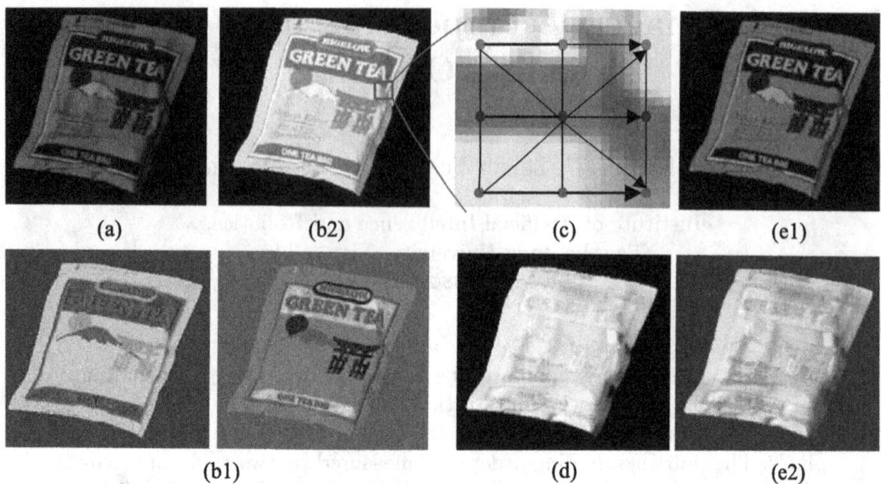

Fig. 1. The flow chart of decomposing a single image into shading and reflectance. (a) The input image; (b1) The projection of the log image onto the 2D shadow-free plane, and pixels with similar reflectance have similar values in this plane; (b2) The brightness map got from projecting the log image along the norm of the shadow-free plane; (c) The pairwise order of the shading intensity. Dots with the same color represent pixels with similar reflectance. The arrows point from the higher shading intensities to the lower ones. The lines without any arrow indicate nearly equal shading intensities. The width of the lines indicate the reliability of the estimations, while thicker ones stand for higher reliability; (d) The shading map in log space, which is the output of Angular Embedding; (e1) and (e2) are the recovered reflectance and shading image, respectively (Color figure online).

An initial work is the Retinex theory proposed by Land and McCann [2]. It assumes that small gradients in images are caused by shading variations, while large gradients are resulted from reflectance changes. By ignoring the edges corresponding to shading changes, a reflectance image can be recovered by integrating over the left gradient field. The edge types is classified by a threshold of the magnitude of gradients. This kind of classification is more-or-less inaccurate. Some shadow edges are quite strong under certain circumstances [10], while the reflectance edges between similar colors are relatively weak. Another way to classify edges is to utilize shadow-free color spaces [9,11–14]. Basically, if an edge appears in the raw image but not the shadow-free image, it should be a shading edge. Other methods for classifying edges include using classifiers trained on representative patches with shading or reflectance changes [15,16], and utilizing texture information [3]. All these edge-based methods suffer from a problem that a single misclassified edge will provoke errors to a wide area of the reflectance image during integration [17].

Another stream of research combines different types of constraints softly by additive energies [3–8,18]. The energy of smoothness constraints are often modeled as the negative log of normal distributions over the gradients of shading and reflectance. The global sparsity of reflectance can be captured by minimizing either the Rényi Entropy of reflectance [8], the cluster-wise variation in a shadow-free space [4,19] or the number of different reflectance values [7]. An energy minimization process ensures that the recovered reflectance and shading image best satisfy the synthesized constraints. Although these methods avoid hard classification of gradients, they bring in a new problem that different kinds of constraints are hinged together and relaxed for compromission. As a result, the element constraints may not be satisfied accurately. More specifically, the normal distribution of shading gradients tend to smooth the intensive shadow edges, while the smoothness of reflectance will blur the texture.

We propose to infer the shading image from shading orders, which capture not only the shading smoothness between nearby pixels but also the difference between distant pixels or those separated by shadow edges. The flow chart of our method is shown in Fig. 1. To estimate the shading orders, we introduce a brightness measure derived from the Bi-illumination Dichromatic Reflection Model (BIDR) [20]. The brightness has a linear relationship to the shading intensity, while the reflectance determines the bias. Combining brightness with different properties of the scene results in different estimation methods. The sparsity of reflectance ensures that the pixels can be clustered to a limited number of categories. For pixels with the same reflectance, the shading orders can be estimated from the brightness orders directly, since their biases will be canceled out. Unlike the edge-based methods, the brightness order does not rely on gradients that are sensitive to noise and image blur. It does not add any prior distribution to the shading either, so it can preserve different kinds of shading changes including those sharp shadow edges. For pixels with different reflectance, we first estimate the difference of biases between different categories. The smoothness of shading implies that within a small patch the shading is nearly constant, so the bias difference equals to the brightness order. For pixel pairs within local areas under smooth shading, their shading orders can also be estimated by low-order (constant or linear) models of the local shading image. Thanks to the linear relation between shading and brightness, the coefficients can be easily got by fitting the local brightness image.

The estimation methods above are complementary, each of which aims at specific image regions that the underlying properties are valid. Unlike the weighted summation used by the MRF models, we select the most reliable estimation for each pair of pixels, so unreliable estimations will not interfere the results. The reliability of the estimations are determined by the validity of the underlying properties, which is evaluated based on multiple cues, not limited to the magnitude of gradients. The densely sampled local shading orders together with their reliability are fed to Angular Embedding (AE) [21], resulting in a globally consistent shading image. AE uses complex matrix to encode pairwise orders and their confidences simultaneously. It uses spectral decomposition to get a near-global optimal solution. Moreover, it adopts a cosine error function, which is proved to be more robust to outliers than the traditional L1 or L2 errors [21].

The paper is organized as follows. In Sect. 2, we begin with projecting the raw image into a shadow-free plane and a brightness dimension. Then we estimate the shading order either from the brightness order or a low-order fitting of the local shading map. The confidences of these estimations are evaluated in Sect. 3, and the process of inferring the global shading orders is described in Sect. 4.

2 Pairwise Order of Shading from Shadow Free Projection

In the log space, a surface with only diffuse reflection can be represented by

$$\log I^i = \log F^i C_b^i L_a^i + \log\left(\frac{\gamma}{M^i} + 1\right) \tag{1}$$

where the superscript $i \in \{r, g, b\}$ indexes the RGB channels. F is the response of the camera sensor. C_b is the body reflection. L_a is the ambient illumination, and $M = L_a/L_d$ is the ratio between the ambient illumination and the direct illumination. BIDR [20] assumes that both of the direct and ambient illuminants are constant across the scene, so the illuminant ratio M is constant. When there are multiple direct illuminants with the same color, their effect can be summed up. $\gamma \in [0, 1]$ is the shading intensity.

The BIDR model [20] delivers a shadow-free plane whose normal direction is:

$$w^i = \frac{\log(\frac{1}{M^i} + 1)}{\sqrt{\sum_i (\log(\frac{1}{M^i} + 1))^2}} \tag{2}$$

It is the direction of the parallel lines pointing from the dark pixels (whose $\gamma = 0$) to the bright ones (whose $\gamma = 1$) with the same body reflectance C_b. We call it the brightening direction. See Fig. 2 for an example. The pixels are projected into the space spanned by the dimension along w and the plane UV perpendicular to it:

$$\begin{aligned} I^w &= \log I \cdot w \\ I^u &= \log I \cdot u = \log F C_b L_a \cdot u \\ I^v &= \log I \cdot v = \log F C_b L_a \cdot v \end{aligned} \tag{3}$$

where u and v are unit base vectors of the UV plane. $\cdot$ is the inner product. We can see that the projections I^u and I^v are invariant to the shading intensity, and pixels with similar reflectance C_b are staying closely together. The brightening direction is assumed to be exactly the direction that the distribution of the pixels in its null space gets the minimum entropy [20,22]. Fast Gaussian Transform is adopted to calculate the Rényi Entropy efficiently [22]. Histogram-based techniques can further accelerate the process [23].

The shading intensity is fully captured by the projection I^w, and we call it the brightness. To further analyze the relation between the brightness and the shading intensity, we first approximate the log function of shading intensity in Eq. 1 by the following linear function:

$$\log(\frac{\gamma}{M^i} + 1) \approx \frac{\gamma}{M^i} \tag{4}$$

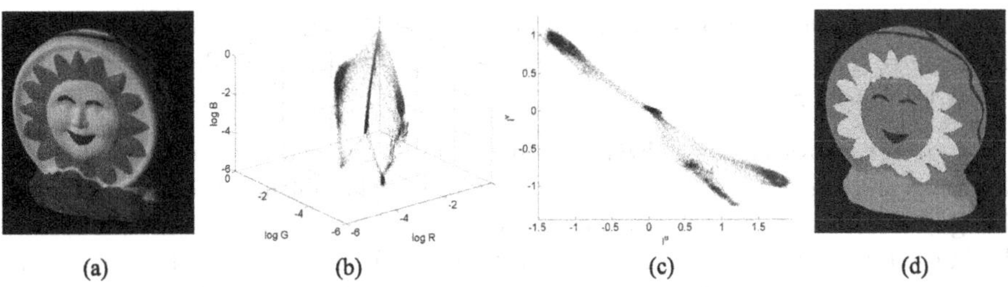

Fig. 2. The brightening direction and shadow-free plane. (a) The raw image; (b) The pixels in log RGB space. The white, orange, blue and dark red pixels form 4 nearly parallel lines; (c) Projections of pixels on the shadow-free plane. The shadow-free plane is perpendicular to the brightening direction. We can see that the pixels fall into 4 groups on the shadow-free plane, each for a distinct color. The red stars indexed by 1$\sim$ 4 are cluster centers for white, orange, blue and dark red pixels, respectively; and (d) The cluster image. The pixels are successfully categorized by reflectance (Color figure online).

which is valid when $\frac{\gamma}{M^i}$ is small. Then the brightness can be rewritten to be:

$$\begin{aligned} I^w &= \log I \cdot w \\ &\approx \sum_i \log FC_b L_a \frac{\frac{1}{M^i}}{\sqrt{\sum_i \frac{1}{(M^i)^2}}} + \sum_i \frac{\frac{\gamma}{M^i}\frac{1}{M^i}}{\sqrt{\sum_i \frac{1}{(M^i)^2}}} \\ &= I^b(C_b) + \tilde{\gamma} \end{aligned} \tag{5}$$

The brightness I^w is composed of two parts: the ambient reflectance $I^b(C_b) = \sum_i \log FC_b L_a \frac{\frac{1}{M^i}}{\sqrt{\sum_i \frac{1}{(M^i)^2}}}$ that is a function of the body reflectance C_b, and the scaled shading intensity $\tilde{\gamma} = \sqrt{\sum_i \frac{1}{(M^i)^2}}\gamma$. The scale factor will not affect the shading order, so we just omit it for now. It will be recovered in Sect. 4.1.

The linear relationship between brightness and shading intensity is the basis for estimating shading orders. Consider a pair of pixels at positions p and q. According to Eq. 5, the shading order can be estimated by:

$$O(p,q) = \tilde{\gamma}(p) - \tilde{\gamma}(q) = (I^w(p) - I^w(q)) - (I^b(p) - I^b(q)) \tag{6}$$

The ambient reflectance I^b are unknown biases varying with the body reflectance C_b. If a pair of pixels have the same body reflectance, their shading order is equal to their brightness order. Otherwise we need to know the difference of their ambient reflectance beforehand. We estimate the difference of ambient reflectance between different categories of pixels according to the sparsity of global reflectance, as described later in this section. However, the difference of ambient reflectance cannot be accurately estimated for some images, then we resort to the shading-smoothness-based methods.

In natural scenes, the shading intensities vary smoothly in most parts of the images. This property suggests that we can fit the local shading map by low-order functions.

First-order Smoothness (FS). The normal directions of flat surfaces change slowly, so the angle between the incident light and the normal direction will not change too much. According to the cosine law of the Lambertian reflection, the shading intensity will not change too much either. We assume that the first-order derivative of the shading field is almost 0 everywhere. Consequently, the adjacent pixels have identical shading intensity. This assumption is valid for nearly flat surfaces, when no shadow boundaries occur on them.

Second-order Smoothness (SS). For a local area of a smooth surface, the normal direction rotated smoothly. As a result, the shading intensity will change smoothly. We assume that the second-order derivative of the shading field is close to 0, so we can fit the local shading field centered at p by a linear function. We further assume that the adjacent pixels of p share the same body reflectance with p. Under this assumption, the slope of the linear model $\frac{\partial \tilde{\gamma}(p)}{\partial p} = \frac{\partial I^w(p)}{\partial p}$, where $\frac{\partial I^w(p)}{\partial p}$ is the first-order derivative of I^w evaluated at p.

Formally, we can estimate the order of shading intensity O between pixels p and q in the following ways:

$$O(p,q) = \begin{cases} I^w(p) - I^w(q) & \text{if } C_b(p) = C_b(q) \\ I^w(p) - I^w(q) - (I^b(p) - I^b(q)) & \text{if } C_b(p) \neq C_b(q) \\ 0 & \text{if } q \in N(p) \\ \frac{\partial I^w(p)}{\partial p} \cdot (p - q) & \text{if } \frac{\partial^2 (I^w(p))}{\partial p^2} \approx 0 \end{cases} \tag{7}$$

where $N(p)$ is the neighborhood of p, and $p - q$ is the spatial distance between p and q. In practice, we calculate the derivative and the spatial distance in horizontal and vertical directions separately. Notice that, the preconditions of the estimations are not mutual exclusive, so different methods may be applicable to the same pair of pixels. We need to choose the most reliable estimation, whose preconditions are best satisfied. See Sect. 3 for details. In the mean time, the preconditions together cover all possible situations, so we can find at least one suitable method for each pair of pixel. The redundancy and completeness of these methods result in robust estimations of pairwise shading orders.

According to Eq. 7, the differences of ambient reflectance I^b are needed for estimating shading order between pixels with different body reflectance. It is infeasible to calculate the absolute value of I^b due to several unknown factors of it (Eq. 5). Instead, we cluster the pixels by body reflectance, and estimate the difference of ambient reflectance between different categories. We assume that pixels within a small patch have similar shading intensities. According to Eq. 6, if the shading intensities $\tilde{\gamma}$ are the same, the difference of ambient reflectance will be equal to the difference of brightness. Figure 3 gives an example with two categories. The image is divided into dense grids with 10 pixels in each side. We calculate the difference of ambient reflectance between the categories within

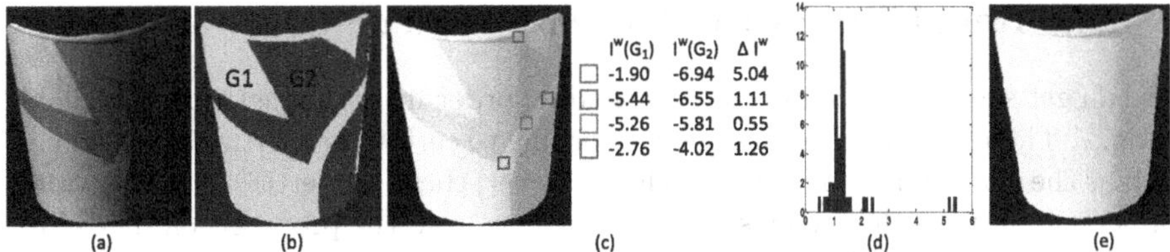

Fig. 3. Estimating the difference of ambient reflectance between categories. (a) The image. (b) The cluster label image. Green: Pixels from category $G1$; and Red: Pixels from category $G2$; (c) Left: The brightness image I^w with some representative patches indicated by the squares. Right: The median brightness of the two categories within each patch as well as their difference. The difference got from the blue square is an outlier, since there is a shadow edge inside it. So does the green one. (d) The histogram of the patch-wise differences of ambient reflectance between the two categories. The grids with only one category of pixels are ignored. The peak of the histogram is selected to be the estimated difference of ambient reflectance, which is 1.3 for this image. (e) The estimated shading intensity. It is got from adding the brightness of category G_2 by the difference of ambient reflectance 1.3 while keeping the brightness of category G_1 unchanged (Color figure online).

each grid. Then we generate a histogram of those grid-wise measures, and take the highest peak to be the final estimation. The reliability of the estimation P is set to be the height of the highest peak accordingly.

When there are multiple categories in the image, we need to estimate the difference of ambient reflectance between each pair of categories. However, some categories are not close enough in the image plane, such that none of the local patches contain pixels from both of these categories. To bridge the gap, we resort to the other categories lying between. We build an undirected graph $G = (V, E)$, where V is the set of nodes representing the categories, and E is the set of edges. The weight of the edge $E_{s,t}$ between node s and t is set to be $1/P_{s,t}$, where $P_{s,t}$ is the confidence of the estimation of their ambient reflectance order as described before. When $P_{s,t}$ is 0, it means category s and t are not adjacent and $E(s,t)$ will be cut off. We can get an estimation of the ambient reflectance difference between any two nodes by summing up the ambient reflectance differences along the path connecting them. To get the most consistent pairwise difference, we extract the Minimum Spanning Tree (MST) of the graph G. The MST ensures that there is one and only one path between any pair of nodes, so the difference of ambient reflectance between the nodes can be uniquely determined. In the mean time, the summation of confidences of the pairwise differences are maximized.

The sparsity of the reflectance spectra within a single image [24] implies that we can cluster the pixels into a small number of categories by their body reflectance. Notice that, pixels on the shadow-free plane UV are well organized by their reflectance (see Fig. 2(c) for an example). A simple k-means is used to cluster the pixels by reflectance in the shadow-free plane UV. The number of clusters is set to be the number of peaks (local maxima) in the 2D histogram of I^u and I^v. The bin size of the histogram is empirically set to be 0.03.

3 The Reliability of the Pairwise Orders

We can get several estimations of the shading order from the methods described in Eq. 7. These methods are designed according to certain properties of the scene, such as the smoothness of shading field. However, these properties may be invalid for certain parts of the scene, so the estimations from the proposed methods are more or less different from the ground-truth. We analyze the robustness of the properties to the perturbations that may happen in the scene or to local areas. Then we evaluate the validity of these properties for each pair of pixels through calculating the joint probability of the occurrences of the perturbations they are not robust to.

The confidence of individual method is calculated by a Noisy-Or model, which is the probability of all its preconditions being satisfied:

$$C_m(p,q) = \prod_{n \in \mathcal{C}_m} 1 - P_n(p,q) \tag{8}$$

where m belongs to the set of methods in Eq. 7, namely the Brightness Order (BO), the Brightness Order minus Bias difference (BOB), the First-order Smoothness (FS) and the Second-order Smoothness (SS) of shading. $\mathcal{C}_m$ is the set of perturbations that the estimation method m is not robust to, as listed in Table. 1. The probability $P_n(p,q)$ measures the probability of the perturbation n occurring between pixel p and q. We first calculate a distance measure between the pair of pixels according to each feature, and translate the distance into probability by a sigmoid function in the form of $sigm(x;w) = \frac{2}{1+e^{-wx}} - 1$. Here w is a positive scalar, which is a parameter of the model.

Table 1. The robustness of the methods for estimating the pair-wise shading orders with respect to different perturbations.

Perturbations	BO	BOB	FS	SS
Clustering Error (CE)	Yes	No	Yes	Yes
Local Reflectance Variation (LRV)	No	No	Yes	No
Reflectance Change (RC)	No	Yes	Yes	Yes
Shadow Edges (SE)	Yes	Yes	No	No
Spatial Distance (SD)	Yes	Yes	No	Moderate

Cluster Error (CE) denotes the uncertainty of the clustering results in the shadow-free plane. When the pixels are incorrectly assigned to the categories, their ambient reflectance cannot be well represented by the estimated ambient reflectance of their categories. We model each cluster as a multivariate normal distribution, and calculate the probability of each pixel belonging to the category that the pixel is assigned to. The Cluster Error for a pair of pixels is represented as the probability that at least one of the pixels does not belong to its assigned category. In addition, the difference of ambient reflectance between color categories are inaccurately estimated sometimes, causing step edges at the boundaries between different categories. The final Cluster Error is calculated by:

$$P_{CE}(p,q) = (1 - P_C(p)P_C(q)) \cdot sigm(e_{\hat{\gamma}}(p,q); w_1) \tag{9}$$

where P_C denotes the probability of a pixel belonging to the category that it is assigned to. The subscript $\hat{\gamma}$ stands for the brightness map I^w minus the categorical ambient reflectance. Inspired by the similarity measure in [25], we set the strength of the step edge $e_{\hat{\gamma}}(p,q)$ to be the largest magnitude of the gradients of $\hat{\gamma}$ evaluated at the pixels along the path connecting p and q.

Local Color Variance (LCV) reflects the textureness of the local regions. In highly textured areas, the blur effect over different colors will produce various mixed colors, whose ambient reflectance are unpredictable. In implementation we represent LCV as follows:

$$P_{LRV}(p,q) = sigm(\max(\sigma(I^{uv}(p)), \sigma(I^{uv}(q))); w_2) \tag{10}$$

where $\sigma(I^{uv}(p))$ is the sum of the standard variations of I^u and I^v within the 3x3 window centered at pixel p.

Reflectance Change (RC) is modeled as follows:

$$P_{RC}(p,q) = sigm(d_{uv}(p,q); w_3) \cdot sigm(e_w(p,q); w_4) \tag{11}$$

where d_{uv} is the geometric distance in shadow-free space UV. Similar to $e_{\hat{\gamma}}(p,q)$, $e_w(p,q)$ is the magnitude of the edge lying between p and q in the brightness image. It is used to distinguish regions with similar color but different reflectance intensities, especially achromatic regions like white and gray. The underlying assumption is that the edges caused by reflectance change are often stronger than those caused by shading changes.

Shadow Edges (SE) are caused by occlusions of the direct light. They are always quite intensive compared to those shading changes caused by surface normal change. We measure the probability of existing a shadow edge between pixel p and q by:

$$P_{SE}(p,q) = sigm(e_{\hat{\gamma}}(p,q); w_5) \tag{12}$$

The biased shading intensities $\hat{\gamma}$ is defined the same as that in Eq. 9, but scaled by a different weight.

Spatial Distance (SD) affects the accuracy of fitting the local shading by low order models. The probability of a pair of pixels being far away from each other is calculated by:

$$P_{SD}(p,q) = sigm(d_s(p,q); w_6) \tag{13}$$

where d_s is the geometric distance.

4 Infer the Global Shading Map from Pairwise Shading Orders

The local estimations from different methods are combined through selecting the most confident one of them, while the confidence is calculated accordingly:

$$C(p,q) = \max_m C_m(p,q) \tag{14}$$

Now we have got a matrix O of the pairwise orders of the shading intensities together with their confidence matrix C. To get a global shading map, we need to align these pairwise measurements. Here we use the Angular Embedding method [21] to embed the shading intensities of the pixels into the angular space, such that the global orders of the embedded points keep their pairwise orders.

Let $Z(p) = e^{i\gamma(p)}$ denote the embedding of the shading intensity of pixel p on the unit circle in the complex plane. Here $i = \sqrt{-1}$. The norm of $Z(p)$ is always 1, and the angle $\Theta(p,q)$ from $Z(p)$ to $Z(q)$ is the order of shading intensity between p and q. It is expected that $\Theta(p,q)$ is consistent with the pairwise shading order $O(p,q)$, when it gets a high confidence. Angular Embedding minimizes the difference between the embedding $Z(p)$ and the estimation of it from its neighbors, $\bar{Z}(p)$ weighted by its total confidence $D(p,p)$:

$$\begin{aligned} &\min_Z \sum_p D(p,p) \cdot \|Z(p) - \bar{Z}(p)\|^2 \\ &\text{s.t. } \|Z(p)\| = 1, \forall p \end{aligned} \tag{15}$$

where D is a diagonal degree matrix:

$$D(p,p) = \frac{\sum_q (C(p,q))}{\sum_{p,q} (C(p,q))} \tag{16}$$

and

$$\bar{Z}(p) = \frac{1}{\sum_q (C(p,q))} \sum_q C(p,q) \cdot Z(q) \cdot e^{iO(p,q)} \tag{17}$$

This optimization problem is hard to solve, since it has n constraints, where n is the number of sampled pixels. In implementation, the constraints are relaxed to be $Z'DZ = 1_n' D 1_n$. To make the optimization tractable, we consider only the orders between nearby pixels. The neighborhood is set to be a square of 30 pixels in each side. The confidence of the orders between a pixel with any pixel outside its neighborhood is set to be 0.

The optimization problem in Eq. 15 is solved by a spectral partitioning algorithm [25] with complex-valued eigenvectors. The solution is the angle of the first eigenvector $\angle Z_0$ which has the smallest eigenvalue. It should be pointed out that the angles of the points on the unit circles are within the scope of $[-\pi, \pi]$. We need to ensure that the angle between any pair of $Z(p)$ and $Z(q)$ is no larger than 2π, otherwise the points may overlap with each other. We scale the brightness image I^w and the the ambient reflectance images I^b by a positive scalar in the beginning, such that the difference of brightness is no larger than 2π. The scaling operation will not disturb the order of Z, and it will be recovered in Sect. 4.1.

The angles $\angle Z_0$ keep the pairwise order of the shading intensities, but the absolute values of the angles have no determined mappings to the shading intensities. Angular Embedding allows the points to rotate as a whole around the original point. Figure 4 gives an example. We can see that the angles of the

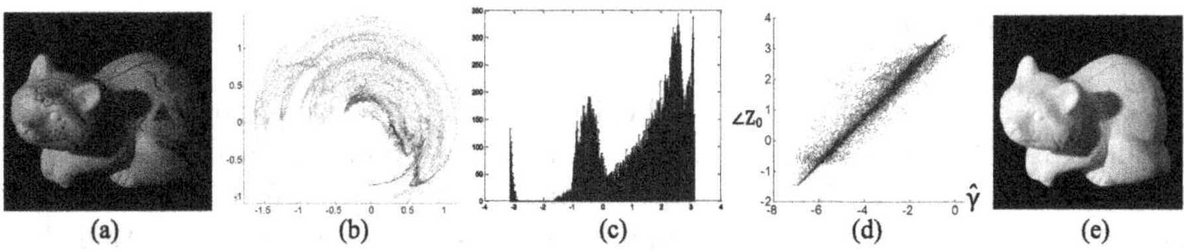

Fig. 4. An example of the Angular Embedding results. (a) The image; (b) The output embedding with the smallest eigenvalue. There is a gap between the brightest and the darkest pixels; (c) The histogram of the angles of embedding. The bins with zero counts are generated by the gap. The pixels fell into the bins to the left of the zero-count bins will be shifted to the right by 2π; (d) The relation between the output angles and the biased shading intensities $\hat{\gamma}$. Most of them stay roughly in a line; and (e) The recovered shading image in log space.

brightest pixels in this image appear in the interval of $[-\pi, -0.5\pi]$, lower than those of the dark pixels. As a result, the brightest pixels will be mistaken to be "shadowed". To solve this problem, their angles need to be increased by 2π instead. Notice that, the darkest pixels and the bright pixels are always separated by a noticeable gap on the circles in the complex plane. The gap can be easily located by the consecutive empty bins of the histogram of the angles $\angle Z_0$. All the pixels whose angles are smaller than the darkest pixels will be increased by 2π. After that, the angles will have a roughly linear relation to the biased shading intensities $\hat{\gamma}$ (See Fig. 4(d)). That is because most of the input pairwise shading orders are calculated by the brightness orders (through the BO or BOB method), while the brightness has a global linear relationship to the shading intensities. We further normalize the angles $\angle Z_0$ to be within the interval of $[0, 1]$, which produce the final shading intensities γ (See Fig. 4(f)).

4.1 Recovering Shading and Reflectance

The reflectance image is regarded to be the brightened image under full direct illumination. That is, the shading intensity γ is 1 for every pixel of the image. From Sect. 4 we have already got the shading intensities, now we can recover the reflectance by raising the shading intensities of all the pixels to 1 along the brightening direction. According to Eqs. 1 and 4, the log image $logI$ is close to a linear function of γ with an unknown slope k. The recovered reflectance image is:

$$R^i = e^{logI^i + kw^i(1-\gamma)} = I^i e^{kw^i(1-\gamma)} \tag{18}$$

while the shading map can be got by:

$$S^i = e^{kw^i(\gamma-1)} \tag{19}$$

We find a reasonable slope k through a voting process. For each channel i and each pixel p, we find the scalar $\tilde{k}^i(p)$ that makes the recovered $R^i(p)$ equal to the maximum value of I^i over the image. Then we calculate the histogram of $\tilde{k}^i(p)$, and record the bin that got the most votes, denoted by $\tilde{k}^i$. Here we empirically set the bin size to be 0.05. We set the slope to be $k = \text{median}_i \tilde{k}^i$.

5 Experiments

We evaluate our method on the MIT Intrinsic Images dataset [26], which is a widely used benchmark for evaluating intrinsic decomposition methods. The images are taken in a controlled environment, where the direct illuminations are always white and the ambient illuminations are limited through painting the background to be black. We further test our method on the UIUC shadow dataset [27], where the direct illuminants and the ambient illuminants are uncontrolled.

To quantitatively evaluate the results, we use both the Mean Squared Error (MSE), the Local Mean Squared Error (LMSE) [26], the absolute LMSE (aLMSE) and the correction [28]. Among these metrics, correlation and MSE measure the error in a global way, while LMSE and aLMSE take an average of local errors on small image windows. For each image, the performance of shading image and reflectance image are calculated separately and the average of them is taken to be the result. The final result is the average of the performances over all the images. The main parameters of our model are the positive weights of the sigmoid function in Sect. 3. In our experiments we set w_1 to be $ln3/0.1$, which ensures that the sigmoid function maps a step edge of strength 0.1 to a probability of 0.5. We set $w_2 \sim w_5$ to be $ln3/0.2$, $ln3/0.08$, $ln3/0.1$ and $ln3/0.1$, respectively. Especially, we set the w_6 of the FS method to be twice as much as that of the SS method. We find the medium of the spatial distances of all the pixel pairs $\bar{d}_s$, and set w_6 to be $6ln3/\bar{d}_s$ for the FS method. These parameters are used for all the images of our experiments.

5.1 Results on MIT Intrinsic Image Dataset

We take the image with only diffuse reflection as input, since specular reflection is out of the scope of this paper. We compare our method to the state-of-art together with some classic approaches as listed in Table 2. For each method, a single group of best parameters are used for all the images. Our method achieves the best performance on the correlation and LMSE metric. The SIRFS model gets the lowest MSE [8], but their method relies on priors got from training images. Weiss [29] gets the best aLMSE, but their method takes image sequences captured under different illuminants as input. Among the single-image based methods without training, our model gets the best performance over all the metrics. Specifically, our method performs much better than the method of Color Retinex [26]. One important reason is that our method explicitly take the ambient illuminant into consideration (although it is very weak in this dataset), which results in a better shadow-free plane than that used by Color Retinex. Figure 5 gives some concrete examples. One important advantage of our method is that we can recover the reflectance of very dark areas. The reason is that our model carries out the local fusion of estimations from different methods by a maximization operation (Eq. 14), which preserves the large shading orders between pixels separated by shadow edges. In comparison, the method of Gehler et al. [4] often smoothes the shading map through adding strong smoothness constraints, leaving residuals of shadows in the recovered reflectance image. This problem is even more serious for the SIRFS model [8], since the smoothed surfaces of the objects in this model always generate smooth shading image. The method of Jiang-HA [28] is based on the global correlation between the mean luminance and luminance amplitude, which recovers the global shading distribution well but not the details in local regions (e.g., the symbols on the raccoon).

Table 2. Results on the MIT Intrinsic Images dataset. Higher correlation and lower MSE, LMSE and aLMSE are better. The method SIRFS is evaluated on 8 images including cup2, deer, frog2, paper2, raccoon, sun, teabag1 and turtle, while the other images are used for training.

	Correlation	MSE	LMSE	aLMSE
Grey Retinex [2]	0.6494	0.1205	0.0329	0.3373
Tappen et al. [16]	-	-	0.0390	-
Color Retinex [26]	0.7146	0.1108	0.0286	0.2541
Jiang-A [28]	0.6184	0.1533	0.0421	0.3988
Jiang-H [28]	0.5829	0.1524	0.0483	0.3476
Jiang-HA [28]	0.6109	0.1579	0.0454	0.3631
Shen-SR [7]	0.7259	0.1223	0.0242	0.2454
Shen-SRC et al. [7]	-	-	0.0204	-
Gehler et al. [4]	0.7748	0.0985	0.0244	0.2544
Serra et al. [17]	0.7862	0.0834	0.0340	0.2958
Li et al. [18]	-	-	0.0190	-
Chang et al. [19]	-	-	0.0229	-
Ours	**0.8582**	0.0684	**0.0189**	0.2252
Weiss [29]	0.7709	0.0900	0.0210	**0.1953**
SIRFS [8]	0.8095	**0.0567**	0.0279	0.2329

5.2 Evaluation Under Chromatic Illuminations

We test our method's ability of handling both direct and ambient illuminants on the UIUC shadow dataset [27]. Figure 6 shows several examples. We compare our method to the method of Jiang-HA [28] and the method proposed by Gehler et al. [4]. We also compare it to the region-pair-based shadow removal method proposed by Guo et al. [27]. For this method the shading map is replaced by a shadow map, in which black pixels indicate shadows and gray ones indicate penumbra. We can see that our method successfully recovers the shading map, not only for the cast shadows but also for the self shading (the first image of Fig. 6). For the image of the cup, only our method recovers the deeply shadowed area inside the cup. In the outdoor scenes (the last 3 columns of Fig. 6), the ambient illuminants are usually the blue sky, which turns the shadowed areas more blueish than the bright areas. Our model recovers their reflectance by

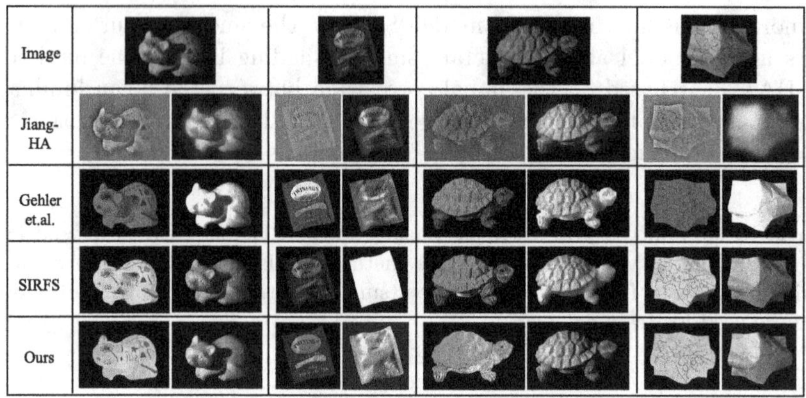

Fig. 5. Typical results on the MIT Intrinsic Images dataset.

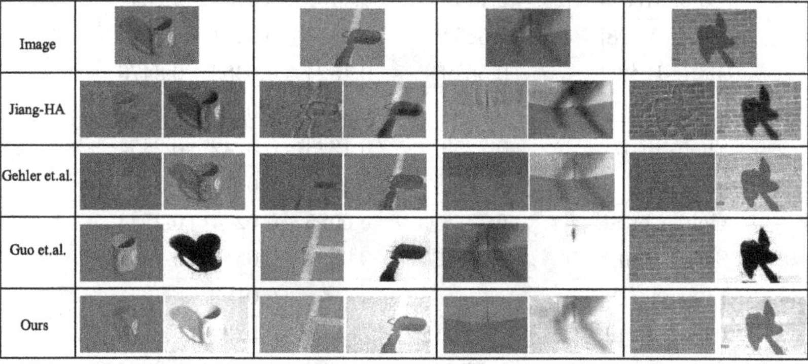

Fig. 6. Typical results on the UIUC shadow dataset.

lighting the dark pixels along the yellowish brightening direction, while the other intrinsic decomposition methods often fail to recover the color of them.

6 Conclusions

We proposed a model to decompose a single image into reflectance and shading by pairwise shading orders. It overcame the limitations of edge-based methods that rely solely on local gradients. The shading orders were estimated by several individual methods, each of which aimed at specific types of image regions. We experimented on different kinds of images, and achieved promising results on most of them. We adopted a new strategy of integrating local cues, that was local competition and global collaboration. The local competition prevented the cues from different sources interfering each other. Especially, it kept the sharp shadow edges from being weaken by the shading smoothness constraints.

Acknowledgement. This work was supported in part by the National Basic Research Program of China under Grant No. 2012CB316400, and the National Natural Science Foundation of China under Grant No. 91120006.

References

1. Barrow, H.G., Tenenbaum, J.M.: Recovering Intrinsic Scene Characteristics from Images. In: Hanson, A.R., Riseman, E.M. (eds.) Computer Vision Systems, vol. 27, pp. 3–26. Academic Press, New York (1978)
2. Land, E.H., McCann, J.J.: Lightness and retinex theory. J. Opt. Soc. Am. **61**, 1–11 (1971)
3. Shen, L., Ping, T., Lin, S.: Intrinsic image decomposition with non-local texture cues. In: IEEE Conference on Computer Vision and Pattern Recognition, pp. 1–7 (2008)
4. Gehler, P., Rother, C., Kiefel, M., Zhang, L., Schölkopf, B.: Recovering intrinsic images with a global sparsity prior on reflectance. In: Shawe-Taylor, J., Zemel, R.S., Bartlett, P.L., Pereira, F.C.N., Weinberger, K.Q. (eds.) Advances in Neural Information Processing Systems, pp. 765–773. MIT press, Massachusetts (2011)
5. Lee, K.J., Zhao, Q., Tong, X., Gong, M., Izadi, S., Lee, S.U., Tan, P., Lin, S.: Estimation of intrinsic image sequences from image+depth video. In: Fitzgibbon, A., Lazebnik, S., Perona, P., Sato, Y., Schmid, C. (eds.) ECCV 2012, Part VI. LNCS, vol. 7577, pp. 327–340. Springer, Heidelberg (2012)
6. Chen, Q., Koltun, V.: A simple model for intrinsic image decomposition with depth cues. In: IEEE International Conference on Computer Vision (2013)
7. Shen, L., Yeo, C.: Intrinsic images decomposition using a local and global sparse representation of reflectance. In: IEEE Conference on Computer Vision and Pattern Recognition, pp. 697–704 (2011)
8. Barron, T.T., Malik, J.: Color constancy, intrinsic images, and shape estimation. In: Fitzgibbon, A., Lazebnik, S., Perona, P., Sato, Y., Schmid, C. (eds.) Computer Vision - ECCV 2012. LNCS, vol. 7575, pp. 57–70. Springer, Berlin (2012)
9. Garces, E., Munoz, A., Lopez-Moreno, J., Gutierrez, D.: Intrinsic images by clustering. Comput. Graph. Forum **31**, 1415–1424 (2012)
10. Huang, X., Hua, G., Tumblin, J., Williams, L.: What characterizes a shadow boundary under the sun and sky? In: IEEE International Conference on Computer Vision, pp. 898–905 (2011)
11. Mark, B.F., Drew, M.S.: Recovering shading from color images. In: Sandini, Giulio (ed.) ECCV 1992. LNCS, vol. 588. Springer, Heidelberg (1992)
12. Gevers, T.: Reflectance-based classification of color edges. In: IEEE International Conference on Computer Vision, p. 856 (2003)
13. Finlayson, G.D., Hordley, S.D., Drew, M.S.: Removing shadows from images. In: Heyden, A., Sparr, G., Nielsen, M., Johansen, P. (eds.) ECCV 2002, Part IV. LNCS, vol. 2353, pp. 823–836. Springer, Heidelberg (2002)
14. Van de Weijer, J., Gevers, T., Geusebroek, J.M.: Edge and corner detection by photometric quasi-invariants. IEEE Trans. Pattern Anal. Mach. Intell. **27**, 625–630 (2005)
15. Tappen, M.F., Freeman, W.T., Adelson, E.H.: Recovering intrinsic images from a single image. IEEE Trans. Pattern Anal. Mach. Intell. **27**, 1459–1472 (2005)
16. Tappen, M.F., Adelson, E.H., Freeman, W.T.: Estimating intrinsic component images using non-linear regression. In: IEEE Conference on Computer Vision and Pattern Recognition, pp. 1992–1999 (2006)

17. Serra, M., Penacchio, O., Benavente, R., Vanrell, M.: Names and shades of color for intrinsic image estimation. In: IEEE Conference on Computer Vision and Pattern Recognition, pp. 278–285 (2012)
18. Li, Y., Brown, M.S.: Single image layer separation using relative smoothness. In: The IEEE Conference on Computer Vision and Pattern Recognition (2014)
19. Chang, J., Cabezas, R., Fisher III, J.W.: Bayesian nonparametric intrinsic image decomposition. In: Proceedings of the European Conference on Computer Vision (2014)
20. Maxwell, B.A., Friedhoff, R.M., Smith, C.A.: A bi-illuminant dichromatic reflection model for understanding images. In: IEEE Conference on Computer Vision and Pattern Recognition (2008)
21. Yu, S.X.: Angular embedding: A robust quadratic criterion. IEEE Trans. Pattern Anal. Mach. Intell. **34**, 158–173 (2012)
22. Finlayson, G., Drew, M., Lu, C.: Entropy minimization for shadow removal. Int. J. Comput. Vis. **85**, 35–57 (2009)
23. Barron, J.T., Malik, J.: Shape, albedo, and illumination from a single image of an unknown object. In: IEEE Conference on Computer Vision and Pattern Recognition, pp. 334–341 (2012)
24. Omer, I., Werman, M.: Color lines: image specific color representation. IEEE Conference on Computer Vision Pattern Recognition. vol. 2, pp. 946–953 (2004)
25. Shi, J., Malik, J.: Normalized cuts and image segmentation. In: IEEE Conference on Computer Vision and Pattern Recognition (1997)
26. Grosse, R., Johnson, M.K., Adelson, E.H., Freeman, W.T.: Ground-truth dataset and baseline evaluations for intrinsic image algorithms. In: IEEE International Conference on Computer Vision, pp. 2335–2342 (2009)
27. Guo, R., Dai, Q., Hoiem, D.: Single-image shadow detection and removal using paired regions. In: IEEE Conference on Computer Vision and Pattern Recognition, pp. 2033–2040 (2011)
28. Jiang, X., Schofield, A.J., Wyatt, J.L.: Correlation-based intrinsic image extraction from a single image. In: Daniilidis, K., Maragos, P., Paragios, N. (eds.) ECCV 2010, Part IV. LNCS, vol. 6314, pp. 58–71. Springer, Berlin Heidelberg (2010)
29. Weiss, Y.: Deriving intrinsic images from image sequences. In: IEEE International Conference on Computer Vision, pp. 68–75 (2001)

Never Get Lost Again: Vision Based Navigation Using StreetView Images

Aparna Taneja(✉), Luca Ballan, and Marc Pollefeys

ETH Zurich, Zurich, Switzerland
aparna.taneja@gmail.com

Abstract. In this paper we propose a simple and lightweight solution to estimate the geospatial trajectory of a moving vehicle from images captured by a cellphone exploiting the map and the imagery provided by Google Streetview.

Images are intelligently compared against the streetview data, and a recursive Bayesian framework is applied to perform continuous localization of the vehicle inside the discrete structure of the streetview graph.

Experiments run on a dataset 10.7 km long, show that the system is able to infer its position and orientation despite the low resolution and limited field of view offered by an off the shelf consumer device. Our method shows to be robust with respect to significant changes in appearance and structure of the environment across the images, obtaining an average accuracy of 13 m in position, and 16° in orientation.

1 Introduction

Consumer navigation devices, such as Tomtom and Garmin, are common tools that assist drivers during their journey, as they provide directions, and help in the navigation of complicated networks of streets. These devices are nowadays available in most of the vehicles, but they heavily rely on the Global Positioning System (GPS), which is in general not very precise (with an accuracy that is at best around 10 m), and its signal may be absent or perturbed, especially in the presence of skyscrapers or inside a tunnel. Although this is not much of an issue for humans, its impact can be catastrophic when used in the context of autonomous or semi-autonomous driving vehicles.

To cope for this, the robotics community has explored the usage of other kinds of sensors, like compasses and inertial sensors, which, not only help in localizing the vehicle, but also provide its orientation. This additional information is very important, and would enable novel types of visualizations, in the context of navigation. Imagine the possibility of seeing an image of the street aligned with the point of view of the driver before a turn at a complicated intersection, or near an exit on a highway: directions can be superimposed on this image to avoid making the wrong turn (see Fig. 1). Such augmented visualizations are only possible if both the location and the orientation are estimated correctly. This is not possible using conventional sensors, since their measurements are highly affected by the environment. For instance, artificial magnetic fields, like

D. Cremers et al. (Eds.): ACCV 2014, Part V, LNCS 9007, pp. 99–114, 2015.
DOI: 10.1007/978-3-319-16814-2_7

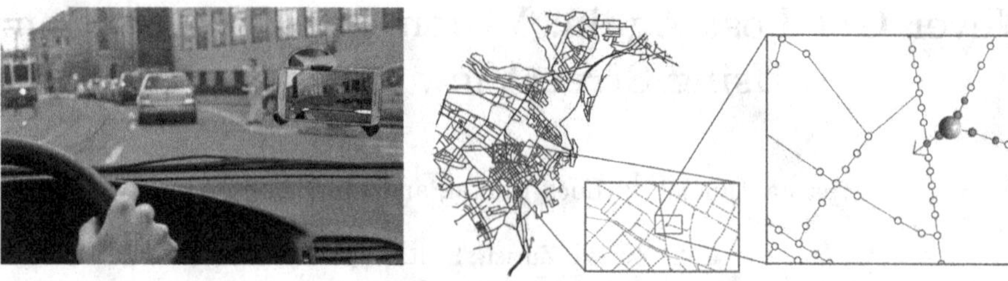

Fig. 1. A device capturing images at low frame rate is mounted on a car driving around an urban environment. Our approach exploits the captured images and the streetview graph to track the movement of the vehicle on the map.

those created by power lines or tram lines, lead to noisy compass measurements with errors as high as 150° at times.

On the other hand, the vision community has developed several algorithms to infer the location of an image exploiting either large collections of geo-tagged images [1–3], or 3D models of urban environments [4–9]. While the availabilty of these 3D models is still restricted to a few cities in the world, large collection of images are becoming increasingly available thanks to services like Flickr and Panoramio. However, even for these collections, majority of the images are actually covering only popular/touristic locations around the world, and the number of images covering residential streets or highways for instance, is still very low.

Recently [10] proposed a method exploiting OpenStreetMaps (OSM) to perform continuous localization on a vehicle driving around a city. The key idea is to use the geometry of this map to align and localize the trajectories obtained from visual odometry [11–13].

Inspired by this work, we propose a method to use a similar map of the environment, in particular Google Streetview. Similarly to OSM, Google Streetview offers a graphical representation of the streets of the world as a network of nodes, each of which represents a specific location, and edges between these nodes represent their relative connectivity via streets. The level of detail of this map is however coarser compared to OSM. In fact, the streets are represented as piecewise linear segments sampled every 10 to 20 m, making it difficult to apply a curve matching based technique. To compensate for this lack of detail, we go one step further, and leverage also the image information available with this graph, i.e., the Google Streetview images.

Unlike the image collections provided by Flickr and Panoramio, Google Streetview offers a much broader and uniform coverage of the streets of the world, although at a relatively sparse sampling rate. This sparsity prohibits the usage of most of the 3D reconstruction techniques used by the large-scale localization approaches based on 3D models.

In this paper we propose a simple and lightweight solution to estimate the geospatial trajectory of a moving vehicle from images captured at 1 fps by an off the shelf consumer mobile device, such as a cellphone, mounted on the windshield of the vehicle. We formulate the problem as a recursive Bayesian estimation of the position and the orientation of the vehicle using as observation the monocular images captured by the device, and the related compass measurements.

In contrast to classic image retrieval based techniques, we exploit the fact that our query images can be aligned almost perfectly with images in the database using a similar concept as proposed in Video Compass [14]. This allows us to maintain low computational requirements, and hence our solution can be easily ported as a client-server application on a mobile device. Therefore, for a person driving from one point to another, even if the GPS loses reception at some point, our system will help the driver localize and orient himself in the environment, by comparing images taken from the phone with those on the database.

In contrast to [10], which showed impressive results on stereo odometry we do not perform structure from motion and use only monocular videos, which was shown to be a challenging scenario even with their approach. Moreover, since we use the additional information provided by streetview images, our approach would in principle also work in a Manhattan world with a monotonous grid like structure.

2 Related Work

Most of the vision based localization approaches formulate the problem as an image retrieval task, typically using bag-of-words representations [15] or vocabulary trees [16] to efficiently search through large datasets of geo-tagged images. These methods rely on pure occurrence-based statistics to retrieve the geo-location of a query image [3,17–20]. In particular, [17] localizes videos taken from the web using Google streetview imagery. However, such methods in general fail in cases where the relative locations of the features on the image are also important. To cope for this, methods like [20–24] perform geometric consistency between the query image and the top ranked matching images from the database. This however becomes quite inefficient in case of repetitive urban structures or high fractions of mismatches, increasing the computationally complexity. Moreover, since these methods rely on RANSAC, their parameters need to be tuned precisely for each scene, as also observed in [25]. In our approach, we also take into account the relative location of the features on the images, but at the same time we aim at a simple lightweight solution, such that the computational load on both the client and the server side is minimal, and not much information has to be stored on the client side.

Methods like [6,8,26,27] instead, first recover the 3D structure of the images in the database and then perform a 2D-to-3D matching with the query image. If the number of inliers is higher than a certain threshold, the image is considered to be localized. 3D reconstruction however, is in itself an extremely difficult problem to solve, and it is even more challenging in a sparse dataset like Google Streetview.

In contrast, [10] performs continuous localization by aligning the trajectory of the vehicle obtained from visual odometry with a map of the environment.

Not only does this method require a highly detailed and accurate map of the environment, but it is also constrained by the fact that the images need to be captured with a sufficient density such that structure from motion can be applied, i.e., enough features can be matched across images.

Our approach instead, performs continuous localization on a coarser graphical representation of the environment using images captured on an average every 7 m by a phone camera with a limited field of view. Hence we cannot rely on visual odometry or curve matching techniques.

3 Algorithm

We model the map of the environment as a streetview graph (V, E), where each node $v \in V$ represents a specific location in the environment (stored as latitude and longitude coordinates), and each edge $e \in E$ between two nodes, indicates that the corresponding locations are connected by a street (see Fig. 1(right)). At each location v, a spherical panoramic image is available, representing the scene at that location. Let P_v denote this image. All of these panoramas are assumed to be aligned with respect to the north direction, and to have fixed roll and pitch angles relative to the tangent plane of the street.

We model the state of the car at time t using two random variables, $s_t \in V$ and $\rho_t \in S^1$, indicating respectively the position and the orientation of the car on the map. While the position is represented discretely as a node index on the streetview graph (V, E), the direction of motion ρ_t is represented as a unit vector in the x-y coordinates of the map. ρ_t is therefore a continuous quantity not necessarily indicating a valid traveling direction on the streetview graph as one might initially assume, i.e., ρ_t does not in general belong to E. This choice is made to account for changes of lane, U-turns, intersections, or in general any motion which is not modeled by the streetview graph.

Our algorithm tracks the state of the car at each time instance on the basis of the images captured by the device and their related compass measurements. Tracking is initialized with s_0 being the starting point of the car journey or being the last position measured by the GPS when the signal was available. The orientation ρ_0 is initialized as being equiprobable over all S^1. In all the subsequent time instances, our algorithm computes a probability map over all the possible car positions and orientations on the map. Precisely, it computes $P(s_t, \rho_t \mid I_t, c_t)$, i.e., the probability of each pair (s_t, ρ_t) given, as observations, the image I_t captured by the mobile device, and the corresponding compass measurement c_t, both measured at time t. Every time a new image is acquired, this probability map is updated on the basis of the new observations and a motion model. The best estimate for the car position is then obtained by selecting the state with maximum probability (maximum a posteriori).

While our approach broadly resembles the particle filtering algorithm, it is not the same, since no approximation on the posterior probability is made and no re-sampling is used. In fact, we exploit the already discrete nature of our model (see Sect. 3.3) to perform an exhaustive inference over all the possible states of the car. At each time instance, all pairs (s_t, ρ_t) with probability different than 0, are stored as an array, and evaluated at the next time instance.

This makes our approach more robust and capable of recovering from tracking failures since it stores all the possible states of the car, even the least probable ones, helping in scenarios where, after some observations, these states turn out to be the correct ones.

3.1 Motion Model

The motion model provides us with a speculation on the position of the car at time t given the position and orientation probabilities $P(s_{t-1}, \rho_{t-1})$ at time $t-1$. It also provides time continuity on our inference, allowing us to cope with situations where the observations (I_t, c_t) are missing or not informative. This is the case when there are strong occlusions in the image, or when there are similar buildings in a row creating ambiguity on the correct location along the street.

We chose to use a constant speed motion model on the streetview graph. The constant speed motion model is defined in literature for continuous spaces, like $\mathbb{R}^2$ or $\mathbb{R}^3$, therefore some adjustments need to be made to make it work on the discrete space of a graph. Precisely, we first assume s_t to be a Markov chain of order one. Therefore,

$$P(s_t) = \sum P(s_t \mid s_{t-1}, \rho_{t-1}) P(s_{t-1}, \rho_{t-1}) \tag{1}$$

where the sum is intended to be over all $V \times S^1$, i.e., over all the possible positions and orientations (s_{t-1}, ρ_{t-1}), for which the probability $P(s_{t-1}, \rho_{t-1})$ is greater than 0. The probability map $P(s_{t-1}, \rho_{t-1})$ is the one provided by the algorithm at time step $t-1$, while $P(s_t \mid s_{t-1}, \rho_{t-1})$ defines the motion model and is described in the following paragraphs.

Precisely, if the car at time $t-1$ is observed to be at position s_{t-1} with an orientation ρ_{t-1}, it is likely that it is moving on the edge $e \in E$ of the streetview graph that is most parallel to the direction ρ_{t-1}. Therefore, at time t, the car must be on one of the nodes reachable from s_{t-1} through the edge e (see Fig. 2(left)). Note that this is independent from the orientation of the other edges along the path connecting s_t and s_{t-1}, since the car orientation ρ might have changed significantly from time $t-1$ to time t. We define the probability of reaching a specific node s_t on this path as

$$P(s_t \mid s_{t-1}, e) = \mathcal{N}_T(d_e(s_t, s_{t-1}), \sigma_m) \tag{2}$$

where $d_e(s_t, s_{t-1})$ is the length of shortest path connecting the nodes s_t and s_{t-1} that passes through the edge e. In the formula, $\mathcal{N}_T(\cdot, \sigma_m)$ denotes the truncated Gaussian distribution centered at zero and truncated for values less than 0. In our implementation, we set the standard deviation σ_m to 12 m, corresponding to the assumption that, in 68 % of the cases, the car is within 12 m of s_{t-1}.

All these probabilities are combined as follows

$$P(s_t \mid s_{t-1}, \rho_{t-1}) = \sum_{e \in inc(s_{t-1})} P(s_t \mid s_{t-1}, e) P(e \mid \rho_{t-1}) \tag{3}$$

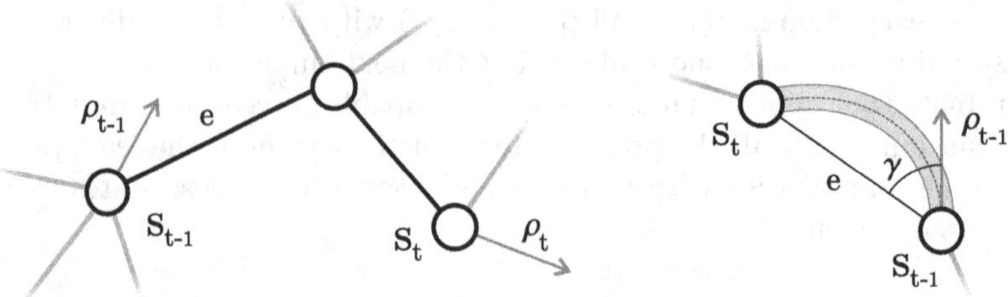

Fig. 2. Motion model on the streetview graph: (left) at position s_{t-1}, the car is likely to move on the edge e since it is the one most parallel to the heading direction ρ_{t-1}; (right) the actual path taken by the vehicle along the physical street might differ significantly from the path on the streetview graph (edge e).

where $inc(s_{t-1})$ represents the set of all edges $e \in E$ incident to node s_{t-1}. Using the Bayes' rule, we define $P(e \mid \rho_{t-1})$ as

$$P(e \mid \rho_{t-1}) = \frac{P(\rho_{t-1} \mid e) P(e)}{P(\rho_{t-1})} = \frac{1}{N} e^{k \cos(\gamma)} \tag{4}$$

where N is a normalization term ensuring that $\sum P(e \mid \rho_{t-1}) = 1$, γ is the angle between the edge e and the direction ρ_{t-1}, and where the concentration parameter k is set to 2.8 corresponding to a circular standard deviation of 40°. Precisely, here we implicitly assume that $P(e)$ is uniform, and $P(\rho_{t-1} \mid e)$ is distributed accordingly to a von-Mises distribution centered at the direction corresponding to the edge e. This is equivalent to assuming that the angle between the actual path taken by the vehicle, and the straight line connecting the two end points of that path, can vary along that path with a standard deviation of 40° (see Fig. 2(right)).

3.2 Observations

Given an image I_t, captured by the device at time t, we aim at inferring how likely is it, that the image was captured in the proximity of a streetview node v. This is performed by comparing the image I_t with the streetview panorama P_v corresponding to the node v.

In contrast to other image based localization techniques, we exploit the fact that, in our scenario, the image I_t and the panorama P_v are already well aligned, or at most they are aligned up to one degree of freedom. This is due to the fact that, in a setup where the device is assumed to be firmly attached to the windshield of the car or to its dashboard, the angle between the camera of the device and the driving direction is fixed over time. Since the driving direction is always parallel to the street, both the tilt and the roll angles of the camera are fixed with respect to the plane tangent to the street, and hence they need to be estimated only once, at the beginning of the journey. This is performed by capturing a few images from the device and by computing the pitch and the roll

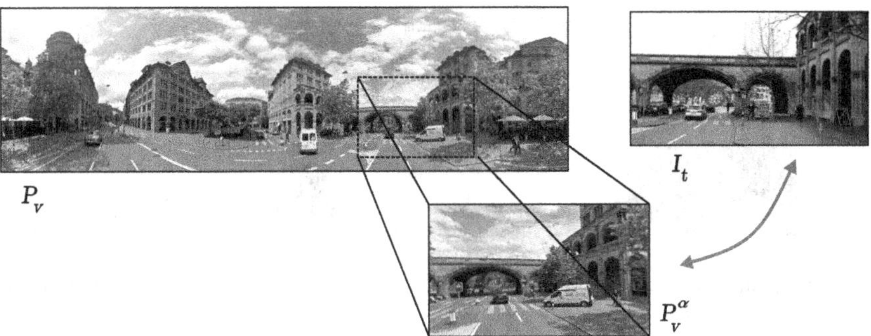

Fig. 3. Street-level vanishing points at an intersection on a panoramic image P_v, and on an image I_t captured by the device. A perspective image P_v^α is extracted for each of the admissible angles, and compared with I_t.

angles which force the vertical vanishing point in I_t to lie on the image y-axis at infinity [28].

The yaw angle of the device instead, measured with respect to the north direction, changes over time and hence has to be estimated every time an image is captured. One might assume that, an initial guess for this orientation can be obtained from the compass. However, this sensor is very sensitive to any artificial magnetic fields present in the environment causing errors as high as 150°. Therefore an exhaustive search for the correct yaw angle needs to be performed.

Fortunately, in a practical scenario, this search can be limited to only those angles which make the forward street-level vanishing point on image I_t match one of the street-level vanishing points on the panoramic image P_v [14]. As an example, the image I_t in Fig. 3, can only have been captured at a yaw angle that makes its forward vanishing point match one of the three possible vanishing points in P_v, each of which correspond to a driving direction. We therefore extract a perspective image from P_v at each of these admissible yaw angles, and compare it to I_t. To be robust to changes in illumination, weather conditions and different camera settings across the images, this comparison is performed on a feature space. Precisely, let P_v^α be the perspective image extracted from panorama P_v at yaw angle α using the same intrinsic parameters as those of image I_t (these are assumed to be known a priori). We subdivide both I_t and P_v^α into blocks of size 30 by 30 pixels, and compute color and gradient descriptors for each of these blocks. We then compare corresponding blocks in each image, and sum up the results of these comparisons to obtain a score indicating how similar I_t and P_v^α are. Precisely, let $d_z(i, I_t)$ denote the descriptor of type z computed for the block i in image I_t, and let $d_z(i, P_v^\alpha)$ denote the corresponding descriptor computed on P_v^α. The similarity measure $o_t^{v,\alpha}$ between image I_t and image P_v^α, is then defined as

$$o_t^{v,\alpha} = \sum_{i,z} w_i^z \left\| d_z(i, I_t) - d_z(i, P_v^\alpha) \right\|_2 \qquad (5)$$

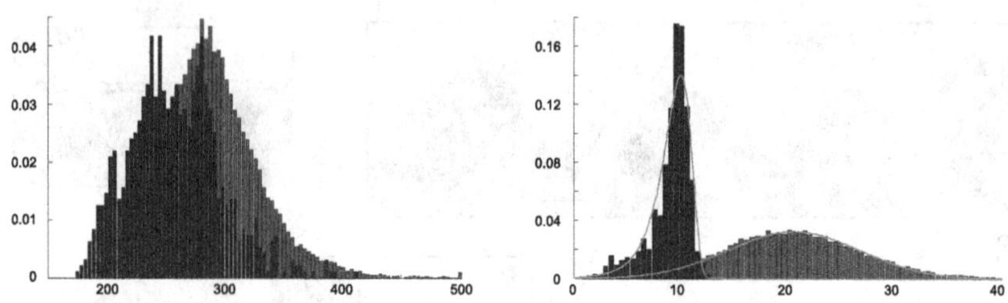

Fig. 4. Distribution of the scores $o_t^{v,\alpha}$ before (left), and after training (right) (Color figure online).

where w_i^z are constants weighing the contribution of each block and the relative influence between the color and the different gradient descriptors.

In our implementation, the color descriptor is simply computed as the average color among all the pixels in block i, hence it is a single triplet in the HSL space. Concerning the gradient descriptor instead, we used HOG [29] descriptors, and computed them as defined in the UoCTTI model [30] which includes the histogram of directed gradients, undirected gradients and a texture information. In addition, for each block we evaluate the entropy of the histogram of directed gradients, indicating how uniform is this distribution. We observed that this provides a sort of contextual information indicating whether the block depicts sky, buildings or road.

To compensate for small misalignments between I_t and P_v^α caused by the fact that, even though the images are aligned with the same orientation, they may have been captured on slightly different positions on the street (lat-long on the map), a window based comparison of the blocks is performed by comparing each block to the 8-neighbouring blocks and returning the minimum score.

Weights: Ideally the score $o_t^{v,\alpha}$ should be close to zero in case of similar images, however, in a first analysis (see Fig. 4(left)), assuming all weights w_i^z equal to 1, the distributions of the scores $o_t^{v,\alpha}$, in case of similar images (blue), and in case of not similar images (red), show a considerable overlap. This is due to the fact that, some feature types and some blocks contribute incoherently to the score, degrading its discriminative property. This happens, for instance, in areas of the image which are often occluded by cars and pedestrians, and in the areas that often contain objects close to the camera, and hence prone to registration artifacts. To cope with this, we learn the weights w_i^z minimizing the overlap between the two distributions. Precisely, we trained a linear Support Vector Machine [31] on a dataset of about 30k images, using 10-fold cross-validation. We then set our weights according to the resulting separating hyperplane.

Figure 4(right) shows the score distribution after the training. It is noticeable that, the score $o_t^{v,\alpha}$ is now sufficiently discriminative to tell us whether the image I_t is similar to P_v^α. To integrate this information into our probabilistic framework, we fit two standard distributions on these two histograms, precisely, a Gaussian distribution for the non matching images, and a generalized extreme value distribution for the matching ones.

3.3 Posterior Probability and Tracking

Given the observed matching scores o_t and the compass measurement c_t, the posterior probability of the car state at time t can be written as

$$P(s_t, \rho_t \mid o_t, c_t) = \frac{1}{N} P(o_t, c_t \mid s_t, \rho_t) P(s_t, \rho_t) \tag{6}$$

$$= \frac{1}{N} P(o_t, c_t \mid s_t, \rho_t) P(\rho_t \mid s_t) P(s_t) \tag{7}$$

where the normalization term $N = P(o_t, c_t)$ is computed by ensuring that the sum $\sum P(s_t, \rho_t \mid o_t, c_t)$ over all pairs of nodes s_t and available directions ρ_t is equal to one. $P(s_t)$ is provided by the motion model, as described in Eq. 1. The probability $P(\rho_t \mid s_t)$ instead is assumed to be uniform over all the yaw angles admissible at node s_t, as described in Sect. 3.2. Precisely, let $\alpha_1, \ldots, \alpha_n$ be the set of all these admissible yaw angles, the probability density of ρ_t given s_t is therefore defined as,

$$P(\rho_t \mid s_t) = \frac{1}{n} \sum_{j=1}^{n} \delta(\rho_t - (\alpha_j - \Delta)) \tag{8}$$

where δ denotes the Dirac delta function, and Δ denotes the angle between the car heading direction and the device yaw direction. Note that Δ is fixed over time, and therefore it needs to be estimated only once, at the beginning of the journey. Equation 8 tells us that, $P(\rho_t \mid s_t)$ is different from zero if and only if ρ_t coincides with one of the admissible α in s_t, minus the correction Δ.

Concerning the likelihood $P(o_t, c_t \mid s_t, \rho_t)$, we assume independence between the compass measurements and the matching scores, therefore

$$P(o_t, c_t \mid s_t, \rho_t) = P(c_t \mid s_t, \rho_t) \prod_{v, \alpha_j} P\left(o_t^{v,\alpha_j} \mid s_t, \rho_t\right). \tag{9}$$

The compass measurements $P(c_t \mid s_t, \rho_t)$ are assumed to be affected by a circular Gaussian noise on S^1, that we approximate using a von-Mises distribution centered at the direction of motion ρ_t plus the correction Δ. Due to the high level of noise affecting this measurement, the standard deviation for this distribution was set to $\sigma_c = 60°$ in our experiments.

Concerning the generative model for the matching scores $P\left(o_t^{v,\alpha_j} \mid s_t, \rho_t\right)$ instead, we define it as

$$P\left(o_t^{v,\alpha_j} \mid s_t, \rho_t\right) = \begin{cases} \mathrm{Gev}(o_t^{v,\alpha_j}, \mu_+, \sigma_+, \xi_+) & s_t = v \wedge \rho_t = \alpha_j - \Delta \\ \mathcal{N}(o_t^{v,\alpha_j}, \mu_-, \sigma_-) & \textit{else} \end{cases} \tag{10}$$

where $\mathrm{Gev}(\cdot, \mu_+, \sigma_+, \xi_+)$ and $\mathcal{N}(\cdot, \mu_-, \sigma_-)$ indicate the generalized extreme value distribution and the Gaussian distribution estimated in Sect. 3.2, for the matching images and the non matching ones, respectively.

Client-Server Framework: All previous operations (feature extraction, color conversion, color averaging and window based comparison) can be quickly performed on the GPU using shaders. Street-level vanishing points for each panorama in the database can be precomputed, and stored on the server side [32]. On the client side instead, only the streetview graph (V, E) is needed, not the panoramas P_v.

Every time a new image I_t is captured by the device, the forward vanishing point at the street level is estimated. We approximate this, by determining amongst all the vanishing points in the image, the one which is closest to the center of the image. Alternatively, this point can be easily tracked along the journey, as it always lies in the same region on the image, except when the car is turning. The descriptors for image I_t are then computed, and this information, along with the coordinates of the forward vanishing point, and the list of probable locations where the motion model is expecting the car to be, are sent to the server for evaluation. The required bandwidth for this communication is around 70 KB.

The server computes the scores o_t^{v,α_j} for each of the requested panoramas and each of the corresponding admissible yaw angles. During our experiments, the number of requested locations per image I_t was on an average 14. The server then sends back the results to the client which performs the inference updating the list of possible states as described above.

Time: For each phone image, vanishing point extraction takes 46ms while computing the descriptor takes 72 ms. Comparing this descriptor with an average of 14 locations and updating the tracked states takes under 0.001 ms.

4 Results

The proposed algorithm was evaluated on three different sequences captured by driving around an urban environment, covering a total distance of 10.7 km. Precisely, we mounted a Samsung Galaxy S4 on the windshield of a car at an estimated angle $\Delta = 20°$ with respect to the driving direction, as shown in Fig. 1. The phone captured images at 1 frame/sec, at a resolution of 960 by 540 pixels, and with a horizontal field of view of 60.3°. We drove at different times of the day and with moderate traffic conditions, at an average speed of 25 km/h with occasional peaks up to 65 km/h. Each image I_t was therefore captured at an average distance of 7 m, with peaks that went up to 18 m. Such a scenario would be quite challenging for a monocular structure from motion based method. Since we are using a low end consumer camera, the captured images suffered from rolling shutter distortion and motion blur. For comparison purposes, GPS information was also recorded.

The streetview graph (V, E) and the corresponding panoramic images were obtained using the Google StreetView API [33]. The error on this data is on an average around 3.7 m in the position, and 1.9° degrees in the orientation [34]. For the explored locations, the streetview data had an average sampling density of 14 m, and it was a few years old, showing structural and appearance changes in

Table 1. (Top) Statistics on the errors obtained in each of the evaluated sequences. (Bottom) Comparison with alternative approaches evaluated on sequence #1: (Geom) geometric verification based approach, (Feat) feature matching based comparison.

		ε_{graph} [nodes]			$\varepsilon_{\|\cdot\|_2}$ [m]			θ_{gps} [deg]		θ_{graph} [deg]	
		mean	median	std	mean	median	std	mean	median	mean	median
Our	**Seq. #1**	0.53	0.0	1.20	10.77	7.10	15.43	14.75	3.87	15.75	3.68
	Seq. #2	0.60	0.0	0.90	9.48	6.14	10.55	12.12	3.87	16.97	4.04
	Seq. #3	1.12	0.0	2.77	17.70	5.67	36.10	20.75	6.87	23.62	8.40
Alt	**Geom**	3.57	2.0	3.59	46.38	40.52	35.51	27.70	26.19	36.35	26.77
	Feat	4.23	2.0	4.70	47.10	34.46	40.46	18.03	4.27	19.58	3.90

the environment like new buildings, new paints/signs on buildings. Also different lighting conditions and seasonal changes (like changes in vegetation) were clearly visible compared to the phone images.

To quantitatively evaluate the performance of our method, we compared the obtained results against the GPS and the streetview graph. Table 1 reports the statistics of this comparison. In particular, we computed the Euclidean distance between our prediction and the GPS measurement, denoted as $\varepsilon_{|\cdot|_2}$ in the table. Since our estimate is constrained to be on the streetview graph, this error is biased by the discretization of the graph. Therefore, we also compute the length of the shortest path on the graph connecting our estimate and the node closest to the GPS position, ε_{graph} in the table. While the Euclidean distance is measured in meters, the distance on the graph is measured in number of nodes. Please note that, although $\varepsilon_{|\cdot|_2}$ might look high, one needs to account also for the sampling rate of the streetview data (14 m on average).

The performance on the orientation was evaluated in a similar way, by comparing our prediction with respect to the bearing direction measured by the GPS when the car was moving, θ_{gps} in the table, and also with the direction of the corresponding edge in the streetview graph, θ_{graph}. Again, this error has to be considered in light of the coarse representation of the streets in the map.

In general the algorithm performs well in all the three sequences. However, the third sequence was quite challenging, because the car drove through some regions which were not covered by the streetview graph. Therefore our estimate, due to this lack of connectivity, hovered around these regions until there were valid observations again, then the correct track was recovered gradually. This happened for 10 % of the frames, increasing the localization error.

Figure 5 shows some of the locations tested during our experiments. For each location, the figure provides the image captured by the phone I_t, the streetview image P_v^α corresponding to the location and the orientation estimated by our algorithm, and the streetview map zoomed in at the corresponding location. The green spheres on the map denote the possible car positions, with their size being proportional to their probabilities. The yellow sphere is the maximum a posteriori estimate with the related orientation shown as a red arrow. The cyan sphere represents the groundtruth GPS position with the related orientation measured by the compass (in blue), and measured by the GPS (in green).

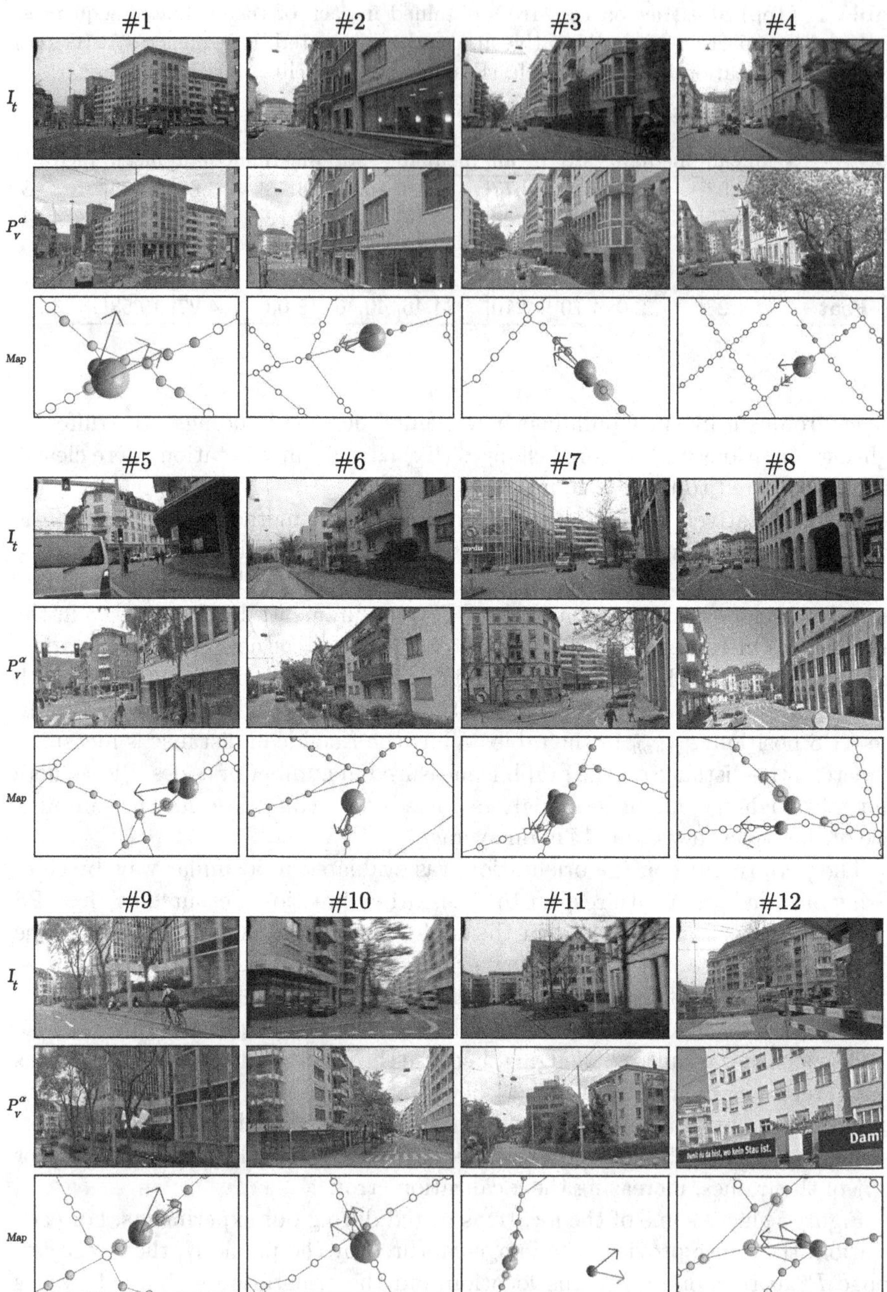

Fig. 5. Some of the evaluated locations: The map indicates the groundtruth GPS position (cyan sphere) displayed together with the bearing direction (green arrow), and the compass direction (blue arrow). Our prediction is displayed as a yellow sphere together with the estimated direction of motion (red arrow) (Color figure online).

Location #1 shows a typical inter ion, with streetside repair in progress in the panoramic image, while locations #2, #3, and #4 show examples of residential streets. In all these cases the alignment was quite accurate. In particular, the algorithm performs well in case #4, despite the strong change in vegetation causing a major occlusion. For both locations #3 and #4, the illumination between I_t and P_v was also quite different, since the latter was captured at a different time of the day. In cases #5, #6, and #7 instead, the scene had changed over time. Particulary, in location #5 the color of the front building and the signs on the building on the right had changed. Similarly in location #6, the building on the right had been repainted, and a new bus stop had been placed. Location #7 shows an example where an old building had been replaced completely with a new construction. Changes like this are quite challenging, despite this, the images were localized correctly. However, this may not happen when there are major changes on both sides of the street for instance. Location #8 shows an example where the GPS location was quite erroneous, whereas our algorithm was able to correctly localize the image on the graph. Such situations occur frequently, as the GPS is generally imprecise. Locations #9 and #10 show two scenarios where the images captured by the phone have significant motion blur. Despite this the algorithm was able to localize them accurately.

Failure Cases: All the above cases demonstrate the robustness of our method with respect to partial appearance and structural changes in the environment. However, failures occurred when the streetview data was extremely incoherent with respect to the current state. This is the case of locations #11 and #12 where in the first case, an entire street was missing, and in the second case, construction work in progress changed the layout of the intersection. Hence the algorithm lost track and recovered only after a while.

Computing the forward vanishing point on the phone image is only possible when enough structure is visible, i.e., when there are no strong occlusions and when the car is not facing only fronto-parallel buildings. However, in our experiments, this succeeded in 89 % of the cases. In the remaining cases, the motion model helps maintain the track.

Comparison with Prior Work: To compare our method with a geometric verification based technique, like the one proposed in [20], we extracted perspective images for each requested panorama at angles corresponding to the street directions in the graph. We then matched SURF [35] features between these images and the phone image I_t. Geometric verification was then performed by estimating the essential matrix relating each pair of images using RANSAC. Non-linear refinement was applied on the resulting matrix in order to minimize the reprojection error. The number of inliers was then recomputed on the basis of the new pose, and used as a feature to discriminate between similar and dissimilar images. We fit two Gaussian distributions on the basis of the statistics of these features. These were then used as generative model for the score $P\left(o_t^{v,\alpha_j} \mid s_t, \rho_t\right)$ in our framework. The fourth row in Table 1 reports the errors obtained with this method on sequence #1. The errors in the position are much higher, and since most of the matched features correspond to objects localized in a small region of the image, it increases the error in orientation as well.

To evaluate our approach with respect to a image retrieval based method, such as [2], we extracted perspective images from each of the requested panoramas at each of the admissible yaw angles, as in our approach. We then performed SURF matching by keeping only those correspondences satisfying the distance-ratio rule of [36]. This number was then used as a feature for our inference, as described before. Such a technique is in principle similar to a standard feature voting based retrieval technique, but deployed in conjunction with our motion model. The fifth row in Table 1, shows the results obtained for sequence #1. As expected, the error on orientation is low, since we used, as input, the already aligned images. The error on position instead, is higher, since this method neglects the geometric disposition of the features in the image. One should also consider that, in this case, the computational time was 7 times higher than in our approach.

5 Conclusions

We presented a method to perform continuous localization of a vehicle from images captured by a cellphone exploiting the map and the imagery provided by Google Streetview.

We formulated the problem as a recursive Bayesian estimation of the position and the orientation of the vehicle on the streetview graph. Differently from classic image retrieval based techniques, we exploit the fact that our query images can be aligned almost perfectly with the images in the database, keeping the computational requirements low.

Unlike sophisticated acquisition systems, we addressed a practical situation and perform continuous localization with a consumer mobile device with a limited field of view, low resolution and low frame rate. Despite the coarse representation of the streetview graph and its possible incoherence with the current structure and appearance of the environment, our algorithm achieved a good accuracy.

In principle, our method can be used on any datasets with street side imagery, such as those of Navteq, Microsoft etc., but we chose to use Google Streetview due to its universal coverage and free availability.

References

1. Schindler, G., Brown, M., Szeliski, R.: City-scale location recognition. In: CVPR (2007)
2. Zamir, A.R., Shah, M.: Accurate image localization based on google maps street view. In: Daniilidis, K., Maragos, P., Paragios, N. (eds.) ECCV 2010, Part IV. LNCS, vol. 6314, pp. 255–268. Springer, Heidelberg (2010)
3. Hays, J., Efros, A.A.: Im2gps: estimating geographic information from a single image. In: CVPR (2008)
4. Baatz, G., Koser, K., Chen, D., Grzeszczuk, R., Pollefeys, M.: Leveraging 3D city models for rotation invariant place-of-interest recognition. IJCV **96**(3), 315–334 (2012)

5. Ramalingam, S., Bouaziz, S., Sturm, P., Brand, M.: Skyline2gps: localization in urban canyons using omni-skylines. In: IROS (2010)
6. Sattler, T., Leibe, B., Kobbelt, L.: Fast image-based localization using direct 2D-to-3D matching. In: ICCV (2011)
7. Irschara, A., Zach, C., Frahm, J.M., Bischof, H.: From structure-from-motion point clouds to fast location recognition. In: CVPR (2009)
8. Li, Y., Snavely, N., Huttenlocher, D., Fua, P.: Worldwide pose estimation using 3D point clouds. In: Fitzgibbon, A., Lazebnik, S., Perona, P., Sato, Y., Schmid, C. (eds.) ECCV 2012, Part I. LNCS, vol. 7572, pp. 15–29. Springer, Heidelberg (2012)
9. Schindler, G., Krishnamurthy, P., Lublinerman, R., Liu, Y., Dellaert, F.: Detecting and matching repeated patterns for automatic geo-tagging in urban environments. In: CVPR (2008)
10. Brubaker, M.A., Geiger, A., Urtasun, R.: Lost! leveraging the crowd for probabilistic visual self-localization. In: CVPR (2013)
11. Wu, C.: Towards linear-time incremental structure from motion. In: 3DV (2013)
12. Kaess, M., Ni, K., Dellaert, F.: Flow separation for fast and robust stereo odometry. In: ICRA (2009)
13. Geiger, A., Ziegler, J., Stiller, C.: Stereoscan: dense 3D reconstruction in real-time. In: IEEE Intelligent Vehicles Symposium (2011)
14. Kosecká, J., Zhang, W.: Video compass. In: Heyden, A., Sparr, G., Nielsen, M., Johansen, P. (eds.) ECCV 2002, Part IV. LNCS, vol. 2353, pp. 476–490. Springer, Heidelberg (2002)
15. Sivic, J., Zisserman, A.: Video google: a text retrieval approach to object matching in videos. In: ICCV (2003)
16. Nistér, D., Stewénius, H.: Scalable recognition with a vocabulary tree. In: CVPR (2006)
17. Vaca, G., Zamir, A.R., Shah, M.: City scale geo-spatial trajectory estimation of a moving camera. In: CVPR (2012)
18. Torii, A., Sivic, J., Pajdla, T., Okutomi, M.: Visual place recognition with repetitive structures. In: CVPR (2013)
19. Cummins, M., Newman, P.: Fab-map: probabilistic localization and mapping in the space of appearance. Int. J. Robot. Res. **27**(6), 647–665 (2008)
20. Zhang, W., Kosecka, J.: Image based localization in urban environments. In: 3DPVT, pp. 33–40 (2006)
21. Galvez-Lopez, D., Tardos, J.D.: Bags of binary words for fast place recognition in image sequences. IEEE Trans. Rob. **28**(5), 1188–1197 (2012)
22. Baatz, G., Köser, K., Chen, D., Grzeszczuk, R., Pollefeys, M.: Handling urban location recognition as a 2D homothetic problem. In: Daniilidis, K., Maragos, P., Paragios, N. (eds.) ECCV 2010, Part VI. LNCS, vol. 6316, pp. 266–279. Springer, Heidelberg (2010)
23. Sunderhauf, N., Protzel, P.: Brief-gist closing the loop by simple means. In: IROS (2011)
24. Raguram, R., Tighe, J., Frahm, J.M.: Improved geometric verification for large scale landmark image collections. In: BMVC (2012)
25. Lee, G.H., Pollefeys, M.: Unsupervised learning of threshold for geometric verification in visual-based loop-closure. In: IEEE International Conference on Robotics and Automation (ICRA) (2014)
26. Lim, H., Sinha, S.N., Cohen, M.F., Uyttendaele, M.: Real-time image-based 6-DOF localization in large-scale environments. In: CVPR (2012)

27. Li, X., Wu, C., Zach, C., Lazebnik, S., Frahm, J.-M.: Modeling and recognition of landmark image collections using iconic scene graphs. In: Forsyth, D., Torr, P., Zisserman, A. (eds.) ECCV 2008, Part I. LNCS, vol. 5302, pp. 427–440. Springer, Heidelberg (2008)
28. Hartley, R., Zisserman, A.: Multiple View Geometry in Computer Vision. Cambridge University Press, Cambridge (2004)
29. Dalal, N., Triggs, B.: Histograms of oriented gradients for human detection. In: CVPR (2005)
30. Vedaldi, A., Fulkerson, B.: VLFeat: An open and portable library of computer vision algorithms (2008). http://www.vlfeat.org/
31. Fan, R.E., Chang, K.W., Hsieh, C.J., Wang, X.R., Lin, C.J.: Liblinear: a library for large linear classification. J. Mach. Learn. Res. **9**, 1871–1874 (2008)
32. Bazin, J.C., Pollefeys, M.: 3-line RANSAC for orthogonal vanishing point detection. In: IROS (2012)
33. https://developers.google.com/maps/documentation/streetview/
34. Taneja, A., Ballan, L., Pollefeys, M.: Registration of spherical panoramic images with cadastral 3D models. In: 3DIMPVT (2012)
35. Bay, H., Tuytelaars, T., Van Gool, L.: SURF: speeded up robust features. In: Leonardis, A., Bischof, H., Pinz, A. (eds.) ECCV 2006, Part I. LNCS, vol. 3951, pp. 404–417. Springer, Heidelberg (2006)
36. Lowe, D.G.: Distinctive image features from scale-invariant keypoints. IJCV **60**, 91–110 (2004)

Qualitative and Quantitative Spatio-temporal Relations in Daily Living Activity Recognition

Jawad Tayyub(✉), Aryana Tavanai, Yiannis Gatsoulis, Anthony G. Cohn, and David C. Hogg

School of Computing, University of Leeds, Leeds LS2 9JT, UK
sc12jbmt@leeds.ac.uk

Abstract. For the effective operation of intelligent assistive systems working in real-world human environments, it is important to be able to recognise human activities and their intentions. In this paper we propose a novel approach to activity recognition from visual data. Our approach is based on qualitative and quantitative spatio-temporal features which encode the interactions between human subjects and objects in an efficient manner. Unlike the state of the art, our approach uses significantly fewer assumptions and does not require knowledge about object types, their affordances, or the sub-level activities that high-level activities consist of. We perform an automatic feature selection process which provides the most representative descriptions of the learnt activities. We validated the method using these descriptions on the CAD-120 benchmark dataset, consisting of video sequences showing humans performing daily real-world activities. The method is shown to outperform state of the art benchmarks.

1 Introduction

One of the most challenging areas of research in the fields of computer vision and pattern recognition is learning and understanding human activities from observed visual data. The research question is, given a sequence of images with one or more people performing various activities, is an intelligent system capable of recognising the activities that are being performed? Despite its long research history [1–4] finding a universal semantic representation for activity analysis is still a difficult challenge due to the complexity of human activities and the variability of how these activities can be performed, even by the same person. Activity analysis is often investigated from a security domain perspective, as automatic recognition of human behaviour in sensitive areas is a critical issue for video surveillance [5–7]. Recently however, understanding daily human activities has also become popular in moving towards smart environments and robotic assistive living, where activity analysis is vital for effective operation.

Electronic supplementary material The online version of this chapter (doi:10.1007/978-3-319-16814-2_8) contains supplementary material, which is available to authorized users.

D. Cremers et al. (Eds.): ACCV 2014, Part V, LNCS 9007, pp. 115–130, 2015.
DOI: 10.1007/978-3-319-16814-2_8

In prior work, two distinct approaches have been adopted, those that first detect objects and then examine the spatial and temporal relationships between these objects [8], and those that examine patterns of image features directly without first detecting the objects [9]. In the object-level based approaches, some use qualitative relations between pairs of objects (e.g. disjoint, partially-overlapping), whilst others work directly with quantitative relations such as distances.

In this paper, we propose a novel method for activity recognition that combines quantitative and qualitative representations, feature selection and a standard multi-class classifier. The method significantly improves on the state of the art performance on the publicly available activity CAD-120 dataset from Cornell.[1] The prior state of the art on this dataset [10,11] learns and recognises human activities by modelling the sub-activities from which they are composed and the affordances of the objects involved, as well as how these change over time and relate to one another. Although the recognition of sub-activities and object types/affordances may be important for some applications, we show that it is possible to achieve a very high level of recognition performance of high level activities without either of these.

The rest of the paper is organised as follows. Section 2 presents related work. Section 3 describes our proposed framework in detail. In Sect. 4 the experimental results are presented and discussed. The conclusions and future work are presented in Sect. 5.

2 Related Work

Qualitative spatio-temporal relations are primarily successful as they capture key spatial and temporal changes in visual data, and have become quite common in representing activities in various approaches. These approaches are analysed in this section.

In previous work [12–14] spatial relations based on the well established RCC spatial calculus [15–17] were combined with temporal relations based on Allen's Interval Algebra [18] to produce a qualitative spatio-temporal graph that represents an activity. Although previous results have demonstrated the effectiveness of this method, its lack of quantitative features that are not encapsulated by the qualitative ones makes the method unable to distinguish between events and activities where these quantitative features are important. In our experiments we demonstrate the importance of using quantitative features together with qualitative features.

The RCC spatial calculus together with Allen's Interval Algebra has also been used in [19], but in that work pre-defined knowledge of the object categories was also exploited and together with the spatio-temporal features and using Inductive Logic Programming (ILP) the developed system was able to learn and recognise observed human activities. Although the system demonstrated successful results and its ability to avoid over-fitting of the training dataset was a key strength, its reliance of prior knowledge about the categories of the objects in conjunction

[1] CAD-120: http://pr.cs.cornell.edu/humanactivities/data.php.

with its strict classification approach due to ILP, causes performance issues when these are missing.

A hierarchical approach using variable length Markov models and taking as observations the contour of a human body in terms of control points has been developed to learn and recognise human activities, and has been evaluated in exercise activities that require no object interactions [20,21]. Given the nature of the feature vector which takes into account the contour of the object rather than actual spatial relations between spatial interest points, it is questionable whether it will be able to deal with activities that involve object interactions.

Other approaches [22,23] have used interest point detectors, extracted a 3D cuboid at each interest point, computed descriptors for each of the cuboids and then clustered similar descriptors together hence forming a feature descriptor codebook similar to the traditional bag-of-words approach. An extension to this method is using a probabilistic approach that combines prior domain knowledge to model each activity as a distribution over the codewords and each video as a distribution over the activities [24]. Although the advantage of these approaches that use image descriptors is that they do not require skeleton or object tracks to describe the activity observed, they are unable to take into account spatio-temporal relations between the different relevant entities in the scene, which are important elements when learning and recognising human activities [17,25]. To address this issue, the concept of a "spatio-temporal phrase" that is defined as a combination of local words in a certain spatial and temporal structure, including their order and relative positions is introduced [26]. This is a very similar approach to the graphical representation described before [12–14], however, the spatio-temporal phrase still does not include qualitative spatial relations and also the temporal relations are much fewer than the Allen's Interval Algebra used in the graphs method.

An alternative approach is using convolutional deep learning methods to learn templates of the patterns of the activities and then be able to recall them [27–29]. Although deep learning methods have demonstrated impressive results in visual pattern matching, they require large training datasets and training is very computationally expensive. Furthermore, like the bag-of-words approaches for activity recognition, deep learning methods have to-date operated at the image level and do not consider rich spatio-temporal relations among the relevant entities in the scene. Other approaches [30,31] make use of low-level optical flow input and build high-level spatio-temporal representations of the activity. Ryoo [30] extracts feature points from a video and describes the scene by modelling spatio-temporal relations between these feature points. Similarly, Brendel [31] builds on representing activities as spatio-temporal graphs generated from pixel intensities and motion properties in the video. These approaches show promising results but suffer from image-level distortions, such as motion-blur, lighting changed etc., and do not capture high-level scene reasoning.

In our approach, we make use of the CAD-120 dataset. Much work has been done using this dataset. Benchmark setting approaches developed by Koppula [10,11], Rybok [32] have focused on modelling activities using generalized description of objects. Koppula [10,11] made use of object affordances, i.e. the purpose of an object, in order to build stronger models of activities, supporting the hypothesis that the use of object affordances instead of specific object descriptions is more beneficial since it is more important to know what an object does rather than what an object is. Rybok [32], similarly, generalizes object modelling by representing regions in a scene where objects are interacting through detection of salient object features rather than complete objects themselves. These approaches, however, still heavily model objects in order to recognize activities. In our work, we give equal weight to modelling all interactions amongst elements (all skeleton joints and objects) in a scene thus removing heavily weighted bias towards object modelling alone.

3 Framework

We propose that in order for an intelligent system to effectively recognise observed human activities, we encode both the qualitative and quantitative spatio-temporal relations of the relevant entities in the scene. For this we research and develop a method that allows an intelligent system to learn and recognise high-level activities by selecting the most important and discriminative features from a set of feature templates that were designed based on qualitative and quantitative spatio-temporal feature representations (QQSTR) of the activities. The resulting selected features are then used to train a multi-class support-vector machine (SVM) for future prediction. These steps are shown in Fig. 1.

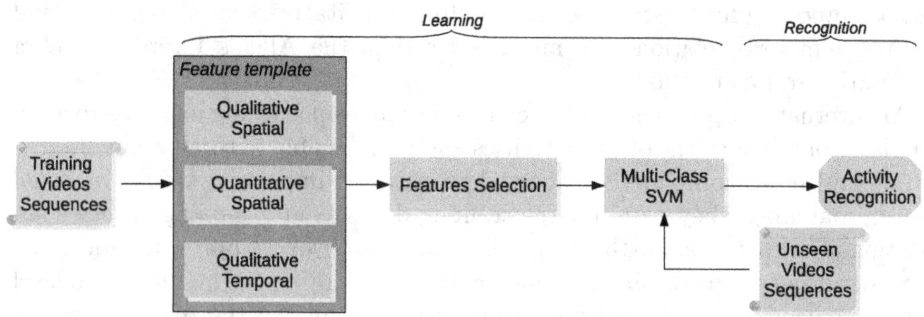

Fig. 1. Flowchart showing the high-level steps of the QQSTR

Before the detailed explanation of the model is given, it is useful to briefly describe the key terms in the QQSTR: spatial, temporal, qualitative and quantitative.

Spatial: These features describe properties and relations between objects that exist in space. Examples of spatial features are poses of objects, relative poses of objects with respect to other objects, absolute and relative direction of motion, etc.

Temporal: These features describe properties and relations of the objects or activities themselves in the time domain. Allen's interval algebra is an example of temporal relation features between two events. Other examples of temporal features are (a) the time an activity starts and its duration, (b) the time before a car runs out of fuel, etc.

Qualitative: The term qualitative is defined as "relating to, measuring, or measured by the quality of something rather than its quantity"[2]. For example a qualitative spatial feature is that two objects are partially overlapping each other without specifying the proportion of overlap. A qualitative temporal feature example is that an activity starts and finishes before another activity starts. Both, RCC and Allen's interval algebra are qualitative relational frameworks.

Quantitative: In contrast to qualitative, the term quantitative is defined as "relating to, measuring, or measured by the quantity of something rather than its quality" (see Footnote 2). An example of a spatial quantitative feature is saying that two objects overlap each other by 30 %; an example of a temporal quantitative feature is saying that an activity finishes 5 min before another activity starts.

Our feature set F consists of three components, namely qualitative spatial, quantitative spatial and qualitative temporal components. All three components comprise of histograms and statistical measures both of which are noise resilient. We have chosen not to include a quantitative temporal component as we found that the qualitative temporal components encodes sufficient temporal information in the domain under consideration and including quantitative component would result is unnecessary additional complexity to the feature space in $\mathbf{F}$.

$$F = \langle F_1, F_2, F_3 \rangle \tag{1}$$

In Eq. 1, F_1 is the set of qualitative spatial features, F_2 is the set of qualitative temporal features and F_3 is the set of quantitative spatial features. The complete feature set F then undergoes minimum-redundancy maximum-relevancy (MRMR) [33] feature selection in order to identify features from each set F_1, F_2 and F_3 that have a significant contribution. This selection step provides the minimal and most discriminative representation of an activity.

3.1 Qualitative Spatial Representations (F_1)

The qualitative spatial representation (QSR) used is based on the well-established Region Connection Calculus-5 (RCC-5) [16], which is a binary mereological calculus containing 5 relations. We use a still coarser representation which we refer to as RCC-3. It contains the relations DR (discrete), PO (partial overlap) and PiP {the union of the RCC-5 relations PPi, PP, EQ} (Part, Part inverse and equality). These form a Jointly Exhaustive and Pairwise Disjoint (JEPD) set of relations and, as with RCC-5, RCC-3 holds between pairs of entities (tracked

---

[2] http://www.oxforddictionaries.com.

objects and human body parts) in n-dimensional Cartesian space. All three relations are symmetric, though in our work we arrange the use of PiP such that the first argument is always a part of the second (or equal to it, however in practice equals rarely occurs). This is effectively the representation used in [13] and for representational convenience we use D and P rather than DR and PiP in the rest of the paper. These RCC-3 relations are graphically shown in Fig. 2 and they are denoted as $R = \{\text{D, PO, P}\}$.

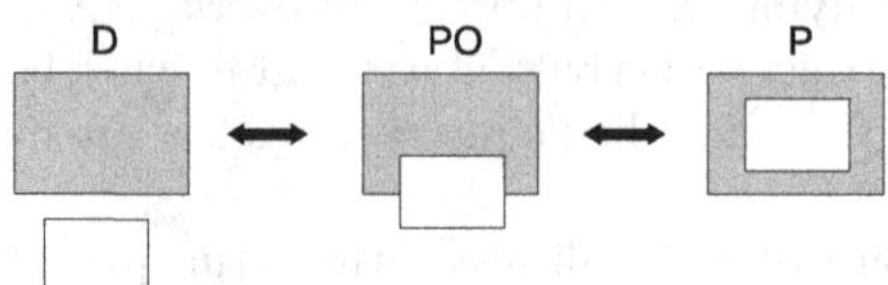

Fig. 2. Region Connection Calculus-3 showing the three distinct relations between a pair of objects

We first compute these pairwise RCC relations from the tracks of the entities, producing sequences of RCC relations for each pairwise combination of entities. A low-pass filter is then applied across the sequences of relations to suppress any jitter caused due to objects and skeleton detection error. An important aspect in QSR activity recognition is to model the relation changes that occur between entities, as these represent the discriminative stages of an activity. In related work [13,14,19], this is achieved by aggregating repeated consecutive occurrences of a relation for each pairwise combination of entities. In other words, by parsing individually every sequence row $S_{e_i,e_j} \in S$ which are the RCC chains (sequences) between any two entities e_i and e_j, each chain is suppressed while $S_{e_i,e_j,t} = S_{e_i,e_j,t-1}$. By only locally focussing on how the RCC relations of a specific pair of objects is evolving, it limits the representative strength of the spatial feature, as it ignores how the changes in S_{e_i,e_j} are affecting the changes in the spatial relations of the rest of the entities; i.e. local segmentation ignores the holistic picture.

We propose an alternative approach to suppress the spatial relation chains in S when only all chains are the same as the ones before. Again in simple terms, instead of looking individually at every S_{e_i,e_j} which are the rows of S, we suppress the RCC relations while $S_t = S_{t-1}$, i.e. if there is a change between column t and $t-1$ of S. An example of local and propagated segmentation is illustrated in Fig. 3 and the benefits of propagated segmentation over local segmentation are demonstrated in the experimental results section. Finally, we compute the number of occurrences of sub-sequences of length 1, 2, 3 and 4 in the propagated segmented RCC sequence, as these sub-sequences represent the minimal blocks that describe an activity in terms of qualitative spatial relations. The histogram of these sub-sequences is our qualitative spatial feature F_1.

Formally this procedure is described as follows. Let E be the set of entities in the scene. Then at each frame, t, we compute between entities $e_i, e_j \in E$

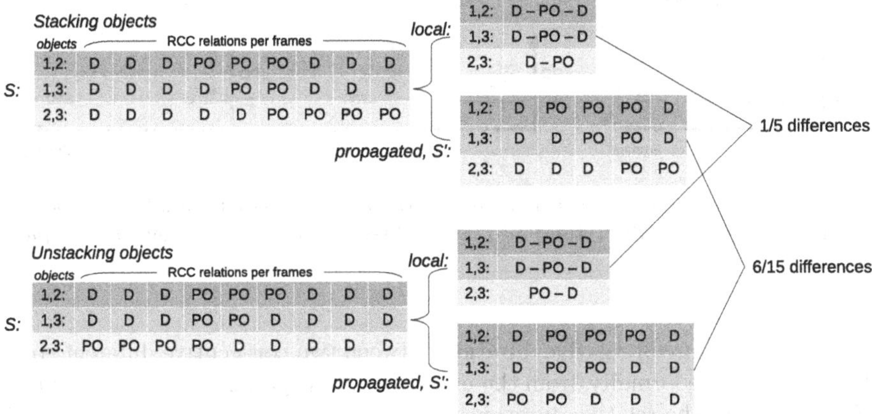

Fig. 3. Example showing the expressive power of propagated segmentation over local segmentation in two activities (stacking and unstacking objects)

$(i \neq j)$, the RCC relation $R_{e_i,e_j,t}$, from the Cartesian positions of these two entities at this frame. This produces a $m \times n$ matrix S of r relations for all m possible pairwise combinations of the entities for each one of the n frames in the video. Propagated segmentation on S is computed by aggregating relation changes that occur in any of the pairwise relations sequences $S_{[t:t+1]}$, producing a new matrix S'. Then, we form a histogram of all possible RCC relation changes with length $l \in [1:4]$ that occur in the whole video represented by S' for all m pairwise combination of entities. The total number of these histogram bins is $m \times \sum_{l=1}^{4} \text{len}(R)^l$, where as previously described $\text{len}(R) = 3$. For example, consider the propagated segmentation S' for *stacking objects* activity shown in Fig. 3. The bins of the histogram for object 1 and 2 would be $\langle D; D\text{-}PO; \ldots; D\text{-}PO\text{-}PO\text{-}D\rangle_{1,2}$ with counts $\langle 2; 1; \ldots; 1\rangle$, and all other possible RCC combinations filled in with zeroes so that the length of the histogram feature has the same length for all activities. This is repeated for the remaining pairwise combinations (1, 3 and 2, 3) and the resulting histograms for each pairwise combination are joined together to form the complete feature representing the activity video. This becomes the qualitative spatial representation feature set F_1, with length of $\mathbb{R}^{120\times m}$.

3.2 Qualitative Temporal Representations (F_2)

Spatial changes in F_1 alone do not capture the notion of time in an activity which, for some activities, are maybe important. For example, there might be similarity of the spatial relations between the *talking on the phone* and *biting an apple* activities; capturing the time dependencies between spatial changes can help in discerning such situations. One commonly used method for describing temporal relations is Allen's Interval Algebra [18]. Since Allen's temporal relations do not encode quantitative duration relations, we expand the *meets* relation, by adding

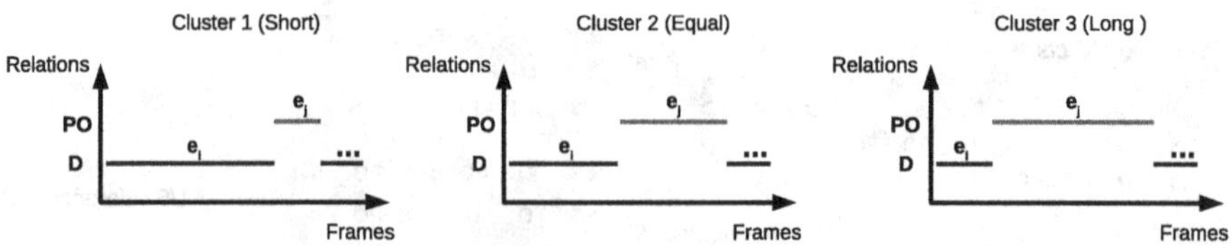

Fig. 4. Ratios computed between relative lengths of two consecutive different spatial relations e_i and e_j, then discretised into one of three clusters representing *short*, *equal* or *long* durations.

a qualitative measure of relative duration between two consecutive different spatial relations. More formally, from the non-segmented spatial relations sequences of S we calculate the relative duration ratio d:

$$d = \frac{\text{len}(e_j)}{\text{len}(e_i)}, \; e_i \text{ meets } e_j \tag{2}$$

To obtain a qualitative measure of the relative duration, the quantitative ratios are clustered together using k-means. In practice, we found that discretisation of the continuous space of ratio values can be sufficiently captured with three clusters ($k = 3$). As illustrated in Fig. 4, these three clusters give the notion of duration ratios as either being *short*, *equal* or *long*[3]. Once the temporal relations are in a qualitative form it is possible to compute their histogram which is our qualitative temporal feature F_2, with a length of $\mathbb{R}^{9 \times m}$. The total number of features in F_2 is given by $m \times (\text{len}(R)^2 - \text{len}(R)) \times k$ where m is the number of all pairwise combination of objects, $\text{len}(R)^2 - \text{len}(R)$ denotes the total number of pairwise combinations of spatial relation changes with no repetition. For example for objects 1 and 3 in S of activity *stacking objects* shown in Fig. 3, the bin $\langle (D\text{-}PO)_{short}; (D\text{-}PO)_{equal}; \ldots; (PO\text{-}D)_{long} \rangle_{1,3}$ provides the counts $\langle 1; 0; \ldots; 1 \rangle$.

3.3 Quantitative Spatial Representations (F_3)

Qualitative spatial representations successfully abstract a good representation of a video scene through capturing interactions. However, due to the coarse representation of space and time, it is often not possible to discern similar looking activities that are performed at a different scale or speed. Quantitative spatial representations, on the other hand, are able to encode such finer motions in an activity as seen in previous work [35]. In our approach we make use of various quantitative spatial representations to aid our model in the recognition problem.

Euclidean distances: We compute the Euclidean distances between the centroid of the bounding boxes of each pair of elements in the scene. An element could be any of the following skeleton parts: head, hands, torso, shoulders,

[3] Note that this is similar to the INDU calculus [34] which extends the interval calculus by discretising whether intervals in a before, meets or overlaps relationship are shorter, equal or longer than each other.

hips, and any of the objects in the scene. Lower body parts are not used due to their high rate of occlusion. For a compact and generic representation we compute the descriptive statistics of this distances distribution, namely we compute the mean (μ), standard deviation (σ), kurtosis (κ) and skewness (γ). We use these statistical measures as quantitative spatial features.

Relative direction of motion: A problem with some qualitative spatial relations is that in some cases they are unable to distinguish mirror activities, e.g. pushing and pulling. To resolve this issue we calculate the relative direction of motion between two objects, i.e. whether two objects are approaching or departing from each other. We calculate this for every possible pair of objects using their timed minimum and maximum Euclidean distances. By knowing how the relative direction of the motions change for pairs of objects in the scene it is possible to distinguish between mirror activities.

The descriptive statistics of the Euclidean distances combined with the relative direction of motion of the entities, form the quantitative spatial representation F_3. The number of total features in F_3 is given by $\mathbb{R}^{5 \times m}$ where m denotes all pairwise combinations of entities and 5 represents the number of statistical metrics of Euclidean distances plus relative directions of motion.

3.4 Feature Selection and Learning

The feature template F is the most generic representation of an activity. However, the importance of each of the features in it is determined by the nature of the activities. We employ a feature selection step that automatically identifies from F the feature set $F^{'}$ that is more discriminating for activity classes c. We apply this by using the *Minimum-Redundancy Maximum-Relevance* (MRMR) feature selection method [33], which is based on mutual information between two random variables, α and β as shown in Eq. 3. Specifically, MRMR is based on two criteria, namely maximum-relevance and minimum-redundancy, which are described below.

$$I(\alpha; \beta) = H(\alpha) + H(\beta) - H(\alpha, \beta) \tag{3}$$

Maximum-Relevance: This criterion approximates Max-Dependency $D(F, c)$, by searching for features using the mean of all mutual information values between feature x_i and classes c, that satisfy Eq. 4.

$$max\ D(F^{'}, c), D = \frac{1}{|F'|} \sum_{x_i \in F'} I(x_i; c). \tag{4}$$

Minimum-Redundancy: If any two features, x_i and x_j, have a high dependency between them, one of them is redundant in the feature set, $F^{'}$, and is therefore removed while still preserving the discriminative-class power of the feature set. Therefore, by using the Minimal-Redundancy criterion, as shown in Eq. 5, mutually exclusive features are chosen.

$$min\ R(F^{'}), R = \frac{1}{|F'|^2} \sum_{x_i, x_j \in F'} I(x_i; x_j). \tag{5}$$

By defining the operator $\phi(D, R)$ to combine these two criteria, as shown in Eq. 6, the minimal most discriminative feature set, $F^{'}$, for a given set of activities classes is obtained.

$$max\ \phi(D, R), \phi = D - R \tag{6}$$

We use the feature set $F^{'}$ to train a multi-class SVM [36] to recognise the high-level activities using a polynomial kernel of degree $d = 2$ and $\gamma = 0.75$.

4 Results and Discussion

We evaluate our framework on the Cornell activity dataset (CAD-120)[4] which we describe in Sect. 4.1. We then describe our experimental setup and evaluation method in Sect. 4.2. In Sect. 4.3 we compare our approach against a state of the art benchmark. Section 4.4 provides an in depth analysis and discussion of the strengths of our approach.

4.1 Description of the Benchmark Dataset

CAD-120 comprises of 120 RGB-D video sequences of four human subjects performing daily living activities which are recorded using a Microsoft Kinect camera. Out of these four subjects two are male and two are female; three are right-handed and one is left-handed. Each video is labelled with a single high-level activity name: *making cereal*, *taking medicine*, *stacking objects*, *unstacking objects*, *microwaving food*, *picking objects*, *cleaning objects*, *taking food*, *arranging objects* and *having a meal*. The dataset provides skeleton tracks of people in the scene, as well as auto and ground truth tracks of the objects present in each one of the videos. Figure 5 shows some sample images of the dataset.

4.2 Experimental Procedure

For validation and comparison, we follow the same evaluation procedure as the one presented in the current state of the art [10]. We adopt a 4-fold cross validation approach where we train on three subjects and test on the fourth new subject. In addition, on the training set we perform a 3-fold cross validation for the feature selection process where we train on two subjects and we use the third subject for feature selection with the method described in Sect. 3.4. We then combine the extracted features of each of the three folds together and remove repetitions to form our final most-discriminative features set.

We then use the new feature set to compute the results of the main testing fold which we take an average across the four folds. We report the micro accuracy, macro precision and macro recall for the activity recognition. Micro accuracy is the average of the percentages of correctly classified labels across the four folds. Macro precision and recall are the averages of precision and recall respectively for all classes.

[4] http://pr.cs.cornell.edu/humanactivities/data.php.

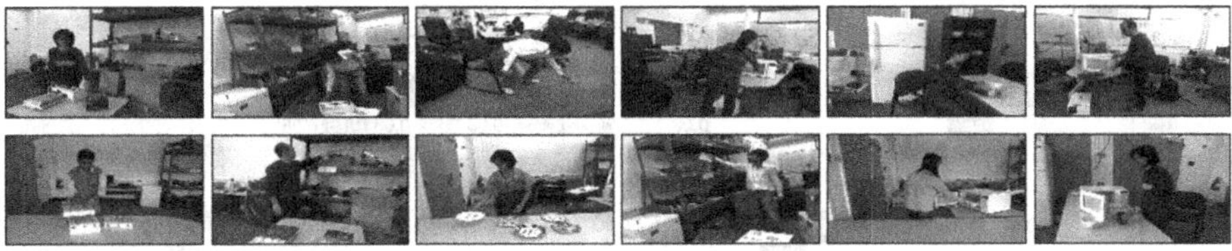

Fig. 5. CAD-120 dataset sample screen shots (see Footnote 4)

4.3 Activity Recognition Results

Table 1 shows the performance of our approach on high-level activity recognition of the CAD-120 dataset. It can be observed that we achieve an accuracy of 95.2 %, precision of 95.2 % and recall of 95.0 %. This is a significant improvement of 12.1 %, 8.2 % and 15.0 % in terms of accuracy, precision and recall when ground-truth temporal segmentation of sub-activities is not known, as well as an improvement of 1.7 %, 0.2 % and 1.7 % when it is known. The assumption of knowing the temporal segmentation of the sub-level activities is not required by our method, but it is needed by the benchmark method. These results demonstrate that our approach efficiently and effectively captures the interactions between the human subjects and the objects without needing any prior knowledge about the types and the affordances of the objects in the scene or knowledge of sub-level activities. Figure 6 presents the confusion matrix obtained with ground truth bounding boxes. From the strong diagonal it is evident that there is nearly no confusion in discriminating different high-level activities.

Table 1. Performance measurements with and without ground-truth temporal segmentation based on accuracy, precision and recall

Method	Accuracy	Precision	Recall
assuming ground-truth temporal segmentation			
Koppula et al. [11]	84.7 ± 2.4	85.3 ± 2.0	84.2 ± 2.5
Koppula, Saxena [10]	93.5 ± 3.0	95.0 ± 2.3	93.3 ± 3.1
assuming no ground-truth temporal segmentation			
Koppula et al. [11]	80.6 ± 1.1	81.8 ± 2.2	80.0 ± 1.2
Koppula, Saxena [10]	83.1 ± 3.0	87.0 ± 3.6	82.7 ± 3.1
QQSTR-gt-tracks	**95.2** ± 2.0	**95.2** ± 1.6	**95.0** ± 1.8
assuming no ground-truth temporal segmentation and no ground-truth object bounding boxes			
Koppula et al. [11]	75.0 ± 4.5	75.8 ± 4.4	74.2 ± 4.6
Rybok et al. [32]	**78.2**	-	-
QQSTR-auto-tracks	75.8 ± 6.8	**77.9** ± 11.0	**75.4** ± 9.1

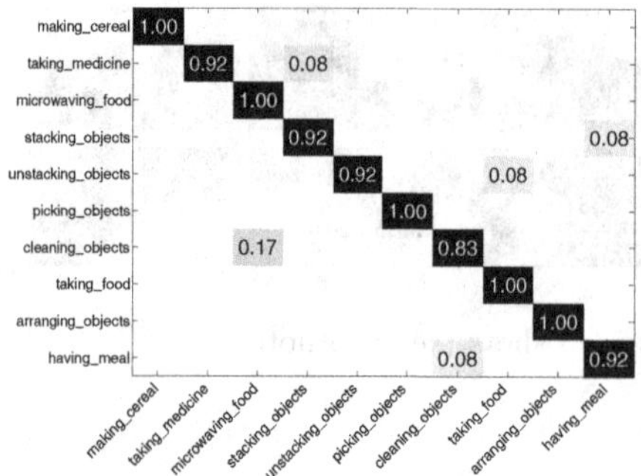

Fig. 6. Confusion matrix with ground-truth object tracks

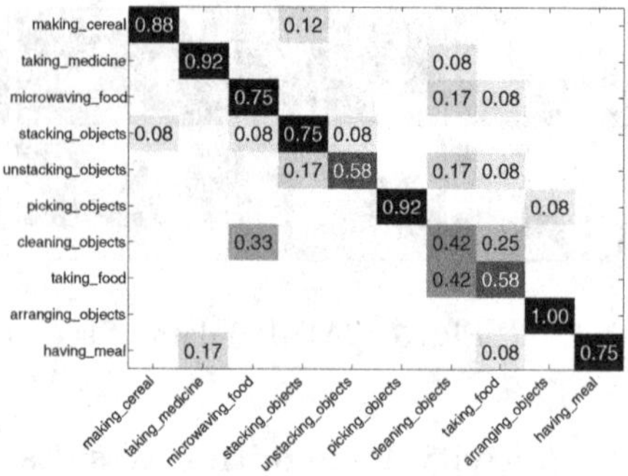

Fig. 7. Confusion matrix with automated object tracks

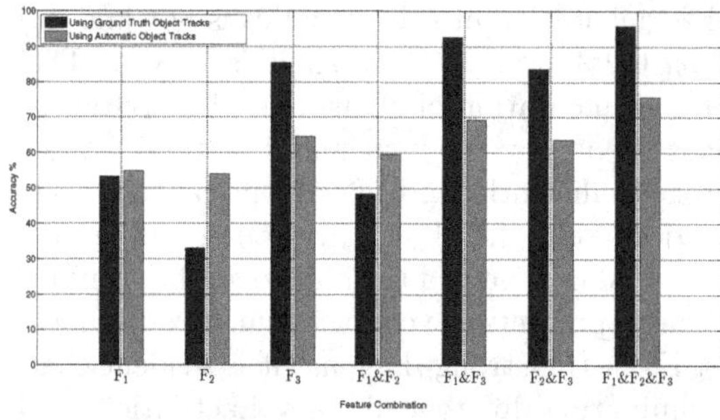

Fig. 8. Accuracy for different combinations of features types

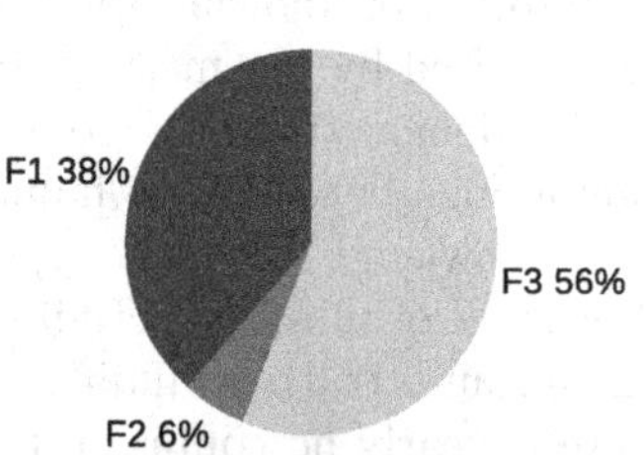

Fig. 9. Ratio of the number of each feature type over the total number of selected features

The results presented so far are obtained using ground-truth object tracks. We evaluate our method on more realistic scenarios by using the noisy automatic object tracks provided by the CAD-120 dataset. We compare our results with [10,32]. Rybok et al. requires no object tracks as their method is based on saliency and optical features. Table 1 shows that our method is robust and achieves comparable results to the other two methods. Specifically, it achieves an accuracy of 75.8 %, which is only 2.4 % lower than the highest performance by Rybok et al. Results also show marginal increase of 0.8 % over results of Koppula et al.

Figure 7 illustrates the confusion matrix for our results using automated object tracks. We can observe that most activities obtain a high accuracy while there is confusion between the *cleaning objects* and *taking food* activities. We suspect that this confusion between these two activities occurs due to potentially high level of noise in the object tracks. This suspicion is supported by Fig. 6 which shows that when the tracks are noiseless a high degree of separation is achieved.

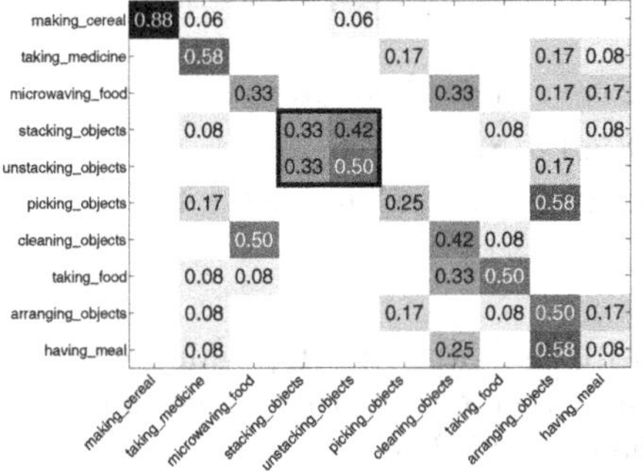

Fig. 10. High confusion between *stacking* and *unstacking* activities, highlighted in red, is evident when using local segmentation (Color figure online)

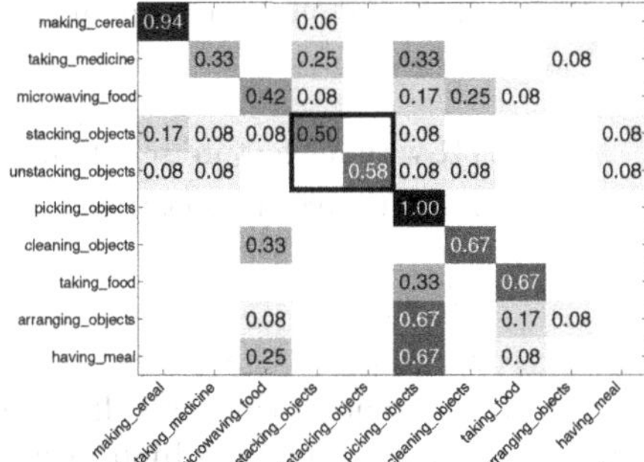

Fig. 11. There is no confusion between *stacking* and *unstacking* activities, highlighted in red, when using propagated segmentation (Color figure online)

4.4 Discriminative Strength of Features Types

We firstly investigate the strength of QQSRT (F) versus using individual and pairwise combinations of the different feature types. Figure 8 shows the accuracies for ground-truth and automatic tracks for F and all the different combinations of F_1, F_2 and F_3. It can be seen that F outperforms all other combinations. However, there are other interesting observations. To begin with, qualitative spatial representation (F_1) and qualitative temporal representation (F_2) seem to be robust to noisy automatic tracks. On the other hand, quantitative spatial representation F_3, although more prone to noisy tracks, achieves a higher performance in the case of smooth tracks. Furthermore it can be seen that F_1 and F_3 when combined together have a higher discriminating ability than when combined with F_2. This is confirmed by Fig. 9 which shows post feature selection performance contributions of F_1, F_2 and F_3. It can be seen that the contribution of F_2 in F is much lower than those of F_1 and F_3. Despite the fact that F_2 is contributing less, it is still an important component of the overall feature set since its inclusion achieves the highest performance.

We next evaluate the benefit of propagated segmentation over local segmentation as described in the methodology section. Figures 10 and 11 show the confusion matrices obtained when using local and propagated segmentation respectively. To objectively investigate the effect of propagated segmentation on the qualitative spatial relations F_1, we perform experimentation as before using F_1 alone. It can be seen that implementing the global propagation eliminates confusion between the mirrored activities of *stacking* and *unstacking*. These results validate our hypothesis that by taking into account the holistic picture and looking at how the spatial relations change at the global level yields much better results than a narrow focus on individual relational changes.

Table 2. Performance measurements with and without feature selection

	Accuracy	Precision	Recall
QQSTR without feature selection	79.8 ± 1.5	82.45 ± 7.4	79.17 ± 7.8
QQSTR with feature selection	95.2 ± 2.0	95.2 ± 1.6	95.0 ± 1.8

Lastly, we evaluate the performance with and without employing feature selection. Table 2 shows these results. It can be seen that feature selection plays a significant role in achieving high performance of 95.2 %.

5 Conclusions and Future Work

In this paper we proposed a novel method of learning and recognising complex human high-level activities from video sequences. The method is based on qualitative and quantitative spatio-temporal features that capture the person-object interactions in the observed scene in a generic and effective manner. From these features we automatically selected the most discriminative ones and trained a multi-class SVM. We showed that the task of finding the most discriminative features from the original set is an important step. Unlike state of the art methods in activity recognition our method makes very few assumptions and does not need knowledge of object types, their affordances or sub-level activities that compose the high-level activity. We validated our method with extensive experiments over a challenging dataset, for which we significantly outperformed the state of the art approach. Specifically, we achieved an accuracy of 95.2 %, precision of 95.2 % and recall of 95.0 %. This is a significant improvement of 12.1 %, 8.2 % and 15.0 % in terms of accuracy, precision and recall when sub-level activities are not used, as well as an improvement of 1.7 %, 0.2 % and 1.7 % when they are used by the state of the art approach; this assumption of knowing the temporal segmentation of the sub-level activities is not required by our method.

Although in this work our focus was in the recognition of high-level activities, recognition of the sub-level activities is also important. We plan to extend our work to recognise these sub-level activities using a top-down approach, where the recognition of the high-level activity helps to infer the sub-level ones. This is in contrast to a bottom-up approach used by the current state of the art where high-level activities are inferred from sub-level ones.

Acknowledgement. The financial support of RACE (FP7-ICT-287752) and STRANDS (FP7-ICT-600623) projects is gratefully acknowledged.

References

1. Turaga, P., Chellappa, R., Subrahmanian, V., Udrea, O.: Machine recognition of human activities: a survey. IEEE Trans. Circ. Syst. Video Technol. **18**, 1473–1488 (2008)

2. Poppe, R.: A survey on vision-based human action recognition. Image Vis. Comput. **28**, 976–990 (2010)
3. Weinland, D., Ronfard, R., Boyer, E.: A survey of vision-based methods for action representation, segmentation and recognition. Comput. Vis. Image Underst. **115**, 224–241 (2011)
4. Xu, X., Tang, J., Zhang, X., Liu, X., Zhang, H., Qiu, Y.: Exploring techniques for vision based human activity recognition: methods, systems, and evaluation. Sensors **13**, 1635–1650 (2013). Basel, Switzerland
5. Collins, R., Lipton, A., Kanade, T.: Introduction to the special section on video surveillance. IEEE Trans. Pattern Anal. Mach. Intell. **22**, 745–746 (2000)
6. Gowsikhaa, D., Abirami, S., Baskaran, R.: Automated human behavior analysis from surveillance videos: a survey. Artif. Intell. Rev., 1–19 (2012)
7. Ko, T.: A survey on behavior analysis in video surveillance for homeland security applications. In: 2008 37th IEEE Applied Imagery Pattern Recognition Workshop, pp. 1–8 IEEE (2008)
8. Chen, J., Cohn, A.G., Liu, D., Wang, S., Ouyang, J., Yu, Q.: A survey of qualitative spatial representations. Knowl. Eng. Rev. FirstView, 1–31 (2013)
9. Laptev, I.: On space-time interest points. Int. J. Comput. Vis. **64**, 107–123 (2005)
10. Koppula, H., Saxena, A.: Learning spatio-temporal structure from RGB-D videos for human activity detection and anticipation. In: Proceedings of the International Conference on Machine Learning (ICML) (2013)
11. Koppula, H., Gupta, R., Saxena, A.: Learning human activities and object affordances from RGB-D videos. Int. J. Robot. Res. **32**, 951–970 (2013)
12. Sridhar, M., Cohn, A.G., Hogg, D.C.: Learning functional object-categories from a relational spatio-temporal representation. In: European Conference on Artificial Intelligence (2008)
13. Sridhar, M., Cohn, A.G., Hogg, D.C.: Unsupervised learning of event classes from video. In: AAAI (2010)
14. Sridhar, M., Cohn, A.G., Hogg, D.C.: Discovering an event taxonomy from video using qualitative spatio-temporal graphs. In: European Conference on Artificial Intelligence (2010)
15. Randell, D., Zhan, C., Cohn, A.G.: A spatial logic based on regions and connection. In: Third International Conference on Knowledge Representation and Reasoning (1992)
16. Cohn, A.G., Hazarika, S.: Qualitative spatial representation and reasoning: an overview. Fundamenta Informaticae **46**, 1–29 (2001)
17. Cohn, A.G., Renz, J.: Qualitative spatial representation and reasoning. In: van Harmelen, F., Lifschitz, V., Porter, B. (eds.) Handbook of Knowledge Representation, pp. 551–596. Elsevier B.V, Amsterdam (2008)
18. Allen, J.: Maintaining knowledge about temporal intervals. Commun. ACM **26**, 832–843 (1983)
19. Dubba, K., Cohn, A.G., Hogg, D.C.: Event model learning from complex videos using ILP. In: European Conference on Artificial Intelligence, pp. 93–98 (2010)
20. Galata, A., Johnson, N., Hogg, D.: Learning behaviour models of human activities. In: British Machine Vision Conference (1999)
21. Galata, A., Johnson, N., Hogg, D.: Learning variable-length markov models of behavior. Comput. Vis. Image Underst. **81**, 398–413 (2001)
22. Dollar, P., Rabaud, V., Cottrell, G., Belongie, S.: Behavior recognition via sparse spatio-temporal features. In: 2005 IEEE International Workshop on Visual Surveillance and Performance Evaluation of Tracking and Surveillance, pp. 65–72. IEEE (2005)

23. Xia, L., Aggarwal, J.: Spatio-temporal depth cuboid similarity feature for activity recognition using depth camera. In: 2013 IEEE Conference on Computer Vision and Pattern Recognition, pp. 2834–2841. IEEE (2013)
24. Zhang, H., Parker, L.: 4-dimensional local spatio-temporal features for human activity recognition. In: 2011 IEEE/RSJ International Conference on Intelligent Robots and Systems, pp. 2044–2049. IEEE (2011)
25. Forbus, K.: Qualitative modeling. In: van Harmelen, F., Lifschitz, V., Porter, B. (eds.) Handbook of Knowledge Representation, pp. 361–393. Elsevier B.V, Amsterdam (2008)
26. Zhang, Y., Liu, X., Chang, M.-C., Ge, W., Chen, T.: Spatio-temporal phrases for activity recognition. In: Fitzgibbon, A., Lazebnik, S., Perona, P., Sato, Y., Schmid, C. (eds.) ECCV 2012, Part III. LNCS, vol. 7574, pp. 707–721. Springer, Heidelberg (2012)
27. Taylor, G.W., Fergus, R., LeCun, Y., Bregler, C.: Convolutional learning of spatio-temporal features. In: Daniilidis, K., Maragos, P., Paragios, N. (eds.) ECCV 2010, Part VI. LNCS, vol. 6316, pp. 140–153. Springer, Heidelberg (2010)
28. Chen, B., Ting, J.A., Marlin, B., de Freitas, N.: Deep learning of invariant spatio-temporal features from video. In: NIPS 2010 Deep Learning and Unsupervised Feature Learning Workshop (2010)
29. Le, Q.V., Zou, W.Y., Yeung, S.Y., Ng, A.Y.: Learning hierarchical invariant spatio-temporal features for action recognition with independent subspace analysis. In: CVPR 2011, pp. 3361–3368. IEEE (2011)
30. Ryoo, M.S., Aggarwal, J.: Spatio-temporal relationship match: video structure comparison for recognition of complex human activities. In: 2009 IEEE 12th International Conference on Computer Vision, pp. 1593–1600 (2009)
31. Brendel, W., Todorovic, S.: Learning spatiotemporal graphs of human activities. In: Proceedings of the 2011 International Conference on Computer Vision, ICCV 2011. IEEE Computer Society (2011)
32. Rybok, L., Schauerte, B., Al-Halah, Z., Stiefelhagen, R.: "Important Stuff, Everywhere!" activity recognition with salient proto-objects as context. In: IEEE Winter Conference on Applications of Computer Vision (WACV) (2014)
33. Peng, H., Long, F., Ding, C.: Feature selection based on mutual information: criteria of max-dependency, max-relevance, and min-redundancy. IEEE Trans. Pattern Anal. Mach. Intell. **27**, 1226–1238 (2005)
34. Pujari, A., Vijaya Kumari, G., Sattar, A.: INDu: an interval & duration network. In: Foo, N. (ed) AI 1999. LNCS, vol. 1747, pp. 291–303. Springer, Heidelberg (1999)
35. Behera, A., Hogg, D.C., Cohn, A.G.: Egocentric activity monitoring and recovery. In: Lee, K.M., Matsushita, Y., Rehg, J.M., Hu, Z. (eds.) ACCV 2012, Part III. LNCS, vol. 7726, pp. 519–532. Springer, Heidelberg (2013)
36. Chang, C.C., Lin, C.J.: LIBSVM: a library for support vector machines. ACM Trans. Intell. Syst. Tech. **2**, 27:1–27:27 (2011)

Blur-Resilient Tracking Using Group Sparsity

Pengpeng Liang[1(✉)], Yi Wu[1,2], Xue Mei[3], Jingyi Yu[4], Erik Blasch[5], Danil Prokhorov[3], Chunyuan Liao[6], Haitao Lang[1,7], and Haibin Ling[1]

[1] Department of Computer and Information Sciences, Temple University, Philadelphia, USA
pliang@temple.edu
[2] Jiangsu Key Laboratory of Big Data Analysis Technology, Nanjing University of Information Science and Technology, Nanjing, China
[3] Toyota Research Institute, North America, Ann Arbor, USA
[4] Department of Computer and Information Sciences, University of Delaware, Newark, USA
[5] Air Force Research Lab, Rome, NY, USA
[6] HiScene Information Technologies, Shanghai, China
[7] Department of Physics and Electronics, Beijing University of Chemical Technology, Beijing, China

Abstract. In this paper, a Blur Resilient target Tracking algorithm (BReT) is developed by modeling target appearance with a groupwise sparse approximation over a template set. Since blur templates of different directions are added to the template set to accommodate motion blur, there is a natural group structure among the templates. In order to enforce the solution of the sparse approximation problem to have group structure, we employ the mixed $\ell_1 + \ell_1/\ell_2$ norm to regularize the model coefficients. Having observed the similarity of gradient distributions in the blur templates of the same direction, we further boost the tracking robustness by including gradient histograms in the appearance model. Then, we use an accelerated proximal gradient scheme to develop an efficient algorithm for the non-smooth optimization resulted from the representation. After that, blur estimation is performed by investigating the energy of the coefficients, and when the estimated target can be well approximated by the normal templates, we dynamically update the template set to reduce the drifting problem. Experimental results show that the proposed BReT algorithm outperforms state-of-the-art trackers on blurred sequences.

1 Introduction

Visual object tracking is an important topic in computer vision and it has many applications, such as automatic surveillance, human computer interaction, vehicle navigation, etc. Designing a useful real-world visual tracking algorithm is very challenging, and tremendous efforts have been made toward handling issues such as illumination changes [1], occlusions [2,3], background clutter [4], and abrupt motions [5]. However, most of the current trackers do not explicitly take motion blur into account, which is pervasive in the real videos when the targets

D. Cremers et al. (Eds.): ACCV 2014, Part V, LNCS 9007, pp. 131–145, 2015.
DOI: 10.1007/978-3-319-16814-2_9

move fast. One possible approach is to deblur the videos first before performing tracking. Nevertheless, though some fast deblurring methods such as [6,7] have been recently developed, they are still computationally expensive. So this approach is not suitable for time sensitive visual tracking tasks. Also, the tracking performance will depend on the quality of deblurred videos directly.

Tracking through blur has been previously studied in [8–10]. In [8], blurred regions are matched with a matching score governed by a cost function in terms of region deformation parameters and two motion blur vectors, where the cost function is optimized with a gradient-based search technique. In [9], a mean-shift tracker is first used to locate the target. When the matching score is low, blur detection and estimation is performed, then mean-shift with blur template is applied. In [10], a blur driven tracker using sparse representation is proposed, which incorporates blur templates of different directions into the template space to model blur degradations. However, though the enhanced appearance space is more expressive, ambiguity also increases. For example, a target candidate that belongs to the background might be well represented by some blur templates. Also, the templates of the blur driven tracker are fixed, therefore when the appearance of the target changes significantly, the tracker is susceptible to drifting.

In this paper, we propose a robust blurred target tracking algorithm using group sparse representation under a particle filter framework with enhanced template space. Three components distinguish our work from previous ones: (1) since blur templates of different directions are added to the template space and the motion blur of the target always tends only one direction in a frame, there is a natural group structure among the templates, i.e., the blur templates of one direction belong to the same group. In order to enforce the solution of the sparse representation of a target candidate to have group structure, we adopt a structured sparsity inducing norm which is a combination of ℓ_1 norm and a sum of ℓ_2 norms over groups of variables [11]; (2) to account for the increase of ambiguity in the template space after enhancing it with blur templates, based on the observation that blur templates of the same direction have much more similar gradient histograms than blur templates in different directions, we use a combination of the reconstruction error and a sum of weighted distances between gradient histograms of a target candidate and each of the non-trivial templates as loss function. The resulting non-smooth convex optimization problem is solved using an accelerated proximal gradient method that guarantees fast convergence; and (3) in order to capture the appearance changes of the target and reduce the drifting problem, we perform blur detection by investigating the energy of the reconstruction coefficients. The template set is updated dynamically when two criteria based on the coefficients associated with templates are satisfied.

In the rest of the paper, related work is reviewed in Sect. 2. In Sect. 3, we present the proposed tracking algorithm and the approach for solving the resulting non-smooth convex optimization problem. Section 4 experimentally compares the proposed tracker with several state-of-the-art trackers over blurred sequences. Section 5 concludes the paper.

2 Related Work

Due to the extensive literature about visual tracking, we only review the typical works and those most related to ours. For a through survey of the tracking algorithms, we refer the readers to [12] or recent tracking evaluation papers [13–16]. Current tracking algorithms can be categorized as either discriminative or generative approaches. Discriminative approaches formulate tracking as a binary classification problem, the aim of which is to distinguish the target from background. Typical discriminative tracking approaches include online boosting [17], semi-online boosting [18], MIL tracking [19] and structured output tracking [20]. Generative approaches are based on appearance model, where tracking is performed by searching for the region most similar to the target model. Typical generative tracking methods include mean shift tracker [21], eigentracker [22], incremental tracker [23], and VTD tracker [24]. The appearance model is usually dynamically updated in order to adapt to the target appearance variations caused by pose and illumination changes.

Sparse representation has been successfully applied to visual tracking in [25], and further exploited in [26–28]. In [25], the tracker represents each target candidate as a sparse linear combination of dynamically updated templates, and the tracking task is formulated as finding the candidate with the minimum reconstruction error. In [26], a real-time L1 tracker is proposed by using accelerated proximal gradient approach to solve a modified ℓ_1 norm related minimization model with ℓ_2 norm regularization of the trivial templates. In [27], dynamical group sparsity is used to explore the spatial relationship among discriminative features and temporal relationship among templates. In [28], multi-task sparse learning is adopted to mine the interdependencies among the target candidates during tracking.

Among the previous works [8–10] on blurred target tracking, the work in [10] is most related to ours in that both incorporate blur templates into the appearance space. Our method is however different in several aspects: (1) our method exploits the natural group structure among the templates by a structured sparsity regularization; (2) our method integrates gradient information in the appearance to boost the tracking robustness; and (3) we update the template set dynamically guided by blur estimation so that our method is more robust to target appearance variations.

3 Blur Resilient Tracking Using Group Sparse Representation

3.1 Review of the Blur-Driven Tracker (BLUT)

We briefly review the blur-driven tracker (BLUT) proposed in [10], which is the main inspiration of the proposed BReT tracker and we inherit its notations as well.

Particle Filter: The particle filter [29] is a Bayesian sequential importance sampling technique for estimating the posterior distribution of state variables

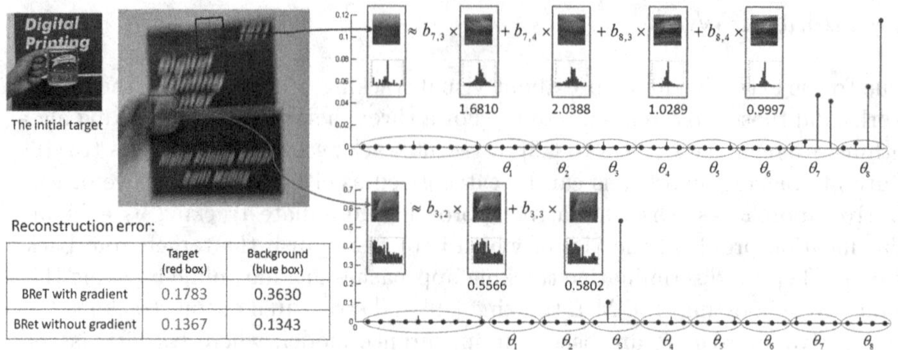

	Target (red box)	Background (blue box)
BReT with gradient	0.1783	0.3630
BRet without gradient	0.1367	0.1343

Fig. 1. Top left: The tracking results of BReT with and without gradient information, indicated by red box and blue box respectively. **Bottom left:** the reconstruction error of the two candidates measured by $0.5||\mathbf{Tc} - \mathbf{y}||_2^2$ using different tracking approaches. **Right:** The group sparse representation of the two candidates using BReT with gradient information, the L1 distance between the gradient histograms of the estimated target and each of the selected templates are also given (Color figure online).

characterizing a dynamic system. It uses finite set of weighted samples to approximate the posterior distribution regardless of the underlying distribution. For visual tracking, we use $\mathbf{x}_t$ as the state variable to describe the location and shape of the target at time t. Given all available observations $\mathbf{y}_{1:t} = \{\mathbf{y}_1, \mathbf{y}_2, \ldots, \mathbf{y}_t\}$ up to time t, the posterior $p(\mathbf{x}_t|\mathbf{y}_{1:t})$ is approximated by a set of N samples $\{\mathbf{x}_t\}_{i=1}^N$ with importance weights w_t^i. The optimal $\mathbf{x}_t$ is obtained by maximizing the approximate posterior probability: $\mathbf{x}_t^* = \arg\max_{\mathbf{x}} p(\mathbf{x}|\mathbf{y}_{1:t})$.

Subspace Representation with Blur Templates: In order to model the blur degradations, blur templates are incorporated into the appearance space in [10]. The appearance of the tracking target $\mathbf{y} \in \mathbb{R}^d$ is represented by templates $\mathbf{T} = [\mathbf{T}_a, \mathbf{T}_b, \eta\mathbf{I}]$,

$$\mathbf{y} = [\mathbf{T}_a, \mathbf{T}_b, \eta\mathbf{I}] \begin{bmatrix} \mathbf{a} \\ \mathbf{b} \\ \mathbf{e} \end{bmatrix} \hat{=} \mathbf{Tc}, \quad \text{s.t.} \quad \mathbf{c}_T \succeq 0, \tag{1}$$

where $\mathbf{T}_a = [\mathbf{t}_1, \cdots, \mathbf{t}_{n_a}] \in \mathbb{R}^{d \times n_a}$ contains n_a normal templates, $\mathbf{T}_b = [\mathbf{t}_{1,1}, \cdots, \mathbf{t}_{1,n_l}, \cdots, \mathbf{t}_{n_\theta,1}, \cdots, \mathbf{t}_{n_\theta,n_l}] \in \mathbb{R}^{d \times n_b}$ contains n_b blur templates, $\mathbf{I}$ is the $d \times d$ identity matrix containing the trivial templates used for modeling image corruption, η is used to control the weight of the trivial templates. Accordingly, $\mathbf{a} = (a_1, a_2, \cdots, a_{n_a})^\top \in \mathbb{R}^{n_a}$, and $\mathbf{b} \in \mathbb{R}^{n_b}$ are called *normal coefficients* and *blur coefficients* respectively, $\mathbf{e} = (e_1, e_2, \cdots, e_d)^\top$ is called *trivial coefficients*, $\mathbf{c} = [\mathbf{a}^\top, \mathbf{b}^\top, \mathbf{e}^\top]^\top$ and $\mathbf{c}_T = [\mathbf{a}^\top, \mathbf{b}^\top]^\top$.

The first normal template $\mathbf{t}_1$ is obtained from the unblurred object patch of the target in the first frame, which is usually selected manually or by detection algorithms, other templates are shifted from it. Given a blur free patch I of the target, different blurred versions I_b of the target can be modeled as convolving

I with different kernels. In our framework, $\mathbf{t}_{i,j} = \mathbf{t}_1 \otimes \mathbf{k}_{i,j}$ is the $(i,j)^{th}$ blur template, where $\mathbf{k}_{i,j}$ is a Gaussian kernel that represents a 2D motion toward direction θ_i with magnitude l_j, where $\theta_i \in \Theta = \{\theta_1, \cdots, \theta_{n_\theta}\}$, and $l_j \in \mathcal{L} = \{l_1, \cdots, l_{n_l}\}$. Consequently, we have $n_b = n_\theta \times n_l$ blur templates. Based on the directions of the blur kernels, we have $\mathbf{b} = [\mathbf{b}_1^\top, \cdots, \mathbf{b}_{n_\theta}^\top]^\top \in \mathbb{R}^{n_b}$, where $\mathbf{b}_i = (b_{i,1}, b_{i,2}, \cdots, b_{i,n_l})^\top \in \mathbb{R}^{n_l}$ are the coefficients for the blur templates toward i^{th} direction.

Blur-Driven Proposal Distribution: In [10], to use the estimated motion information from the sparse representation to guide the particle sampling process, estimated motion information from different sources are integrated into the proposal distribution, which is a combination of the first-order Markov transition $p(\mathbf{x}_t|\mathbf{x}_{t-1})$, the second-order Markov transition $p(\mathbf{x}_t|\mathbf{x}_{t-1}, \mathbf{x}_{t-2})$, and $q_i(\mathbf{x}_t|\mathbf{x}_{t-1}, \mathbf{y}_{t-1})$ based on the blur motion estimation along direction θ_i.

3.2 Loss Function with Gradient Information

Incorporating blur templates into the appearance space allows for a more expressive appearance space to model blur degradations. However, with the augmented template space, ambiguity also increases, and some background might be well represented by some blur templates, especially when only grayscale information is used, as shown in Fig. 1. In order to make the tracking algorithm more robust, based on the observation that though motion blur significantly changes the statistics of the gradients of the templates, the blur templates in the same direction have much more similar gradient histograms than blur templates of different directions, we propose to use the combination of the reconstruction error and a sum of weighted distances between the target candidate and each of the non-trivial templates as loss function.

For each template of $[\mathbf{T}_a, \mathbf{T}_b]$, we calculate its gradient histogram by letting each pixel vote for an gradient histogram channel, and get $\mathbf{D} = [\mathbf{d}_1, \mathbf{d}_2, \cdots, \mathbf{d}_{n_a+n_b}] \in \mathbb{R}^{h \times (n_a+n_b)}$, where h is the number of bins of the gradient histogram; and for the target candidate, we calculate its gradient histogram $\mathbf{g} \in \mathbb{R}^h$. Since we don't consider the trivial templates when calculating the sum of weighted distances, we let $\mathbf{d} = [||\mathbf{d}_1 - \mathbf{g}||_1, ||\mathbf{d}_2 - \mathbf{g}||_1, \cdots, ||\mathbf{d}_{n_a+n_b} - \mathbf{g}||_1, 0, \cdots, 0] \in \mathbb{R}^{(n_a+n_b+d)}$ indicate the distance between $\mathbf{g}$ and the gradient histogram of each element in $\mathbf{T}$. $||\mathbf{dc}||_2^2$ is used to measure the sum of the weighted distances, and

$$\frac{1}{2}||\mathbf{Tc} - \mathbf{y}||_2^2 + \beta||\mathbf{dc}||_2^2 \tag{2}$$

is used as the loss function.

3.3 Group Sparsity via $\ell_1 + \ell_1/\ell_2$ Mixed Norm

For the augmented template set with blur templates of different directions, since the motion blur of the target is always toward only one direction at time t, there is a natural group structure among the templates. The representation of the target candidate should not only be sparse, but also have group structure, i.e., the coefficients should also be sparse at the group level. In our tracking framework, we divide the templates into $n_g = n_\theta + d + 1$ groups $\mathcal{G} = \{G_1, G_2, \cdots, G_{n_\theta+d+1}\}$ using the following scheme: the normal templates are in one group; the blur templates in the same direction forms a group; and each trivial template is an individual group. In order to capture the group information among the templates and achieve sparsity at the same time, we employ a structured sparsity inducing norm which combines the ℓ_1 norm and a sum of ℓ_2 norms over groups of variables [11]. The mixed norm is known as "sparse group Lasso".

Combining the loss function (2) and the $\ell_1 + \ell_1/\ell_2$ mixed norm results in the following non-smooth convex optimization problem:

$$\min_{\mathbf{c}} \frac{1}{2}\|\mathbf{Tc}-\mathbf{y}\|_2^2 + \beta\|\mathbf{dc}\|_2^2 + \lambda_1\|\mathbf{c}\|_1 + \lambda_2\sum_{i=1}^{n_g}\|\mathbf{c}_{G_i}\|_2,$$
$$\text{s.t.} \quad \mathbf{c}_T \succeq 0 \tag{3}$$

where $\mathbf{c}_{G_i}$ are coefficients associated with G_i.

Once (3) is solved, the observation likelihood can be derived from the reconstruction error of $\mathbf{y}$ as $p(\mathbf{y}_t|\mathbf{x}_t) \propto \exp\{-\alpha\|\mathbf{Tc}-\mathbf{y}\|_2^2\}$, where α is a constant used to control the shape of the Gaussian kernel.

3.4 Solve (3) by Accelerated Proximal Gradient

To solve the non-smooth convex optimization problem in Eq. (3), we adopt the accelerated proximal gradient method FISTA [30] which has convergence rate of $O(\frac{1}{k^2})$, where k is the number of iterations. FISTA is designed for solving the following unconstrained optimization problem:

$$\min_{\mathbf{z}} F(\mathbf{z}) = f(\mathbf{z}) + g(\mathbf{z}) \tag{4}$$

where f is a smooth convex function with Lipschitz continuous gradient, and g is a continuous convex function which is possibly non-smooth.

In order to solve Eq. (3) with FISTA, we let $\mathbf{z} = [z_1, z_2, \cdots, z_{n_a+n_b+d}]^\top$ and make the substitution $\mathbf{c} = [z_1^2, z_2^2, \cdots, z_{n_a+n_b}^2, z_{n_a+n_b+1}, \cdots, z_{n_a+n_b+d}]^\top$ to incorporate the explicit constraint in Eq. (3) into the objective function, and solve the following optimization problem:

$$\min_{\mathbf{z}} \frac{1}{2}\|\mathbf{Tc}-\mathbf{y}\|_2^2 + \beta\|\mathbf{dc}\|_2^2 + \lambda_1\|\mathbf{z}\|_1 + \lambda_2\sum_{i=1}^{n_g}\|\mathbf{z}_{G_i}\|_2 \tag{5}$$

where $\mathbf{z}_{G_i}$ is associated with group G_i. Then, Eq. (5) can be re-expressed as Eq. (4), where

$$f(\mathbf{z}) = \frac{1}{2}\|\mathbf{Tc}-\mathbf{y}\|_2^2 + \beta\|\mathbf{dc}\|_2^2 \tag{6}$$

and

$$g(\mathbf{z}) = \lambda_1\|\mathbf{z}\|_1 + \lambda_2\sum_{i=1}^{n_g}\|\mathbf{z}_{G_i}\|_2 \tag{7}$$

To develop a proximal gradient method, the following quadratic approximation of $F(\mathbf{z})$ at a given point $\mathbf{z}^{(k)}$is considered, for $L > 0$

$$\begin{aligned} Q_L(\mathbf{z}, \mathbf{z}^{(k)}) =& f(\mathbf{z}^{(k)}) + \langle \mathbf{z} - \mathbf{z}^{(k)}, \nabla f(\mathbf{z}^{(k)}) \rangle \\ &+ \frac{L}{2} \|\mathbf{z} - \mathbf{z}^{(k)}\|_2^2 + g(\mathbf{z}) \end{aligned} \tag{8}$$

where $\nabla f(\mathbf{z}^{(k)})$ is the gradient function of $f(\cdot)$ at point $\mathbf{z}^{(k)}$.

Lemma 1 [30]. *Let f be a continuously differentiable function with Lipschitz continuous gradient and Lipschitz constant $L(f)$. Then, for any $L \geq L(f)$,*

$$F(\mathbf{z}) \leq Q_L(\mathbf{z}, \mathbf{z}^{(k)})$$

According to Lemma 1, given $L \geq L(f)$, a unique solution of $F(\mathbf{z})$ can be obtained by minimizing $Q_L(\mathbf{z}, \mathbf{z}^{(k)})$,

$$p_L(\mathbf{z}^{(k)}) = \arg \max_{\mathbf{z}} \frac{1}{2} ||\mathbf{z} - \hat{\mathbf{z}}|| + \frac{1}{L} g(\mathbf{z}) \tag{9}$$

where $\hat{\mathbf{z}} = \mathbf{z}^{(k)} - \frac{1}{L} \nabla f(\mathbf{z}^{(k)})$, and

$$\nabla f(\mathbf{z}) = \text{diag}(\mathbf{w})(\mathbf{T}^\top \mathbf{T}\mathbf{c} - \mathbf{T}^\top \mathbf{y}) + 2\beta \text{diag}(\mathbf{w})\mathbf{d}^\top \mathbf{d}\mathbf{c} \tag{10}$$

where $\mathbf{w} = [2z_1, 2z_2, \cdots, 2z_{n_a+n_b}, 1, \cdots, 1] \in \mathbb{R}^{n_a+n_b+d}$. Equation (9) just ignores the constant $z^{(k)}$ in Eq. (8), and the minimum of Eq. (8) can be obtained by solving Eq. (9). Algorithm 1 describes FISTA with backtracking.

Algorithm 1. FISTA with backtracking [30]

Input: $L_0 > 0$, $\tau > 1$, $\mathbf{v}^{(1)} = \mathbf{z}^{(0)}$, $t_1 = 1$

1: **for** k=1,2,..., iterate until convergence **do**
2: set $L = L_{k-1}$
3: **while** $F(p_L(\mathbf{v}^{(k)})) > Q_L(p_L(\mathbf{v}^{(k)}), \mathbf{v}^{(k)})$ **do**
4: $L = \tau L$
5: **end while**
6: set $L_k = L$ and update
7: $\mathbf{z}^{(k)} = p_{L_k}(\mathbf{v}^{(k)})$,
8: $t_{k+1} = \frac{1+\sqrt{1+4t_k^2}}{2}$,
9: $\mathbf{v}^{(k+1)} = \mathbf{z}^{(k)} + (\frac{t_k - 1}{t_{k+1}})(\mathbf{z}^{(k)} - \mathbf{z}^{(k-1)})$
10: **end for**

A critical step of Algorithm 1 is to solve Eq. (9) efficiently. Since the $\ell_1 + \ell_1/\ell_2$-norm is a special case of the tree structured group Lasso, Eq. (9) can be converted to

$$p_L(\mathbf{z}^{(k)}) = \arg \max_{\mathbf{z}} \frac{1}{2} ||\mathbf{z} - \hat{\mathbf{z}}|| + \sum_{i=0}^{m} \sum_{j=1}^{n_i} w_j^i ||\mathbf{z}_{G_j^i}||_2 \tag{11}$$

where m is the depth of the index tree defined in [31], n_i is the number of groups at depth i, $w_j^i \geq 0 (i = 0, 1, \cdots, m, j = 1, 2, \cdots, n_i)$ is the pre-defined weight for group G_j^i. We apply the $\text{MY}_{\text{tgLasso}}$ algorithm [31] to solve Eq. (11) efficiently. $\text{MY}_{\text{tgLasso}}$ algorithm maintains a working variable $\mathbf{u}$ initialized with $\hat{\mathbf{z}}$, then it traverses the index tree in the reverse breadth-first order to update $\mathbf{u}$ with $\mathbf{u}^i_{G^i_j} = \mathbf{u}^{i+1}_{G^i_j} \max\left(0, 1 - w^i_j / \|\mathbf{u}^{i+1}_{G^i_j}\|\right)$.

The time complexity of $\text{MY}_{\text{tgLasso}}$ algorithm is $O(mn)$, where n is the dimension of $\mathbf{z}$. After converting Eqs. (9)–(11), the index tree has a constant depth 2, so the time complexity for solving Eq. (9) is $O(n)$, where $n = n_a + n_b + d$.

3.5 Template Update with Blur Detection

In order to capture the appearance variations of the target caused by illumination or pose changes, the template set needs to be updated during tracking. Since the appearance of the target is corrupted when heavy blur appears, updating the template set with heavily blurred target cannot capture the appearance changes of the target. So we propose to perform blur detection of the tracking result before updating the template set.

To detect blur, we investigate the response of both normal coefficients and blur coefficients obtained from solving the optimization problem Eq. (3). If the target is not blurred, the energy of the normal coefficients will be dominant. One criterion for updating the template set is $\frac{E(\mathbf{a})}{E(\mathbf{a})+E(\mathbf{b})} > 0.9$, where $E(\cdot)$ represents the energy which is the sum of the absolute value of the corresponding coefficients. Also, trivial templates are activated when the target cannot be well approximated by the template set. In order to avoid contaminating the template set, another criterion for updating template set is $\frac{E(\mathbf{e})}{E(\mathbf{a})+E(\mathbf{b})+E(\mathbf{e})} < 0.1$. When the target is not similar to any of the normal templates, and both of the above two criteria are satisfied, we replace the normal template having lowest response with the target template.

Algorithm 2. BReT: Blur resilient tracker

Input: Current frame F_t, sample set $\mathbf{S}_{t-1}$, template set $\mathbf{T}_{t-1}$

1: **for** $i = 1$ to N **do**
2: Draw N particles $\mathbf{x}_t^i$ with the blur driven proposal distribution
3: Obtain the candidate patch $\mathbf{y}_t^i$ of $\mathbf{x}_t^i$
4: Solving the optimization problem (3)
5: Calculate the observation likelihood $p(\mathbf{y}_t^i|\mathbf{x}_t^i)$
6: **end for**
7: Locate the target $\mathbf{x}_t^*$ with the maximum observation likelihood
8: Estimate motion from blur via the blur coefficients of the estimated target
9: Update the template set $\mathbf{T}_t$ with blur detection
10: Update the sample set $\mathbf{S}_t$ by resampling with p

4 Experiments

We implemented the proposed algorithm with MATLAB R2011b, and the SLEP package [32] is used to solve Eq. (11). In our tracking framework, the state variable $\mathbf{x}_t$ is modeled by four parameters $\mathbf{x}_t = (t_x, t_y, s, \theta)$, where (t_x, t_y) are the 2D translation parameters, s is the scale variation parameter, and θ is the rotation variation parameter. In our experiment, $n_a = 10$ normal templates are used, and we set $n_\theta = 8$, $n_l = 4$, so there are $10 + 8 \times 4 = 42$ non-trivial templates in total. For the optimization problem Eq. (3), we set $\beta = 0.35$, $\lambda_1 = 0.03$, $\lambda_2 = 0.03$; for the number of bins of the gradient histogram, we set $h = 19$; and for the weight of trivial templates, we set $\eta = 0.15$. These parameters are kept the same for all the sequences.

To evaluate the performance of the blurred target tracking algorithm, we compile a set of 12 challenging blurred tracking sequences, denoted as *owl, face, body, car1, car2, car3, car4, jumping, running, cola, dollar* and *cup*. The sequences *owl, face, body, car1, car2, car3* and *car4* were used in [10] and can be downloaded from an online source including the ground truth.[1] The sequence *jumping* and the associated ground truth can be downloaded from an online source.[2] For the sequences *running, cola, dollar* and *cup*, we collected them ourselves and labeled the ground truth manually, and these four sequences contain 2400 frames. In total we use 6235 frames for the experiments.

We compared the proposed BReT algorithm with seven state-of-the-art visual trackers: VTD [24], L1APG [26], IVT [23], MIL [19], OAB [17], Struck [20] and BLUT [10]. We use the publicly available source codes or binaries from the referenced authors with the same initialization of the target in the first frame. We first used the default parameter settings of the above trackers to evaluate them. Nevertheless, all but the BLUT [10], which is specifically designed for blurred target tracking, failed on most of the sequences. One critical reason for the failure of these trackers is that the search radius is not large enough or the variance of the motion model under the particle filter framework is not large enough to cover the fast motion in these blurred sequences. So we tuned each of these trackers specifically. We increased the search radius of Struck from 30 to 100, and the search radius of MIL and OAB from 25 to 100. For L1APG, VTD, IVT and BReT which use the particle filter technique, we set the number of particles to $N = 600$. For L1APG and IVT, we set the variance of the motion model the same as BReT. For VTD, since the binary code has a predefined value for the variance of the motion model and only allows the user to specify how many times to enlarge or shrink this value, we set the variance ten times as large as the predefined one. For BLUT, the parameter setting provided in the original code works better, so we kept it unchanged. Among all these trackers, only VTD uses color information, while the others only use grayscale information.

[1] http://www.dabi.temple.edu/~hbling/data/TUblur.zip.

[2] http://cvlab.hanyang.ac.kr/tracker_benchmark/seq/Jumping.zip.

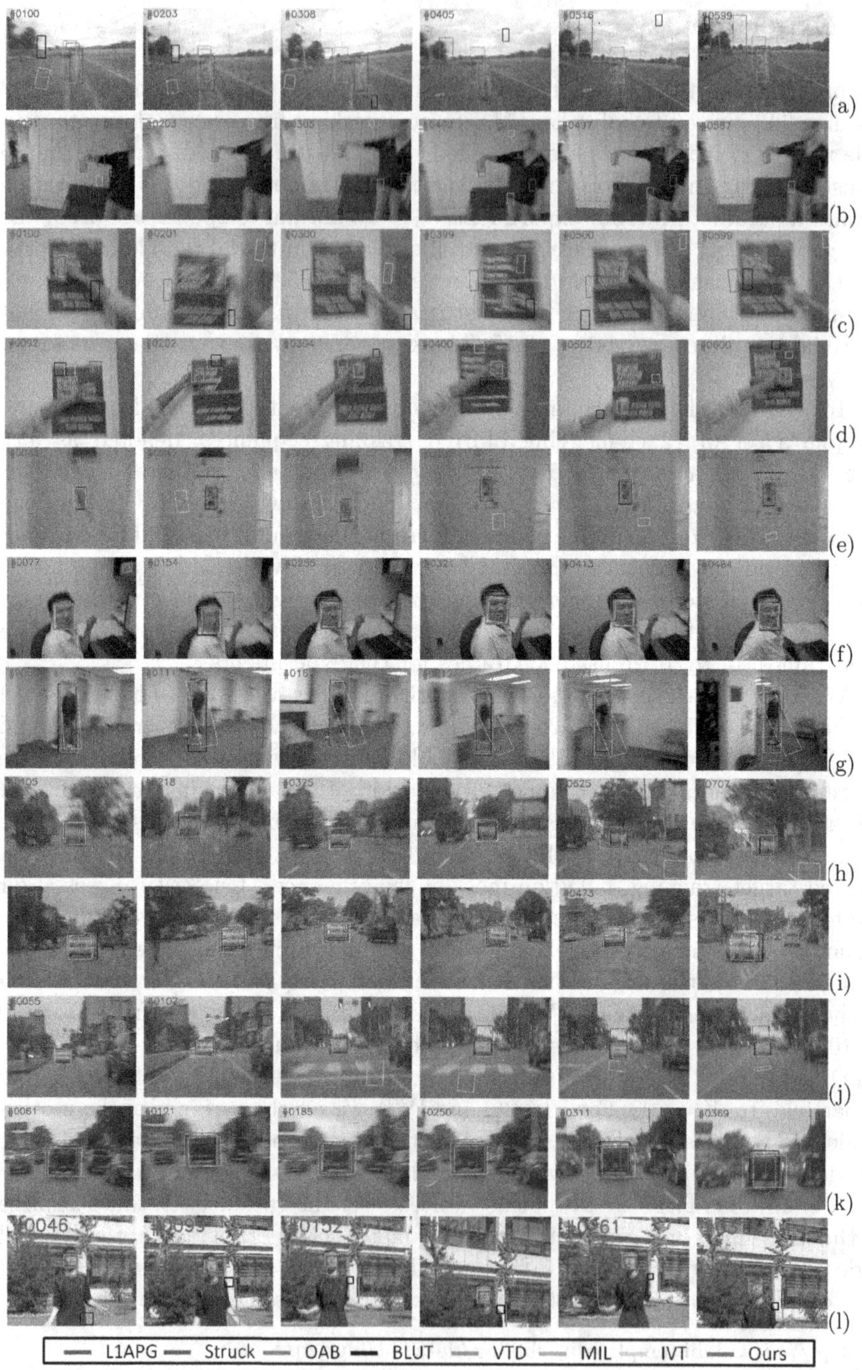

Fig. 2. Tracking results of eight algorithms on 12 sequences. The name of the sequences are (a) running, (b) cola, (c) dollar, (d) cup, (e) owl, (f) face, (g) body, (h) car1, (i) car2, (j) car3, (k) car4 and (l) jumping.

4.1 Qualitative Evaluation

The sequence *running* was captured outdoors, a person is running on the playground while being videotaped by another person who is also running. Some tracking results are shown in Fig. 2(a). Both our tracker and VTD track the target well. Without using color information, the target is very similar to the grass, especially when blur appears. We believe that the success of VTD on this sequence can be attributed to the use of color information.

In the sequence *cola*, a moving cola can was tracked, as shown in Fig. 2(b). When blur appears, it is hard to distinguish the target from the sofa and the clothes of the person with only grayscale information. The appearance of the target also changed slightly by rotation. Our tracker and VTD perform well on this sequence, while the other trackers start to fail when heavy blur appears.

Results on the sequence *dollar* are shown in Fig. 2(c), in which a paper dollar was tracked. Our tracker is capable of tracking the target for most frames of the sequence. MIL also exhibits comparable results, but starts to lose the target completely at frame 505.

Figure 2(d) demonstrates the results of the *cup* sequence. Our tracker, Struck and MIL can track the target for almost all frames. Other trackers often locate the area near the edge between the indicator board and the wall as target. A possible reason is that there is a white stripe containing characters in the top of cup surface, and the rest of the surface of the cup is blue in general.

In the sequence *owl*, a plane object was tracked as shown in Fig. 2(e). VTD starts to fail at frame 46 and locates a sign that has similar color as the target. IVT starts to fail at frame 183. Our tracker, BLUT, Struck, L1APG can track the target accurately through the whole sequence. MIL and OAB also obtain comparable results on this sequence.

Results on the sequence *face* are shown in Fig. 2(f), in which the target is not only blurred but also has slight pose variation. All the trackers except OAB perform well on this sequence, while OAB meets problems from frame 68.

Results on the sequence *body* are given in Fig. 2(g). A person is walking in this sequence, and most of the frames are severely blurred. IVT cannot correctly obtain the direction of the target. Though OAB does not completely lose the target through the sequence, for most of the sequence, it cannot get the accurate position of the target. Other trackers works well on this sequence and get comparable results.

The sequences *car1, car2, car3, car4* are captured from outdoor traffic scenes. The results for *car*1 are shown in Fig. 2(h). OAB starts to drift at frame 100, MIL, IVT and L1APG start to drift at frame 533 when very heavy blur appears. Our tracker, BLUT, Struck and VTD can track the target successfully for most of the frames. Figure 2(i) shows the results on *car2*, MIL and OAB perform poorly, and start to drift at frame 107 and frame 77 respectively. Other trackers work well on this sequence, and our tracker, BLUT, L1APG, VTD, IVT perform a little better than Struck. Figure 2(j) gives the results on *car3*. IVT lost the target at frame 121, Struck lost the target at frame 186 and the sky was tracked as the target by Struck. Results of sequence *car4* are given in Fig. 2(k), where OAB

Table 1. Success rate of the trackers (median). The best, second and third bests are in red, blue and green respectively.

Video	MIL	OAB	VTD	IVT	Struck	L1APG	BLUT	Ours
running	0.03	0.05	0.88	0.07	0.45	0.16	0.07	0.85
cola	0.10	0.07	0.73	0.06	0.14	0.04	0.06	0.81
dollar	0.78	0.42	0.43	0.33	0.17	0.17	0.09	0.90
cup	0.95	0.11	0.65	0.11	0.97	0.42	0.11	0.99
owl	0.71	0.68	0.07	0.28	0.99	0.98	1.00	1.00
face	0.76	0.14	1.00	0.95	1.00	0.96	0.98	0.99
body	0.59	0.09	0.56	0.20	0.88	0.65	0.67	0.77
car1	0.72	0.15	0.99	0.70	0.99	0.69	0.99	0.99
car2	0.41	0.12	0.94	0.96	0.88	0.98	0.97	0.99
car3	0.74	0.93	0.89	0.33	0.54	0.99	0.94	1.00
car4	0.68	0.11	1.00	0.75	0.99	0.71	0.69	0.97
jumping	0.92	1.00	0.11	1.00	1.00	1.00	0.03	0.99
median	0.72	0.13	0.81	0.33	0.93	0.70	0.68	0.99

Table 2. Success rate of the trackers (mean ± standard deviation). The best, second and third bests are in red, blue and green respectively.

Video	MIL [19]	OAB [17]	VTD [24]	IVT [23]	Struck [20]	L1APG [26]	BLUT [10]	Ours
running	0.06±0.05	0.07±0.04	0.91±0.04	0.07±0.02	0.45±0.00	0.17±0.08	0.07±0.01	0.70±0.28
cola	0.12±0.04	0.09±0.04	0.72±0.06	0.05±0.02	0.15±0.06	0.04±0.02	0.07±0.03	0.78±0.12
dollar	0.74±0.13	0.33±0.13	0.47±0.07	0.33±0.00	0.30±0.32	0.29±0.27	0.10±0.04	0.73±0.32
cup	0.82±0.24	0.27±0.37	0.68±0.09	0.20±0.21	0.80±0.33	0.42±0.19	0.11±0.01	0.99±0.00
owl	0.77±0.18	0.64±0.34	0.07±0.00	0.27±0.03	0.98±0.00	0.91±0.17	1.00±0.00	1.00±0.00
face	0.79±0.06	0.13±0.06	1.00±0.00	0.95±0.03	1.00±0.00	0.77±0.29	0.98±0.01	0.99±0.00
body	0.53±0.21	0.09±0.03	0.55±0.10	0.17±0.09	0.88±0.01	0.60±0.20	0.68±0.03	0.77±0.03
car1	0.71±0.19	0.18±0.06	0.99±0.01	0.80±0.15	0.99±0.00	0.69±0.00	0.99±0.00	0.99±0.00
car2	0.41±0.15	0.11±0.06	0.78±0.36	0.93±0.08	0.88±0.00	0.98±0.01	0.97±0.01	0.99±0.00
car3	0.71±0.21	0.80±0.29	0.91±0.08	0.60±0.37	0.53±0.01	0.86±0.30	0.95±0.05	1.00±0.00
car4	0.74±0.13	0.16±0.12	0.95±0.11	0.75±0.03	0.99±0.00	0.74±0.09	0.67±0.05	0.97±0.02
jumping	0.89±0.15	1.00±0.00	0.18±0.10	0.92±0.18	1.00±0.00	1.00±0.00	0.03±0.02	0.98±0.03
mean	0.61±0.27	0.32±0.31	0.68±0.31	0.50±0.36	0.75±0.31	0.62±0.32	0.55±0.43	0.91±0.12

starts to locate the target inaccurately from frame 34. Our tracker, VTD and Struck get excellent results on this sequence.

Figure 2(l) shows the results of *jumping*, in which the target was jumping and causing obvious motion blur. Compared with other sequences, the motion in *jumping* is relatively simple, mainly includes up and down motion. All the trackers except BLUT and VTD perform well on this sequence.

4.2 Quantitative Evaluation

We use two criteria to evaluate these trackers quantitatively. We first use the percentage of frames for which the estimated target location is within a threshold distance from the ground truth to measure the success rate of each tracker, and

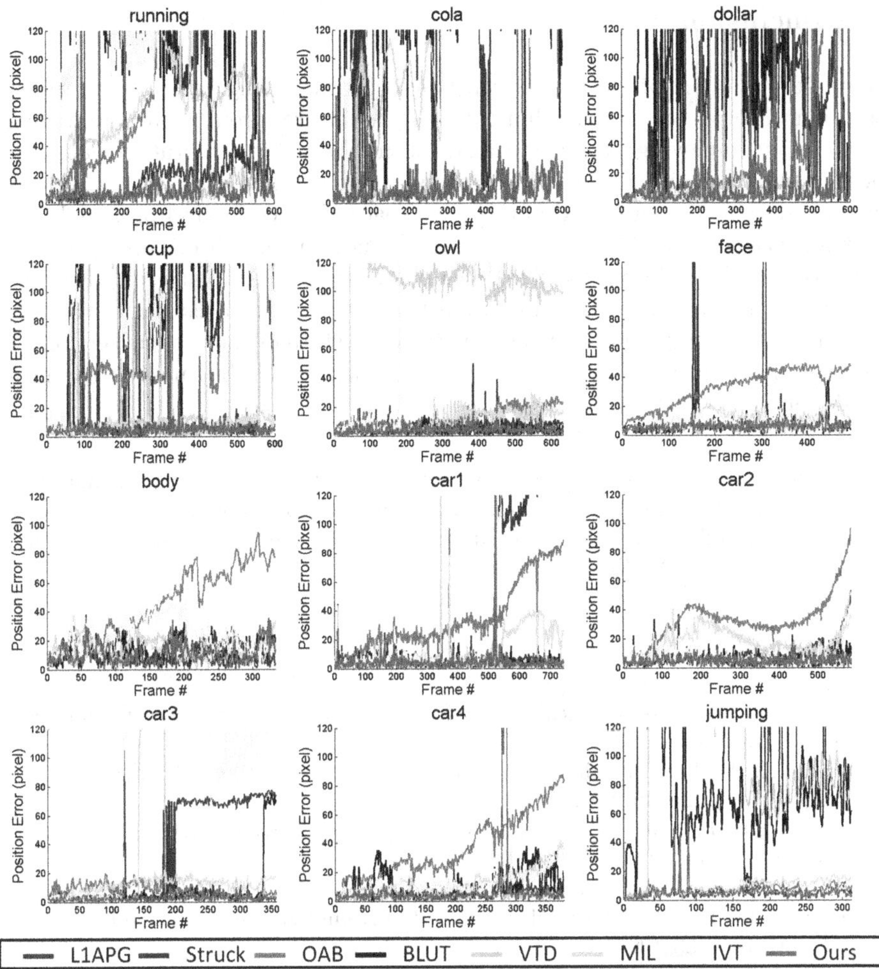

Fig. 3. Quantitative comparison of the trackers in terms of position errors (in pixel).

we use 15 pixels as the threshold. Since all these trackers involve randomness, we run each tracker five times on all the sequences, and report both the median result and the average result with standard deviation. Table 1 summarizes the results using median, and the results of mean with standard deviation are given in Table 2. We also plot the center location error of each tracker on all the sequences over time according to the median results, as shown in Fig. 3. From the results, we can see that our tracking algorithm works favorably against state-of-the-art methods. The good performance can be attributed to the use of group sparse representation to approximate the target candidate and incorporating gradient information to the loss function to reduce the ambiguity of the enhanced appearance space.

5 Conclusion

We propose a robust blurred target tracking algorithm using group sparse representation. The proposed algorithm exploits the natural group structure among templates by employing a $\ell_1+\ell_1/\ell_2$ mixed norm. We also incorporate the appearance information from gradient histograms in a loss function that helps reduce the ambiguity of the enhanced appearance space. An accelerated proximal gradient approach is adopted to solve the resulting non-smooth convex optimization problem. In addition, we dynamically update the template set with blur detection to make the tracker more robust to appearance variations of the target. Finally, we compared our tracker with seven state-of-the-art trackers on 12 blurred sequences to demonstrate the effectiveness and robustness of the proposed tracker.

Acknowledgement. This work was supported in part by the US NSF Grants IIS-1218156 and IIS-1350521. Wu was supported in part by NSFC under Grants 61005027 and 61370036, and Lang was supported by "Beijing Higher Education Young Elite Teacher Project" (No.YETP0514).

References

1. Silveira, G.F., Malis, E.: Real-time visual tracking under arbitrary illumination changes. In: CVPR (2007)
2. Adam, A., Rivlin, E., Shimshoni, I.: Robust fragments-based tracking using the integral histogram. In: CVPR (2006)
3. Jia, X., Lu, H., Yang, M.H.: Visual tracking via adaptive structural local sparse appearance model. In: CVPR (2012)
4. Hu, W., Li, X., Zhang, X., Shi, X., Maybank, S.J., Zhang, Z.: Incremental tensor subspace learning and its applications toforeground segmentation and tracking. IJCV **91**, 303–327 (2011)
5. Kwon, J., Lee, K.M.: Wang-landau monte carlo-based tracking methods for abrupt motions. PAMI **35**, 1011–1024 (2013)
6. Cho, S., Lee, S.: Fast motion deblurring. ACM Trans. Graph. **28**, 145:1–145:8 (2009)
7. Xu, L., Zheng, S., Jia, J.: Unnatural l0 sparse representation for natural image deblurring. In: CVPR (2013)
8. Jin, H., Favaro, P., Cipolla, R.: Visual tracking in the presence of motion blur. In: CVPR (2005)
9. Dai, S., Yang, M., Wu, Y., Katsaggelos, A.K.: Tracking motion-blurred targets in video. In: ICIP (2006)
10. Wu, Y., Ling, H., Yu, J., Li, F., Mei, X., Cheng, E.: Blurred target tracking by blur-driven tracker. In: ICCV (2011)
11. Bach, F., Jenatton, R., Mairal, J., Obozinski, G.: Convex optimization with sparsity-inducing norms. In: Sra, S., Nowozin, S., Wright, S. (eds.) Optimization for Machine Learning, pp. 19–53. MIT Press, Cambridge (2011)
12. Yilmaz, A., Javed, O., Shah, M.: Object tracking: a survey. ACM Comput. Surv. **38**, 13 (2006)

13. Wu, Y., Lim, J., Yang, M.H.: Online object tracking: a benchmark. In: Proceedings of IEEE Conference on Computer Vision and Pattern Recognition, pp. 2411–2418 (2013)
14. Pang, Y., Ling, H.: Finding the best from the second bests-inhibiting subjective bias in evaluation of visual tracking algorithms. In: Proceedings of IEEE International Conference on Computer Vision, pp. 2784–2791 (2013)
15. Kristan, M., Pflugfelder, R., Leonardis, A., Matas, J., Porikli, F., Khajenezhad, A., Salahledin, A., Soltani-Farani, A., Zarezade, A., Petrosino, A., et al.: The visual object tracking vot2013 challenge results. In: IEEE Workshop on visual object tracking challenge (2013)
16. Smeulders, A.W.M., Chu, D.M., Cucchiara, R., Calderara, S., Dehghan, A., Shah, M.: Visual tracking: an experimental survey. IEEE Trans. Pattern Anal. Mach. Intell. **36**, 1428–1441 (2014)
17. Grabner, H., Grabner, M., Bischof, H.: Real-time tracking via on-line boosting. In: BMVC (2006)
18. Grabner, H., Leistner, C., Bischof, H.: Semi-supervised on-line boosting for robust tracking. In: Forsyth, D., Torr, P., Zisserman, A. (eds.) ECCV 2008, Part I. LNCS, vol. 5302, pp. 234–247. Springer, Heidelberg (2008)
19. Babenko, B., Yang, M.H., Belongie, S.: Robust object tracking with online multiple instance learning. PAMI **33**, 1619–1632 (2011)
20. Hare, S., Saffari, A., Torr, P.H.S.: Struck: structured output tracking with kernels. In: ICCV (2011)
21. Comaniciu, D., Ramesh, V., Meer, P.: Kernel-based object tracking. PAMI **25**, 564–577 (2003)
22. Black, M.J., Jepson, A.D.: Eigentracking: robust matching and tracking of articulated objects using a view-based representation. IJCV **26**, 63–84 (1998)
23. Ross, D.A., Lim, J., Lin, R.S., Yang, M.H.: Incremental learning for robust visual tracking. IJCV **77**, 125–141 (2008)
24. Kwon, J., Lee, K.M.: Visual tracking decomposition. In: CVPR (2010)
25. Mei, X., Ling, H.: Robust visual tracking and vehicle classification via sparse representation. PAMI **33**, 2259–2272 (2011)
26. Bao, C., Wu, Y., Ling, H., Ji, H.: Real time robust l1 tracker using accelerated proximal gradient approach. In: CVPR (2012)
27. Liu, B., Yang, L., Huang, J., Meer, P., Gong, L., Kulikowski, C.: Robust and fast collaborative tracking with two stage sparse optimization. In: Daniilidis, K., Maragos, P., Paragios, N. (eds.) ECCV 2010, Part IV. LNCS, vol. 6314, pp. 624–637. Springer, Heidelberg (2010)
28. Zhang, T., Ghanem, B., Liu, S., Ahuja, N.: Robust visual tracking via structured multi-task sparse learning. IJCV **101**, 367–383 (2013)
29. Doucet, A., De Freitas, N., Gordon, N., et al.: An introduction to sequential Monte Carlo methods. In: Doucet, A., De Freitas, N., Gordon, N. (eds.) Sequential Monte Carlo Methods in Practice. Statistics for Engineering and Information Science, vol. 1, pp. 3–14. Springer, New York (2001)
30. Beck, A., Teboulle, M.: A fast iterative shrinkage-thresholding algorithm for linear inverse problems. SIAM J. Imag. Sci. **2**, 183–202 (2009)
31. Liu, J., Ye, J.: Moreau-Yosida regularization for grouped tree structure learning. In: NIPS (2010)
32. Liu, J., Ji, S., Ye, J.: SLEP: Sparse Learning with Efficient Projections. Arizona State University (2009)

Visual Tracking via Supervised Similarity Matching

Ji Zhang(✉), Jie Sheng, and Ankur Teredesai

Center for Data Science, Institute of Technology,
University of Washington Tacoma, Tacoma, USA
zhangj32@uw.edu

Abstract. Supervised learning algorithms have been widely applied in tracking-by-detection based methods for object tracking in recent years. Most of these approaches treat tracking as a classification problem and solve it by training a discriminative classifier and exhaustively evaluating every possible target position; problems thus exist for two reasons. First, since the classifier describes the common feature of samples in an implicit way, it is not clear how well the classifier can represent the feature of the desired object against others; second, the brute-force search within the output space is usually time consuming, and thus limits the competence for real-time application. In this paper, we treat object tracking as a problem of similarity matching for streaming data. We propose to apply unsupervised learning by Locality Sensitive Hashing (LSH) and use LSH based similarity matching as the main engine for target detection. In addition, our method applies a Support Vector Machine (SVM) based supervised classifier cooperating with the unsupervised detector. Both the proposed tracker and several selected trackers are tested on some well accepted challenging videos; and the experimental results demonstrate that the proposed tracker outperforms the selected other trackers in terms of the effectiveness as well as the robustness.

1 Introduction

Object tracking in unconstrained scenarios is one of the fundamental problems of computer vision. The challenge in this topic lies mainly in the complexity of tracking environments such as severe illumination change, target deformation, background clutter, partial occlusion, to name just a few. Inspired by the tracking-by-detection framework [1], which has been proposed to treat object tracking as a detection problem and solve it by supervised learning and prediction, a major research axis has been focused on building online classifiers to describe the dynamic target with discriminative power against the background. Among this group, Garbner et al. [2,3] and Stalder et al. [4] applied boosting algorithm for the classification task. Babenko [5] extended the idea by using

Electronic supplementary material The online version of this chapter (doi:10.1007/978-3-319-16814-2_10) contains supplementary material, which is available to authorized users.

D. Cremers et al. (Eds.): ACCV 2014, Part V, LNCS 9007, pp. 146–161, 2015.
DOI: 10.1007/978-3-319-16814-2_10

a more sophisticated sampling strategy to alleviate ambiguity among training data. Meanwhile, SVM has been deeply exploited; for example, the method proposed in [6] exploits an online-SVM algorithm called Larank [7,8] and solves the curse of kernelization by maintaining a fixed-sized set of support vectors [9,10]. Aiming at improved performance of that idea, several SVM-based trackers [11–13] has been proposed in three aspects respectively: increasing the sensitivity to new samples, strengthening the adaptive ability on target deformation, and fusing multiple features by binary code to build a better target model.

In spite of demonstrated success in previous research, classification-based trackers often suffer drifting problems where a tracker confidently tracks a position that covers the true target location in part and can hardly correct itself once it starts to make such mistake. This is mainly because that treating tracking problem as a classification task is not straightforward and has inevitable defects. For most supervised algorithms [2,5,6,14,15], the basic idea is to train a function $h : X \rightarrow R$, where X is feature space and h returns a classification confidence score evaluating how likely a sample would be the target. The function h acts as a summary of target appearance so far from the beginning, and is updated online by continuously adding more training samples frame by frame. This is where severe drifting problems may occur because training samples at different time are equally treated in those algorithms, i.e., old samples have the same influence on h as new samples do, while the new ones in fact should have more influence in order to keep h up-to-date. Previous research has been done to alleviate this problem by weighting more on the new data [11]. However, underrating old data may lead to incomplete view of the target and the fragility to noise. The dilemma is due to the inherent flaw of supervised methods, that is, trying to train an implicit function describing common feature of all the training samples at the cost of each samples uniqueness. According to that implicit function, however, it is difficult to evaluate how well the trained function can represent the varying target and how confident it is to track.

The main contribution of this paper is that we propose a novel tracking algorithm based on unsupervised learning and similarity search. Using a new framework for incorporating unsupervised learning with supervised learning, our algorithm is carefully designed to prevent drifting problems and to improve the overall accuracy. Later we will show the effectiveness of our method by experimental results; here, we want to highlight the advantages of our algorithm over supervised approaches in the following two aspects.

First, an intuitive understanding of tracking by human vision has helped us come up with better ideas. After confirming a target, what a human being does is to keep memorizing new appearance of the target while detecting it according to the memory. This mechanism can be well exported to computer vision system by applying unsupervised learning and similarity matching based on it. Specifically, the process of unsupervised learning corresponds to the human keeping memorizing target, and similarity matching acts like human eye detection based on the learned data. We claim that our novel tracking framework overcomes the main flaw of supervised methods. On the one hand, thanks to the large capacity provided by hash tables, all possible appearance of the target can be learned, and this ensures complete knowledge of all possible appearance of the target; on the other hand, the uniqueness of a sample is well preserved because each sample is individually stored without information loss, and the proposed detection strategy is able to output a clear path to find the target based on this complete set of samples rather than a vague summary of them.

Second, our method avoids the redundancy of brute-force search in the detection steps of supervised methods. Suppose $X \in R^d$ is the feature space where d is the feature dimension, and Y is the search space with all possible target positions, then the new target position is estimated by the following function

$$y = \underset{y \in Y}{\operatorname{argmax}}\, h(x_t^{p_{t-1} \circ y}) \tag{1}$$

where $p_{t-1} \in P$ is the target position on $t-1$ with $t = 1, 2, \ldots, T$ being the discrete time instants, $y_t \in Y$ is the transformation such that the new position is approximated by the composition defined as $p_t = p_{t-1} \circ y_t$, and $x_t^p \in X$ is the feature of a sample at position p at time t. It is usually in a brute force manner to find y_t and is usually time costly but inevitable due to the fact that supervised classification or regression merely predicts a value rather than a vector or a structure that explicitly represents the desired transformation. Therefore, every potential sample needs to be enumerated to find the optimal one. In contrast, our method returns the specific sample that is the most similar to the query. That means, the output of our core engine is not a value but a datum in the same format with the query. If we record each datum's relative location to the target, then after similarity searching, we can consider the most similar sample's relative position as the query's and easily get the target position by its inverse. Specifically, the position estimation function in our approach becomes

$$y_t = g(x_t^{p_{t-1}}) \tag{2}$$

where g retrieves the nearest neighbor of $x_t^{p_{t-1}}$ and returns the associated attribute, without checking every possible transformation in the output space. Therefore, brute-force searching in the output space is avoided and time complexity is reduced from $O(n)$ to $O(1)$ where N is the amount of candidates in the output space Y.

The remaining of this paper is organized as follows. In Sect. 2 we will discuss the learning and detection steps of our algorithm respectively, and the proposed cooperation strategy between LSH and SVM will be described in details. In this section we also present the implementation procedures of our approach and two algorithms are provided; one for the learning step and the other for the detection step of the proposed approach. Experiments to examine the difference between our proposed tracker and 13 other selected trackers are conducted in Sect. 3. Both the quantitative and qualitative performance evaluations will be discussed, according to experimental results. Effectiveness and robustness of our tracker will be demonstrated. Section 4 concludes the paper.

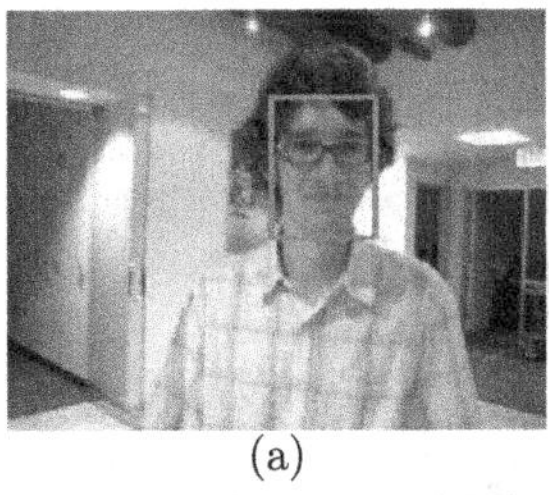
(a)

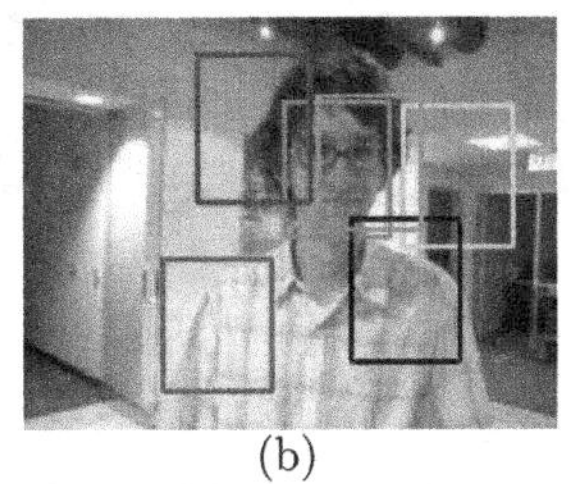
(b)

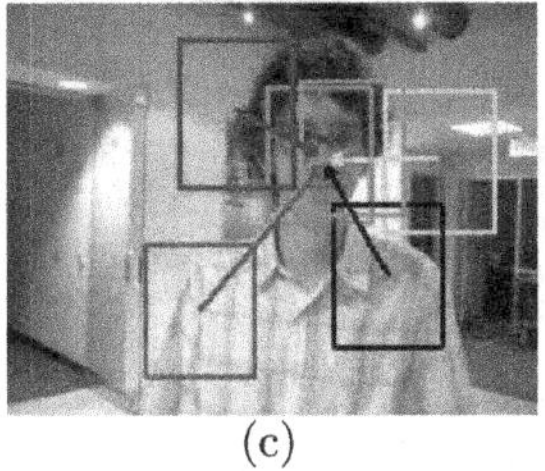
(c)

Fig. 1. Illustration of our learning strategy: (a) a random frame from a test video; (b) a certain number of boxes are generated around the current target box (in green) for sampling; (c) for each sample (in colors other than green), a transformation structure is associated with it. Since only translation is considered, the transformation structure here is a 2D vector indicating the offset from the sample to the target (Color figure online)

2 Technical Details

2.1 Learning

Benefiting from the key-value indexing architecture of LSH tables, the value domain can be filled with a structure that directly represents the transformation. Specifically, as shown in Fig. 1, in frame $f_t \in F$, we take a fixed number of samples within a preset radius centered at the target position $p = p_t \circ y$ by transformation $y \in Y$. We extract the sample feature x_t^p and generate a key-value pair $< x_t^p, y^{-1} >$ where y^{-1} is the inverse of y such that $p \circ y^{-1} = p_t \circ y \circ y^{-1} = p_t$, and insert it into the hash tables. By doing this, the tracker learns how each sample can be transformed back to the center, and this is the foundation of our detection step, to be described later.

Without loss of generality, we only consider targets 2D translation to simplify the problem, and therefore the transformation between two boxes can be represented as a vector $y \in R^n$ indicating 2D displacement from one to another. Extension to more complex transformation is straightforward and can be realized by simply substitute y with a more sophisticated structure that describes the enriched transformation model.

2.2 Detection

Figure 2 illustrates the detection step with an example in two consecutive frames. As mentioned earlier, the position estimation function g in Eq. (1) searches for a querys nearest neighbor by its key and returns the corresponding value. Given a previous target position p_{t-1} at time t, the task of detection is to estimate a transformation y_t according to Eq. (1) such that the new target position is achieved by the composition $p_t = p_{t-1} \circ y_t$. However, a simple calculation by Eq. (1) is not sufficient to get accurate results, since similarity searching is an approximation method with random errors and they may accumulate along

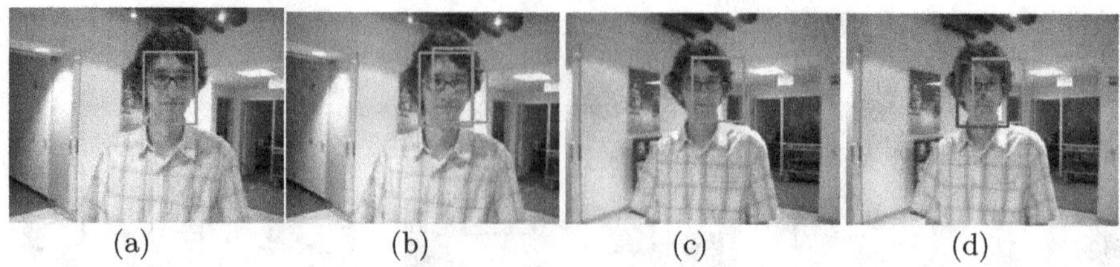

Fig. 2. Illustration of our detection strategy. (a) is one frame of the video at time $t-1$ and the green box is the target position, while the orange box in (b) is one of the training samples learned at $t-1$. Then the target moves towards left and (c) is the frame at time t, but the target box still stays where it was in (a). To detect the new target position, a similarity searching is done on the sample in green box in (c), and the result indicates that the green sample in (c) is in similar situation of the orange sample in (b). Given that, the tracker retrieves the transformation associated with the orange box, and moves the green one towards left to the blue one, which is the new target position at time t as shown in (d) (Color figure online)

the tracking. We propose two ways to minimize the potential error. The first is to do the position estimation in a gradient-descent-like way. The second is to cooperate with supervised classification. We describe the former in this section, and details about the latter will be discussed in the next section.

We refer to the mechanism of gradient descending and propose to do similarity searching in an iterative manner. In frame f_t, we apply Eq. (1) for at most M rounds rather than only once. On each round $m = 1, 2, \dots, M$, we obtain a new estimated target position by $p_t^m = p_t^{m-1} \circ y^m$, where we define $p_t^0 = p_{t-1}$ as the target position in f_{t-1}, and $y^m = g(X_t^{p_t^{m-1}})$ means the transformation y^m in round M is obtained according to the output of round $m-1$. The iteration stops either when it reaches M rounds or when the transformation y^m is small enough. Since only 2D translation is considered in this paper, we define that y^m is sufficiently small when $\|y^m\|_2$ decreases to less than a preset threshold δ. Ideally, this condition should be as strict as $\|y^m\|_2$ being exactly zero which corresponds to the exact expected target position. However, since our calculation is discrete and based on feature similarity rather than real gradient, convergence on $\|y^m\|_2$ is not guaranteed. Considering the high flexibility of tracking environment, it may be the most case where $\|y^m\|_2$ shakes around a small value around zero. That is why we set a small threshold δ to stop iteration softly. On the other hand, if the computation fails to converge into the threshold, it probably means the target just suffered a large change on appearance and a certain number of iteration would suffice for a good estimation. Eventually, we have the final transformation $y_t = y^m, 1 \leq m \leq M$.

2.3 Cooperation with Supervised Classification

Collaboration between tracker and validator has been successfully applied in the previous research [4,16]. In [16], an independent fern-like structure is used

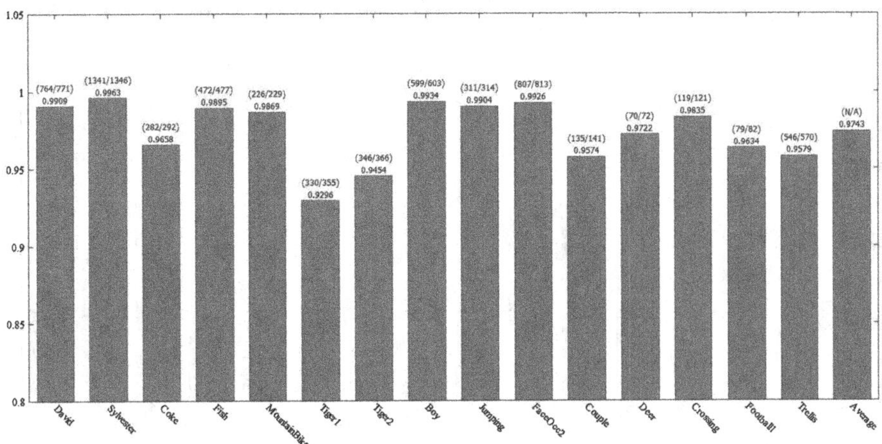

Fig. 3. Number of frames containing positive neighbors and their percentages

to learn a binary classifier in a supervised manner, and the tracking results are verified by it in order to ensure high accuracy. In [4], an online supervised recognizer is trained as an adaptive prior for tracking. The proposed method in this paper applies the similar idea, and we note that our supervised classifier can greatly improve the tracker, in the following two points of view.

Firstly, a potential issue of similarity matching is that the nearest neighbor may not be associated with the best transformation. This could be ascribed to large appearance variation of the target and the intrinsic approximation of similarity matching. Inspired by [16], we propose to use the classifier verification strategy to solve this problem. In the detection step, we retrieve K nearest neighbors instead of only one, and sort them in descending order according to the similarity with the query. Then we make a temporal transformation based on each of these neighbors associated models. The image patch within the transformed box is sent to the classifier for a verification. If the feedback is positive, it means the transformation is good. We do such verification from the most similar neighbor to the least, and it stops once the classifier reports the first positive one. If there is no such neighbor then we consider the LSH detection to be plausible, and simply pick the first one regardless of its verification result. Plausible LSH detection doesn't necessarily mean tracking failure but only indicates conflict between the tracker and the verifier, and when it happens we always choose the trackers output. In fact, during our experiment such conflict occurs for very few times. Figure 3 shows the percentage of frames where positive nearest neighbors exist for each of our 15 test videos. As shown, successful cooperation between LSH tracker and SVM verifier occurs for the most time and the average percentage of verified detection is above 97 %.

Secondly, in most supervised approaches, new data is sampled once per frame to update the classifiers. It is beneficial to do learning so often in supervised setting, since more data can provide richer information about the target and

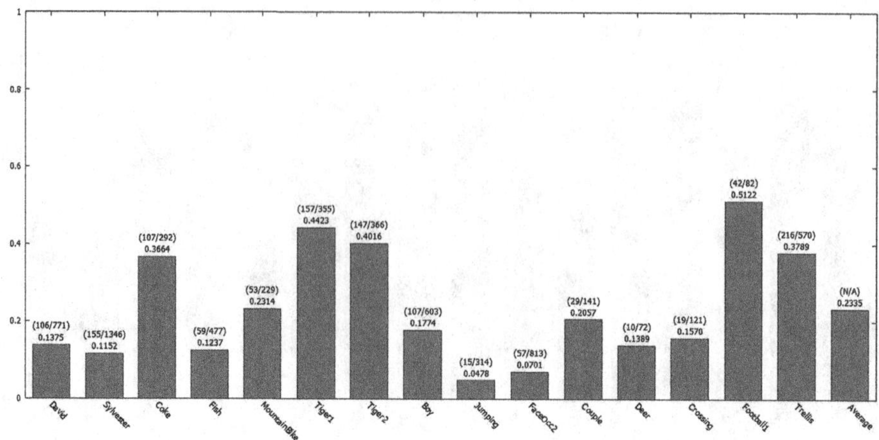

Fig. 4. Number of frames where new positive support vectors are added and their percentages

alleviate the ambiguity of the classifier. In contrast, our LSH based algorithm may suffer from frequent updating. The main reason is that LSH tables preserve each individual sample rather than integrate all of them. Therefore, with a higher updating frequency, consecutive samples would be closer on the timeline and they would become more similar. As a result, similarity matching is more likely to be confused when selecting the nearest neighbor, leading to inaccurate output. Ideally, learning should run faster when the target changes significantly and slower when it doesnt. That is to say, the frequency is controlled by the level of target variation.

Now we need a way to determine when the target is undergoing fast change. We notice that well-structured classifiers may also be efficient tools to detect data novelty, and SVM is one of them [17,18]. The support vectors can be regarded as a brief description of all previous samples, and increment of support vectors during learning is usually associated with large adjustment of the split hyperplan. This is a sign of singular data among the training data set. In the tracking scenario, it can be interpreted as significant appearance change of the target. Inspired by this, we propose a simple novelty detection strategy: variation occurs only when there are new positive support vectors added. Since we update the SVM classifier in every frame, support vectors increase simultaneously with the targets change, but the frequency is much less than once per frame. Figure 4 shows the percentage of frames where new positive support vectors occur for all the 15 test videos. As we can see, the value varies from 4.78 % to 51.22 %, which is mainly due to the different levels of target variation in different videos. Meanwhile, the average percentage is only 23.35 %, indicating that less than one fourth of frames have the necessity to update the LSH database. Both the variance in percentage and the low mean value demonstrate the effectiveness and efficiency of our dynamic strategy.

2.4 Implementation Details

The streaming form of image data requires the algorithm to be in an online manner. It is intuitive to implement LSH online, since we only need to periodically insert new sample and do queries based on current data. When the size of data reaches the maximum capacity of hash tables, we simply delete the oldest data to create space. For the online SVM, some research has been done on this topic [6–8, 10]. We refer to Struck [6] and take advantage of the accuracy and speed of Larank [7] by using it only in 2-class setting. Similar with [6], we also apply a budget strategy to maintain a maximum number of support vectors in order to keep the computational cost acceptable.

The concept of LSH was firstly introduced by Indyk and Motwani in [19]. The main property of LSH is that similar items have high probability to be collided being mapped into the same buckets. During the past decade many variants have been proposed and their success has been demonstrated [20–24]. In this research we use Multi-Probe Locality Sensitive Hashing (MPLSH) [22] as the implementation of LSH. MPLSH is based on p-stable distribution hashing [20], where each hash function is defined by:

$$h_{\mathbf{a},\mathbf{b}}(\mathbf{v}) = \lfloor \frac{\mathbf{a} \cdot \mathbf{v} + \mathbf{b}}{W} \rfloor \tag{3}$$

where a is a normalized d-dimensional random vector generated by a Gaussian distribution, W is a real number and b is a random number chosen in [0, W]. The multi-probe strategy aims at generating a probing sequence of buckets that are most likely to contain the most similar items, in order to obtain as many nearest neighbors as possible within an acceptable computing expense.

Algorithm 1. Learning step of our tracking algorithm (from the second frame)

Input:

the new target position p_t in the t-th frame f_t;

1: Obtain a set $S_pos = (s_j, y_i)|i = 1, 2, \ldots, L$ by sampling at each position within a radius $R1$ centered at p_t, then obtain the negative set $S_neg = (s_j, y_j)|j = 1, 2, \ldots M$ by randomly selecting M samples out of a radius R_2 with $R_1 < R_2$;

2: Update the SVM classifier by S_pos and S_neg, check if there is new positive support vector added;

3: **if** there is new positive support vector added **or** it is at the update period point, **then**

4: Obtain a set $S = (s_i, y_i)|i = 1, 2, \ldots, N$ containing all the N samples within a radius R_2 centered at p_t, with y_i being the associated transformation of s_i. Then insert each s_i into the LSH database;

5: **end if**

The main workflow of the learning step is described in Algorithm 1. For the first frame we conduct learning for both the LSH database and the SVM classifier. For the rest frames, we update the SVM classifier and check if any

Algorithm 2. Detection step of our tracking algorithm

Input:

t-th frame f_t; target position in the $t-1$-th frame p_{t-1};

Output:

target position p_t in the t-th frame $f-t$;

$p^0 = p_{t-1}$;
for $i = 1$ to M **do**
  Do similarity searching on p^{i-1} and get the neighbor set $P = p_k|k = 1, 2, \ldots, k$ containing K nearest neighbors in descending order of similarity with p^{i-1};
  for $j = 1$ to K **do**
    Obtain the temporal target position $p_j^{'} = p_j \circ y_j$ where y_j is the transformation associated with p_j;
    Extract the image patch I_j at $p_j^{'}$ and do a verification $SVM(I_j)$;
    if $SVM(I_j) = true$ **then**
      break;
    end if
  end for
  if there is one patch I_j that is verified to be valid **then**
    $p^i \leftarrow p_j^{'}$;
    $y^i \leftarrow y_j$;
  else
    $p^i \leftarrow p_1^{'}$;
    $y^i \leftarrow y_1$;
  end if
end for
$p_t = p^i$;

new positive support vector is added. If so, or if not but it is at the period point for static update, we update the LSH database. The sampling strategy for the SVM classifier is similar to [15] with a little modification, where positive samples are taken at every possible position that is close to the target, while negative samples are randomly chosen within an area far away from the target.

Algorithm 2 summarizes the detection step. As it states, estimation of the new target position is done for M rounds iteratively. For each round, K nearest neighbors are retrieved and sorted in descending order. SVM is then applied to verify each of them in order to pick the first valid one. The iteration stops either when it reaches M rounds or the most recent transformation y^i is smaller than a threshold δ. In this paper we set δ as 5 in pixels.

3 Experiments

3.1 Experiment Setup

We implement our algorithm by C++ in Linux-32 bit on a PC with an Intel Core i5 2.5 GHz CPU and 4 GB RAM. Similar with [6], we use Haar-like feature and generate a 192-dimension vector for each image patch. The Multi-Probe Locality

Table 1. The VOC overlap ratio (VOR) comparison results of 14 trackers over 15 sequences with an average value for each tracker. Numbers are represented in percentage. The best and the second best in each row is shown in bold and underlined, respectively

	Ours	MTT	CT	Frag	DFT	BSBT	L1APG	IVT	MIL	Struck	LSH	TLD	ASLA	VTD
Deer	**45.77**	21.30	2.73	11.73	45.58	13.29	39.61	13.71	37.85	44.86	4.93	34.63	4.87	41.27
Sylvester	73.63	71.17	60.79	60.35	25.43	62.14	35.68	54.60	8.46	**73.66**	62.17	61.36	63.89	61.24
Fish	**87.67**	64.51	66.92	49.21	65.86	60.60	86.18	81.54	61.92	82.19	85.70	67.71	84.73	51.46
Coke	**67.09**	59.28	26.91	3.69	15.01	27.04	21.66	10.56	3.25	56.55	16.30	17.04	18.56	12.06
Crossing	**71.18**	17.53	60.15	30.06	59.92	20.93	17.43	22.76	64.73	54.95	35.77	28.34	70.56	27.86
Couple	**68.28**	37.48	5.39	60.24	8.73	5.70	34.85	7.27	42.11	50.89	9.10	50.83	18.58	8.88
David	**55.49**	43.19	18.29	2.33	24.82	41.54	54.80	9.37	5.35	47.19	32.42	49.74	53.74	14.23
FaceOcc2	77.21	75.65	59.21	66.19	**77.94**	57.20	70.45	71.77	58.81	77.46	72.12	61.69	74.74	44.73
Football1	74.49	56.91	28.59	28.59	74.34	11.96	38.89	51.76	25.52	56.58	72.90	37.34	57.62	**77.62**
Boy	**78.02**	40.42	41.73	41.73	19.39	67.51	35.13	25.75	2.21	74.96	33.97	49.21	72.72	75.19
Jumping	64.31	6.96	31.52	**65.08**	5.96	26.25	42.22	20.25	28.31	60.84	12.11	57.20	24.26	10.47
MountainBike	77.14	71.08	12.95	10.59	**77.25**	63.20	67.98	39.79	12.60	70.80	73.51	18.52	69.59	34.03
Tiger1	64.11	32.44	13.40	34.95	58.17	27.37	42.48	12.96	4.95	63.90	12.41	47.19	31.83	**64.50**
Tiger2	55.00	46.58	41.79	7.66	34.39	21.50	58.94	17.86	12.52	**60.48**	12.97	54.94	18.46	25.29
Trellis	**71.91**	60.74	34.22	35.71	41.74	15.27	42.56	16.73	26.70	70.89	40.53	39.61	71.47	38.95
Average	**68.75**	47.02	33.64	33.87	42.30	34.77	45.92	30.45	26.35	63.08	38.46	45.02	49.04	39.19

Sensitive Hashing(MPLSH) is implemented by lshkit, a publicly available C++ library of the MPLSH algorithm, with the parameters where W is 1.0, the number of hash tables L is 4, the probing step level T is 5, and the nearest neighbors number K is 10. The online SVM algorithm, Larank, is implemented by our own code with reference to [6] but under the two-class setting, and we set the support vector budget as 200. A Gaussian kernel is applied and the slack value is set as 100. The learning radius for LSH database is 20. The positive sample radius R_1 for classifier update is set as 2 and the negative radius R_2 is 50. The static update frequency F is set as one per 4 frames for all the sequences.

Three evaluation metrics are applied here: VOC overlap ratio (VOR), center location error (CLE) and tracking success rate (SR), all calculated between algorithm output boxes B_o and ground truth boxes B_g. VOR is defined by $\frac{area(B_o \cap B_g)}{area(B_o \cup B_g)}$, CLE is defined as the average distance between the centers of B_o and B_g, and SR is defined as the ratio of frames whose VOR are larger than 50 % among all frames.

3.2 Quantitative Performance Evaluation

In this section we evaluate the performance of our algorithm by comparison with other 13 trackers. Among them, [4,15,16,25–30] have Matlab implementation in [31] and we use it directly in our experiment. For [5,6,32,33], we use the code posted on their corresponding websites. Fifteen publicly available sequences from [31] are selected for the comparison, and we use each sequence with its original length. The chosen sequences contain challenges such as illumination variation, fast motion, partial occlusion, in-plane and out-of-plane rotation, to name just a few. The ground truth data for the sequences are also collected from [31] except *David*, where we use the ground truth of all the frames from frame No. 1 to frame No. 771 given by [16] instead of from 300 to 771. The longer one contains larger illumination change and we regard it as a higher evaluation standard

Table 2. The center location error (CLE) comparison results of 14 trackers over 15 sequences with an average value for each tracker. Numbers are represented in pixels. The best and the second best in each row is shown in bold and underlined, respectively

	Ours	MTT	CT	Frag	DFT	BSBT	L1APG	IVT	MIL	Struck	LSH	TLD	ASLA	VTD
Deer	**12.35**	26.80	114.12	82.35	12.48	43.25	17.84	40.24	14.99	12.87	55.84	27.94	93.26	15.41
Sylvester	**5.78**	6.51	15.48	14.75	53.96	12.01	28.02	37.58	82.73	6.00	13.00	12.01	9.60	21.06
Fish	**2.86**	13.26	13.51	25.41	12.71	31.75	3.69	3.70	15.08	4.74	3.79	9.10	4.21	19.21
Coke	**5.81**	8.53	21.52	66.97	31.12	18.01	22.98	43.94	59.91	7.77	33.30	29.31	29.44	37.09
Crossing	2.26	40.20	5.52	37.52	7.88	45.82	53.37	3.01	4.19	6.66	25.43	22.97	**2.07**	39.32
Couple	**4.59**	36.51	103.84	9.54	112.79	88.10	27.45	96.20	37.75	33.32	111.77	18.37	89.91	105.88
David	**6.12**	17.75	41.67	114.50	41.97	18.51	11.69	220.06	75.50	14.01	24.28	15.11	6.83	76.53
FaceOcc2	6.96	9.18	17.69	14.71	7.47	31.03	9.06	6.91	19.37	**6.79**	10.02	14.75	8.34	51.35
Football1	3.35	11.90	18.75	18.75	5.76	46.82	13.94	19.12	17.46	7.04	3.76	78.81	6.50	**2.69**
Boy	1.34	24.23	29.85	29.85	76.43	5.48	35.10	51.80	26.84	1.92	19.38	2.45	1.47	**1.21**
Jumping	5.53	53.03	16.92	**4.50**	63.35	27.36	23.33	36.73	16.89	6.18	40.39	7.41	48.83	56.01
MountainBike	**3.14**	5.09	113.18	120.07	3.62	7.23	5.32	43.25	112.80	5.30	3.82	102.00	4.98	67.28
Tiger1	7.49	33.44	48.15	28.24	11.81	30.51	22.84	119.08	56.28	7.66	57.42	14.87	31.78	**7.32**
Tiger2	9.19	13.09	14.39	71.30	24.93	31.12	8.23	37.08	42.81	**7.19**	52.25	11.65	84.61	31.71
Trellis	7.35	13.42	39.43	56.25	48.22	80.69	38.69	122.35	54.70	8.53	59.14	16.89	**5.82**	37.48
Average	**5.61**	20.86	40.93	46.31	34.30	34.51	21.44	58.74	42.49	9.07	34.24	25.58	28.51	37.97

for algorithm performance. Tables 1, 2, and 3 show the results of performance comparison under the three criteria. Figure 3 provides a complete view of performance by plotting CLE frame-by-frame for all the 11 trackers on 15 sequences. As we can see, our algorithm has overall better performance over others, and even for the ones where our tracker does not get the best, its performance is still close to the best. For a concise display, we only show CLE plots here. VOR and SR plots can be found in our supplementary material.

3.3 Qualitative Performance Evaluation

In this section we discuss several key components of our algorithm and illustrate their contribution to the overall performance of our tracker. We treat our algorithm with different components as different algorithms and we do the similar experiments as the ones conducted in the last section. Similarly, we use the three same criteria to evaluate the overall performance on all the 15 sequences.

Table 3. The success rate (SR) comparison results of 14 trackers over 15 sequences with an average value for each tracker. Numbers are represented in pixels. The best and the second best in each row is shown in bold and underlined, respectively

	Ours	MTT	CT	Frag	DFT	BSBT	L1APG	IVT	MIL	Struck	LSH	TLD	ASLA	VTD
Deer	26.76	7.04	1.41	7.04	22.54	11.27	**33.80**	9.86	16.90	21.13	2.82	9.86	4.23	30.99
Sylvester	**96.65**	84.98	84.76	70.71	28.55	72.27	33.80	67.88	0.37	93.98	76.28	80.97	78.44	71.52
Fish	**100.00**	81.09	71.22	41.81	60.29	65.34	**100.00**	**100.00**	83.19	**100.00**	**100.00**	94.96	**100.00**	55.04
Coke	**89.00**	85.57	13.06	3.44	9.62	24.74	22.68	13.40	1.37	57.73	15.12	15.12	15.81	12.71
Crossing	**100.00**	22.50	76.67	40.83	66.67	23.33	22.50	23.33	86.67	70.83	41.67	23.33	95.00	38.33
Couple	**76.43**	32.86	5.00	70.00	10.00	7.14	32.86	8.57	57.14	61.43	10.00	55.71	23.57	10.71
David	76.62	53.90	7.79	0.13	13.38	36.88	**84.42**	15.97	0.13	64.16	12.34	57.79	71.17	7.01
FaceOcc2	**100.00**	96.06	71.31	75.25	100.00	65.02	96.31	92.36	77.83	99.75	98.03	73.77	94.58	51.23
Football1	**100.00**	59.46	25.68	25.68	87.84	10.81	33.78	63.51	9.46	54.05	97.30	51.35	51.35	**100.00**
Boy	**99.34**	48.01	53.16	53.16	23.59	87.21	43.85	30.90	0.33	98.50	32.89	42.86	97.84	**99.67**
Jumping	**98.72**	6.39	16.29	96.81	8.63	31.31	64.22	25.56	1.28	93.61	12.46	77.96	33.23	14.38
MountainBike	**100.00**	**100.00**	16.67	11.84	**100.00**	89.04	89.91	52.63	16.23	90.35	98.25	25.44	93.86	42.11
Tiger1	**87.29**	37.57	2.54	40.11	72.88	25.14	43.50	15.54	2.82	86.72	10.45	55.65	38.14	79.10
Tiger2	63.84	51.23	33.70	9.59	39.18	13.15	75.34	20.82	11.51	**77.81**	14.25	69.86	22.74	20.27
Trellis	**95.61**	67.66	37.08	42.18	51.14	11.25	51.14	17.93	31.99	93.67	43.76	50.44	89.81	44.99
Average	**87.35**	55.62	34.42	39.24	46.29	38.26	55.21	37.22	26.48	77.58	44.37	52.34	60.65	45.20

Table 4. Comparison results of our algorithm with different frequency values on 15 sequences based on VOC overlap rate (VOR), center location error (CLE), and success rate (SR). We only display the best result in bold under each criterion for clarity and conciseness

	VOR					CLE					SR				
Sequences	F=1	F=2	F=4	F=8	F=inf	F=1	F=2	F=4	F=8	F=inf	F=1	F=2	F=4	F=8	F=inf
Deer	**47.03**	46.31	45.77	46.11	45.47	**11.98**	12.25	12.35	12.24	12.42	**33.80**	23.94	26.76	28.17	28.17
Sylvester	66.95	58.33	**73.63**	62.13	64.95	9.78	33.21	**5.78**	15.02	11.99	82.16	80.45	**96.65**	72.19	80.00
Fish	49.32	85.77	**87.67**	86.40	86.40	27.06	3.76	**2.86**	3.54	3.54	59.45	**100.00**	**100.00**	**100.00**	**100.00**
Coke	50.91	56.16	**67.09**	66.17	66.17	9.25	8.05	5.81	**5.60**	**5.60**	52.58	72.16	**89.00**	83.51	83.51
Crossing	36.64	28.32	71.18	**71.34**	19.30	25.78	54.94	**2.26**	2.61	64.34	48.33	38.33	**100.00**	**100.00**	24.17
Couple	54.75	65.73	**68.28**	27.92	47.88	17.83	5.55	**4.59**	70.95	42.61	64.29	75.71	**76.43**	32.86	64.29
David	54.34	43.74	**55.49**	53.39	53.39	6.61	16.74	**6.12**	8.71	8.71	75.32	52.21	**76.62**	74.42	74.42
Faceocc2	69.79	**78.44**	77.21	77.09	75.85	12.88	**6.27**	6.96	6.56	7.10	86.70	**100.00**	**100.00**	**100.00**	**100.00**
Football1	43.24	41.66	**74.49**	66.30	50.91	26.42	49.78	**3.35**	5.01	10.64	51.35	51.35	**100.00**	74.32	54.05
Boy	70.53	67.06	**78.02**	69.74	26.76	2.46	3.35	**1.34**	2.53	20.87	97.67	88.04	**99.34**	95.51	31.73
Jumping	62.51	**64.79**	64.31	19.76	63.68	5.86	**5.35**	5.53	54.23	5.77	97.44	98.40	98.72	29.71	**99.36**
MountainBike	33.74	62.82	**77.14**	55.43	20.35	63.72	6.73	**3.14**	48.80	105.07	40.35	91.23	**100.00**	69.74	26.32
Tiger1	23.34	28.12	**64.11**	54.29	9.57	58.52	62.94	**7.49**	10.84	55.84	19.77	36.16	**87.29**	50.28	5.08
Tiger2	21.48	46.18	**55.93**	19.65	18.02	36.75	18.61	**9.60**	60.29	79.96	24.38	48.22	**63.84**	24.93	22.19
Trellis	47.42	28.76	**71.91**	57.66	21.22	29.60	82.90	**7.35**	18.38	74.28	50.79	36.20	**95.61**	69.42	25.48

For each of the following two components, we tune one at a time and control the other by setting it as the default value. The defaults values are $F = 4$ and $K = 20$.

Static LSH Update Frequency *F*. The static LSH update frequency determines the regular learning pace and therefore ensures the sufficiency of information. We set this parameter as 1, 2, 4, 8, infinite, respectively, meaning that the LSH database is updated every 1, 2, 4, 8 frames in addition to the dynamic strategy and infinite means there is no static frequency and updating only depends on the dynamic control. Table 4 shows the comparative performance under the

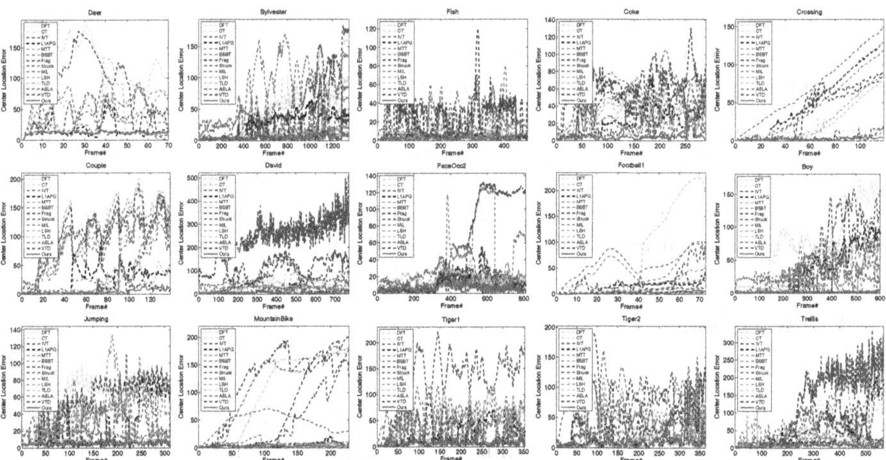

Fig. 5. The frame-by-frame center location error (CLE) plots for all the 15 sequences. Our method is drawn in red (Color figure online).

Table 5. Comparison results of our algorithm with different numbers of nearest neighbors on 15 sequences based on VOC overlap rate (VOR), center location error (CLE), and success rate (SR). We only display the best result in bold under each criterion for clarity and conciseness

	VOR				CLE				SR			
Squences	K=1	K=5	K=10	K=20	K=1	K=5	K=10	K=20	K=1	K=5	K=10	K=20
Deer	41.95	**45.77**	**45.77**	**45.77**	20.25	**12.35**	**12.35**	**12.35**	**29.58**	26.76	26.76	26.76
Sylvester	72.62	73.17	**73.63**	**73.63**	6.22	5.97	**5.78**	**5.78**	95.76	95.76	**96.65**	**96.65**
Fish	84.34	87.63	**87.67**	**87.67**	4.58	**2.85**	2.86	2.86	**100.00**	**100.00**	**100.00**	**100.00**
Coke	**70.01**	63.83	67.09	17.74	**4.69**	6.44	5.81	52.27	87.29	82.47	**89.00**	23.37
Crossing	69.00	**71.18**	**71.18**	**71.18**	3.66	**2.26**	**2.26**	**2.26**	95.00	**100.00**	**100.00**	**100.00**
Couple	56.30	**68.28**	**68.28**	**68.28**	38.49	**4.59**	**4.59**	**4.59**	72.14	**76.43**	**76.43**	**76.43**
David	53.35	53.56	**55.49**	**55.49**	8.38	8.23	**6.12**	**6.12**	71.82	71.69	**76.62**	**76.62**
Faceocc2	**77.78**	77.21	77.21	77.10	**6.71**	6.97	6.96	7.01	**100.00**	**100.00**	**100.00**	**100.00**
Football1	30.12	55.28	**74.49**	**74.49**	83.71	10.54	**3.35**	**3.35**	32.43	62.16	**100.00**	**100.00**
Boy	76.96	76.96	**78.02**	**78.02**	1.56	1.56	**1.34**	**1.34**	99.00	99.00	**99.34**	**99.34**
Jumping	19.79	**64.31**	**64.31**	**64.31**	56.70	**5.53**	**5.53**	**5.53**	30.03	**98.72**	**98.72**	**98.72**
MountainBike	53.57	**77.14**	**77.14**	**77.14**	48.82	**3.14**	**3.14**	**3.14**	66.23	**100.00**	**100.00**	**100.00**
Tiger1	8.04	64.01	**64.11**	24.30	52.65	7.88	**7.49**	56.60	8.47	84.75	**87.29**	30.79
Tiger2	**60.43**	56.41	55.93	30.03	7.85	9.17	9.60	61.02	**73.97**	64.38	63.84	36.99
Trellis	64.78	65.09	**71.91**	46.21	12.31	11.58	**7.35**	57.03	73.99	85.59	**95.61**	54.13

three metrics on all the 15 sequences. As we can observe, for each of the three criteria, our algorithm performs best in terms of overall accuracy when F is 4, which is a proper value to keep the learning pace reasonably slow and satisfy the purpose of preventing data redundancy.

Number of Retrieved Nearest Neighbors *K*. Intuitively, the larger this parameter is, the more positive neighbors there will be, and correspondingly the more confident the results will be. However, a neighbor set with larger size also contains more weak neighbors, which may increase the risk of false verification by the classifier. Here, we aim to evaluate the effect of this factor by setting K as 5, 10, 15, and 20 and apply the same experiments on each of them. Table 5 shows the comparative performance under the three metrics on the 15 sequences. As shown, 10 is the best value for K in terms of overall performance. It is worth noticing that for most of the sequences the results of $K = 10$ and $K = 20$ are the same. This is a desirable property because it indicates that most positive nearest neighbor is among the top 10 in the neighbors list. Thus, it is not necessary to retrieve large amount of neighbors to achieve promising performance.

4 Conclusion

In this paper we propose a novel tracking framework based on cooperation of unsupervised similarity searching and supervised classification. We regard tracking as a problem of similarity matching on streaming data, and use an SVM based classifier to improve its accuracy and control the LSH learning frequency. From a learning view of point, this strategy is an innovative variant of the well-studied classification-based tracking, which assigns each sample with a confidence value while our method directly assigns the transformation structure. Benefiting from that, our method avoids the brute-force search within the output space and successfully alleviates the intrinsic obscurity of supervised approaches in describing targets. We show experimentally that our tracker has superior performance over state-of-art trackers.

We do believe that the proposed tracking framework contributes to a brand new field where more unsupervised strategies could be introduced into tracking. Future studies can be done based on this framework, such as using other unsupervised structures for similarity matching and applying more sophisticated novelty detection algorithms for controlling updating frequency. Besides, transformation model can also be enriched in order to include more variation types such as rotation and scale changes.

References

1. Avidan, S.: Support vector tracking. IEEE Trans. Pattern Anal. Mach. Intell. **26**, 1064–1072 (2004)
2. Grabner, H., Grabner, M., Bischof, H.: Real-time tracking via online boosting. In: BMVC, pp. 47–56 (2006)
3. Grabner, H., Leistner, C., Bischof, H.: Semi-supervised on-line boosting for robust tracking. In: Forsyth, D., Torr, P., Zisserman, A. (eds.) ECCV 2008, Part I. LNCS, vol. 5302, pp. 234–247. Springer, Heidelberg (2008)
4. Stalder, S., Grabner, H., Gool., L.V.: Beyond semi-supervised tracking: tracking should be as simple as detection, but not simpler than recognition. In: 2009 IEEE 12th International Conference on Computer Vision Workshops (ICCV Workshops), pp. 1409–1416 (2009)
5. Babenko, B., Yang, M.H., Belongie., S.: Visual tracking with online multiple instance learning. In: Computer Vision and Pattern Recognition 2009, pp. 983–990 (2009)
6. Hare, S., Saffari, A., Torr., P.H.: Struck: structured output tracking with kernels. In: 2011 IEEE International Conference on Computer Vision (ICCV), pp. 263–270 (2011)
7. Bordes, A., Bottou, L., Gallinari, P., Weston., J.: Solving multiclass support vector machines with larank. In: Proceedings of the 24th International Conference on Machine Learning, pp. 89–96 (2007)
8. Bordes, A., Usunier, N., Bottou, L.: Sequence labelling SVMs trained in one pass. In: Daelemans, W., Goethals, B., Morik, K. (eds.) ECML PKDD 2008, Part I. LNCS (LNAI), vol. 5211, pp. 146–161. Springer, Heidelberg (2008)
9. Crammer, K., Kandola, J.S., Singer., Y.: Online classification on a budget. In: Neural Information Processing Systems (NIPS), vol. 2, 5 (2003)
10. Wang, Z., Crammer, K., Vucetic., S.: Multi-class pegasos on a budget. In: Proceedings of the 27th International Conference on Machine Learning (ICML 2010), vol. 2, pp. 1143–1150 (2010)
11. Yao, R., Shi, Q., Shen, C., Zhang, Y., van den Hengel, A.: Robust tracking with weighted online structured learning. In: Fitzgibbon, A., Lazebnik, S., Perona, P., Sato, Y., Schmid, C. (eds.) ECCV 2012, Part III. LNCS, vol. 7574, pp. 158–172. Springer, Heidelberg (2012)

12. Yao, R., Shi, Q., Shen, C., Zhang, Y., van den Hengel., A.: Part-based visual tracking with online latent structural learning. In: Computer Vision and Pattern Recognition (CVPR) 2013, pp. 2363–2370 (2013)
13. Li, X., Shen, C., Dick, A., van den Hengel., A.: Learning compact binary codes for visual tracking. In: Computer Vision and Pattern Recognition (CVPR) 2013, pp. 2419–2426 (2013)
14. Saffari, A., Leistner, C., Santner, J., Godec, M., Bischof., H.: On-line random forests. In: Computer Vision Workshops (ICCV Workshops) 2009, pp. 1393–1400 (2009)
15. Zhang, K., Zhang, L., Yang, M.-H.: Real-time compressive tracking. In: Fitzgibbon, A., Lazebnik, S., Perona, P., Sato, Y., Schmid, C. (eds.) ECCV 2012, Part III. LNCS, vol. 7574, pp. 864–877. Springer, Heidelberg (2012)
16. Kalal, Z., Mikolajczyk, K., Matas, J.: Tracking-learning-detection. IEEE Trans. Pattern Anal. Mach. Intell. **34**, 864–877 (2012)
17. Schlkopf, B., Williamson, R.C., Smola, A.J., Shawe-Taylor, J., Platt., J.C.: Support vector method for novelty detection. In: Neural Information Processing Systems(NIPS), vol. 12, pp. 582–588 (1999)
18. Gmez-Verdejo, V., Arenas-Garca, J., Lazaro-Gredilla, M., Navia-Vazquez, A.: Adaptive one-class support vector machine. IEEE Trans. Signal Process. **59**, 2975–2981 (2011)
19. Indyk, P., Motwani., R.: Approximate nearest neighbors: towards removing the curse of dimensionality. In: Proceedings of the Thirtieth Annual ACM Symposium on Theory of Computing, pp. 604–613 (1998)
20. Datar, M., Immorlica, N., Indyk, P., Mirrokni., V.S.: Locality-sensitive hashing scheme based on p-stable distributions. In: Proceedings of the Twentieth Annual Symposium on Computational Geometry, pp. 253–262 (2004)
21. Weiss, Y., Torralba, A., Fergus., R.: Spectral hashing. In: Neural Information Processing Systems (NIPS), vol. 9, 6 (2008)
22. Lv, Q., Josephson, W., Wang, Z., Charikar, M., Li., K.: Multi-probe LSH: efficient indexing for high-dimensional similarity search. In: Proceedings of the 33rd International Conference on Very large Data Bases, pp. 950–961 (2007)
23. Kulis, B., Grauman., K.: Kernelized locality-sensitive hashing for scalable image search. In: 2009 IEEE 12th International Conference on Computer Vision, pp. 2130–2137 (2009)
24. Heo, J.P., Lee, Y., He, J., Chang, S.F., Yoon., S.E.: Spherical hashing. In: 2012 IEEE Conference on Computer Vision and Pattern Recognition (CVPR), pp. 2957–2964 (2012)
25. Zhang, T., Ghanem, B., Liu, S., Ahuja., N.: Robust visual tracking via multi-task sparse learning. In: 2012 IEEE Conference on Computer Vision and Pattern Recognition (CVPR), pp. 2042–2049 (2012)
26. Adam, A., Rivlin, E., Shimshoni., I.: Robust fragments-based tracking using the integral histogram. In: 2012 IEEE Conference on Computer Vision and Pattern Recognition (CVPR), pp.798–805 (2006)
27. Sevilla-Lara, L., Learned-Miller., E.: Distribution fields for tracking. In: 2012 IEEE Conference on Computer Vision and Pattern Recognition (CVPR), pp.1910–1917 (2012)
28. Bao, C., Wu, Y., Ling, H., Ji., H.: Real time robust l1 tracker using accelerated proximal gradient approach. In: 2012 IEEE Conference on Computer Vision and Pattern Recognition (CVPR), pp.1830–1837 (2012)
29. Ross, D.A., Lim, J., Lin, R.S., Yang, M.H.: Incremental learning for robust visual tracking. International Journal of Computer Vision (IJCV) **77**, 125–141 (2012)

30. Jia, X., Lu, H., Yang., M.H.: Visual tracking via adaptive structural local sparse appearance model. In: 2012 IEEE Conference on Computer Vision and Pattern Recognition (CVPR), pp. 1822–1829 (2012)
31. Wu, Y., Lim, J., Yang., M.H.: Online object tracking: A benchmark. In: 2013 IEEE Conference on Computer Vision and Pattern Recognition (CVPR), pp. 2411–2418 (2013)
32. He, S., Yang, Q., Lau, R.W., Wang, J., Yang., M.H.: Visual tracking via locality sensitive histograms. In: 2013 IEEE Conference on Computer Vision and Pattern Recognition (CVPR), pp. 2427–2434 (2013)
33. Kwon, J., Lee., K.M.: Visual tracking decomposition. In: 2010 IEEE Conference on Computer Vision and Pattern Recognition (CVPR), pp. 1269–1276 (2010)

Multi-state Discriminative Video Segment Selection for Complex Event Classification

Prithviraj Banerjee(✉) and Ram Nevatia

University of Southern California, Los Angeles, USA
pbanerje@usc.edu

Abstract. Recognizing long range complex events composed of a sequence of primitive actions is a challenging task, as videos may not be consistently aligned in time with respect to the primitive actions across video examples. Moreover, there can exist arbitrary long intervals between, and within the execution of primitive actions. We propose a novel multistate segment selection algorithm, which pools features from the discriminative segments of a video. We present an efficient linear programming based solution, and introduce novel linear constraints to enforce temporal ordering between segments from different states. We also propose a regularized version of our algorithm, which automatically determines the optimum number of segments to be selected in each video. Furthermore, we present a new, provably faster $O(N \log N)$ algorithm for the single state K-segment selection problem. Our results are validated on the Composite Cooking Activity dataset, containing videos of cooking recipes.

1 Introduction

Human activity recognition is a fundamental problem in computer vision. The difficulty of the task varies greatly based on the complexity of the actions themselves, and the imaging conditions. It is useful to characterize the activities as falling into three broad classes. Firstly, is the class of relatively short period activities consisting of primitive actions such as shake, hug and wave [1], and snippets of sport activities like diving, golf-swing [2] *etc.* A second category of activities consist of complex events naturally described as a composition of simpler and shorter term primitive actions; examples include videos of cooking recipes and assembly instructions, which take place in a structured environment consisting of fixed camera and consistent background structures, such as kitchen tops and shelves. Lastly, there is the category of *videos in the wild*, such as amateur video uploads on YouTube, where there is significant variety in camera pose and challenging background environments.

The focus of this work lies on the second category of activities. Even though the three categories face common challenges caused by ambiguities inherent to

We thank Marcus Rohrbach for his help in providing the MP2 Cooking Composite Activities dataset. This research was supported, in part, by the Office of Naval Research under grant #N00014-13-1-0493.

D. Cremers et al. (Eds.): ACCV 2014, Part V, LNCS 9007, pp. 162–177, 2015.
DOI: 10.1007/978-3-319-16814-2_11

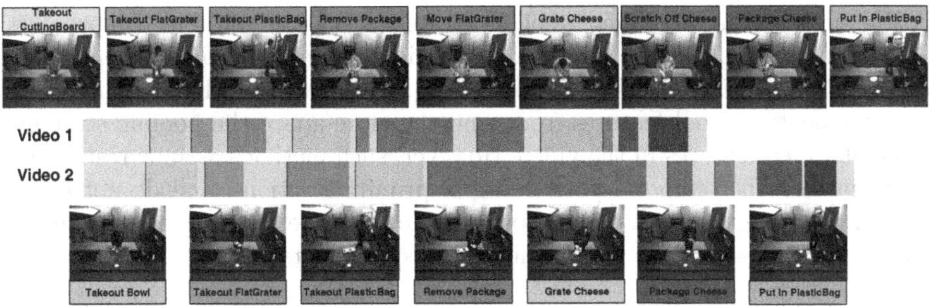

Fig. 1. Composite event *Grating Cheese* is composed of numerous primitive actions which occur with varying durations and arbitrary gaps between them, making it a challenge to learn a composite event classifier.

images and variations in the actor clothing, style and background variations, there are also significant differences. For the shorter-term activities, local features such as STIPs or Dense Trajectory (DT) features aggregated by methods such as Bag of Words [3,4] or Fisher Vectors [5] have been found to give good performance. However, such methods are not adequate for the more complex events due to the much larger variations possible in such activities. Consider the example of *grating cheese* illustrated in Fig. 1, where the relatively straightforward task of retrieving cheese from the refrigerator, unwrapping it, grating it and replacing the cheese back, is performed in varying styles by two different actors. Some actors retrieve a bowl (or a tray) before (or after) retrieving the grater, resulting in only a loose temporal ordering between the primitive states of the activity, making it difficult to estimate a fixed temporal distribution of the states in a video sequence. Moreover, there are significant variations in the duration of each state due to different speeds and styles of the actors, and optional actions like *moving the grater* may cause large gaps between the essential states of the event. The task becomes even more challenging due to gaps appearing within the execution of a state, as actors tend to take breaks during long actions, like *grating cheese*, and hence violating the usual assumption of temporal continuity with respect to primitive action executions. However, we note that certain long range temporal relationships are not violated, such as retrieving the cheese before grating it, and a composite event recognizer should learn such relationships.

Furthermore, such videos may contain many intervals that are not of direct relevance to the activity of interest, for example, resting in between parts of the task. Some of these variations may be captured by spatio-temporal feature pooling strategies [3,6], where the video is divided into spatio-temporal grids of histograms. However, rigid grid quantizations are not likely to be sufficient for un-aligned and un-cropped videos [4], and are sensitive to temporal variations in action executions. There has been work representing such activities by dynamical graphical models such as Dynamic Bayesian Networks [7,8]; however, these representations can be highly sensitive to varying time intervals and spurious intervening activities.

We suggest that dynamic pooling strategies offer a suitable compromise between static pooling and the rigid dynamical models. Dynamic pooling has been used in previous works, such as [2,9,10], which identify the discriminative video segments to pool features from, and therefore adapt the pooling strategy to the observed features in the video. However, such methods assume restrictive constraints on the temporal positioning of primitive actions, and do not allow for arbitrary length inter-action gaps, and furthermore restrict the hypothesis space for primitive actions to continuous video segments only.

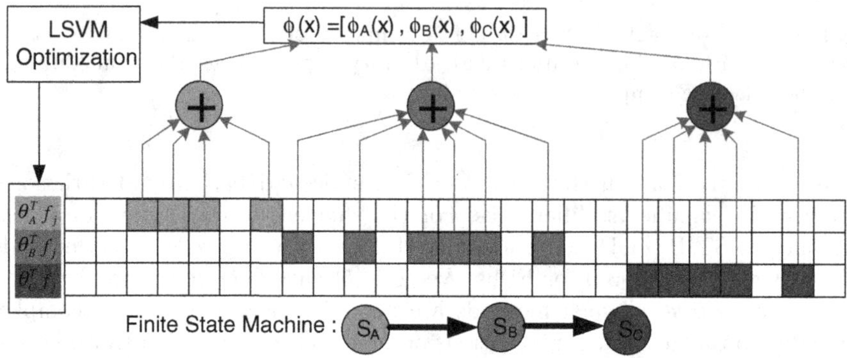

Fig. 2. Flow diagram for multistate dynamic feature pooling algorithm. A 3-state finite state machine is assumed, which specifies a temporal ordering as $S_A < S_B < S_C$. Segment classification scores are computed $w.r.t$ each state, and the discriminative segments are selected by solving a linear programe. The aggregate feature statistics from the selected segments are pooled to compute a global feature statistic $\Phi(x)$. which is used for training a Latent-SVM classifier, and hence learn the optimal activity classification weights θ. The weight learning and feature poolling is repeated iteratively till convergence.

Our work is closest in spirit to [11], which proposed a dynamic pooling algorithm that treats the locations of characteristic segments of the video as latent variables which are inferred for each video sequence in a LSVM framework. The possible set of segment selections is combinatorial in size, and they propose a fractional integer linear programming based solution to obtain the exact solution. However, [11] does not distinguish between the primitive actions in a video during pooling, and incorporates only weak pair-wise temporal associations by considering an exhaustive set of segment pairs during both training and testing phase, making it unsuitable for long-term complex event recognition.

We are motivated to extend the segment selection algorithm [11] to incorporate learning of temporal relationships between primitive actions, and propose a novel temporal segment selection algorithm for complex event recognition. We formulate the task of multi-state dynamic feature pooling as a linear programming optimization problem, where the discriminative weights for feature classification are learned iteratively in a latent support vector machine (LSVM). Figure 2 presents an overview of our approach while assuming a three state model. Aggregate statistics, such as histograms of spatio-temporal features are computed from overlapping segments of the video, and a classification score is assigned to each segment *w.r.t* each state. The discriminative segments are identified on a per-state basis, and a global feature vector Φ is pooled from the selected segments, which is used to train the LSVM classifier. Our algorithm is simultaneously (1) robust to arbitrary gaps between primitive states while respecting their temporal ordering, (2) robust to gaps within primitive states caused by varying durations of primitive action executions, and (3) selects the discriminative sub-segments of the video for classifying the composite event. Our algorithm eschews any manual annotations of the states during training, and instead automatically infers the important states from the training data.

Our key contributions are multi fold: (1) We present a new provably fast solution to the K-segment selection problem, which improves the running time of the previously proposed [11] fractional linear program based solution to $O(N \log N)$, (2) we present a regularized linear programming optimization for multi-state K-segment selection for dynamic feature pooling, and finally (3) propose a novel extension to our linear program for automatically determining the number of discriminative segments in a video, and hence avoiding pooling features from non-informative (*w.r.t* to the complex event label) video segments.

We validate our algorithm on the recently introduced Composite Cooking Dataset [12], which consists of a collection of cooking recipe demonstrations performed by multiple actors while following a weakly enforced script. Each recipe is a long term composite event, consisting of a series of primitive actions like opening cupboard, taking out toaster, peeling vegetables *etc*, and we show significantly improved results on the dataset, along with an analysis of the discriminative segments selected by our algorithm.

2 Related Work

We focus our survey on classification algorithms using different feature pooling strategies, and also briefly review algorithms modeling temporal structure of complex activities.

Static pooling algorithm model the (x, y, t) distribution of features in the 3-dimensional video volume, and fix the pooling strategy before commencing classifier training, and do not adapt dynamically to the features statistics observed during training. A popular class of pooling strategy divides the video into multiple spatio-temporal grids [3,6], and concatenates the feature statistics computed from each of the grids into a global video-wide feature vector, while other approaches construct interest point centric histograms [4,13,14], where feature statistics are accumulated from static spatio-temporal grids centered around each detected interest point. However, the *static* nature of the feature pooling grids assumes that the underlying action is consistently aligned with the video, and makes it sensitive to time and duration shifts in action instances.

In real life videos, the actions of interest might occur in only small a fraction of the frames. Restricting the classifier to the important video segments [15,16] has been shown to improve recognition accuracy, emphasizing the importance of *dynamic* feature pooling algorithms, which only compute feature statistics from the important segments of a video, determined dynamically during training. While some algorithms ignore the temporal structure, and select only a single continuous subsequence [15,17] of the video, others represent the video as a sequence of atomic segments [2,9,10] and either learn or manually define temporal relationships between the segments. A variety of atomic segment representations have been proposed such as histogram of codewords over temporal [2] and spatio-temporal volumes [10], poselet based representation of human actions [18], and scene context based video decomposition [19]. However they either ignore temporal ordering [19], or assume well cropped videos without arbitrary gaps between the atomic segments [2,10], while [18] selects only a small number of discrete frames, and requires a manually defined set of relevant poselets, further restricting it to primitive single-human actions.

A popular class of approaches represent the complex event as a sequence of state transition of a finite state machine, where the state definitions can be semantic, such as human key-poses [7] or linear interpolations between 3D joint positions [8]. Other approaches favor non semantic state definitions based on low level feature, such as discriminative motion patches [20] and histogram of gradient/flow features [21]. The event label is inferred using either logic models [22], or generative [23] and conditional [8,24] probabilistic graphical models like HMM and CRF. Such methods have shown robust performance on short duration activities like walking, jumping *etc.*, however due to their inherent Markovian nature, they are unable to handle long range dependencies between primitive action segments, and are sensitive to variations in duration and style of action execution. Recently, [21] proposed a conditional variable duration HMM model for action classification on youtube videos, however it does not distinguish between video segments based on relevance to the composite event, and instead attempts to model every segment as a valid state, making it susceptible to spurious features from unimportant segments.

3 Pooling Interest Point Features for Event Classification

Classical framework for event recognition using low level image features consists of a three stage process: detection, pooling and classification. The detection stage consists of computing a set of descriptors $\mathbf{x}_i = \{\boldsymbol{x}_k\}$ from spatio-temporal interest point detections in the ith video. The pooling stage involves combining the multiple local feature descriptors into a single global feature $\Phi(\mathbf{x}_i)$ representation of the video. Lastly in the classification stage, discriminative classifiers like support vector machines are trained using the global features as training data.

Our contributions are in the feature pooling stage of the framework. We present a new, provably faster, algorithm to a previous segment selection algorithm by Li et al. [11]. We further propose a novel algorithm for pooling features from the discriminative time intervals of a video, while modeling the temporal dynamics present in the activity in a joint optimization framework. We also present an extension to our algorithm which automatically determines the optimum number of segments to select.

3.1 Discriminative Segment Selection

We first describe the basic framework of discriminative segment selection, where the video is divided into N equal-length temporal segments. Let $\mathbf{f}_j$ be the locally pooled feature computed from the jth segment, where the pooling criteria can be as simple as computing a histogram of codewords detected within the segment. The global feature descriptor is computed by pooling a subset of the segments:

$$\Phi(\mathbf{x}, \mathbf{h}) = \frac{\sum_j \mathbf{f}_j h_j}{\sum_j e_j h_j} \quad , \quad \Phi^*_{\boldsymbol{\theta},\mathbf{x}} = \max_{\boldsymbol{h}} \boldsymbol{\theta}^T \Phi(\mathbf{x}, \boldsymbol{h}) = \max_{\boldsymbol{h}} \frac{\sum_j \boldsymbol{\theta}^T \mathbf{f}_j h_j}{\sum_j e_j h_j} \qquad (1)$$

where h_j is a binary variable indicating the selection of the jth segment, and e_j is a strictly positive constant which normalizes the $\Phi(\cdot)$ with respect to the number of segments selected. A variety of representations can be chosen for $\mathbf{f}_j$ and e_j, for example, setting $\mathbf{f}_j$ as the histogram of codewords and e_j as the sum of codewords appearing in the jth segment results in the classical BoW feature.

The discriminative weight vector $\boldsymbol{\theta}$ computes the score c_j corresponding to each segment, where the score is proportional to the importance of the segment in classifying the given event. The weight vector $\boldsymbol{\theta}$ is learned using a Latent-SVM optimization [25,26]:

$$\min_{\boldsymbol{\theta}} \frac{1}{2}\|\boldsymbol{\theta}\|_2^2 + C\sum_{i\in\mathcal{P}} \max\left(1, \Phi^*_{\boldsymbol{\theta},\mathbf{x}_i}\right) + C\sum_{i\in\mathcal{N}} \max\left(0, 1+\Phi^*_{\boldsymbol{\theta},\mathbf{x}_i}\right) - C\sum_{i\in\mathcal{P}} \Phi^*_{\boldsymbol{\theta},\mathbf{x}_i} \quad (2)$$

where $\mathcal{P}$ and $\mathcal{N}$ are the set of positive and negative training examples.

3.2 $\mathcal{K}$-Segment Selection (KSS)

Inference of the latent variable $\boldsymbol{h}$ in Eq. 1 determines the important segments in a video, and the inference algorithm can be stated as a $\mathcal{K}$-segment selection problem, where the objective is to select the $\mathcal{K}$ most optimum segments from a video for classification purpose, and is equivalent to solving the following fractional integer linear program:

$$\text{KSS}(\mathcal{K}): \quad \text{maximize} \frac{\sum_{j=1}^N c_j h_j}{\sum_{j=1}^N e_j h_j} \quad \text{s.t.} \quad \sum_{j=1}^N h_j = \mathcal{K} \quad , \quad \forall_j h_j \in \{0,1\} \quad (3)$$

where $c_j = \boldsymbol{\theta}^T \mathbf{f}_j$ is the classification score value corresponding to the feature vector $\mathbf{f}_j$, pooled from the jth segment. Li et al. [11] proposed a relaxed linear programming solution to solve the above integer problem, where the fractional linear program is transformed to an equivalent standard linear program [27]. An optimal solution to the linear program is computed using the standard simplex algorithm, which has exponential worst case complexity, and on average polynomial time complexity. We next present a provably faster algorithm to solve the $\mathcal{K}$-segment selection problem.

3.3 Linear Time Subset Scanning

Our key observation is that selecting the optimum $\mathcal{K}$ segments in a video by optimizing Eq. 3, is equivalent to solving the Linear Time Subset Scanning (LTSS) problem [28]. We give a brief introduction to the LTSS problem, and refer the readers to [28] for the details. Let us define a subset $\mathcal{S} = \{j \ni h_j = 1\}$, and define the following two additive statistics over the subset: $X(\mathcal{S}) = \sum_{j \in \mathcal{S}} c_j$ and $Y(\mathcal{S}) = \sum_{j \in \mathcal{S}} e_j$. We further define a subset scoring function $F(\mathcal{S}) = F(X, Y) = \frac{X(\mathcal{S})}{Y(\mathcal{S})}$ according to which we want to select the best possible subset. For all scoring functions $F(\mathcal{S})$ satisfying the LTSS property, the optimal subset $\mathcal{S}$ maximizing the score can be found by ordering the elements of the set according to some *priority* function $G(j)$, and selecting the top $\mathcal{K}$ highest priority elements.

A scoring function $F(\mathcal{S})$ satisfies the LTSS property (Theorem 1 [28]) with priority function $G(j) = \frac{c_j}{e_j}$, if (1) $F(\mathcal{S}) = F(X, Y)$ is a quasi-convex function of two additive sufficient statistics of subset $\mathcal{S}$, (2) $F(\mathcal{S})$ is monotonically increasing with $X(\mathcal{S})$, and (3) all additive elements of $Y(\mathcal{S})$ are positive. In our case, the scoring function $F(\mathcal{S}) = \frac{\sum_{j \in \mathcal{S}} c_j}{\sum_{j \in \mathcal{S}} e_j} = \frac{\sum_j c_j h_j}{\sum_j e_j h_j} = F(\boldsymbol{h})$ is a ratio of linear functions in the segment selector variable vector $\boldsymbol{h}$, and hence can be shown to be quasi-convex [27] using a simple analysis of its α-sublevel sets. Monotonicity of $F(\boldsymbol{h})$ w.r.t. $X(\mathcal{S})$ is shown due to them being linearly related, and furthermore, e_j are strictly positive by design, as they represent the normalization factor for each segment. Hence, the $\mathcal{K}$-Segment Selection problem satisfies the LTSS property with priority function $G(j) = \frac{c_j}{e_j}$. To select the optimum $\mathcal{K}$ segments, we sort the set of segment scores: $\left\{\frac{c_j}{e_j}\right\}_{j=1}^{N}$, and select the segments corresponding to the top $\mathcal{K}$ scores. Therefore our algorithm reduces the $\mathcal{K}$-segment selection problem to a simple sorting problem with a time complexity of $O(N \log N)$, which is an order of magnitude faster than solving a linear program. Note, that we only require an unordered list of the top $\mathcal{K}$ segments, and hence, one can select the $\mathcal{K}^{th}$ largest element using the linear time median-of-medians selection algorithm, and select the top $\mathcal{K}$ segments through a linear traversal over all the segments, which solves the problem in $O(N)$ linear time.

4 Multistate K-Segment Selection (MKSS)

The $\mathcal{K}$-segment selection algorithm [11] does not consider the temporal relationships between the selected segments, and hence ignores the temporal ordering of primitive action sequences composing a complex event. In effect, it can be viewed as a *single state* segment selection. We are motivated to extend the $\mathcal{K}$-segment selection algorithm to a multi-state formulation, where each state corresponds to discriminative primitive actions present in the video. Let us consider a two state problem, where our objective is to select the optimum sub-segments for both state A and state B, such that state A occurs in the video before state B. This is equivalent to a finite state machine where state A transitions to state

B. We define $\mathbf{h}^A, \mathbf{h}^B \in \{0,1\}^N$ as the segment selection indicator vectors corresponding to the two states. To ensure the temporal ordering in the selected subsegments, we construct the following constraint:

$$\mathcal{K}h_j^B + \sum_{t=j}^{N} h_t^A \leq \mathcal{K} \qquad 1 \leq j \leq N \tag{4}$$

The linear equation defines a mutual exclusion constraint on states A and B, such that if the jth segment is assigned to state B, then all temporal successor segments appearing after j cannot be assigned to state A. Similar constraints can be placed on predecessor segments of state B when selecting the jth segment for state A. Using Eq. 4, we can build any left to right transition finite state machine with arbitrary number of states. Note, that self transitions are implicitly modeled, as the selected segments of a particular state can be arbitrarily separated.

State duration models specify the expected time a Markovian system will spend in a particular state. Similar duration constraints can be placed on our state models by specifying a compactness constraint:

$$\mathcal{K}h_j^A + \sum_{t=1}^{j-\delta} h_t^A + \sum_{t=j+\delta}^{N} h_t^A \leq \mathcal{K} \qquad 1 \leq j \leq N \tag{5}$$

The compactness constraint specifies that all the segments selected for the state A, must lie within a temporal window of length 2δ, by placing a mutual exclusion constraint on the jth segment and all other segments lying outside the 2δ window. We combine both the temporal constraints and the compactness constraints with the $\mathcal{K}$-segment selection problem, and formulate it as a relaxed linear programming optimization:

$$\begin{aligned}
\text{MKSS}(\mathcal{K}) = \quad & \text{Maximize} \quad \frac{\sum_{s\in\mathcal{S}} \sum_{j=1}^{N} c_j^s h_j^s}{\sum_{s\in\mathcal{S}} \sum_{j=1}^{N} e_j^s h_j^s} \qquad +a \log \sum_{s\in\mathcal{S}} \|\mathbf{h}^s\|_1 && (6)\\
\text{s.t.} \quad C1: \ & 0 \leq h_j^s \leq 1 && \forall s \in \mathcal{S}, \quad 1 \leq j \leq N\\
C2: \ & \sum_{j=1}^{N} h_j^s = \mathcal{K} && \forall s \in \mathcal{S}\\
C3: \ & \mathcal{K}h_j^{s_b} + \sum_{k=j}^{N} h_k^{s_a} \leq \mathcal{K} && \forall (s_a, s_b) \in \mathcal{T}, \quad 1 \leq j \leq N\\
& \mathcal{K}h_j^{s_a} + \sum_{k=1}^{j} h_k^{s_b} \leq \mathcal{K} && \forall (s_a, s_b) \in \mathcal{T}, \quad 1 \leq j \leq N\\
C4: \ & \sum_{s\in\mathcal{S}} h_j^s \leq 1 && 1 \leq j \leq N\\
C5: \ & \mathcal{K}h_j^s + \sum_{k=1}^{j-\delta} h_k^s + \sum_{k=j+\delta}^{N} h_k^s \leq \mathcal{K} && \forall s \in \mathcal{S}, \quad 1 \leq j \leq N
\end{aligned}$$

where $\mathcal{S}$ is the set of states in our model, and $(s_a, s_b) \in \mathcal{T}$ is the set of temporal order constraints where state s_b appears only after state s_a. C1 is the linear relaxation constraint over the binary indicator variables. C2 specifies that exactly $\mathcal{K}$ segments should be selected corresponding to each state. C3 and C5 correspond to the temporal and compactness constraints respectively. C4 ensures that no segment is counted twice during state assignments. The resulting optimization is a fractional linear program, where the objective function is a ratio of linear functions. Solving fractional linear programs is a well explored problem in operations research, and can be solved using a simple transformation [27] to an equivalent standard linear program:

$$\begin{array}{ll} \text{Maximize } \frac{\mathbf{c}^T\mathbf{h}+d}{\mathbf{e}^T\mathbf{h}+f} & \\ \quad G\mathbf{h} \preceq \mathbf{m} & \\ \quad A\mathbf{h} = \mathbf{b} & \\ \quad \mathbf{e}^T\mathbf{h} + f > 0 & \end{array} \iff \begin{array}{l} \text{Maximize } \mathbf{c}^T\mathbf{y} + dz \\ \quad G\mathbf{y} - \mathbf{m}z \preceq 0 \\ \quad A\mathbf{y} - \mathbf{b}z = 0 \\ \quad \mathbf{e}^T\mathbf{y} + fz = 1, \quad z \geq 0 \end{array}$$

where $\mathbf{y} = \frac{\mathbf{h}}{\mathbf{e}^T\mathbf{h}+f}$ and $z = \frac{1}{\mathbf{e}^T\mathbf{h}+f}$. The standard linear program can be efficiently solved using off the shelf solvers[1], as it consists of $O(N|\mathcal{S}|)$ variables and $O(N|\mathcal{S}|^2)$ constraints, which is polynomial in the number of segments and states.

The optimal $\mathbf{h}^s$ vector obtained by solving the linear program in Eq. 6 identifies the selected segments for pooling features corresponding to each state $s \in \mathcal{S}$. The global feature descriptor $\Phi(\mathbf{x})$ is defined as a concatenation of features pooled from the individual states. Assuming a 3-state model such as in Fig. 2, the global feature vector is computed as: $\Phi(\mathbf{x}) = [\Phi_A, \Phi_B, \Phi_C] = \left[\frac{\sum_j \mathbf{f}_j h_j^A}{\sum_j e_j h_j^A}, \frac{\sum_j \mathbf{f}_j h_j^B}{\sum_j e_j h_j^B}, \frac{\sum_j \mathbf{f}_j h_j^C}{\sum_j e_j h_j^C}\right]$, which is used to train an latent-SVM classifier.

5 Selecting Optimal Parameter $\mathcal{K}$

The parameter $\mathcal{K}$ in the $\mathcal{K}$-segment selection problem specifies the number of segments to be selected. However the appropriate $\mathcal{K}$ value can vary from video to video, and there is little intuition on how to compute an appropriate value. One feasible criteria is to select the best $\mathcal{K}$ value by iteratively solving the $\mathcal{K}$-segment selection problem: $\mathcal{K}^* = \text{argmax}_{\mathcal{K}}\text{KSS}(\mathcal{K})$. It can be shown that the optimum value of such an iterative procedure will always be $\mathcal{K}^* = 1$, *i.e.* only selecting the segment with the largest $\frac{c_i}{d_i}$ ratio. Consider the following inequality: $\frac{a_2}{b_2} \leq \frac{a_2+a_1}{b_2+b_1} \leq \frac{a_1}{b_1}$, which can be verified for all $b_1, b_2 \geq 0$ using simple algebraic operations. The inequality shows that any combination of multiple segments will always have a lower ratio value than the single segment with the highest $\frac{c_i}{d_i}$ ratio. A similar theoretical argument cannot be made for MKSS, however in our experiments we observe that the optimum solution is for each state to select a single best segment.

Previously, [11] addressed the problem by adding a logarithmic regularization function : $a \log(\|h\|_1)$, which favors choosing a larger number of segments. However choosing appropriate values of the hyper-parameter a is again non-trivial, and it is estimated through cross-validation for each action category. In effect, the regularization parameter a indirectly chooses the appropriate $\mathcal{K}^*$ value, and is equivalent to selecting $\mathcal{K}^*$ through cross-validation. We next present an extension to our multistate segment selection algorithm for automatically selecting the optimum number of segments.

[1] http://www.gnu.org/software/glpk/.

5.1 Regularized Multistate Segment Selection (RMSS)

The segment selection criteria used in KSS and MKSS are such that the negatively scored segments will never be selected. On the other hand, the segments contributing a positively weighted score corresponds to the discriminative (*w.r.t* classifying the composite event) segments in the video, and hence an appropriate segment selection criteria should maximize the number of positively weighted segments selected while satisfying the multi-state constraints. We define a vector $r_j^{s_a} = 0.5 \times \left(c_j^{s_a} + |c_j^{s_a}|\right)$ which contains all the positive valued scores computed from the segments for state s_a, while the negative valued scores are set to zero. We further define a segment selection constraint $\sum_{j=1}^{N} r_j^{s_a} h_j^{s_a} \geq \Delta \sum_{j=1}^{N} r_j^{s_a}$ which ensures that at least a Δ fraction of the positively weighted segments will be selected as part of the optimum solution. The linear programming optimization for regularized multistate segment selection takes only the positive weight fraction Δ as input parameter, and is defined as follows:

$$\text{RMSS}\,(\Delta) = \text{Maximize} \ \frac{\sum_{s\in\mathcal{S}} \sum_{j=1}^{N} c_j^s h_j^s}{\sum_{s\in\mathcal{S}} \sum_{j=1}^{N} e_j^s h_j^s} \quad , \quad \tilde{K} = \left\lfloor \frac{N}{\|\mathcal{S}\|} \right\rfloor \tag{7}$$

$$\begin{aligned}
\text{s.t.} \quad C1: &\quad 0 \leq h_j^s \leq 1 && \forall s \in \mathcal{S}, \quad 1 \leq j \leq N \\
C2b: &\quad \sum_{j=1}^{N} h_j^s \leq \tilde{K} && \forall s \in \mathcal{S} \\
C3: &\quad \tilde{K} h_j^{s_b} + \sum_{k=j}^{N} h_k^{s_a} \leq \tilde{K} && \forall (s_a, s_b) \in \mathcal{T}, \quad 1 \leq j \leq N \\
&\quad \tilde{K} h_j^{s_a} + \sum_{k=1}^{j} h_k^{s_b} \leq \tilde{K} && \forall (s_a, s_b) \in \mathcal{T}, \quad 1 \leq j \leq N \\
C4: &\quad \sum_{s\in\mathcal{S}} h_j^s \leq 1 && 1 \leq j \leq N \\
C5: &\quad \tilde{K} h_j^s + \sum_{k=1}^{j-\delta} h_k^s + \sum_{k=j+\delta}^{N} h_k^s \leq \tilde{K} && \forall s \in \mathcal{S}, \quad 1 \leq j \leq N \\
C6: &\quad \sum_{j=1}^{N} r_j^{s_a} h_j^{s_a} \geq \Delta \sum_{j=1}^{N} r_j^{s_a} && \forall s \in \mathcal{S} \\
&\quad r_j^{s_a} = 0.5 \times (c_j^{s_a} + |c_j^{s_a}|) && \forall s \in \mathcal{S}, \quad 1 \leq j \leq N \\
C7: &\quad \sum_{j=1}^{N} h_j^{s_a} \geq (1-\theta) \sum_{j=1}^{N} h_j^{s_b} && \forall s_a, s_b \in \mathcal{S} \\
&\quad \sum_{j=1}^{N} h_j^{s_a} \leq (1+\theta) \sum_{j=1}^{N} h_j^{s_b} && \forall s_a, s_b \in \mathcal{S}
\end{aligned}$$

where the parameter $\tilde{K}$ is the maximum number of segments which can be selected per state in a video with N frames. The optimization does not restrict each state to a constant $\tilde{K}$ number of segment selections; instead it relaxes the equality constraint C2 with C2b in Eq. 7, which only places an upper bound on the number of segments selected. It is also desirable that the number of segments selected corresponding to each state is equally balanced across states, so that a single state does not dominate the solution of segment selection. An additional constraint C7 is added to ensure a balanced selection of segments across states, within a margin of $\pm\theta$.

The parameter Δ determines the number of segments selected in the optimum solution. However the constraints in the $RMSS(\Delta)$ optimization can be rendered infeasible for certain values of Δ, in particular, if the Δ value is too high, it is likely that the state transition constraints cannot be satisfied for any combination of segment selection. We further observe that there exists a $\Delta_0 \geq 0$ such that $RMSS(\Delta)$ has a feasible solution for all $\Delta \geq \Delta_0$, and hence the optimization problem is monotonic in Δ with respect to its feasibility. The monotonic behavior suggests a simple binary search over Δ to find the optimal Δ_0 within an error margin of ϵ in $O\left(\log \frac{1}{\epsilon}\right)$ iterations.

6 Experiments and Results

We evaluate our algorithm on the recently introduced Composite Cooking Dataset [12]. The dataset contains 41 cooking recipe demonstrations like *prepare ginger*, *seperate an egg*, *make coffee* etc., where the videos are recorded with a fixed elevated camera recording the actors from the front preparing the dishes inside a kitchen. There are a total of 138 videos of ~16 h containing actions performed by 17 different actors, and are shot at 29.4 fps with 1624 × 1224 pixel resolution. In our experiments, we use the pre-computed histogram of codeword features for each frame, provided with the dataset. The codewords are computed over HoG, HoF, motion boundary histograms and trajectory shape features, extracted from densely sampled interest point tracks [29] in the videos.

We divide each video into overlapping segments of 100 frames each, as primitive events like opening cupboard/refrigerator, retrieving utensils can be reasonably captured using a 100 frame overlapping window. Next, we sum the histogram of codewords from each frame within the jth segment, to construct a single accumulated histogram feature $\boldsymbol{f}_j$. To setup the fractional linear programming problems MKSS and RMSS, we normalize the features from each segment using its L1 norm, and compute the scores values $c_j^s = \theta_s \boldsymbol{f}_j$ for each state s using the current value of the weight vector from the LSVM classifier. The normalization constants e_j^s are set to 1, and in effect, normalize the features based on the number of segments selected. In our experiments, we avoided any action or dataset specific tunning and set the regularization parameter as $a = 5$ for all events, which we empirically observed to select a larger fraction of positively scored segments in the video, and hence contributing more towards classifying the composite event.

6.1 Comparisons with Baselines

To establish a baseline, we implemented a bag of words based SVM classifier, where the codewords in the video are globally pooled into a single histogram. Figure 3 presents our results on the 41 composite cooking actions using a 6-fold cross validation as suggested by [12]. As the BoW features compute only globally aggregated statistics, their performance is quite low on complex long range activities. We also implement a temporally binned BoW classifier, as the

Action Labels	BoW	TB-3	TB-5	TB-7	MKSS-3	MKSS-5	MKSS-7	RMSS-3	RMSS-5	RMSS-7
Chopping a cucumber	0.11	0.14	0.11	0.15	0.12	0.15	0.11	0.12	0.16	0.12
Prepare carrots	0.19	0.33	0.39	0.42	0.39	0.39	0.45	0.38	0.39	0.42
Prepare a peach	0.23	0.11	0.20	0.09	0.10	0.13	0.08	0.17	0.13	0.11
Slice a loaf of bread	0.58	0.61	0.73	0.66	0.75	0.71	0.87	0.77	0.72	0.85
Prepare cauliflower	0.40	0.43	0.42	0.36	0.60	0.65	0.35	0.34	0.63	0.33
Prepare an onion	0.16	0.46	0.26	0.10	0.42	0.19	0.10	0.35	0.20	0.09
Prepare an orange	0.14	0.68	0.47	0.38	0.30	0.42	0.36	0.61	0.44	0.37
Prepare fresh herbs	0.38	0.24	0.14	0.18	0.24	0.20	0.22	0.22	0.22	0.18
Prepare garlic	0.18	0.31	0.12	0.07	0.31	0.32	0.14	0.31	0.16	0.30
Prepare asparagus	0.02	0.03	0.04	0.04	0.03	0.04	0.05	0.04	0.05	0.05
Prepare fresh ginger	0.14	0.37	0.23	0.09	0.12	0.19	0.08	0.14	0.21	0.07
Prepare a plum	0.41	0.18	0.11	0.09	0.36	0.18	0.22	0.61	0.21	0.61
Zest a lemon	0.14	0.20	0.20	0.20	0.20	0.20	0.20	0.25	0.17	0.20
Prepare leeks	0.23	0.33	0.32	0.46	0.42	0.34	0.43	0.34	0.33	0.38
Extract lime juice	0.42	0.48	0.49	0.53	0.44	0.49	0.50	0.46	0.47	0.43
Prepare a pomegranate	0.39	0.81	0.94	0.56	0.53	0.65	0.78	0.48	0.70	0.78
Prepare broccoli	0.20	0.40	0.42	0.47	0.45	0.45	0.46	0.45	0.45	0.60
Prepare potatoes	0.23	0.11	0.15	0.11	0.23	0.22	0.14	0.24	0.23	0.17
Prepare a pepper	0.10	0.16	0.08	0.09	0.14	0.11	0.10	0.18	0.11	0.12
Prepare a pineapple	0.55	0.37	0.48	0.51	0.56	0.74	0.61	0.73	0.77	0.62
Prepare spinach	0.10	0.28	0.31	0.36	0.58	0.58	0.58	0.50	0.28	0.44
Prepare a fresh chilli	0.23	0.05	0.05	0.06	0.09	0.14	0.20	0.10	0.14	0.20
Cook pasta	0.26	0.53	0.45	0.54	0.38	0.49	0.64	0.53	0.47	1.00
Separate an egg	0.65	0.47	0.60	0.63	0.52	0.63	0.57	0.63	0.63	0.56
Prepare broad beans	0.14	0.68	0.18	0.29	0.68	0.51	0.68	0.47	0.52	0.52
Prepare a kiwi fruit	0.15	0.23	0.23	0.10	0.11	0.18	0.11	0.22	0.10	0.12
Prepare an avocado	0.13	0.07	0.13	0.07	0.05	0.08	0.07	0.05	0.10	0.07
Prepare a mango	0.06	0.16	0.30	0.22	0.15	0.29	0.32	0.21	0.29	0.33
Prepare figs	0.30	0.06	0.07	0.07	0.09	0.13	0.22	0.10	0.14	0.21
Use box grater	0.42	0.75	0.49	0.39	0.65	0.63	0.57	0.73	0.71	0.57
Sharpen knives	0.75	0.63	1.00	0.75	0.67	0.67	0.75	0.75	1.00	1.00
Use speed peeler	1.00	0.10	0.10	0.10	0.20	0.33	0.25	0.20	0.20	0.20
Use a toaster	0.16	0.57	0.39	0.35	0.42	0.43	0.31	0.52	0.34	0.20
Use a pestle-mortar	0.55	0.55	0.59	0.65	0.63	0.60	0.63	0.65	0.60	0.50
Use microplane grater	0.20	0.49	0.23	0.20	0.18	0.26	0.29	0.21	0.25	0.27
Make scrambled egg	0.22	0.45	0.57	0.56	0.50	0.65	0.61	0.53	0.78	0.72
Prepare orange juice	0.64	0.65	0.81	0.69	0.81	0.83	0.83	0.81	0.83	0.78
Make hot dog	0.05	0.30	0.18	0.59	0.21	0.21	0.44	0.40	0.40	0.44
Pour beer	0.56	0.10	0.06	0.03	0.56	0.53	0.53	0.53	0.55	1.00
Make tea	0.28	0.46	0.33	0.35	0.53	0.51	0.61	0.50	0.56	0.75
Make coffee	0.53	0.88	0.75	0.88	0.71	0.75	0.71	0.75	0.75	0.71
Splitwise Average MAP	0.30	0.40	0.36	0.35	0.39	0.41	0.41	0.42	0.41	0.41

Fig. 3. MAP result table for the Composite Cooking dataset. Column TB presents the MAP scores from a temporally binned BoW classifier [3] with 3, 5 and 7 temporal partitions. MAP scores for MKSS and RMSS algorithm for different number of states (3, 5 and 7) is also given for each action. The highest MAP score across states is highlighted (Color figure online).

one proposed by [3]. We experiment with three types of binning structures, where the video is divided into 3, 5 and 7 equal length partitions, and histogram of codewords computed from each partition are concatenated together. We observe considerable improvement in MAP values compared to the BoW classifier, which we attribute to the temporal pooling of features which is important for complex event detection. However, the performance starts decreasing as the number of partitions is increased, which we attribute to the static nature of the partitions, making them sensitive to variations in the temporal location of primitive actions.

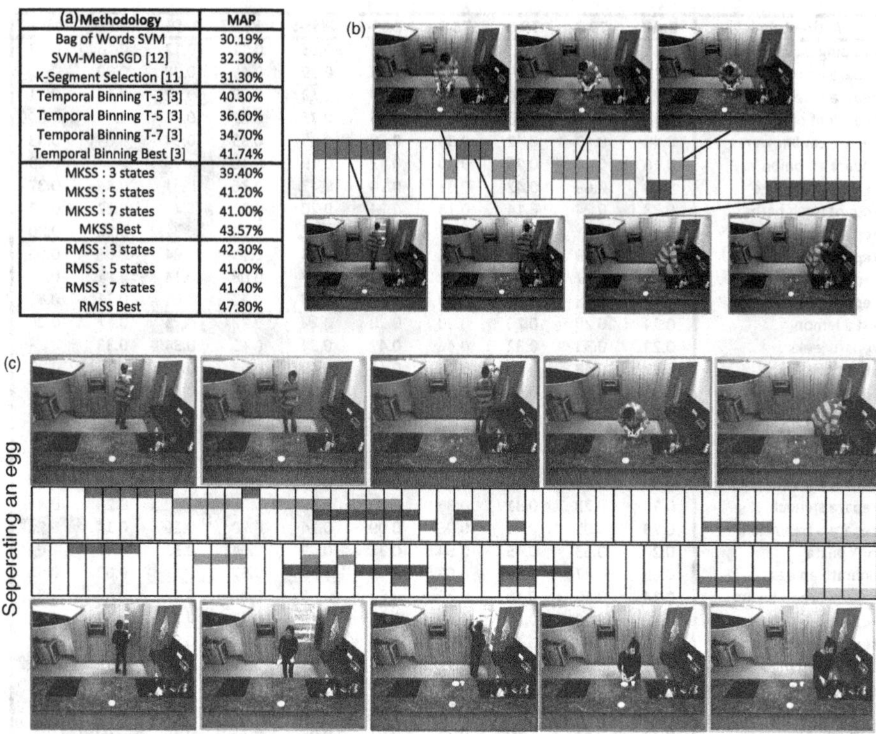

(a) Methodology	MAP
Bag of Words SVM	30.19%
SVM-MeanSGD [12]	32.30%
K-Segment Selection [11]	31.30%
Temporal Binning T-3 [3]	40.30%
Temporal Binning T-5 [3]	36.60%
Temporal Binning T-7 [3]	34.70%
Temporal Binning Best [3]	41.74%
MKSS : 3 states	39.40%
MKSS : 5 states	41.20%
MKSS : 7 states	41.00%
MKSS Best	43.57%
RMSS : 3 states	42.30%
RMSS : 5 states	41.00%
RMSS : 7 states	41.40%
RMSS Best	47.80%

Fig. 4. (a) MAP result table. (b) 3-State segment selection result for *Seperating an egg* with representative frames of the selected segments. (c) 5-State segment selection result with comparisons of the frames selected by each state (Color figure online).

We next evaluate both the MKSS and RMSS algorithms for three different number of states: 3, 5 and 7. The optimal number of states is a function of the complexity of the underlying event in the video, and also the amount of variety present across videos of the same event class. Figure 4(a) shows the average MAP over all classes of the MKSS and RMSS algorithm for the different number of states, and also the average of the best performance. The MKSS and RMSS algorithms achieve on average an MAP score of 41.47 % and 47.80 % respectively. Our method outperforms the SVM-MeanSGD [12] algorithm, which learns a SVM classifier using chi-square kernels and reports a score of 32.30 %. We note, that [12] also reports an MAP score of 53.9 % using external textual scripts to guide the classifier training, however our focus is on purely computer vision based approaches, and expect our algorithm to also benefit from similar complimentary modalities. We also implemented the $\mathcal{K}$-segment selection [11] algorithm and evaluated it on the dataset. We observe only a minor improvement in performance over traditional BoWs, which we attribute to its lack of temporal structure modeling, which is crucial for classifying long term composite events.

6.2 Segment Selection Results

Solving the MKSS and RMSS algorithms provides us with the optimum segment selection indicator vector $\boldsymbol{h}$, whose elements are real valued numbers between 0 and 1. For visualizing the segments assigned higher selection weights, we threshold the indicator values $\boldsymbol{h}$ such that atleast 40 % of $\|\boldsymbol{h}\|_1$ is retained. Figure 4(b) shows the results of the multistate segment selection algorithm for 3 states on a *seperate an egg* video. We note the clear decomposition of the selected segments into three temporal states, where state-A (red) appears before state-B (green), which is followed by state-C (blue). The states are learned automatically from the training data, and it is difficult to associate a single primitive action with each state. However, we can discern some interesting trends through visual inspection of the results. For example, state-B seems to correspond to working at the counter station, and as the video contains extended periods at the counter, our model only selects some parts of the video. State-A seems to correspond to moving to back of the room and opening a door, and is detected twice in the video where the person approaches the cupboard and the refrigerator. The intervening frames are not important to state-A and are ignored in its score computation. State-C seems to correspond to the person moving to the side to wash the dishes, or to keep them away.

Figure 4 (c,d) compares the segment selection applied to two different videos of the: *separate an egg* activity, where the algorithm assumes a 5-state model, and we see a correlation between the types of primitive actions each of states correspond to across the videos. We note that each state can represent a cluster of features, and hence may correspond to multiple primitive actions and scenes. This becomes more apparent in videos where the actor interchanges the actions of approaching the refrigerator and approaching the cupboard. As our states do not have a semantic understanding of what a refrigerator or a cupboard is, it only recognizes the gross spatio-temporal motions occurring in the scene.

7 Conclusions

We presented a novel multistate segment selection algorithm for pooling features from the discriminative segments of a video. We presented a solution based on efficiently solving a linear programming optimization, and formulate linear constraints to enforce temporal ordering among the states representing the primitive actions of an event. We also presented a provably faster solution to the single state K-segment selection problem [11] and improve the computation time to $O(N \log N)$. Finally, we presented a regularized version of the multi-state segment selection algorithm, which automatically determines the number of segments to be selected for each state in a given video. We evaluated our algorithm on the Composite Cooking Activity dataset [12], and showed significantly improved results compared to other static and dynamic pooling algorithms. One promising approach for future work is to extend the algorithm to incorporate semantic mappings between the states and the underlying feature distributions, and explore automated methods of determining the optimal number of states.

References

1. Ryoo, M., Aggarwal, J.: Spatio-temporal relationship match: video structure comparison for recognition of complex human activities. In: ICCV (2009)
2. Niebles, J.C., Chen, C.-W., Fei-Fei, L.: Modeling temporal structure of decomposable motion segments for activity classification. In: Daniilidis, K., Maragos, P., Paragios, N. (eds.) ECCV 2010, Part II. LNCS, vol. 6312, pp. 392–405. Springer, Heidelberg (2010)
3. Laptev, I., Marszalek, M., Schmid, C., Rozenfeld, B.: Learning realistic human actions from movies. In: CVPR (2008)
4. Kovashka, A., Grauman, K.: Learning a hierarchy of discriminative space-time neighborhood features for human action recognition. In: CVPR (2010)
5. Oneata, D., Verbeek, J., Schmid, C.: Action and event recognition with Fisher vectors on a compact feature set. In: ICCV (2013)
6. Sun, J., Wu, X., Yan, S., Cheong, L., Chua, T., Li, J.: Hierarchical spatio-temporal context modeling for action recognition. In: CVPR (2009)
7. Lv, F., Nevatia, R.: Single view human action recognition using key pose matching and viterbi path searching. In: CVPR (2007)
8. Natarajan, P., Singh, V., Nevatia, R.: Learning 3D action models from a few 2D videos. In: CVPR (2010)
9. Gaidon, A.: Actom sequence models for efficient action detection. In: CVPR (2011)
10. Tian, Y., Sukthankar, R., Shah, M.: Spatiotemporal deformable part models for action detection. In: CVPR (2013)
11. Li, W., Yu, Q., Divakaran, A.: Dynamic pooling for complex event recognition. In: ICCV (2013)
12. Rohrbach, M., Regneri, M., Andriluka, M., Amin, S., Pinkal, M., Schiele, B.: Script data for attribute-based recognition of composite activities. In: Fitzgibbon, A., Lazebnik, S., Perona, P., Sato, Y., Schmid, C. (eds.) ECCV 2012, Part I. LNCS, vol. 7572, pp. 144–157. Springer, Heidelberg (2012)
13. Fathi, A., Mori, G.: Action recognition by learning mid-level motion features. In: CVPR. IEEE (2008)
14. Gilbert, A., Illingworth, J., Bowden, R.: Fast realistic multi-action recognition using mined dense spatio-temporal features. In: ICCV (2009)
15. Schindler, K., Van Gool, L.: Action snippets: how many frames does human action recognition require? In: CVPR (2008)
16. Satkin, S., Hebert, M.: Modeling the temporal extent of actions. In: Daniilidis, K., Maragos, P., Paragios, N. (eds.) ECCV 2010, Part I. LNCS, vol. 6311, pp. 536–548. Springer, Heidelberg (2010)
17. Nowozin, S., Bakir, G., Tsuda, K.: Discriminative subsequence mining for action classification. In: CVPR. IEEE (2007)
18. Raptis, M., Sigal, L.: Poselet key-framing: a model for human activity recognition. In: CVPR (2013)
19. Vahdat, A., Cannons, K., Mori, G., Oh, S., Kim, I.: Compositional models for video event detection: a multiple kernel learning latent variable approach. In: ICCV (2013)
20. Wang, Y., Mori, G.: Hidden part models for human action recognition: probabilistic vs. max-margin. PAMI **33**, 1310–1323 (2011)
21. Tang, K., Fei-Fei, L., Koller, D.: Learning latent temporal structure for complex event detection. In: CVPR, pp. 1250–1257. IEEE (2012)

22. Brendel, W., Fern, A., Todorovic, S.: Probabilistic event logic for interval-based event recognition. In: CVPR, Number I, pp. 3329–3336 (2011)
23. Duong, T., Bui, H., Phung, D., Venkatesh, S.: Activity recognition and abnormality detection with the switching hidden semi-markov model. In: CVPR (2005)
24. Sminchisescu, Kanaujia, A., Li, Dimitris, M.: Conditional models for contextual human motion recognition. In: ICCV (2005)
25. Yu, C.N.J., Joachims, T.: Learning structural SVMs with latent variables. In: ICML (2009)
26. Felzenszwalb, P., McAllester, D.: A discriminatively trained, multiscale, deformable part model. In: CVPR (2008)
27. Boyd, S., Vandenberghe, L.: Convex Optimization. Cambridge University Press, Cambridge (2004)
28. Neill, D.: Fast subset scan for spatial pattern detection. J. Roy. Stat. Soc. Ser. B **74**, 337–360 (2012)
29. Wang, H., Klaser, A.: Action recognition by dense trajectories. In: CVPR, pp. 3169–3176 (2011)

Action Recognition in the Presence of One Egocentric and Multiple Static Cameras

Bilge Soran(✉), Ali Farhadi, and Linda Shapiro

Department of Computer Science and Engineering,
University of Washington, Seattle, USA
{bilge,ali,shapiro}@cs.washington.edu

Abstract. In this paper, we study the problem of recognizing human actions in the presence of a single egocentric camera and multiple static cameras. Some actions are better presented in static cameras, where the whole body of an actor and the context of actions are visible. Some other actions are better recognized in egocentric cameras, where subtle movements of hands and complex object interactions are visible. In this paper, we introduce a model that can benefit from the best of both worlds by learning to predict the importance of each camera in recognizing actions in each frame. By joint discriminative learning of latent camera importance variables and action classifiers, our model achieves successful results in the challenging CMU-MMAC dataset. Our experimental results show significant gain in learning to use the cameras according to their predicted importance. The learned latent variables provide a level of understanding of a scene that enables automatic cinematography by smoothly switching between cameras in order to maximize the amount of relevant information in each frame.

1 Introduction

Activities that people perform in their daily lives span a wide spectrum of actions. Recognizing some actions requires reasoning about complex human-object interactions and detailed observation of the actions. For example, recognizing the cracking of an egg requires observations about the state change of the egg and characteristic postures of the hand. Some other actions, like walking to a refrigerator, are better recognized when a holistic view of an actor is visible. The movement of the human body provides strong cues for these kinds of activities.

The conventional setting of activity recognition involves studying the behavior of an actor from one or multiple static cameras [1]. There has been significant improvement over the last decade on recognizing actions that require observing the movements of the human body. However, in this setting, there are major challenges in recognizing actions that require subtle movements/gestures. This is

Electronic supplementary material The online version of this chapter (doi:10.1007/978-3-319-16814-2_12) contains supplementary material, which is available to authorized users.

D. Cremers et al. (Eds.): ACCV 2014, Part V, LNCS 9007, pp. 178–193, 2015.
DOI: 10.1007/978-3-319-16814-2_12

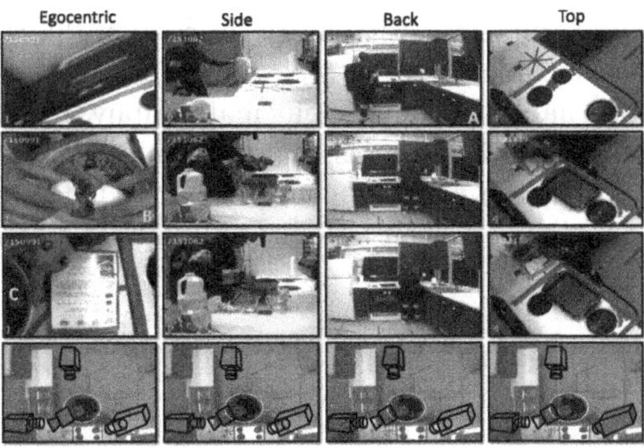

Fig. 1. We study action recognition in the presence of a single egocentric camera and multiple static cameras. The bottom row in Fig. 1 illustrates settings where videos of people making brownies have been recorded from an egocentric camera (first column) and three static cameras (columns 2, 3, 4). Actions like cracking an egg (image B) are better recognized using an egocentric camera where information about subtle movements and complex interaction is available. However, information about holistic body movements is typically missing in egocentric cameras. Actions like walking are better recognized from a static camera (image A). Furthermore, people tend to look away when they perform actions that become procedural memories to them. For example the subject in image C looks at the recipe (instead of looking at the bowl) while stirring the brownie mix. This results in missing valuable action information in egocentric cameras. In this paper, we show a model that can benefit from both egocentric and static cameras by reasoning about the importance of each camera for each action.

mainly due to severe occlusions and distractions from image regions where the actual action is taking place.

An alternative is to use egocentric cameras (also called first-person or wearable cameras), with which the actions are observed from the actor's perspective [2]. Although less susceptible to occlusion, egocentric cameras provide their own set of challenges. For example, the human body, which is one of the main cues for some actions, is not visible in an egocentric camera. The camera has complex motion resulting in frequent blurs and appearance distortions. Furthermore, people tend to look away when they perform actions they are comfortable with. This results in losing major parts of signals that correspond to the main action. For example, when stirring a food mixture, people look around to determine what ingredients they need next, check the time, or read the next step in the recipe. The image marked with "C" in Fig. 1 corresponds to a sample frame from a stirring action in which the actor is actually reading the recipe.

Our goal in this paper is to study the problem of understanding human actions in the presence of a single egocentric and multiple static cameras. If an oracle provides information about the importance of each camera, then the problem of recognizing human actions becomes a multi-modal classification problem. In our formulation we use a latent variable to encode the importance of each camera for each frame and introduce a model to jointly learn the latent camera variables and the action classifiers.

Our experimental results show significant success on the challenging CMU-MMAC dataset that includes both static and egocentric cameras. As a side product, our method enables automatic cinematography. In the presence of an egocentric and multiple static cameras, our method can automatically select a camera through which the action is better observed. By enforcing smooth transitions between cameras, we can automatically direct a scene with multiple cameras.

2 Related Work

Human activity recognition has attracted several researchers over the last decade. Comprehensive surveys are provided in [1,3]. We categorize related work in multi-view action recognition, egocentric activity recognition and a brief summary of virtual cinematography.

Egocentric Action Recognition typically refers to studying human actions from a camera that is mounted on the body (head to chest). To address the challenges and characteristic constraints of egocentric action recognition, [2] uses a SIFT-based representation. Taralova at al. [4] used source constrained clustering to classify actions from egocentric videos. Hand-object interactions are used by [5], where an object-based representation for action recognition that jointly models the objects and actions is proposed. A generative probabilistic model that recognizes actions while predicting gaze locations is proposed by [6]. Hand motion and gaze information for egocentric activity recognition is used by [7]. A novel activities-of-daily-living (ADL) dataset is provided by [8], on which the change in the appearance of the objects in interaction for recognizing activities is explicitly modeled. The problem of understanding simple social interactions in egocentric settings is studied by [9], while [10] examines action recognition in sports videos using egocentric cameras. Ogaki et al. [11] uses eye movements and ego-motions to better recognize indoor activities. Sundaram and Mayol-Cuevas [12] utilizes egocentric action recognition for the purpose of contextual mapping. Sundaram and Mayol-Cuevas [13] studies the problem of activity recognition using low resolution wearable cameras. The affect of gaze prediction in action recognition is explored by [14]. Actions can also be modeled through state transitions as suggested by [15]. From a different perspective, [16] handles a different action recognition problem: trying to understand the other person's interaction with the camera wearer with respect to an egocentric camera.

Multi-view Action Recognition: Multi-view action recognition has been approached by learning latent variables that encode the change in the appearance of actions or view points of actions [17–19], by joint learning of shared structures across multiple views [20], by hierarchical models of spatio-temporal features [21], by local partitioning and hierarchical classification of 3D HOG descriptors [22], by transfer learning [23–25] and by using spatio-temporal self-similarity descriptors [26]. Multiple datasets exists for multi-view action recognition: i3dpost [27], IXMAS [22,28], and CMU-MMAC [29]. We use static and egocentric recordings of the CMU-MMAC dataset in this paper. Spriggs et al. [30] and Fisher and Reddy [31] have studied action recognition by combining egocentric cameras with IMU sensors using the CMU-MMAC dataset. McCall et al. [32] and Zhao et al. [33] used IMU sensors in the same dataset to recognize actions. To the best of our knowledge, there has been no study for activity recognition using an egocentric camera and multiple static cameras. Note that approaches that require 3D reconstruction of the subject or visual hull are not directly applicable to our settings that uses egocentric cameras.

Virtual Cinematography: The majority of the work has focused on active and interactive cinematography, where one has control over the position of the cameras and other parameters such as lighting conditions [34,35]. We are mainly concerned with a passive case where multiple videos of a scene exist, and one needs to decide which camera to use for each frame. Virtual cinematography is not the main focus of this paper, and our model does not address the principles of cinematography. We merely show that our model provides a level of understanding that enables camera selection.

3 Approach

Our task is to recognize human actions in the presence of a single egocentric and multiple static cameras. Our intuition is that each camera plays a different role in predicting an action and should be weighted according to its importance. Given the importance of all cameras for recognizing the action in a frame, the problem of action recognition reduces to a multi-modal classification problem. Unfortunately, the camera importance information is not available. We jointly learn the importance of cameras along with the action classifiers.

During training we are given videos from a single egocentric and multiple static cameras and action labels for each frame. At test time, the task is to assign an action label to each frame given the observations from all the cameras. To set up notation, let us assume that there are C cameras, N frames, and M different actions. Frame i from camera j is represented by a d-dimensional feature vector x_i^j where $i \in \{1:N\}$, and $j \in \{1:C\}$. Each frame i is also labeled with the action label y_i where $y_i \in \{1:M\}$. The importance of each camera j in correctly understanding the action in frame i is represented by $\alpha_i^j \in [0,1]$. Our model aims at coupling the tasks of predicting action classifiers and camera importance variables.

Intuitively, the choice of α should depend on both the observations from all cameras and the action of interest. For example, the static side camera may be more informative than the egocentric camera in encoding walking, while for cracking an egg an egocentric camera is preferred. The importance of cameras may vary during actions. For example, at the beginning of an action like "taking a pan out of an oven" where the movement of the person toward the oven is informative, one might assign more weight to the side static camera. Toward the end of the action where the actor is reaching for the pan inside the oven, the egocentric camera becomes more important. Our model takes the importance of each camera into account while making predictions about actions.

The best estimate of the camera importance variables is the one that maximizes the accuracy of action prediction. We adopt a bi-linear multi-class max margin formulation where the importance of each camera is modeled by an element-wise product operator $\odot$ and a vector A of all latent camera importance variables. We stack all the observations across all cameras into an observation vector $\mathcal{X}_i = [x_i^1, \ldots, x_i^C]$ which is a $(C * d)$-dimensional representation of frame i, where C is the total number of cameras and x_i^j is a d-dimensional vector of each frame i in camera j. To simplify the notation, we assume that the feature vectors have the same dimensionality across cameras. The action classifier $\mathcal{W}_a$ for action a is a $(C * d)$-dimensional classifier. For each frame i, the latent camera importance variable A_i is also a $(C * d)$-dimensional vector, where $A_i = [A_i^1, A_i^2, \ldots, A_i^j, \ldots, A_i^C]$, $j \in \{1 : C\}$. For each camera j, $A_i^j = \alpha_i^j * \mathbf{1}^d$ is a d-dimensional indicator vector that ensures all the dimensions of the feature vector corresponding to a camera are weighted equally.

Our bi-linear max margin model searches for the best camera importance variables that maximize the action prediction accuracy by:

$$
\begin{aligned}
&\min_{A,\mathcal{W},\xi} \sum_{a=1}^{m} \| \mathcal{W}_a \|_2^2 + \lambda \sum_{i=1}^{N} \xi_i^a \qquad (1)\\
&\text{such that}\\
&(A_i^T \odot \mathcal{W}_{y_i})^T (A_i \odot \mathcal{X}_i) > (A_i^T \odot \mathcal{W}_a)^T (A_i \odot \mathcal{X}_i) + 1 - \xi_i^a \quad \forall a \neq y_i, i\\
&A_i = [A_i^1, A_i^2, \ldots, A_i^C]\\
&A_i^j = \alpha_i^j * \mathbf{1}^d \quad j \in \{1 : C\}\\
&\sum_{j=1}^{C} \alpha_i^j = 1, \quad \alpha_i^j \in [0,1], \quad \xi_i \geq 0 \ \ \forall i,
\end{aligned}
$$

where $\mathcal{W}$ is the matrix of all action classifiers across all cameras ($\mathcal{W} = [\mathcal{W}_1 \mathcal{W}_2 \ldots \mathcal{W}_m]$), and ξ is the standard slack variable in max margin formulations.

The first constraint encourages the model to make correct predictions. This constraint pushes for (W, A) of an action to score higher for instances of that action compared to any other action model. The other constraints push the latent variable to be similar for all dimensions within a camera, and contributions of cameras form a convex combination.

Bi-linear relations between the importance variables and action classifiers does not allow direct applications of standard latent max margin methods [36]. To optimize for $A, \mathcal{W}, \xi$ we use block coordinate descent. This involves estimating $\mathcal{W}$ for fixed A and optimizing for A given fixed $\mathcal{W}$. Optimizing for $\mathcal{W}$ given a fixed A reduces to a standard max margin model and can be solved with quadratic programming in dual. We initialize $\mathcal{W}$ by independently trained classifiers for each action. We calibrate these classifiers using the methods of [37].

To encode higher-order correlations in the feature space, we also consider different combinations of cameras, where each combination of cameras can be though of as a new dummy camera. Section 4 shows the benefits of considering such higher order correlations via camera combinations.

Table 1. The comparison of our model with two of the state-of-the-art latent CRF models: Latent Dynamic CRF and Hidden Unit CRF. Our model outperforms both of these methods.

Approach	Avg. Acc.	Avg. per Class Acc.
Latent Dynamic CRF [38]	41.55	33.57
Hidden Unit CRF [39]	24.13	26.22
Our method	**54.62**	**45.95**

4 Experiments

We evaluate our model on how accurately it can predict actions in the settings where an egocentric camera plus multiple static cameras observe human activities. We compare our method with state-of-the-art methods for multi-view activity recognition, such as the Latent Dynamic CRF and the Hidden Unit CRF, and several baselines that aim at evaluating different components of our model. To qualitatively evaluate the quality of the learned camera indicator variables (α), we utilize them in a virtual cinematography task.

In this paper, we are interested in learning to predict human actions in the presence of one egocentric camera plus multiple static cameras. Our experiments are designed to support this task.

4.1 Multiple Static and an Egocentric Camera

Dataset: We chose the challenging CMU Multi-Modal Activity dataset (CMU-MMAC) [29] because it has multiple static and one egocentric videos of subjects performing kitchen activities. We use brownie-making videos, because frame-level annotations of actions are provided. 11 out of 39 actions of the dataset are "unique" to different subjects, therefore it is impossible to recognize those actions with leave-one-subject-out cross validation. After discarding videos of subjects that have synchronization problems due to dropped frames in some cameras (in order to use all 4 cameras) and removing unique actions, we obtain a dataset of 28 different actions, for 5 different subjects, recorded from one egocentric and 3 static cameras in 1/30 sample rate. The final actions include close fridge, crack egg, open brownie bag, pour brownie bag into big bowl, pour oil into measuring cup small, twist on/off cap, stir, take fork, walk to fridge, switch on, open drawer and more. We will make the list of dropped frames and the list of subjects for whom all four cameras can be used publicly available for the CMU-MMAC dataset.

Features: Similar to the creators of the CMU-MMAC dataset [30], we use the GIST [40] features for all the methods and baselines in our experiments on the CMU-MMAC dataset. Eight orientations per scale and four blocks per direction resulting in 512 dimensional GIST features are used with PCA (99 % of data coverage: 80–121 dimensional features). In another study Taralova et al. [4] used

STIP features and showed improvements over GIST features when using only the egocentric data in a bag of words approach (average precision of 0.734 vs. 0.478). In their setting they merged similar action categories into one class and ended up with 15 categories (vs. 28 categories in our experiments) and used 14 subjects for training and 2 for testing having 4 random disjoint sets (vs. our use of 4 subjects for training and a fifth for testing). We choose to use GIST features, because they were originally used on the CMU-MMAC dataset and are suitable for making the comparisons of methods in this paper, where emphasis is not on the feature engineering.

Experimental Setup: Our action model uses a sampling, where negatives are sampled in a 1:3 ratio. The same sampling is preserved across all comparisons. We use leave-one-subject-out as our experimental protocol and both average accuracy and average per class accuracy (Avg. Acc. and Avg. per Class Acc.) as our evaluation metrics. Our model achieves an average accuracy of 54.62 and average per class accuracy of 45.95.

According to our knowledge, this paper is the first attempt to fuse the information from an egocentric and multiple static cameras. We are the first to use the data from all 4 cameras from the CMU-MMAC dataset. Therefore, there is no existing baseline using the egocentric and static views of CMU-MMAC. For this reason, we compared our model with the existing state-of the art methods such as different latent CRF's besides providing our own baselines by modifying different parts of the model.

Comparisons to State-of-the-Art Methods: We compared our method with state-of-the-art methods in multi-view, temporal classification. We selected state of the art methods that are applicable to the settings of an egocentric and multiple static cameras. Note that methods that rely on 3D estimates of the visual hull of the subjects are not directly applicable to egocentric cameras.

Different versions of latent model CRFs have been successfully used in multi-view action recognition. In particular, we compare our method with the Latent Dynamic CRF and the Hidden Unit CRF. The Latent Dynamic CRF [38] is a discriminative method with a strong track record for multi-view activity recognition. It models the sub-structure of action sequences by introducing hidden state variables. In our experiments the best results are obtained by using one hidden node per label. Table 1 shows that our model outperforms the Latent Dynamic CRF on the challenging task of action recognition with one egocentric and multiple static cameras. We also compare our model with the Hidden Unit CRF [39] where there are hidden nodes between action classes and features. Those hidden nodes can reveal the latent discriminative structure in the features. For each frame a Hidden Unit CRF can represent nonlinear dependencies. The best results in our experiments are obtained by using a total number of 100 hidden units. Table 1 shows that our method also outperforms the Hidden Unit CRF.

Both the Latent Dynamic CRF and the Hidden Unit CRF approach the problem of action recognition by joint reasoning over time. In the case of combining egocentric and static cameras, coupling joint temporal reasoning with

Table 2. We compare our method with several baselines. Removing temporal smoothing, considering binary alphas, not considering camera combinations, and encoding per-action α hurts the performance of our model. This supports our intuitions about different parts of our model.

Approach	Avg. Acc.	Avg. per Class Acc.
Baseline 1	41.80	44.05
Baseline 2	52.00	41.55
Baseline 3	47.93	42.45
Baseline 4	44.58	35.01
Baseline 5	48.83	45.89
Baseline 6	43.55	39.81
Baseline 7	48.75	45.66
Baseline 8	35.04	36.97
Our method	**54.62**	**45.95**

discovering the latent structure in the high-dimensional feature space makes the problem extremely challenging. We postulate that separating temporal reasoning from discovering the latent structure might result in more accurate estimates of the latent structure.

Baselines: To further analyze our model, we examine the effects of each component in our model with several baselines designed to challenge different components in our formulation. Except for baseline 1, which measures the effect of Viterbi smoothing, all other baselines use a final Viterbi smoothing stage.

Baseline 1: To examine the importance of encoding temporal information, we remove the Viterbi temporal smoothing at inference and compare it with our full model. Table 2 shows that encoding temporal information helps action recognition in our setting.

Baseline 2: To verify the effects of binary versus continuous α (camera selection vs using all cameras with respect to their calculated importance), we train our model with the binary α constraint, where $\alpha_i^j \in \{0, 1\}$. This forces our model to pick only one camera combination. Table 2 shows results when binary α is used.

Baseline 3: To challenge the observation about encoding higher-order correlations using camera combinations, we compare our method with a version that uses only four cameras (no combination). This baseline uses continuous α. Results in Table 2 show that leveraging higher-order relations of cameras (camera combination) in our latent discriminative model improves action recognition.

Baseline 4: This baseline is similar to the previous one, with one modification: using binary α (camera selection). Table 2 shows that both higher-order correlations of features (camera combination) and using all cameras according to their importance improves the recognition accuracy.

Table 3. To evaluate the importance of each camera in our formulation we remove a camera from our model (with binary α) one at a time, and report the drop in the accuracy. The egocentric camera is the most informative camera in this setting and the back static camera is the least useful one.

Camera combinations	Avg. Acc.	Acc. drop %
Ego + Side + Back + Top	44.58	0
No Side	42.97	3.6
No Top	40.56	9.0
No Back	43.54	2.3
No Ego	**27.99**	**37.2**

Baseline 5: Our optimization learns an α for each frame. One could reasonably worry about a large number of parameters to learn. An alternative is to search for an α for each action. This implies that the importance of the cameras are fixed for all frames during the course of an action. Baseline 5 corresponds to experiments with a per-action α model. The results in Table 2 support our intuition that the importance of the cameras changes during an action.

Baseline 6: Examines the need for latent variables while learning to recognize actions across multiple cameras. In this baseline, we fuse multiple cameras without the latent variable. This late fusion baseline uses action models trained independently for different cameras and fuses them by a second layer RBF SVM. This baseline uses higher-order correlation of features(camera combination) and Viterbi smoothing. Our model differs from this baseline in using the latent α to explicitly encode the relationships across cameras in a discriminative manner. Table 2 shows the importance of our latent variable.

Baseline 7: Instead of learning latent variables, this late fusion baseline combines multiple cameras by equal weights and uses Viterbi smoothing.

Baseline 8: Another way to combine multiple cameras is to combine all the observations at the feature level and expect the classifiers to discover complex relationships in this high-dimensional data. Baseline 7 corresponds to this early fusion model. The results in Table 2 imply that complex relationships cannot be reliably discovered by just fitting a classifier to the combination of features. This baseline also uses Viterbi smoothing.

Besides the given state-of-the-art models and the eight baselines, we also experiment with per-frame classifiers of Logistic Regression (LR) and Nearest Neighbor (NN), and both underperform our model (Avg. Acc. LR = 31.1, NN = 37.1, c.f. 54.6 of ours).

As a sanity check, we also determine if there is apparent discriminative information in any single cameras that can bias the recognition performance on the CMU-MMAC dataset. To do that, we train RBF-SVMs action classifiers with Viterbi using only one camera. Using egocentric, static back, static side, and

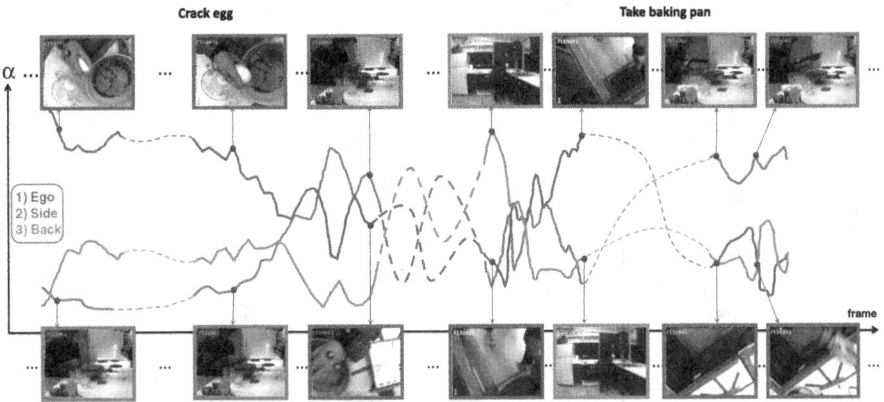

Fig. 2. The distribution of the learned α for "crack egg" and "take baking pan" actions: Our model learns that the egocentric camera contains maximum information for cracking an egg (highest α) when the subject interacts with the egg. Toward the end of the action when the subject looks away from the action, our model assigns more weight to the side static camera that represent the action best. For the "take baking pan" action our model allocated more weight to the static back camera when the subject walks to the cabinet. After opening the cabinet door, our model assigns more weights to the egocentric camera. This is followed by putting more weights on the side camera, when the subject is about to put the pan on the counter top.

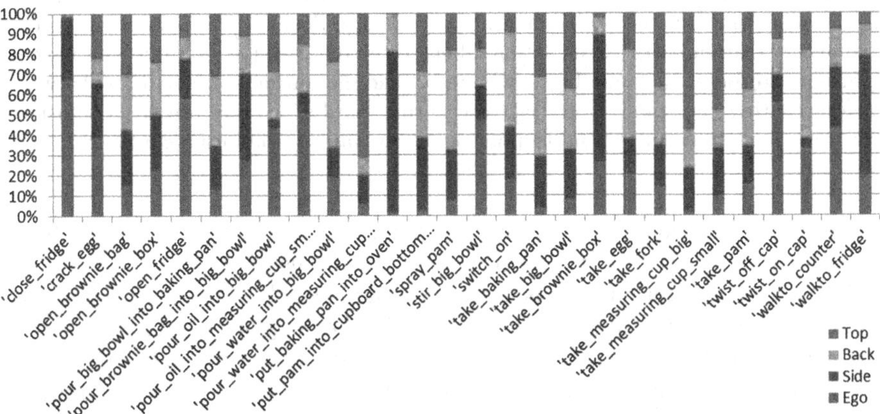

Fig. 3. The preference of our model in terms of cameras for each action. Actions like closing and opening fridge, cracking an egg, pouring oil into bow or measuring cup are better encoded in egocentric camera. For actions such as walking to the fridge, taking a brownie box, and putting a baking pan into oven our model prefers the side view camera where the body movements are visible.

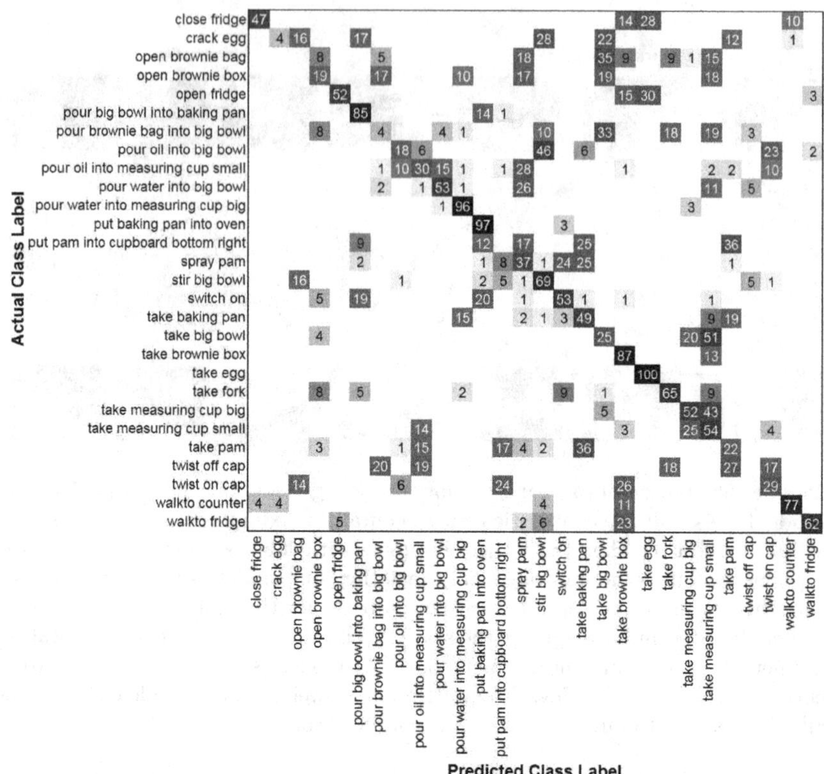

Fig. 4. Confusion matrix resulting from the experiments on the CMU-MMAC dataset. The numbers are rounded and represent percentages. Several off-diagonal confusions are due to the granularity of the action labels in the dataset. For example, the biggest confusions are between "take big bowl" and "take measuring cup small" or between "take measuring cup small" and "take measuring cup big". There are also confusions between actions that correspond to pouring either water or oil into a container.

static top cameras alone results in average accuracies of 37.92, 22.07, 21.26, 20.86, respectively (compared to average accuracy of 54.62 using our full model).

Although our main purpose is not to determine the best type of camera and position in recognizing actions, in order to further explore the importance of each camera in our model, we remove one camera at a time using binary α, and report the percentage drop in the performance numbers. Table 3 compares the accuracies and also the percentage drop in removing each of the cameras. The most informative camera in our setup is the egocentric one, and the least informative one is the back camera. This result is consistent with the nature of the dataset, where most of the actions that require hand-object interactions are best encoded in the subject's viewpoint using an egocentric camera.

To qualitatively evaluate the learned α's, we depict the distribution of α for some frames belonging to the "crack egg" and "take baking pan" actions in Fig. 2.

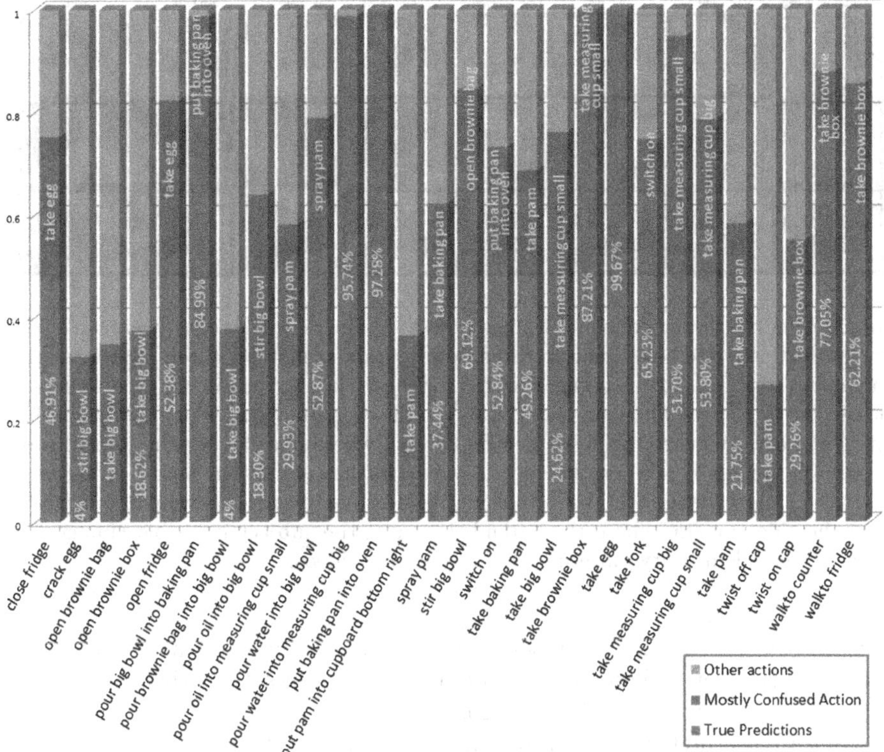

Fig. 5. Analysis of the action recognition on the CMU-MMAC dataset.

When the subject is cracking the egg, our method assigns high weights to the egocentric camera and once the subject's head is turning (and the egocentric camera is not informative) then our method assigns more weights to the side static camera. For the "take baking pan" action our method assigns more weights to the back camera when the subject is moving toward the cabinet. Once the cabinet door is open and the subject starts searching for the baking pan, the egocentric camera claims more weight. Toward the end of this action, the side static camera becomes more informative, and our method assigns more weight to that camera.

Figure 3 shows our model's preference for cameras for each action. Actions like closing and opening fridge, cracking an egg, pouring oil into bow or measuring cup are better encoded by the egocentric camera. For actions such as walking to the fridge, taking a brownie box, and putting a baking pan into the oven, our model prefers the side view camera where the body movements are visible.

Figure 4 shows the confusion matrix we obtained from our experiments on the CMU-MMAC dataset. The numbers are rounded and represent percentages. Several off-diagonal confusions are due to the granularity of the action labels in the dataset. For example, the biggest confusions are between "take big bowl" and

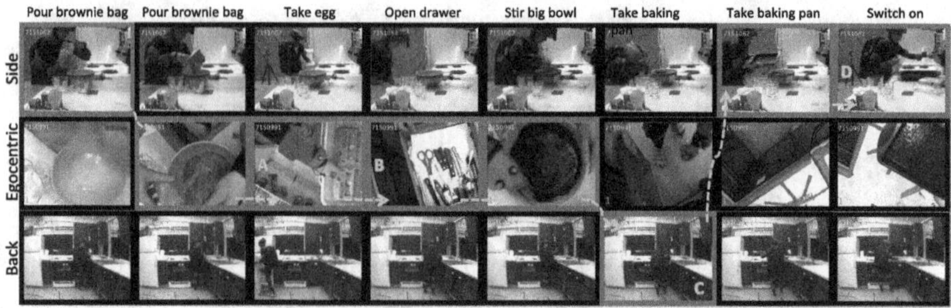

Fig. 6. This figure depicts some frames across 3 cameras (side, ego, back) for eight different actions. Red boxes indicated the frames that our method selects for the virtual cinematography. It is interesting to see that for the "take egg" action our model chooses the egocentric camera where one can clearly see the eggs (Image A). For "taking a fork", our model also switches to the egocentric camera where one can see the items inside the drawer (Image B). When the subject walks to the cabinet our model switches to the back camera (Image C). When the subject is about to turn the oven on our model picks the side camera, where the extended arm of the subject is visible (Image D). Please see supplementary material for the resultant videos.

"take measuring cup small" or between "take measuring cup small" and "take measuring cup big". There are also confusions between actions that correspond to pouring either water or oil into a container.

Figure 5 interprets the confusions in a different way. It shows per-class action recognition accuracies and the most confusing action for all actions in the CMU-MMAC dataset. Like the confusion matrix in Fig. 4 shows, the most confusion comes from very similar actions. The top three actions in terms of their recognition accuracy are "take egg", "put baking pan into oven", and "pour water into big cup". The three most difficult actions for our model are "twist off cap" and "put pan into cupboard bottom right", and "open brownie bag". Another source of confusion stems from the fact that some actions share very similar settings. For example, "open fridge" and "take egg" are frequently confused because the majority of the scene in the "take egg" action corresponds to the half-open door of the fridge. In addition, some actions share very similar body movements. For example, reaching for the same cabinet to take a PAM or a baking pan.

In addition to the experiments with the CMU-MMAC dataset, we have also run some experiments with static cameras on the IXMAS dataset, where the performances of the other methods are already available. Our method performed on-par-with the state of the art on the IXMAS dataset w/o any fine tuning. The details will be reported in a future paper.

4.2 Using α to Direct a Video Scene

To qualitatively evaluate our inferred α, we also use them to direct the scene of "making brownies" recorded from multiple static and an egocentric camera from CMU MMAC dataset. The task is to select which cameras to use for each frame.

We use our learned α to select one camera per frame. Picking the camera with maximum α value results in undesirable frequent switches between cameras. To avoid that we use segmented least squares to smooth the camera transitions. Figure 6 shows examples of the frames across 3 cameras: static side, static back, and egocentric camera. Frames with red boxes are selected by our method. It is interesting to see that when the subject searches for the fork in a drawer, our method switches to the egocentric camera where all the items inside the drawer are visible (Image B in Fig. 6). When the subject moves toward the cabinet to take a baking pan, our method switches to the back camera where human movements are clearly visible (Image C in Fig. 6). When the subject switches on the oven, our method picks the side static camera where the extended arm of the subject is visible (Image D in Fig. 6).

The video in the supplementary material shows examples of the results of directing a scene using the learned α in our model. To avoid undesirable frequent camera switches, we use segmented least squares with 10–20 frames for smoothing. We do not switch between the cameras for inconsistent actions. We encourage the readers to watch the video in the supplementary material.

5 Conclusion

We introduce a model that, for each query frame, discriminatively predicts the importance of different cameras and fuses the information accordingly. We show that our model outperforms state-of-the-art methods that jointly reason across time and actions. Our hypothesis is that joint reasoning across camera importance and actions followed by temporal smoothing is a more manageable learning problem than joint reasoning over time. By being more focused on frame-level discrimination, our model learns meaningful latent variables and can discriminatively suggest the importance of each camera for each frame. The next step involves extending our explicit latent variable formulation to also perform joint reasoning over time. Our learned camera indicator variable provides a level of understanding of the scene that enables meaningful camera selection for automatic cinematography. Our model does not take into account the principles of cinematography.

Our method shows very successful results on the challenging CMU-MMAC dataset by fusing the information from the egocentric and static cameras as needed. To the best of our knowledge, this is the first attempt in combining egocentric action recognition and conventional static camera action recognition.

References

1. Poppe, R.: A survey on vision-based human action recognition. Image Vis. Comput. (2010)
2. Ren, X., Philipose, M.: Egocentric recognition of handled objects: benchmark and analysis. In: CVPR (2009)

3. Aggarwal, J., Ryoo, M.: Human activity analysis: a review. ACM Comput. Surv. **43**, 1–43 (2011)
4. Taralova, E., De la Torre, F., Hebert, M.: Source constrained clustering. In: ICCV (2011)
5. Fathi, A., Farhadi, A., Rehg, J.M.: Understanding egocentric activities. In: ICCV (2011)
6. Fathi, A., Li, Y., Rehg, J.M.: Learning to recognize daily actions using gaze. In: Fitzgibbon, A., Lazebnik, S., Perona, P., Sato, Y., Schmid, C. (eds.) ECCV 2012, Part I. LNCS, vol. 7572, pp. 314–327. Springer, Heidelberg (2012)
7. Kanade, T., Hebert, M.: First-person vision. In: Proceedings of the IEEE (2012)
8. Pirsiavash, H., Ramanan, D.: Detecting activities of daily living in first-person camera views. In: CVPR (2012)
9. Fathi, A., Hodgins, J.K., Rehg, J.M.: Social interactions: a first-person perspective. In: CVPR (2012)
10. Kitani, K.M.: Ego-action analysis for first-person sports videos. IEEE Pervasive Comput. **11**, 92–95 (2012)
11. Ogaki, K., Kitani, K.M., Sugano, Y., Sato, Y.: Coupling eye-motion and ego-motion features for first-person activity recognition. In: CVPR Workshops (2012)
12. Sundaram, S., Mayol-Cuevas, W.: What are we doing here? egocentric activity recognition on the move for contextual mapping. In: ICRA (2012)
13. Sundaram, S., Mayol-Cuevas, W.: High level activity recognition using low resolution wearable vision. In: CVPR (2009)
14. Li, Y.L., Fathi, A., Rehg, J.M.: Learning to predict gaze in egocentric video. In: ICCV (2013)
15. Fathi, A., Rehg, J.M.: Modeling actions through state changes. In: CVPR (2013)
16. Ryoo, M.S., Matthies, L.: First-person activity recognition: what are they doing to me? In: CVPR (2013)
17. Farhadi, A., Tabrizi, M.K., Endres, I., Forsyth, D.A.: A latent model of discriminative aspect. In: ICCV (2009)
18. Wu, X., Jia, Y.: View-invariant action recognition using latent kernelized structural SVM. In: Fitzgibbon, A., Lazebnik, S., Perona, P., Sato, Y., Schmid, C. (eds.) ECCV 2012, Part V. LNCS, vol. 7576, pp. 411–424. Springer, Heidelberg (2012)
19. Gu, C., Ren, X.: Discriminative mixture-of-templates for viewpoint classification. In: Daniilidis, K., Maragos, P., Paragios, N. (eds.) ECCV 2010, Part V. LNCS, vol. 6315, pp. 408–421. Springer, Heidelberg (2010)
20. Song, Y., Morency, L.P., Davis, R.: Multi-view latent variable discriminative models for action recognition. In: CVPR (2012)
21. Wu, C., Khalili, A.H., Aghajan, H.: Multiview activity recognition in smart homes with spatio-temporal features. In: ACM/IEEE International Conference on Distributed Smart Cameras (2010)
22. Weinland, D., Özuysal, M., Fua, P.: Making action recognition robust to occlusions and viewpoint changes. In: Daniilidis, K., Maragos, P., Paragios, N. (eds.) ECCV 2010, Part III. LNCS, vol. 6313, pp. 635–648. Springer, Heidelberg (2010)
23. Farhadi, A., Tabrizi, M.K.: Learning to recognize activities from the wrong view point. In: Forsyth, D., Torr, P., Zisserman, A. (eds.) ECCV 2008, Part I. LNCS, vol. 5302, pp. 154–166. Springer, Heidelberg (2008)
24. Liu, J., Shah, M., Kuipers, B., Savarese, S.: Cross-view action recognition via view knowledge transfer. In: CVPR (2011)

25. Huang, C.-H., Yeh, Y.-R., Wang, Y.-C.F.: Recognizing actions across cameras by exploring the correlated subspace. In: Fusiello, A., Murino, V., Cucchiara, R. (eds.) ECCV 2012 Ws/Demos, Part I. LNCS, vol. 7583, pp. 342–351. Springer, Heidelberg (2012)
26. Junejo, I., Dexter, E., Laptev, I., Perez, P.: View-independent action recognition from temporal self-similarities. PAMI **33**, 172–185 (2011)
27. Gkalelis, N., Kim, H., Hilton, A., Nikolaidis, N., Pitas, I.: The i3DPost multi-view and 3D human action/interaction database. In: CVMP (2009)
28. Weinland, D., Ronfard, R., Boyer, E.: Free viewpoint action recognition using motion history volumes. CVIU **104**, 249–257 (2006)
29. De la Torre, F., Hodgins, J., Montano, J., Valcarcel, S., Macey, J.: Guide to the carnegie mellon university multimodal activity (CMU-MMAC) database. Technical report, CMU, RI (2009)
30. Spriggs, E.H., De la Torre, F., Hebert, M.: Temporal segmentation and activity classification from first-person sensing. In: IEEE Workshop on Egocentric Vision (2009)
31. Fisher, R., Reddy, P.: Supervised multi-modal action classification. Technical report, Carnegie Mellon University (2011)
32. McCall, C., Reddy, K.K., Shah, M.: Macro-class selection for hierarchical k-nn classification of inertial sensor data. In: PECCS (2012)
33. Zhao, L., Wang, X., Sukthankar, G., Sukthankar, R.: Motif discovery and feature selection for CRF-based activity recognition. In: ICPR (2010)
34. Elson, D.K., Riedl, M.O.: A lightweight intelligent virtual cinematography system for machinima production. In: AIIDE (2007)
35. He, L.W., Cohen, M.F., Salesin, D.H.: The virtual cinematographer: a paradigm for automatic real-time camera control and directing. In: Computer Graphics and Interactive Techniques (1996)
36. Felzenszwalb, P.F., Girshick, R.B., McAllester, D.A., Ramanan, D.: Object detection with discriminatively trained part-based models. PAMI **32**, 1627–1645 (2010)
37. Scheirer, W.J., Rocha, A., Michaels, R., Boult, T.E.: Meta-recognition: the theory and practice of recognition score analysis. PAMIs **33**, 1689–1695 (2011)
38. Morency, L., Quattoni, A., Darrell, T.: Latent-dynamic discriminative models for continuous gesture recognition. In: CVPR (2007)
39. van der Maaten, L.J.P., Welling, M., Saul, L.K.: Hidden-unit conditional random fields. In: IJCAI (2011)
40. Oliva, A., Torralba, A.: Building the gist of a scene: the role of global image features in recognition. In: Martinez-Conde, S., Macknik, S., Martinez, L., Alonso, J.-M., Tse, P. (eds.) Progress in Brain Research. Elsevier, Amsterdam (2006)

Robust Online Visual Tracking with a Single Convolutional Neural Network

Hanxi Li[1,3](✉), Yi Li[1,2], and Fatih Porikli[1,2]

[1] Canberra Research Laboratory, NICTA, Sydney, Australia
lihanxi2001@gmail.com

[2] Research School of Engineering, Australian National University, Canberra, Australia

[3] School of Computer and Information Engineering, Jiangxi Normal University, Nanchang, China

Abstract. Deep neural networks, albeit their great success on feature learning in various computer vision tasks, are usually considered as impractical for online visual tracking because they require very long training time and a large number of training samples. In this work, we present an efficient and very robust online tracking algorithm using a single Convolutional Neural Network (CNN) for learning effective feature representations of the target object over time. Our contributions are multifold: First, we introduce a novel truncated structural loss function that maintains as many training samples as possible and reduces the risk of tracking error accumulation, thus drift, by accommodating the uncertainty of the model output. Second, we enhance the ordinary Stochastic Gradient Descent approach in CNN training with a temporal selection mechanism, which generates positive and negative samples within different time periods. Finally, we propose to update the CNN model in a "lazy" style to speed-up the training stage, where the network is updated only when a significant appearance change occurs on the object, without sacrificing tracking accuracy. The CNN tracker outperforms all compared state-of-the-art methods in our extensive evaluations that involve 18 well-known benchmark video sequences.

1 Introduction

Image features play a crucial role in many challenging computer vision tasks such as object recognition and detection. Unfortunately, in many *online* visual trackers features are manually defined and combined [1–4]. Even though these methods report satisfactory results on individual datasets, hand-crafted feature representations would limit the performance of tracking. For instance, normalized cross correlation, which would be discriminative when the lighting condition is favourable, might become ineffective when the object moves under shadow.

Electronic supplementary material The online version of this chapter (doi:10.1007/978-3-319-16814-2_13) contains supplementary material, which is available to authorized users.

D. Cremers et al. (Eds.): ACCV 2014, Part V, LNCS 9007, pp. 194–209, 2015.
DOI: 10.1007/978-3-319-16814-2_13

This necessitates good representation learning mechanisms for visual tracking that are capable of capturing the appearance effectively changes over time.

Recently, deep neural networks have gained significant attention thanks to their success on learning feature representations. Different from the traditional hand-crafted features [5–7], a multi-layer neural network architecture can efficiently capture sophisticated hierarchies describing the raw data [8]. In particular, the Convolutional Neural Networks (CNN) has shown superior performance on standard object recognition tasks [9–11], which effectively learn complicated mappings while utilizing minimal domain knowledge.

However, the immediate adoption of CNN for online visual tracking is not straightforward. First of all, CNN requires a large number of training samples, which is often not be available in visual tracking as there exist only a few number of reliable positive instances extracted from the initial frames. Moreover, CNN tends to easily overfit to the most recent observation, *e.g.*, most recent instance dominating the model, which may result in drift problem. Besides, CNN training is computationally intensive for online visual tracking. Due to these difficulties, CNN has been treated only as an offline feature extraction step on predefined datasets [12,13] for tracking applications so far.

In this work, we propose a novel tracking algorithm using CNN to automatically learn the most useful feature representations of particular target objects while overcoming the above challenges. We employ a tracking-by-detection strategy – a three-layer CNN model to distinguish the target object from its surrounding background. We update this CNN model in an online manner. Our CNN generates scores for all possible hypotheses of the object locations (object states) in a given frame. The hypothesis with the highest score is then selected as the prediction of the object state in the current frame.

Typically, tracking-by-detection approaches rely on predefined heuristics to sample from the estimated object location to construct a set of positive and negative samples. Often these samples have binary labels, which leads to a few positive samples and a large negative training set. As a result, the model deterioration in case of a slight inaccuracy during tracking might happen [4]. Besides, the object locations, except the one on the first frame, is not always reliable as they are estimated by the visual tracker and the uncertainty is unavoidable [14]. To address these two issues, our CNN model employs a special type of loss function that consists of a robust term, a structural term, and a truncated norm. The structural term makes it possible to obtain a large number of training samples that have different significance levels considering the uncertainty of the object location at the same time. The robust term enables considering multiple object location estimates during the tracking process rather than being confined into the single, best location estimates at each frame. The truncated norm is applied on the CNN response to reduce the number of samples in the back-propagation [9,10] stage to significantly accelerate the training process.

We employ the Stochastic Gradient Decent (SGD) method to optimize the parameters in the CNN model. Since the standard SGD algorithm is not tailored for online visual tracking, we propose the following two modifications. First, to prevent the CNN model from overfitting to occasionally detected false positive instances, we introduce a *temporal sampling mechanism* to the batch generation in the SGD algorithm. This temporal sampling mechanism assumes that the object patches shall stay longer than those of the background in the memory. Therefore, we store all the observed image patches into training sample pool, and we choose the positive samples from a temporal range longer than the negative ones. In practice, we found this is a key factor in the robust CNN-based tracker, because discriminative sampling strategy successfully regularizes the training for effective appearance model.

Second, we use multiple image *cues* (low-level image features, such as normalized gray-scale image and image gradient) as independent channels as network input. We update the CNN parameters by iteratively training each channel independently followed by a joint training using their fully-connected layers. This makes the training efficient and empirically we observed that this two-stage iterative procedure is more accurate than jointly training for all cues.

Finally, in order to increase the tracking speed of the CNN-based tracker to a practical level, we propose to update the CNN model in a "lazy" style. The intuition behind this lazy updating strategy is that we assume that the object appearance is more consistent over the video, compared with the background appearances. The CNN-model is only updated when a significant appearance change occurs on the object. In practice, this lazy updating strategy increases the tracking speed significantly without causing any observable accuracy loss.

To summarize, our main contributions include:

- A visual tracker based on online adapting CNN is proposed. As far as we are aware, this is the first time a single CNN is introduced for learning the best features for object tracking in an online manner.
- A robust, structural, and truncated loss function is exploited for the online CNN tracker. This enables us to achieve very reliable (best reported results in the literature) and robust tracking while achieving tracking speeds up to 2.2 fps.
- An iterative SGD method with a temporal sampling mechanism is introduced for competently capturing object appearance changes.

Our experiments on an extensive dataset of 18 videos from recent benchmarks demonstrate that our method outperforms 9 state-of-the-art algorithms and rarely loses the track of the objects. In addition, it achieves a practical tracking speed (from 0.8 fps to 2.2 fps depending on the sequence and settings), which is comparable to many other visual trackers.

2 CNN Architecture

2.1 CNN with Multiple Image Cues

Our CNN consists of two convolutional layers, corresponding sigmoid functions as activation neurons and average pooling operators. The dark gray block in

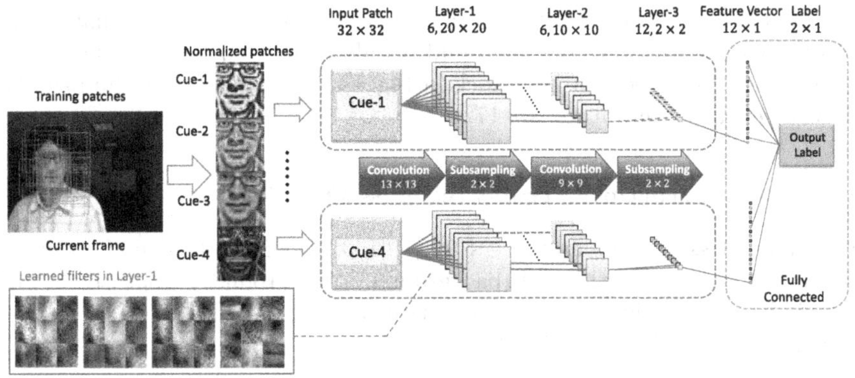

Fig. 1. The architecture of our CNN tracker with multiple image cues.

Fig. 1 shows the structure of our network, which can be expressed as $(32 \times 32) - (10 \times 10 \times 6) - (1 \times 1 \times 12) - (2)$ in conventional neural network notation.

The input is locally normalized 32×32 image patches, which draws a balance between the representation power and computational load. The first convolution layer contains 6 kernels each of size 13×13 (an empirical trade-off between overfitting due to a very large number of kernels and discrimination power), followed by a pooling operation that reduces the obtained feature map (filter response) to a lower dimension. The second layer contains 72 kernels with size 9×9. This leads to a 12 dimensional feature vector in the second layer, after the pooling operation in this layer.

The fully connected layer is a logistic regression operation. It takes the 12D vector computed by the first two layers and generates the score vector $\boldsymbol{s} = [s_1, s_2]^{\mathrm{T}} \in \mathcal{R}^2$, with s_1 and s_2 corresponding to the positive score and negative score, respectively. In order to increase the margin between the scores of the positive and negative samples, we calculate the CNN score of the patch n as

$$f(\boldsymbol{x}_n; \Omega) = S_n = s_1 \cdot \exp(s_1 - s_2), \tag{1}$$

where $\boldsymbol{x}_n$ denotes the input and the CNN is parameterized by the weights Ω.

Effective object tracking requires multiple cues, which may include color, image gradients and different pixel-wise filter responses. These cues are weakly correlated yet contain complementary information. Local contrast normalized cues are previously shown [10] to produce accurate object detection and recognition results within the CNN frameworks. The normalization not only alleviates the saturation problem but also makes the CNN robust to illumination change, which is desired during the tracking. In this work, we use 4 image cues generated from the given gray-scale image, *i.e.*, three locally normalized images with different parameter configurations[1] and a gradient image. We let CNN to

[1] Two parameters r_μ and r_σ determine a local contrast normalization process. In this work, we use three configurations, *i.e.*, $\{r_\mu = 3, r_\sigma = 1\}$, $\{r_\mu = 3, r_\sigma = 3\}$ and $\{r_\mu = 5, r_\sigma = 5\}$, respectively.

select the most informative cues in a data driven fashion. By concatenating the final responses of these 4 cues, we build a fully connected layer to the binary output vector (the green dashed block in Fig. 1). Note that we can find similar architectures in the literature [15–17].

2.2 Robust, Structural, Truncated Loss Function

Structural Loss. Let $\boldsymbol{x}_n$ and $\boldsymbol{l}_n \in \{[0,1]^{\mathrm{T}}, [1,0]^{\mathrm{T}}\}$ denote the cue of the input patch and its ground truth label (background or foreground[2]) respectively, and $f(\boldsymbol{x}_n; \Omega)$ be the predicted score of $\boldsymbol{x}_n$ with network weights Ω, the objective function of N samples in the batch is

$$\mathcal{L} = \frac{1}{N}\sum_{n=1}^{N} \|f(\boldsymbol{x}_n; \Omega) - \boldsymbol{l}_n\|_2 \tag{2}$$

when the CNN is trained in the batch-mode. Equation 2 is a commonly used loss function and performs well in binary classification problems. However, for object localization tasks, usually higher performance can be obtained by 'structurizing' the binary classifier. The advantage of employing the structural loss is the larger number of available training samples, which is crucial to the CNN training. In the ordinary binary-classification setting, one can only use the training samples with high confidences to avoid class ambiguity. In contrast, the structural CNN is learned based upon all the sampled patches.

We modify the original CNN's output to $f(\phi\langle\Gamma, \boldsymbol{y}_n\rangle; \Omega) \in \mathbb{R}$, where Γ is the current frame, $\boldsymbol{y}_n \in \mathbb{R}^o$ is the motion parameter vector of the target object, which determines the object's location in Γ and o is the freedom degree[3] of the transformation. The operation $\phi\langle\Gamma, \boldsymbol{y}_n\rangle$ suffices to crop the features from Γ using the motion $\boldsymbol{y}_n$. The associated structural loss is defined as

$$\mathcal{L} = \frac{1}{N}\sum_{n=1}^{N} [\Delta(\boldsymbol{y}_n, \boldsymbol{y}^*) \cdot \|f(\phi\langle\Gamma, \boldsymbol{y}_n\rangle; \Omega) - \boldsymbol{l}_n\|_2], \tag{3}$$

where $\boldsymbol{y}^*$ is the (estimated) motion state of the target object in the current frame. To define $\Delta(\boldsymbol{y}_n, \boldsymbol{y}^*)$ we first calculate the overlapping score $\Theta(\boldsymbol{y}_n, \boldsymbol{y}^*)$ [18] as

$$\Theta(\boldsymbol{y}_n, \boldsymbol{y}^*) = \frac{\text{area}(r(\boldsymbol{y}_n) \bigcap r(\boldsymbol{y}^*))}{\text{area}(r(\boldsymbol{y}_n) \bigcup r(\boldsymbol{y}^*))} \tag{4}$$

where $r(\boldsymbol{y})$ is the region defined by $\boldsymbol{y}$, $\bigcap$ and $\bigcup$ denotes the intersection and union operations respectively. Finally we have

$$\Delta(\boldsymbol{y}_n, \boldsymbol{y}^*) = \left| \frac{2}{1 + \exp(-(\Theta(\boldsymbol{y}_n, \boldsymbol{y}^*) - 0.5))} - 1 \right| \in [0, 1]. \tag{5}$$

[2] Here we follow the labeling style in conventional CNN training.

[3] In this paper $o = 3$, i.e., the bounding box changes in its location and the scale.

And the sample label $\boldsymbol{l}_n$ is set as.

$$\boldsymbol{l}_n = \begin{cases} [1,0]^{\mathrm{T}} & \text{if} \quad \Theta(\boldsymbol{y}_n, \boldsymbol{y}^*) > 0.5 \\ [0,1]^{\mathrm{T}} & \text{elsewise} \end{cases}$$

From Eq. 5 we can see that $\Delta(\boldsymbol{y}_n, \boldsymbol{y}^*)$ actually measures the importance of the training patch n. For instance, patches that are very close to object center and reasonably far from it may play more significant roles in training the CNN, while the patches in between are less important.

Structural Loss with a Robust Term and the Truncated Norm. In visual tracking, when a new frame $\Gamma_{(t)}$ comes, we predict the object motion state $\boldsymbol{y}^*_{(t)}$ as

$$\boldsymbol{y}^*_{(t)} = \arg\max_{\boldsymbol{y}_n \in \mathcal{Y}} \left(f(\phi\langle \Gamma_{(t)}, \boldsymbol{y}_n \rangle; \Omega) \right), \tag{6}$$

where $\mathcal{Y}$ contains all the test patches in the current frame. Among all motion states $\boldsymbol{y}^*_{(t)}$, $\forall t = 1, 2, \ldots, T$, only the first one $\boldsymbol{y}^*_{(1)}$ is always reliable as it is manually defined. Other motion states are estimated based on the previous observations. Thus, the uncertainty of the prediction $\boldsymbol{y}_{(t)}$, $\forall t > 1$ is usually unavoidable. Recall that, the structural loss defined in Eq. 4 could change significantly if a minor perturbation is imposed on $\boldsymbol{y}_{(t)}$, one requires a accurate $\boldsymbol{y}_{(t)}$ in every frame, which is, unfortunately, not feasible.

The Multiple-Instance-Learning (MIL) based approaches [14,19] use the instance bags, rather than individual instances as training samples, and the learning goal is to maximize the maximum score in the positive bag while minimize those in the negative bags [14,19]. Inspired by this idea, we regularize the ordinary structural loss using a set of positive instances rather than only one positive instance, which is novel in the state-of-the-art tracking-by-detection methods. In frame t ($t > 1$), we define the positive instance set as

$$\mathcal{Y}^* = \{\boldsymbol{y}_j \mid \Theta(\boldsymbol{y}_j, \boldsymbol{y}^*) < 0.5,\ f(\phi\langle \Gamma, \boldsymbol{y}_j \rangle; \Omega) > \eta f(\phi\langle \Gamma, \boldsymbol{y}^* \rangle; \Omega)\}. \tag{7}$$

It is easy to see that this set contains all the test samples with high scores and far away from the prediction $\boldsymbol{y}^*$. Here, we set $\eta = 0.975$, which is high enough to eliminate most of the true negatives. Then, we define a robust term based on $\boldsymbol{y}_n$ and $\mathcal{Y}^*$ as

$$r(\boldsymbol{y}_n, \mathcal{Y}^*) = \max\left(0,\ \max_{\boldsymbol{y}_j \in \mathcal{Y}^*} \frac{2}{1 + \exp(-(\Theta(\boldsymbol{y}_n, \boldsymbol{y}_j) - 0.5))} - 1\right). \tag{8}$$

We obtain the structural loss regularized by the positive set $\mathcal{Y}^*$ as

$$\mathcal{L} = \frac{1}{N} \sum_{n=1}^{N} [(\Delta(\boldsymbol{y}_n, \boldsymbol{y}^*) - r(\boldsymbol{y}_n, \mathcal{Y}^*)) \cdot \| f(\phi\langle \Gamma, \boldsymbol{y}_n \rangle; \Omega) - \boldsymbol{l}_n \|_2], \tag{9}$$

We can treat the above structural loss function as a robust version of the loss defined in Eq. 3. The weights of the training samples which have high CNN score

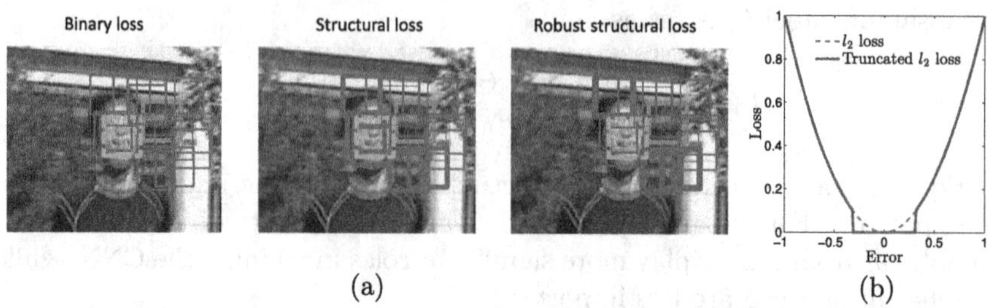

Fig. 2. (a) Illustration of the effects of different loss functions on negative samples. The green block stands for the object location while the blue block is the prediction of the visual tracker. The red blocks are the negative samples labeled according to the prediction (which is incorrect). The thickness of the red blocks represent their importance scores in the following training procedure. (b) Truncated l_2 norm (Color figure online).

but far away from the prediction $\boldsymbol{y}^*$ will be reduced significantly. In practice, we observed this structural loss reduces error accumulation, which usually starts from an incorrectly predicted $\boldsymbol{y}^*$.

The effect of proposed robust structural loss is shown in Fig. 2a, comparing with other two conventional loss functions, *i.e.*, the binary loss and the normal structural loss. We can see that, for a binary loss function, all the negative blocks (in red) share the same training weight. For the normal structural loss, those negative patches that overlap with the prediction (blue block) are assigned smaller weights than those far away from the prediction. As a result, the real object (green block) will be treated as a negative sample with a high importance, which might confuse the classifier. In contrast, the robust structural loss will reduce the weight around the green block as the prediction score for green block is also high, which is, in practice, usually true. Consequently, the incorrectly labeled object block will not play a dominant role in the consecutive training stages, and thus the learned tracker achieve more robustness.

Finally, we speed up the CNN training by employing a truncated l_2-norm in our model. We empirically observe that patches with very small error does not contribute much in the back propagation. Therefore, we can approximate the loss by counting the patches with errors that are larger than a threshold. Motived by this, we define a truncated l_2 norm as

$$\|e\|_{\mathbb{T}} = \|e\|_2 \cdot (1 - \mathbb{1}[\|e\|_2 \leq \beta]), \tag{10}$$

where $\mathbb{1}[\cdot]$ denotes the indicator function while e is the prediction error, *e.g.*, $f(\phi\langle \Gamma, \boldsymbol{y}_n\rangle; \Omega) - \boldsymbol{l}_n$ for patch-n. This truncated norm is visualized in Fig. 2b and now Eq. 9 becomes:

$$\mathcal{L} = \frac{1}{N}\sum_{n=1}^{N} [(\Delta(\boldsymbol{y}_n, \boldsymbol{y}^*) - r(\boldsymbol{y}_n, \mathcal{Y}^*)) \cdot \|f(\phi\langle \Gamma, \boldsymbol{y}_n\rangle; \Omega) - \boldsymbol{l}_n\|_{\mathbb{T}}], \tag{11}$$

It is easy to see that with the truncated norm $\|\cdot\|_{\mathbb{T}}$, the backpropagation [9] process only depends on the training samples with large errors, *i.e.*, $\|f(\phi\langle\Gamma, \boldsymbol{y}_n\rangle; \Omega) - \boldsymbol{l}_n\|_{\mathbb{T}} > 0$. Accordingly, we can ignore the samples with small errors and the backpropagation procedure is significantly accelerated. In this work, we use $\beta = 0.03$.

3 Optimization of CNN for Tracking

3.1 Online Learning: Iterative SGD with Temporal Sampling

Temporal Sampling. Following other CNN-based approaches [9,10], we used Stochastic Gradient Decent (SGD) for the learning of the parameters Ω. However, the SGD we employ is specifically tailored for visual tracking.

Different from detection and recognition tasks, the training sample pool grows gradually as new frames come in visual tracking. Moreover, it is desired to learn a consistent object model over *all* the previous frames and then use it to distinguish the object from the background in the *current* frame. This implies that we can effectively learn a discriminative model on a long-term positive set and a short-term negative set.

Based on this intuition, we tailor the SGD method by embedding in a temporal sampling process. In particular, given that the positive sample pool is $\mathbb{Y}^+_{1:t} = \{\boldsymbol{y}^+_{1,(1)}, \boldsymbol{y}^+_{2,(1)}, \cdots, \boldsymbol{y}^+_{N-1,(t)}, \boldsymbol{y}^+_{N,(t)}\}$ and the negative sample pool is $\mathbb{Y}^-_{1:t} = \{\boldsymbol{y}^-_{1,(1)}, \boldsymbol{y}^-_{2,(1)}, \cdots, \boldsymbol{y}^-_{N-1,(t)}, \boldsymbol{y}^-_{N,(t)}\}$, when generating a mini-batch for SGD, we sample the positive pool with the probability

$$\mathrm{Prob}(\boldsymbol{y}^+_{n,(t')}) = \frac{1}{tN}, \tag{12}$$

while sample the negative samples with the probability

$$\mathrm{Prob}(\boldsymbol{y}^-_{n,(t')}) = \frac{1}{Z}\exp\left[-\sigma(t-t')^2\right], \tag{13}$$

where $\frac{1}{Z}$ is the normalization term and we use $\sigma = 10$ in this work.

In a way, the above temporal selection mechanism can be considered to be similar to the "multiple-lifespan" data sampling [20]. However, [20] builds three different codebooks, each corresponding to a different lifespan, while we learn one discriminative model based on two different sampling distributions.

Iterative Stochastic Gradient Descent (IT-SDG). Recall that we use multiple image cues as the input of the CNN tracker. This leads to a CNN with higher complexity, which implies a low training speed and a high possibility of overfitting. By noticing that each image cue may be weakly independent, we train the network in a iterative manner. In particular, we define the model parameters as $\Omega = \{\mathbf{w}^1_{cov}, \cdots, \mathbf{w}^K_{cov}, \mathbf{w}^1_{fc}, \cdots, \mathbf{w}^K_{fc}\}$, where $\mathbf{w}^k_{cov}$ denotes the filter parameters in cue-k while $\mathbf{w}^k_{fc}$ corresponds to the fully-connected layer. After

Algorithm 1. Iterative SGD with temporal sampling

Inputs: Frame image $\mathit{\Gamma}_{(t)}$; Two sample pools $\mathbb{Y}^+_{1:t}$, $\mathbb{Y}^-_{1:t}$;

CNN model (K cues) $f(\phi\langle\mathit{\Gamma}_{(t)},\cdot\rangle;\mathit{\Omega}=\{\mathbf{w}^1_{cov},\cdots,\mathbf{w}^K_{cov},\mathbf{w}^1_{fc},\cdots,\mathbf{w}^K_{fc}\})$.

Estimated/given $\boldsymbol{y}^*$;

Learning rates $\hat{r}=\frac{r}{K}$; minimal loss ε; training step budget $M \gg K$.

procedure IT-SGD($\mathbb{Y}^+_{1:t}$, $\mathbb{Y}^-_{1:t}$, f, $\boldsymbol{y}^*$, $\hat{r}$, r, M)

Sample samples from $\mathbb{Y}^+_{1:t}$ and $\mathbb{Y}^-_{1:t}$, according to 12 and 13.

Save the selected samples in $\mathbb{Y}=\{\boldsymbol{y}_1,\boldsymbol{y}_2,\cdots,\boldsymbol{y}_N\}$ with labels $\boldsymbol{l}_1,\boldsymbol{l}_2,\cdots,\boldsymbol{l}_N$.

for $m \leftarrow 1,\ M-1$ **do**

Calculate loss $\mathcal{L}_m=\frac{1}{N}\sum_{n=1}^{N}\left[(\Delta(\boldsymbol{y}_n,\boldsymbol{y}^*)-r(\boldsymbol{y}_n,\mathcal{Y}^*))\cdot\left\|f_m(\phi\langle\mathit{\Gamma}_{(t)},\boldsymbol{y}_n\rangle;\mathit{\Omega})-\boldsymbol{l}_n\right\|_{\mathbb{T}}\right]$

If $\mathcal{L}\leq\varepsilon$, **break**;

$k=\mathrm{mod}(m,K)+1$;

Update $\mathbf{w}^k_{cov}$ using SGD with learning rate r for f_m;

Jointly update $\{\mathbf{w}^1_{fc},\cdots,\mathbf{w}^K_{fc}\}$ for f_m, with step length $\hat{r}$;

Save $f_{m+1}=f_m$;

end for

end procedure

Outputs: New CNN model $f^*=f_{m^*}, m^*=\arg\max_m \mathcal{L}_m$.

we complete the training on $\mathbf{w}^k_{cov}$, we evaluate the filter responses from all the cues in the fully-connected layer and then jointly update $\{\mathbf{w}^1_{fc},\cdots,\mathbf{w}^K_{fc}\}$ with a small learning rate (see Algorithm 1). This can be regarded as a coordinate-descent variation of SGD. In practice, we found out both the temporal sampling mechanism and the IT-SDG significantly curb the overfitting problem.

3.2 Lazy Update and the Overall Work Flow

It is straightforward to updating the CNN model using the IT-SGD algorithm at each frame. However, this could be computationally expensive as the complexity of training processes would dominate the complexity of the whole algorithm. On the other hand, in case the appearance of the object is not always changing, a well-learned appearance model can remain discriminant for a long time.

Motivated by this, we propose to update the CNN model in a lazy manner. When tracking the object, we only update the CNN model when the training loss $\mathcal{L}_1$ is above 2ε. Once the training start, the training goal is to reduce $\mathcal{L}$ below ε. As a result, usually $\mathcal{L}_1 < 2\varepsilon$ holds in a number of the following frames, and thus no training is required for those frames. This way, we accelerate the tracking algorithm significantly (Fig. 3).

4 Experiments

Video Sequences and Algorithms Compared. We evaluate our method on 18 benchmark video sequences that cover most challenging tracking scenarios such as scale changes, illumination changes, occlusions, cluttered backgrounds and fast motion. The first frames of these sequences are shown in Fig. 4.

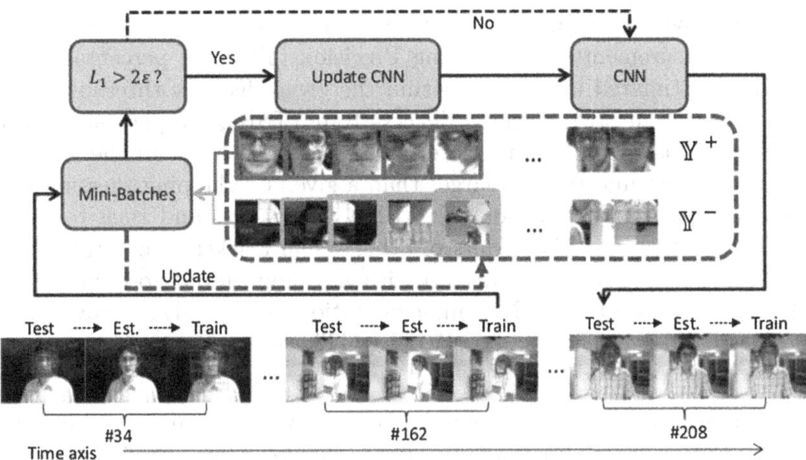

Fig. 3. Work flow of proposed algorithm. The bottom row shows the three-stages operations on a frame: test, estimation and training. In the training frames, the green bounding-boxes are the negative samples while the red ones denote the positive samples. The dashed block covers the positive sample pool $\mathbb{Y}^+$ (red) and negative sample pool $\mathbb{Y}^-$ (green). In each pool, the edges of the sample patches indicate their sampling importances. The thicker the edge, the more possible it will be selected for training (Color figure online).

We compare our method with 5 other state-of-the-art trackers including TLD [21], CXT [22], ASLA [23], Struck [4], SCM [24], and 4 classical tracking algorithms, *e.g.*, Frag [3], CPF [1], IVT [25] and MIL [14].

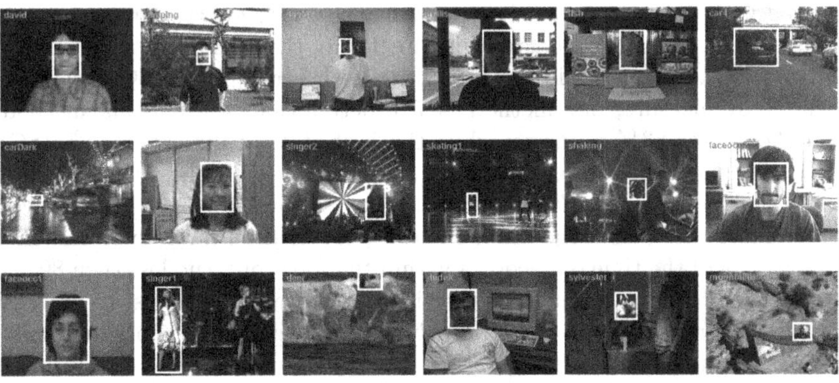

Fig. 4. The first frames of the selected video sequences. From top left to bottom right: David, Jumping, David2, Trellis, Fish, Car4, CarDark, Girl, Singer2, Skating1, Shaking, FaceOcc2, FaceOcc1, Singer1, Deer, Dudek, Sylvester, MountainBike. The red blocks are the initialization in the first frame (Color figure online).

Performance Measurements. The tracking results are evaluated via the following two measurements: (1) Tracking Precision (TP), the percentage of the frames whose estimated location is within the given distance-threshold (τ_d) to the ground truth, and (2) Tracking Success Rate (TSR), the percentage of the frames in which the overlapping score defined in Eq. 4 between the estimated location and the ground truth is larger than a given overlapping-threshold (τ_o). For a fair comparison, we run our algorithm for 5 times and then report the average TP/TSR scores. The results of other visual trackers are obtained from [26]. We run our algorithm in Matlab with an unoptimized code mixed with CUDA-PTX kernels for the CNN implementation. The hardware environment includes one quad-core CPU and a NVIDIA GTX580.

Parameter Setting. Most parameters of the CNN tracker are given in Sects. 2 and 3. In addition, there are some motion parameters for sampling the image patches. In this work, we only consider the displacement Δ_x, Δ_y and the relative scale s of the object[4]. In a new frame, we sample 1500 random patches in a Gaussian Distribution which centers on the previous predicted state. The standard deviation for the three dimensions are 10, 10 and 0.02, respectively. Note that, all parameters are fixed for all videos for most objective evaluation; no parameter tuning is performed for any specific video sequence.

Main Comparison Results. Firstly, we evaluate all algorithms using fixed thresholds, i.e. $\tau_d = 15$, $\tau_o = 0.5$, which is a common setting in tracking evaluations. Results are given in Table 1. Specifically, the score of TP and TSR are shown in each table block. The average performance is also reported for each tracker.

We can see that, our method achieves much better overall average results compared with other trackers. The performance gap between our method and the reported best result in the literature are 9 % for the TP measure: our method achieves 83 % accuracy while the best state-of-the-art is 74 % (SCM method). For the TSR measure, our method is 7 % better than the existing methods: our method gives 83 % accuracy while the best state-of-the-art is 76 % (SCM method). Furthermore, our CNN tracker have ranked as the best method for 17 times. These numbers for Struck, ASLA and SCM are 16, 13, 9, respectively. Another observation from the Table 1 is that, our method rarely performs inaccurately; 89 % of the time our score is within the top scores (no less then 80 % of the highest score for one sequence). As visible, our tracker is robust to dramatic appearance changes, e.g. due to motion blurs (Jumping and Deer) or illumination variations (Fish, Trellis and Singer2).

In fact, the superiority of our method becomes more clear when the experiments with different measurement criteria (different τ_d, τ_o) are conducted. In specific, for TP, we evaluate the trackers with the thresholds $\tau_d = 1, 2, \cdots, 50$ while for TSR, we use the thresholds $\tau_o = 0$ to 1 at the step of 0.05. According

[4] $s = h/32$, where h is object's height.

Table 1. The tracking scores of the proposed method and other visual trackers. The reported results are shown in the order of "TP/TSR". The top scores are shown in red for each row. For CNN tracker, a score is shown in blue if it is higher than 80 % of the highest value in that row.

	CNN	TLD	CXT	ASLA	Struck	SCM	Frag	CPF	IVT	MIL
david	0.84/0.80	1.00/0.97	1.00/0.83	1.00/0.96	0.32/0.24	1.00/0.91	0.13/0.12	0.11/0.03	0.95/0.79	0.42/0.23
jumping	1.00/1.00	0.98/0.85	0.86/0.29	0.29/0.17	1.00/0.80	0.14/0.12	0.96/0.85	0.14/0.11	0.18/0.10	0.76/0.48
david2	1.00/1.00	1.00/0.95	1.00/1.00	1.00/0.95	1.00/1.00	1.00/0.91	0.31/0.30	1.00/0.46	1.00/0.93	0.69/0.32
trellis	0.99/0.98	0.48/0.47	0.88/0.81	0.86/0.86	0.83/0.78	0.86/0.85	0.35/0.36	0.22/0.17	0.32/0.31	0.17/0.24
faceocc2	0.90/0.92	0.69/0.83	0.98/0.95	0.67/0.81	0.99/1.00	0.74/0.87	0.54/0.75	0.29/0.35	0.91/0.91	0.55/0.94
faceocc1	0.59/1.00	0.04/0.83	0.19/0.77	0.13/0.31	0.24/1.00	0.65/1.00	0.83/1.00	0.18/0.52	0.34/0.98	0.15/0.76
dudek	0.19/0.33	0.50/0.84	0.73/0.92	0.61/0.90	0.78/0.98	0.80/0.98	0.48/0.59	0.45/0.69	0.84/0.97	0.57/0.86
singer1	0.74/0.89	0.98/0.99	0.80/0.32	1.00/1.00	0.56/0.30	1.00/1.00	0.23/0.22	0.94/0.32	0.81/0.48	0.33/0.28
deer	1.00/1.00	0.73/0.73	0.94/0.92	0.03/0.03	1.00/1.00	0.03/0.03	0.18/0.21	0.04/0.04	0.03/0.03	0.08/0.13
fish	1.00/1.00	0.98/0.96	1.00/1.00	1.00/1.00	1.00/1.00	0.84/0.86	0.52/0.55	0.09/0.10	1.00/1.00	0.34/0.39
car4	1.00/0.85	0.86/0.79	0.30/0.30	1.00/1.00	0.97/0.40	0.97/0.97	0.18/0.21	0.03/0.02	1.00/1.00	0.35/0.28
carDark	0.92/0.88	0.61/0.53	0.71/0.69	1.00/1.00	1.00/1.00	1.00/1.00	0.39/0.25	0.11/0.02	0.77/0.70	0.27/0.18
singer2	0.87/0.91	0.04/0.10	0.05/0.04	0.03/0.04	0.03/0.04	0.11/0.16	0.16/0.20	0.08/0.14	0.04/0.04	0.18/0.48
sylvester	0.82/0.58	0.94/0.93	0.76/0.75	0.78/0.75	0.93/0.93	0.89/0.89	0.68/0.68	0.79/0.71	0.68/0.68	0.54/0.55
girl	0.94/0.84	0.87/0.76	0.74/0.64	1.00/0.91	1.00/0.98	1.00/0.88	0.63/0.54	0.69/0.54	0.36/0.19	0.51/0.29
mountainbike	0.55/0.68	0.25/0.26	0.28/0.28	0.78/0.86	0.86/0.90	0.86/0.96	0.13/0.14	0.08/0.15	0.87/0.98	0.52/0.57
shaking	0.79/0.93	0.33/0.40	0.05/0.11	0.25/0.38	0.08/0.17	0.70/0.90	0.07/0.07	0.14/0.12	0.01/0.01	0.18/0.23
skating1	0.77/0.34	0.26/0.23	0.20/0.12	0.76/0.69	0.29/0.37	0.72/0.42	0.14/0.12	0.20/0.19	0.08/0.07	0.12/0.10
Overall	0.83/0.83	**0.64/0.69**	**0.64/0.60**	**0.68/0.70**	**0.71/0.71**	**0.74/0.76**	**0.38/0.40**	**0.31/0.26**	**0.57/0.56**	**0.37/0.41**

to the scores under different criteria, we generate the precision curves and the success-rate curves for each tracking method, which is shown in Fig. 5.

From the score plots we can see that, overall the CNN tracker ranks the first (red curves) for both TP and TSR evaluations. Our algorithm is very robust when $\tau_o < 0.68$ and $\tau_d > 7$ as it outperform all other trackers. The CNN tracker rarely misses the target completely. Having mentioned that when the overlap thresholds are tight (*e.g.* $\tau_o > 0.8$ or $\tau_d < 5$), our tracker has similar response to rest of the trackers we tested.

In many applications, it is more important to not to loose the target object than very accurately locate its bounding box. As visible, our tracker rarely looses the object. Usually the object is much smaller than the frame and there is no big difference between 68 % overlapping and 90 % for users in this scenario.

Verification for Loss Function and the Temporal Sampling. Here we verify the two proposed modifications to the CNN model. We rerun the whole experiment using the CNN tracker without one or both of the modifications. The scores of our CNN tracker with different settings are reported in Table 2.

From the table we can see that, both the robust structural loss and the temporal sampling method contribute the success of our CNN tracker. In particular, the temporal sampling plays a more important role and the robust structural loss further increase the accuracy by 5 %. Similar to the previous evaluation, we plot the precision-curves and the success-rate curves for the CNN tracker with different settings. The curves consistently go up when the components are added into the CNN model. That indicates the validity of the propose modifications (Fig. 6).

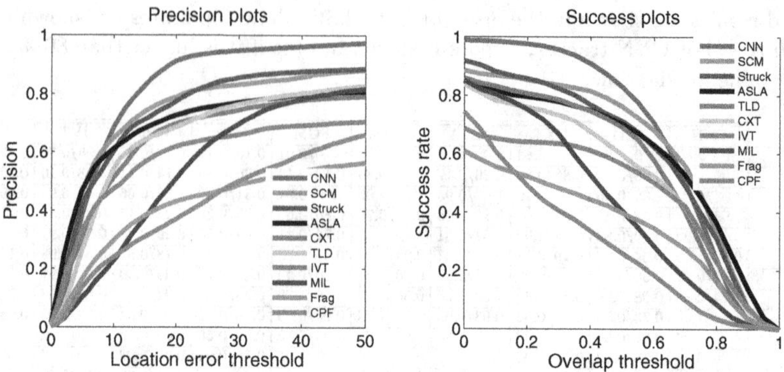

Fig. 5. The Precision Plot (left) and the Success Plot (right). The color of one curve is determined by the rank of the corresponding trackers, not their names (Color figure online).

Table 2. The performance comparison between CNN tracker variations.

	david	*Jumping*	*david2*	*trellis*	*faceOcc2*	*faceocc1*	*dudek*	*singler1*	*deer*	
CNN-std	0.67/0.64	0.05/0.05	0.27/0.26	0.76/0.79	0.93/0.95	0.46/0.88	0.01/0.21	0.95/0.91	0.95/1.00	
CNN-NoTemp	0.65/0.62	0.29/0.28	0.65/0.63	0.78/0.79	0.79/0.72	0.35/0.81	0.06/0.22	0.83/0.97	0.99/1.00	
CNN-NoStruct	0.88/0.69	0.68/0.68	1.00/0.99	0.97/0.96	0.79/0.72	0.40/0.99	0.12/0.27	0.68/0.81	1.00/1.00	
CNN-ours	0.84/0.80	1.00/1.00	1.00/1.00	0.99/0.98	0.90/0.92	0.59/1.00	0.19/0.33	0.74/0.89	1.00/1.00	
	fish	*car4*	*carDark*	*singer2*	*sylvester*	*girl*	*mountainbike*	*shaking*	*sylvester*	**overall**
CNN-std	1.00/1.00	0.15/0.18	1.00/0.99	0.54/0.60	0.54/0.44	0.08/0.08	0.93/0.92	0.43/0.50	0.61/0.09	**0.57/0.58**
CNN-NoTemp	0.97/1.00	0.85/0.66	0.88/0.67	0.54/0.59	0.67/0.50	0.52/0.35	0.85/0.81	0.22/0.32	0.39/0.08	**0.63/0.61**
CNN-NoStruct	1.00/1.00	1.00/0.87	1.00/1.00	0.83/0.90	0.86/0.75	0.85/0.63	0.59/0.82	0.75/0.84	0.54/0.28	**0.77/0.79**
CNN-ours	1.00/1.00	0.99/0.85	0.92/0.88	0.87/0.91	0.82/0.58	0.94/0.84	0.55/0.68	0.79/0.93	0.77/0.34	**0.83/0.83**

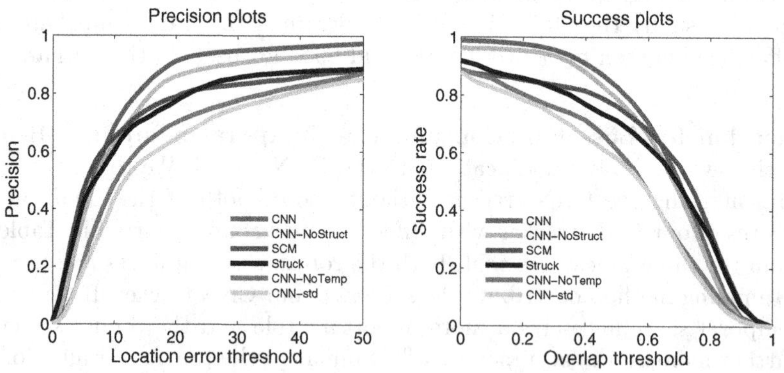

Fig. 6. The Precision Plot (left) and the Success Plot (right). The color of one curve is determined by the rank of the corresponding trackers, not their names (Color figure online).

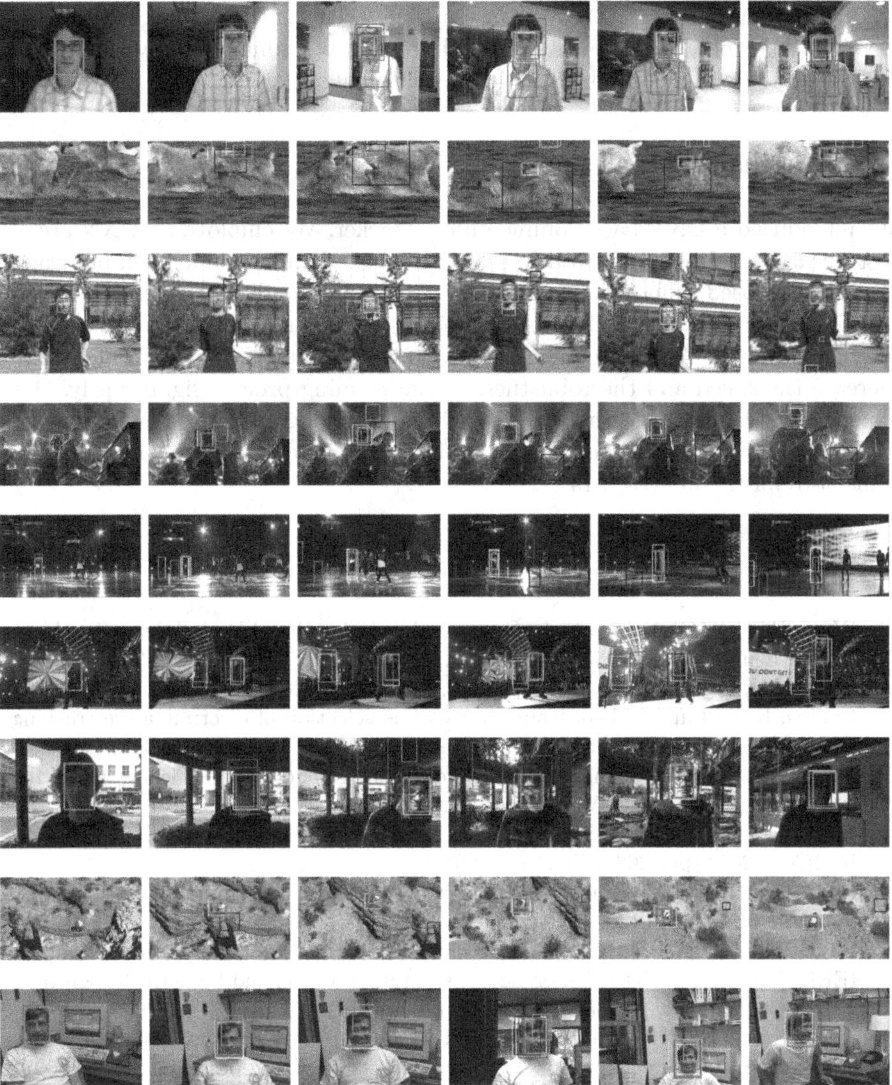

Fig. 7. Tracking results of the CNN tracker compared with other 6 visual trackers. The tracker are shown in different colors: green–CNN tracker; red–Struck; blue–SCM; black–CPF; yellow–ASLA; cyan–IVT; magenta–MIL; white–ground-truth. In each row, the 6 frames roughly span the whole sequence (Color figure online).

Some Tracking Examples. In Fig. 7 we show the tracking results of our CNN tracker comparing with three state-of-the-art trackers (SCM, Struck and ASLA) and three classical tracking methods (IVT, MIL, CPF), on 9 video sequences. Here we show some good results obtained by using our algorithm (row 1 to row 7) and some sequences on which the CNN tracker is outperformed by the other trackers (the last two rows). We can see that, even for the "failure" cases, the CNN tracker does not lose the target while is only "kidnapped" by some local part of the object (the human for the *mountainbike*).

5 Conclusion

We introduced a CNN based online object tracker. We employed a CNN architecture and a robust structural loss function that handles multiple input cues. We also proposed to modify the ordinary Stochastic Gradient Descent for visual tracking by iteratively update the parameters and add a temporal sampling mechanism in the mini-batch generation. This tracking-tailored SGD algorithm increase the speed and the robustness of the training process significantly. Our experiments demonstrate that the CNN-based tracking algorithm performs very well on 18 benchmark sequences and achieves the comparable tracking speed to some state-of-the-art trackers.

References

1. Pérez, P., Hue, C., Vermaak, J., Gangnet, M.: Color-Based Probabilistic Tracking. In: Heyden, A., Sparr, G., Nielsen, M., Johansen, P. (eds.) ECCV 2002, Part I. LNCS, vol. 2350, pp. 661–675. Springer, Heidelberg (2002)
2. Collins, R.T., Liu, Y., Leordeanu, M.: Online selection of discriminative tracking features. IEEE Trans. Pattern Anal. Mach. Intell. **27**, 1631–1643 (2005)
3. Adam, A., Rivlin, E., Shimshoni, I.: Robust fragments-based tracking using the integral histogram. In: CVPR 2006, vol. 1 (2006)
4. Hare, S., Saffari, A., Torr, P.H.: Struck: structured output tracking with kernels. In: ICCV 2011, pp. 263–270. IEEE (2011)
5. Lowe, D.G.: Distinctive image features from scale-invariant keypoints. Int. J. Comput. Vis. **60**, 91–110 (2004)
6. Dalal, N., Triggs, B.: Histograms of oriented gradients for human detection. In: IEEE Computer Society Conference on Computer Vision and Pattern Recognition, CVPR 2005, vol. 1, pp. 886–893. IEEE (2005)
7. Ahonen, T., Hadid, A., Pietikainen, M.: Face description with local binary patterns: application to face recognition. IEEE Trans. Pattern Anal. Mach. Intell. **28**, 2037–2041 (2006)
8. Bengio, Y., Courville, A., Vincent, P.: Representation learning: a review and new perspectives. IEEE Trans. Pattern Anal. Mach. Intell. **35**, 1798–1828 (2013)
9. Kavukcuoglu, K., Sermanet, P., Boureau, Y.L., Gregor, K., Mathieu, M., LeCun, Y.: Learning convolutional feature hierachies for visual recognition. In: NIPS 2010
10. Krizhevsky, A., Sutskever, I., Hinton, G.: Imagenet classification with deep convolutional neural networks. In: NIPS 2012 (2012)
11. Ciresan, D.C., Meier, U., Schmidhuber, J.: Multi-column deep neural networks for image classification. In: CVPR 2012 (2012)
12. Fan, J., Xu, W., Wu, Y., Gong, Y.: Human tracking using convolutional neural networks. Trans. Neural Netw. **21**, 1610–1623 (2010)
13. Wang, N., Yeung, D.Y.: Learning a deep compact image representation for visual tracking. In: NIPS 2013 (2013)

14. Babenko, B., Yang, M.H., Belongie, S.: Visual tracking with online multiple instance learning. Transactions on Pattern Analysis and Machine Intelligence (2011)
15. Zheng, Y., Liu, Q., Chen, E., Ge, Y., Zhao, J.L.: Time series classification using multi-channels deep convolutional neural networks. In: Li, F., Li, G., Hwang, S., Yao, B., Zhang, Z. (eds.) WAIM 2014. LNCS, vol. 8485, pp. 298–310. Springer, Heidelberg (2014)
16. Ciresan, D., Meier, U., Schmidhuber, J.: Multi-column deep neural networks for image classification. In: 2012 IEEE Conference on Computer Vision and Pattern Recognition (CVPR), pp. 3642–3649. IEEE (2012)
17. Cireşan, D., Meier, U., Masci, J., Schmidhuber, J.: Multi-column deep neural network for traffic sign classification. Neural Netw. **32**, 333–338 (2012)
18. Everingham, M., Van Gool, L., Williams, C.K., Winn, J., Zisserman, A.: The pascal visual object classes (voc) challenge. Intl J. Comput. Vis. **88**, 303–338 (2010)
19. Viola, P., Platt, J., Zhang, C., et al.: Multiple instance boosting for object detection. In: NIPS, vol. 2, p. 5 (2005)
20. Xing, J., Gao, J., Li, B., Hu, W., Yan, S.: Robust object tracking with online multi-lifespan dictionary learning. In: 2013 IEEE International Conference on Computer Vision (ICCV), pp. 665–672. IEEE (2013)
21. Kalal, Z., Matas, J., Mikolajczyk, K.: Pn learning: bootstrapping binary classifiers by structural constraints. In: CVPR 2010, pp. 49–56. IEEE (2010)
22. Dinh, T.B., Vo, N., Medioni, G.: Context tracker: exploring supporters and distracters in unconstrained environments. In: CVPR 2011, pp. 1177–1184. IEEE (2011)
23. Jia, X., Lu, H., Yang, M.H.: Visual tracking via adaptive structural local sparse appearance model. In: CVPR 2012, pp. 1822–1829. IEEE (2012)
24. Zhong, W., Lu, H., Yang, M.H.: Robust object tracking via sparsity-based collaborative model. In: CVPR 2012, pp. 1838–1845. IEEE (2012)
25. Ross, D.A., Lim, J., Lin, R.S., Yang, M.H.: Incremental learning for robust visual tracking. Intl. J. Comput. Vis. **77**, 125–141 (2008)
26. Wu, Y., Lim, J., Yang, M.H.: Online object tracking: a benchmark. In: CVPR 2013 (2013)

Bi-Stage Large Point Set Registration Using Gaussian Mixture Models

Junfen Chen[1], Munir Zaman[2(✉)], Iman Yi Liao[3], and Bahari Belaton[1]

[1] School of Computer Sciences, Universiti Sains Malaysia, Glugor, Malaysia
cj11_com079@student.usm.my, bahari@cs.usm.my

[2] Faculty of Engineering, University of Nottingham Malaysia Campus, Semenyih, Malaysia
munir.zaman@nottingham.edu.my

[3] School of Computer Science, University of Nottingham Malaysia Campus, Semenyih, Malaysia
iman.liao@nottingham.edu.my

Abstract. Point set registration is to determine correspondences between two different point sets, then recover the spatial transformation between them. Many current methods, become extremely slow as the cardinality of the point set increases; making them impractical for large point sets. In this paper, we propose a bi-stage method called bi-GMM-TPS, based on Gaussian Mixture Models and Thin-Plate Splines (GMM-TPS). The first stage deals with global deformation. The two point sets are grouped into clusters independently using K-means clustering. The cluster centers of the two sets are then registered using a GMM based method. The point sets are subsequently aligned based on the transformation obtained from cluster center registration. At the second stage, the GMM based registration method is again applied, to fine tune the alignment between the two clusters to address local deformation. Experiments were conducted on eight publicly available datasets, including large point clouds. Comparative experimental results demonstrate that the proposed method, is much faster than state-of-the-art methods GMM-TPS and QPCCP (Quadratic Programming based Cluster Correspondence Projection); especially on large non-rigid point sets, such as the swiss roll, bunny and USF face datasets, and challenging datasets with topological ambiguity such as the banana dataset. Although the Coherent Point Drift (CPD) method has comparable computational speed, it is less robust than bi-GMM-TPS. Especially for large point sets, under conditions where the number of clusters is not extreme, a complexity analysis shows that bi-GMM-TPS is more efficient than GMM-TPS.

1 Introduction

Point set registration has become an active research topic due to its wide applications in object tracking, motion recovery, 3D image reconstruction, stereo matching, to name a few. Registration between two point sets is to find out the meaningful correspondences between the points among the two sets and

D. Cremers et al. (Eds.): ACCV 2014, Part V, LNCS 9007, pp. 210–225, 2015.
DOI: 10.1007/978-3-319-16814-2_14

to recover the underlying spatial transformation that warps one point set onto another [2,14]. A point set is a collection of the spatial coordinates (locations), while other information such as mesh structure and texture information may not be involved.

In recent years, several state-of-the-art algorithms have greatly influenced the field, including robust point matching algorithm based on thin-plate splines (RPM-TPS) [5], coherent point drift algorithm (CPD) [14] and Jian's method [8,9], amongst others. For convenience, we call Jian's method GMM-TPS in this paper, which is an extension of a correlation-based point set registration proposed by Tsin and Kanade [17]. Jian and Vemuri represented two point sets as two separate Gaussian Mixture Models (GMMs), and formulated point sets registration as aligning two distribution functions via minimizing their dissimilarity. However, registration speed slows down dramatically as the number of points increases, especially in the case of non-rigid point sets registration. Another problem with GMM-TPS is that it is not reliable when topological ambiguity is exhibited in the data (e.g., see the banana dataset plotted in Fig. 5(a)).

In this paper, we propose a bi-stage point set registration framework to address the above problems. The first stage is a coarse alignment that deals with global deformation. A clustering method is applied to divide the two point sets into clusters separately. The two cluster centers are then registered using a GMM-based method, the transformation of which is subsequently extended to the entire point sets. At the fine registration stage, each pair of clusters between the two point sets is registered also using a GMM-based method to accommodate any local deformation. The alignment problem is solved by minimizing the dissimilarity of two GMMs with respect to thin-plate splines (TPS) transformation. As our proposed method applies GMM-TPS method at both stages in the implementation, we conveniently name it as bi-GMM-TPS.

The proposed bi-GMM-TPS method can deal with point set registration in following situations that are not well handled otherwise: (i) the deformation appears uneven in different parts of the data, and (ii) the two data sets present global misalignment caused by topological ambiguity. It is also worth noting that the proposed method presents a concept of a general top-down hierarchical framework for large point set registration, where the specific registration method in each stage may be methods other than GMM-TPS.

The rest of this paper is organized as follows. An overview of point sets registration is presented in Sect. 3. A hierarchical bi-stage point sets registration framework and implementation details are described in Sect. 4. In Sect. 5, we evaluate the performances of the proposed algorithm. Section 6 concludes the paper and recommends possible future works.

2 Related Works

Point sets registration involves three main topics: (i) the modelling of the point set registration, (ii) the correspondences between the points among the two sets, and (iii) the transformation that aligns one point set onto the other. As for the modelling, Joshi and Lee [10], Luo and Hancock [13] and Myronenko and Song [14,15], formulated point set registration as a maximum likelihood (ML) estimation problem forcing the GMM centroids to approach the data points; where one point set denotes the GMM centroids and the other represents the data points in a Gaussian mixture. While Tsin and Kanade [17], Jian and Vemuri [8,9] also considered registration as an alignment of two Gaussian mixtures, they represent the two point sets as two separate GMMs centroids. By considering structure information of a point set as a weighted neighborhood graph, the point matching problem can be formulated as a probabilistic graphical model that can be solved by maximizing its associated probability [3,6]. A Riemannian framework of point cloud matching was first proposed by Deng et al. [21]. They treated point clouds matching as a shape matching problem where the point cloud is represented by a Schrödinger Distance Transform (SDT) shape representation.

Chui [4] considered the latter two components of registration as two variables. All registration methods can be categorized into two types, according to the methods handling these two variables. One type of registration method attempts to determine the transformation without needing to establish the explicit point correspondences. This category includes density-based alignment approaches and TPS based registration algorithms [8,9]. Under a similarity transformation, instead of the complex non-rigid transformation in points matching, when the transformation variables are eliminated, the least squares optimization problem with respect to correspondences constraints decomposes into a concave optimization with global optimality [22]. In [23], the concave optimization problem is further studied to reduce the complexity of computing the lower bound by a k-cardinality linear assignment.

The other type of point set registration method attempts to solve correspondences and transformation simultaneously via some alternative updating scheme such as expectation maximization (EM) [1]. Examples include iterative closest point (ICP) algorithm and its variations [7,12], robust point matching algorithm (RPM-TPS) [5], and coherent point drift algorithm (CPD) [14,15].

Recently, clustering methods have also been incorporated in some approximation schemes to deal with large point sets registration problems. A quadratic programming based cluster correspondence projection (QPCCP) algorithm was proposed to pursue the approximate solution by relaxing the correspondences to a continuous value [11]. A farthest-point clustering was used to group point set X into N clusters and point set Y into M clusters [19]. Here, computational complexity decreases by considering the relatively fewer cluster correspondences instead of dense point correspondences. Subsequently, the recovery of point correspondences from cluster correspondences is carried out by a simple substitution.

A further approximation of the point registration algorithm is based on clusters and a generalized radial basis function [20]. This approach was a variant of RPM-TPS where Gaussian kernel function replaces TPS to construct a non-rigid mapping. Deterministic annealing was adopted to update the weight matrix and the correspondence matrix. K-means clustering [1] was used to group one set into a number of clusters, while the other set remains untouched. The number of clusters is gradually increased leading to a coarse-to-fine matching. The proposed method is efficient and beneficial for large and unevenly distributed data. However, it is sensitive to missing and rough correspondences.

Although the proposed method is also based on clustering, it is different from the aforementioned approximation methods in that (i) the result from registering the cluster centers is not the end but the input to a second fine alignment stage; (ii) all points in both point sets are involved in the registration process, and (iii) it is insensitive to missing or rough correspondences (inherited from GMM-TPS).

3 Gaussian Mixture Models-Thin Plate Splines (GMM-TPS)

This section provides a summary of GMM-TPS [9]. TPS is an effective radial basis function (RBF) for representing coordinate mappings $\mathbb{R}^d \rightarrow \mathbb{R}^d$ (d=2 or 3). Given a control point set $Q = \{q_1, q_2, \ldots, q_t\}$, The TPS mapping function is defined as:

$$T(p) = pA_1 + h + \sum_{i=1}^{t} w_i U(\|p - q_i\|) \tag{1}$$

where A_1 is a $d \times d$ rigid transformation parameter, $p, q_i \in \mathbb{R}^d$, and $U(r)$ is the radial basis function.

A homogeneous coordinates trick (a point denoting as $[1, p_x, p_y]$) is introduced to lead to the following form of the TPS mapping function

$$T(p) = pA + UW \tag{2}$$

where $A = \begin{bmatrix} h \\ A_1 \end{bmatrix}$ is a $(d+1) \times d$ global affine parameters, W is a $t \times d$ local non-rigid warping parameters and U is a row vector describing structure information between point p and control set Q.

Given two finite point sets $M = \{m_1, m_2, \ldots, m_a\}$, and $S = \{s_1, s_2, \ldots, s_b\}$, where $m_i, s_j \in \mathbb{R}^d$. Develop two Gaussian mixtures for M and S respectively:

$$f(x) = \sum_{i=1}^{a} \alpha_i \phi(x; T(m_i), \Sigma_i^2) \tag{3}$$

$$g(x) = \sum_{j=1}^{b} \beta_j \phi(x; s_j, \Pi_j^2) \tag{4}$$

where x is a spatial point (a vector); α_i, β_j are weights for Gaussian function ϕ; Σ_i^2, Π_j^2 are covariances, and T denotes the TPS transformation. The model can be simplified by assuming equal weights and isotropic covariances in (3) and (4).

Jian and Vemuri [9] have also pointed out that the final registration results were similar for most reasonable selections of covariance in their experiments.

The two point sets registration problem can be formulated as aligning two Gaussian mixtures. If two point sets are aligned sufficiently accurately, the corresponding two mixtures would be expected to be highly similar. A cost function for this is given by:

$$J = \int f^2 dx - 2\int fg\, dx + \frac{\lambda}{2}\|LT\|^2 \tag{5}$$

The first two terms measure the similarity between two Gaussian mixtures via a L2 distance. The last term is a regularization term to control the smoothness of TPS mapping function. Parameter λ balances the regularization strength. The resulting bending energy is $trace(W^T KW)$, where the kernel matrix $K = K_{i,j} = U(|q_i - q_j|)$, describes the internal structure information among the control point set. An elegant closed-form solution is provided by a gradient-based numerical optimization algorithm L-BFGS-B in [18].

4 Bi-Stage Point Sets Registration Framework

4.1 The Bi-Stage Registration Framework

K-means clustering is a popular unsupervised learning algorithm. It groups similar spatial points to form a cluster, thus its center represents the spatial structure of the cluster to a certain degree. Motivated by it, the first stage alignment is designed to obtain a global and coarse TPS transformation on cluster centers. $X = \{x_1, x_2, \dots, x_m\}$ is clustered into k clusters denoting as $X_i = \{x^i_1, x^i_2, \dots, x^i_{n_i}\}$, $i = 1, 2, \dots, k$, and the centers set is $C = \{c_1, c_2, \dots, c_k\}$. Similarly, $Y = \{y_1, y_2, \dots, y_n\}$ is clustered into k clusters as $Y_j = \{y^j_1, y^j_2, \dots, y^j_{n_j}\}$, $j = 1, 2, \dots, k$, and centers set is $S = \{s_1, s_2, \dots, s_k\}$. For registration, there is no specific requirement on the number of clusters. Without loss of generality, we therefore set the number of clusters in both point sets to be the same.

Two Gaussian mixtures are generated for C and S respectively. A TPS mapping function $u(A^{(1)}, W^{(1)})$ is computed by minimizing the divergence of two Gaussian mixtures using gradient-based optimization L-BFGS-B. We update set X and its clusters $X_1, X_2, \dots, X_k$ and denote them as $\tilde{X}$ and $\tilde{X}_1, \tilde{X}_2, \dots, \tilde{X}_k$ respectively. The resultant alignment is capable of effectively removing the influence of global misalignment.

In addition, this coarse alignment provides a finer initialization for further local registration, as the resultant TPS function $u(A^{(1)}, W^{(1)})$ can be extended to the whole set X, by replacing U with a $m \times t$ matrix describing the structure information of set X and control point set Q. The correspondences between the cluster centers are recovered through a bijection function from center set C to S using a nearest neighbour scheme.

At the fine registration stage, dense point registration is conducted on each cluster pair $(\tilde{X}_i, Y_j)$. The resulting TPS function $u(A^{(2)}_i, W^{(2)}_i)$ is used to warp cluster $\tilde{X}_i$ onto Y_j. According to GMM-TPS implemented in the proposed framework, it is obvious that the registration result is influenced only by the points within a cluster, its corresponding cluster, and the control points. The method of aligning two distribution functions based on TPS reduces any possible interference between two clusters X_i and X_j, $i \neq j$. This inherent attribute greatly benefits the division-based alignment for large point sets. A larger number of control points yield a more flexible deformation, however, this will increase computation time. In this paper, less control points obtained from a sparse spacing are used at the coarse alignment stage, with more control points from a dense spacing introduced at the fine registration stage.

Our bi-stage point sets registration algorithm (bi-GMM-TPS) is summarized as follows:

Algorithm 1. Bi-Stage Point Set Registration with K-means Clustering

procedure BI-GMM-TPS
  $X \leftarrow$ moving model point set X
  $Y \leftarrow$ fixed scene point set Y
  $Q \leftarrow$ control point set Q
  $k \leftarrow$ no. of clusters
  Clustering:
  $(C1, \mu 1) \leftarrow$ (indices, locations) of cluster centres X
  $(C2, \mu 2) \leftarrow$ (indices, locations) of cluster centres Y
  Global Alignment:
  $A^{(1)}, W^{(1)} \leftarrow$ align $\mu 1$ onto $\mu 2$ using GMM-TPS
  $\tilde{X} \leftarrow$ update X with TPS parameters $A^{(1)}, W^{(1)}$ using TPS warping
  $f \leftarrow$ bijection: assign each element of $\mu 1$ to its nearest neighbour in $\mu 2$
  Local Fine Registration:
  for i=1 to k **do**
    $x \leftarrow \tilde{X}_i$
    $y \leftarrow \tilde{Y}_{f(i)}$
    $A_i^{(2)}, W_i^{(2)} \leftarrow$ align x onto y using GMM-TPS

4.2 Computational Complexity Analysis

GMM-TPS. In GMM-TPS, the computational cost is:

1. Computing two integral values $\int f^2 dx$ and $\int fg dx$: $\mathcal{O}(m^2) + \mathcal{O}(mn)$; and
2. Computing kernel matrices U and K: $\mathcal{O}(mt) + \mathcal{O}(t^2)$.

Thus, the total computational cost for GMM-TPS is

$$d1 = \mathcal{O}(m^2) + \mathcal{O}(mn) + \mathcal{O}(mt) + \mathcal{O}(t^2). \tag{6}$$

BI-GMM-TPS. Assume the number of control points in our bi-GMM-TPS be t (the same as in GMM-TPS). The number of clusters is k. The computing cost is:

1. K-means clustering on point sets X and Y: $\mathcal{O}(km) + \mathcal{O}(kn)$;
2. Initial matching process: $\mathcal{O}(k^2) + \mathcal{O}(k^2) + \mathcal{O}(kt) + \mathcal{O}(t^2)$;
3. Building bijection function from $\mu 1$ to $\mu 2$: $\mathcal{O}(k^2)$, and
4. Local fine registration: $\mathcal{O}\left(\frac{m^2}{k}\right) + \mathcal{O}\left(\frac{mn}{k}\right) + \mathcal{O}(mt) + \mathcal{O}(kt^2)$.

The total cost for bi-GMM-TPS is therefore

$$d2 = \mathcal{O}(km) + \mathcal{O}(kn) + \mathcal{O}(k^2) + \mathcal{O}(kt) + \mathcal{O}(t^2) + \mathcal{O}\left(\frac{m^2}{k}\right) + \mathcal{O}\left(\frac{mn}{k}\right) + \mathcal{O}(mt) + \mathcal{O}(kt^2). \tag{7}$$

Without loss of generality, let $m = \min(m,n)$, $d1 = (m^2 + mn + mt + t^2)$, $d2 = (km + kn + k^2 + kt + t^2 + \frac{m^2}{k} + \frac{mn}{k} + mt + kt^2)$. When $k = 1$ or $k = m$, we can obtain $d2 > d1$. That is to say, two extreme situations lead to a higher computational cost for bi-GMM-TPS.

Comparison Between GMM-TPS and Bi-GMM-TPS. When the computation time of the initial matching process is negligible, and the number of clusters k, satisfies $\frac{m-\sqrt{m^2-4m}}{2} < k < \frac{m+\sqrt{m^2-4m}}{2}$ $(m > 4)$; $d2 < d1$ holds.

Furthermore, we consider the general case. With increasing value of k, $d2$ decreases initially and then increases. Suppose, when $k = k_0$, the minimum of $d2$ is reached, denoted as $\tilde{d2}$. We can see from (7), as t increases $\tilde{d2}$ increases, leading to $d2 > d1$. In practice, the control points will not be too great, otherwise this will increase the computational complexity and the risk of over-fitting. Thus the decision to disregard the computational time for the initial alignment stage can be justified.

5 Experimental Results and Discussion

In this section, extensive experiments are carried out to investigate the performance of the proposed method (bi-GMM-TPS) on various data sets. Quantitative and qualitative comparisons with state-of-the-art registration methods are also presented. All experiments were performed on Matlab, on a PC with 4 GB of RAM and a 2.8 GHz Intel Xeon W3530 CPU running Windows 7 (64-bit).

5.1 Data Analysis

There are eight public data sets being used in the experiments. Four of them are obtained from cited literature in computer vision [9,14]. Three are challenging data sets used in machine learning such as banana, Gaussian and swiss roll data. The last one is obtained from the USF 3D face database representing a very large point set [24]. The descriptions of the datasets are in Table 1.

Table 1. The eight datasets used in our experiments.

Dataset name	Size (points x dimension)	Description
Dolphin	91×2	2D shape edge
Fish	98×2	2D shape edge
Synthetic face	392×3	3D surface
Gaussian	1800×2	2D points cloud
Banana	8000×2	2D shape edge points cloud
Swiss roll	8000×3	3D points cloud
Bunny	8171×3	3D laser range scan
USF face	75972×3	3D laser range scan

To quantitatively evaluate the performance of the registration methods, three metrics are defined in this paper. First, *registration error* is defined as a mean L2 distance between the transformed point set and the scene point set

$$\text{registration error} = \frac{1}{mn}\sum_{i=1}^{m}\sum_{j=1}^{n}\|x_i - y_j\|_{L2} \tag{8}$$

Another measurement is the *number of correspondences*. If the distance between a point in one set and its nearest neighbour in another set is less than a predefined threshold, it is considered that this point has found its correspondence. This metric is defined as:

$$\text{number of correspondences} = |C_X| \tag{9}$$

where $|\cdot|$ is the cardinality of a finite point set; and the correspondences set C_X is generated by

$$C_X = \{y_k, i = 1, 2, \ldots, m |\ d(x_i, y_k) < \tau;\ \text{where } d(x_i, y_k) = \min_j d(x_i, y_j)\} \tag{10}$$

The third metric is *recall*, that was first used in [16] and adopted in [9]. Recall is defined as the proportion of the number of the true-positive correspondences to the total number of ground truth correspondences. Under a reasonable assumption that one-to-one correspondence happens in two clean point sets with the same cardinality. The number of ground truth correspondences is equivalent to the cardinality of the point set. Thus, recall is computed as

$$\text{recall} = \frac{\text{The number of true-positive correspondences}}{\text{Total number of ground truth correspondences}}. \tag{11}$$

5.2 Performance Evaluation of Bi-GMM-TPS

Experiments on Choice of Clustering Methods. Two clustering methods, K-means and K-medoids, are used in the experiments to compare the performance of bi-GMM-TPS on different choices of clustering methods. The results

Table 2. Comparison of registration performance based on K-means and K-medoids.

Dataset	Registration error		Number of correspondences		Recall		Time(s)	
	k-means	k-medoids	k-means	k-medoids	k-means	k-medoids	k-means	k-medoids
Dolphin	0.0342	0.1588	79	39	0.7143	0.1538	0.2148	0.3291
Fish	0.0212	0.0731	93	71	0.4794	0.1327	0.3910	0.2612
Synthetic face	0.0926	0.3077	336	275	0.4388	0.0638	1.20	1.9939
Gaussian	1.0651	1.2007	1771	1780	0.0139	0.0100	1.7197	2.6628

are shown in Table 2. One can choose other clustering methods according to the actual problem one is dealing with.

Due to out of memory problem when computing the k-medoids, we do not have results for swiss roll, banana, bunny and USF 3D face data.

We can see from Table 2 that for bi-GMM-TPS method:

1. K-means can provide lower registration errors than K-medoids on the given data;
2. The recalls based on K-means are higher than those based on K-medoids.
3. For the given distance threshold, K-means found more correspondences on the first three data sets. However, K-medoids obtained higher number of correspondences on Gaussian points cloud;
4. K-means based algorithm runs faster than K-medoids based algorithm on dolphin and Gaussian data, while it is slightly slower on the synthetic face data.

The recall for points cloud data (i.e. Gaussian data) is lower than the recalls for shapes and surface data (i.e., dolphin, fish, and synthetic face data), although the number of correspondences of the former is higher. Furthermore, note that K-medoids finds cluster centers in $\mathcal{O}(N^2)$ time while K-means takes $\mathcal{O}(N)$ time. Based on the above, we find that bi-GMM-TPS using K-means is better than using K-medoids, and therefore K-means is used in all of the following experiments.

Experiments on Number of Clusters, Number of Control Points. Without loss of generality, face data and Gaussian data are chosen for the two groups experiments that are carried out here. The registration results with varying the number of clusters and the number of control points are shown in Fig. 1. The size of the control points is computed by $t = (\text{interval})^d \times d,\ d = 2 \text{ or } d = 3$. The higher the interval value, the larger the number of control points.

Figure 1(a) shows the registration errors (i.e. mean L2 distance) of bi-GMM-TPS on synthetic face data. Figure 1(b) displays the registration errors on Gaussian data. The x-axis is the number of clusters (k) varying from 2 to 15 for (a) and from 2 to 10 for (b) respectively. For each k value, we have conducted 10 runs due to the random initialization for K-means, and the optimal results are shown here. The reason is that our main objective is to evaluate the bi-stage registration framework with a valid clustering result. There may be other clustering

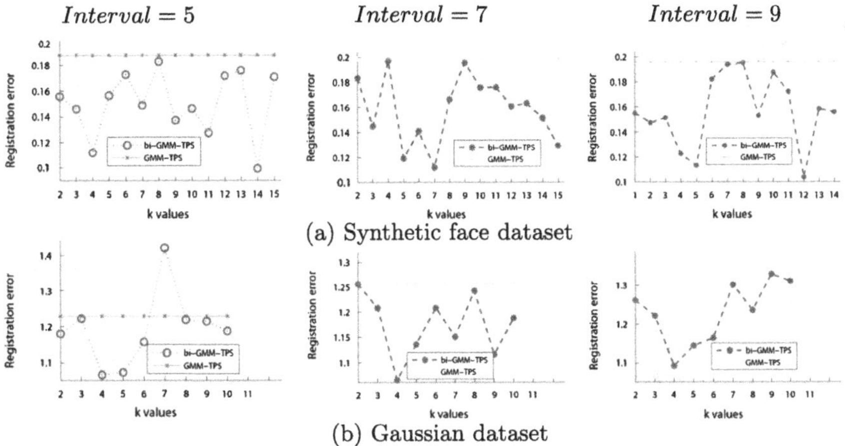

Fig. 1. Registration error of bi-GMM-TPS with respect to k and control points. The horizontal line represents the registration error of GMM-TPS, while the scatter plot represents the registration error of bi-GMM-TPS.

methods that can produce more stable cluster centres than K-means, however, it is out of the scope of this paper and can be addressed in our future work.

As for synthetic face data (see Fig. 1(a)), registration errors for all interval values and all k values in this experiment are less or no greater than the registration errors of the original GMM-TPS. The average registration error with interval value 5 is the smallest. There is no apparent trend between the registration error and the k values. However, as for Gaussian data (see Fig. 1(b)), it is observed that the registration error has an approximately increasing trend when k is larger than 4, especially when interval is 9. Furthermore, when k is 4, the optimal alignment is arrived at for all three intervals. This is due to the fact that Gaussian data has four peaks. When the k value is larger than 4, it is more likely to result in larger registration errors than the GMM-TPS method as evident in $k = 7$ with interval = 5; and $k = 7, 9, 10$ with interval = 9. It is easy to understand as Gaussian data has a clear clustered pattern and any incorrect clustering result would result in larger registration errors. In comparison with Gaussian data, one may see that for synthetic face center of the clusters, greater stability is shown to be concurrent with structure in the data. It is also evident that the computation complexity of our method rises sharply with an increase in the intervals (shown in Fig. 2).

Fluctuation of the registration errors is due to the randomness of the initialization of K-means, that may lead to different center locations each time the bi-GMM-TPS algorithm runs. Deeper studies on this shall be carried out in the future.

Experiments on Choice of Initial Alignments. Bi-GMM-TPS is a general hierarchical framework for large point set registration, the registration methods

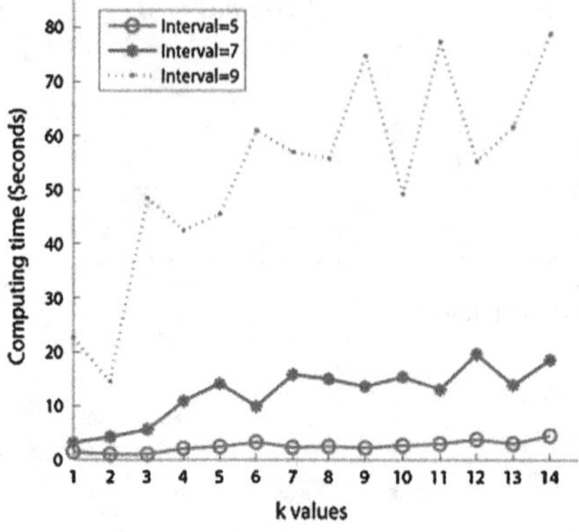

Fig. 2. Computing time on synthetic face data.

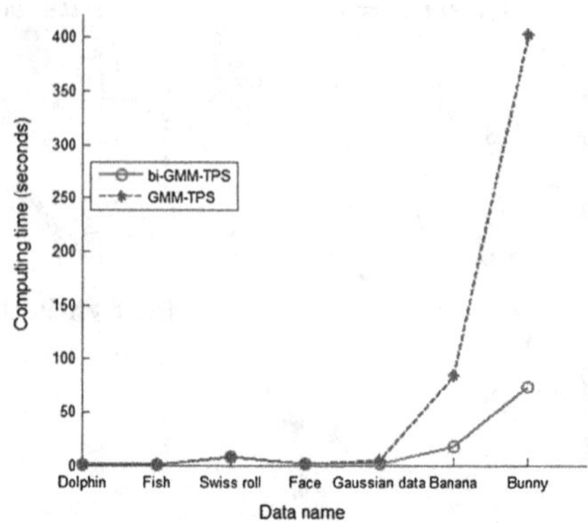

Fig. 3. Comparison of computing times on seven datasets.

in each stage may be other choices than GMM-TPS. ICP-GMM-TPS algorithm refers to the alignment method being iterative closest point (ICP) at the first stage on two clustered centers sets. ICP-GMM-TPS method is tested on synthetic face and banana dataset without any preference and the only intention is to validate the registration performances.

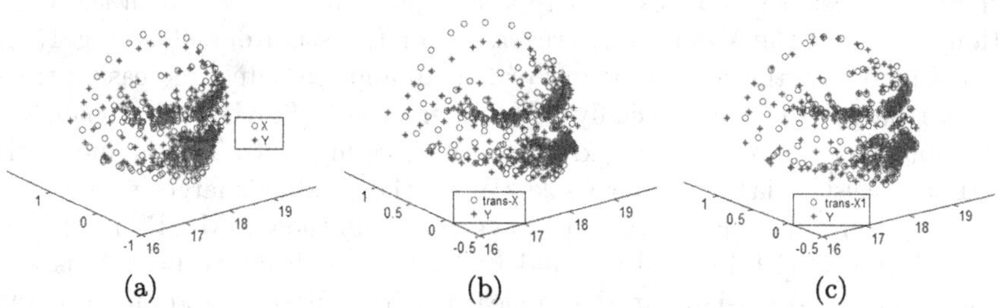

Fig. 4. Point sets registration on synthetic face data. (a) The synthetic face dataset (input data); (b) ICP-GMM-TPS registration; (c) Bi-GMM-TPS registration.

For synthetic face dataset, comparison results between bi-GMM-TPS and ICP-GMM-TPS are shown in Fig. 4 and Table 3. For banana dataset, we have compared ICP and GMM-TPS by registering two clustered center sets. The registration error of GMM-TPS is 8.1924 and the registration error of ICP is 8.8993. More importantly, GMM-TPS remedies the topological ambiguity of banana data, while ICP failed to do so.

Both quantitative performance and visualization of bi-GMM-TPS outperform those of ICP-GMM-TPS. The comparisons on these two datasets demonstrate

Table 3. Comparison of registration performance on synthetic face data.

Algorithm	Registration error	Time (s)
Bi-GMM-TPS	0.0933	8.24
ICP-GMM-TPS	0.1229	9.02

that bi-GMM-TPS is more reliable and flexible than ICP-GMM-TPS when dealing with non-rigid registration.

5.3 Comparisons with GMM-TPS, CPD and QPCCP

The above three comparators are chosen for comparing with the proposed bi-GMM-TPS since

1. GMM-TPS is the basis of the specific implementation in the framework, and
2. CPD is an alternative comparable non-rigid registration method especially for large point sets, and
3. QPCCP has used a clustering method for approximate registration, and is therefore a suitable comparator.

Comparison results between bi-GMM-TPS and GMM-TPS are shown in Figs. 1 and 3. The computational time of two algorithms on seven data sets are plotted in Fig. 3. When the size of the input point set is small, bi-GMM-TPS is slower than GMM-TPS. However, bi-GMM-TPS outperforms GMM-TPS on large data sets such as the Gaussian, banana and bunny data. A comparison of registration errors is carried out on face and Gaussian data in Fig. 1. The horizontal lines are the registration errors of GMM-TPS. All registration errors of bi-GMM-TPS are less than those of GMM-TPS on face data, and most of the registration errors of bi-GMM-TPS are smaller on Gaussian data.

Registration results on banana data shown in Fig. 5, where we set $k = 12$ and interval as 5, clearly demonstrate that bi-GMM-TPS is able to rectify any global misalignment caused by topological ambiguity in the data (Fig. 5(d)), when GMM-TPS failed to do so (Fig. 5(b)). Although we notice that CPD can also remedy topological ambiguity in the data, the transformed point set has been unevenly warped (Fig. 5(c)). Quantitative comparison is shown in Table 4. Although the difference in the registration error between bi-GMM-TPS and GMM-TPS is negligible, the alignment by GMM-TPS is clearly wrong. Furthermore, the bi-GMM-TPS is much faster than GMM-TPS on registering the banana data, while CPD provides the worst registration error and longest computing time among these three methods.

Two 3D face scans chosen at random from the USF 3D face database [24] are used to evaluate the efficiency of bi-GMM-TPS algorithm on large point sets registration. An interval value 5 is used to set the size of the control points. The registration error is 6.3569 and 4.5885 for bi-GMM-TPS and GMM-TPS respectively. There is not much visual difference in terms of registration accuracy.

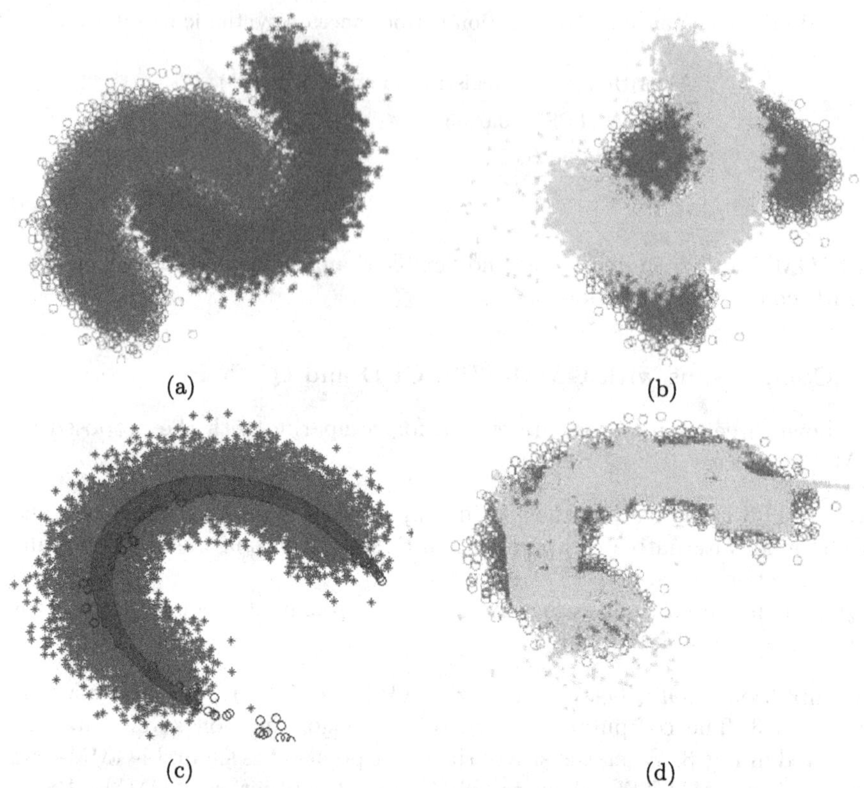

Fig. 5. Point sets registration on banana data. (a) The banana dataset (input data); (b) GMM-TPS registration; (c) CPD registration; (d) bi-GMM-TPS registration

However, the computational time for bi-GMM-TPS is 4.55×10^3 s (~1.26 h), which is much shorter than that of GMM-TPS 67.11×10^3 (~18.64 h). GMM-TPS becomes impractical in dealing very large point sets. CPD method is also carried out on this large dataset and the registration error is 7.7654 with a computational time of 4.42×10^3 s (~1.22 h). CPD is marginally quicker but has the lowest registration accuracy.

QPCCP is compared with the proposed bi-GMM-TPS, for QPCCP has also used clustering methods for approximate registration. As it has been reported that QPCCP demonstrates less registration accuracy in terms of distance-based metrics as compared to GMM-TPS [20], we compared our method with QPCCP using not only the mean L2 distance but also the number of correspondences (refer to Sect. 5.1) on fish data. From Table 5, we can see that bi-GMM-TPS can provide a lower registration error and more correspondences than QPCCP.

Table 4. Comparison of registration performance on banana data.

Algorithm	Registration error	Time (s)
Bi-GMM-TPS	5.8493	17.4
GMM-TPS	5.8450	84.4
CPD	7.8130	97.3

Table 5. Comparison of registration performance on fish data.

Algorithm	Registration error	No. of correspondences
Bi-GMM-TPS	0.0212	93
QPCCP	0.0457	81

6 Conclusion

In this paper, a hierarchical bi-stage registration framework bi-GMM-TPS for large point sets has been proposed. K-means clustering is employed to group large point sets into the same number of clusters respectively. First stage alignment was done on two cluster center sets, where the resultant thin-plate splines (TPS) transformation is applied to the entire point set. Before further registration is conducted on the cluster pairs, the points of one center set find their nearest neighbors in the other center set. Thus, fine registration is performed within the clusters and their corresponding clusters. Extensive experimental results have demonstrated the computational efficiency and robustness of our proposed method. Results have shown that our bi-GMM-TPS method outperforms some of the state-of-the-art point set registration methods GMM-TPS and CPD and QPCCP.

However, registration accuracy of the proposed method depends on the accuracy and reliability of clustering. A clustering method that is robust to point set deformation, and more stable to random initialization will be studied in the future.

Acknowledgement. This work is supported by Postgraduate Research Grant Scheme of Universiti Sains Malaysia (1001-PKOMP-846050) and National Natural Science Foundation of China (61473111).

References

1. Bishop, C.M.: Pattern Recognition and Machine Learning. Springer, New York (2006)
2. Bookstein, F.L.: Principal warps: thin-plate splines and the decomposition of deformations. IEEE Trans. Pattern Anal. Mach. Intell. **11**(6), 567–585 (1989)
3. Caetano, T.S., Caelli, T., Schuurmans, D., Barone, D.A.C.: Graphical models and point pattern matching. IEEE Trans. Pattern Anal. Mach. Intell. **28**(10), 1646–1663 (2004)

4. Chui, H.L.: Non-rigid Point Matching: Algorithm, Extensions and Applications. Yale University, New Heaven (2001)
5. Chui, H.L., Rangarajan, A.: A new point matching algorithm for non-rigid registration. J. Comput. Vis. Image Underst. **89**(3), 114–141 (2003)
6. Conte, D., Foggia, P., Sansone, C., Vento, M.: Thirty years of graph matching in pattern recognition. Int. J. Pattern Recogn. Artif. Intell. **18**(3), 265–298 (2004)
7. Granger, S., Pennec, X.: Multi-scale EM-ICP: a fast and robust approach for surface registration. In: Heyden, A., Sparr, G., Nielsen, M., Johansen, P. (eds.) ECCV 2002, Part IV. LNCS, vol. 2353, pp. 418–432. Springer, Heidelberg (2002)
8. Jian, B., Vemuri, B.C.: A robust algorithm for point set registration using mixture of gaussians. In: 10th IEEE International Conference on Computer Vision (ICCV05), pp. 1246–1251 (2005)
9. Jian, B., Vemuri, B.C.: Robust point set registration using gaussian mixture models. IEEE Trans. Pattern Anal. Mach. Intell. **33**(8), 1633–1645 (2011)
10. Joshi, A., Lee, C.-H.: On the problem of correspondence in range data and some inelastic uses for elastic nets. IEEE Trans. Neural Netw. **6**(3), 716–726 (1995)
11. Lian, W., Zhang, L., Liang, Y., Pan, Q.: A quadratic programming based cluster correspondence projection algorithm for fast point matching. Comput. Vis. Image Underst. **114**, 322–333 (2010)
12. Liu, Y.: Automatic registration of overlapping 3D point clouds using closest points. Image Vis. Comput. **24**(7), 762–781 (2006)
13. Luo, B., Hancock, E.R.: A unified framework for alignment and correspondence. Comput. Vis. Image Underst. **92**(1), 26–55 (2003)
14. Myronenko, A., Song, X.: Point set registration: coherent point drift. IEEE Trans. Pattern Anal. Mach. Intell. **32**(12), 2262–2275 (2010)
15. Myronenko, A., Song, X., Carreira-Perpinan, M.A.: Non-rigid point set registration: coherent point drift. In: Schölkopf, B., Platt, J., Hoffman, T. (eds.) Advances in Neural Information Processing Systems (NIPS), vol. 19, pp. 1009–1016. The MIT Press, Cambridge (2007)
16. Starck, J., Hilton, A.: Correspondence labelling for wide-timeframe free-form surface matching. In: 11th International Conference on Computer Vision (ICCV07), pp. 1–8 (2007)
17. Tsin, Y., Kanade, T.: A correlation-based approach to robust point set registration. In: Pajdla, T., Matas, J.G. (eds.) ECCV 2004. LNCS, vol. 3023, pp. 558–569. Springer, Heidelberg (2004)
18. Zhu, C., Byrd, R.H., Lu, P., Nocedal, J.: Algorithm 778: L-BFGS-B: fortran subroutines for large-scale bound-constrained optimization. ACM Trans. Math. Softw. **23**(4), 550–560 (1997)
19. Gonzalez, T.F.: Clustering to minimize the maximum intercluster distance. Theor. Comput. Sci. **38**, 293–306 (1985)
20. Xu, H., Liu, J., Smith, C.D.: Robust and efficient point registration based on clusters and generalized radial basis functions (C-GRBF). In: IEEE International Conference on Image Processing, pp. 1669–1672 (2012)
21. Deng, Y., Rangarajan, A., Eisenschenk, S., Vemuri, B.C.: A Riemannian framework for matching point clouds represented by the Schrdinger distance transform. In: IEEE Conference on Computer Vision and Pattern Recognition, pp. 1–8 (2014)
22. Lian, W., Zhang, L.: Robust point matching revisited: a concave optimization approach. In: Fitzgibbon, A., Lazebnik, S., Perona, P., Sato, Y., Schmid, C. (eds.) ECCV 2012, Part II. LNCS, vol. 7573, pp. 259–272. Springer, Heidelberg (2012)

23. Lian, W., Zhang, L.: Point matching in the presence of outliers in both point sets: a concave optimization approach. In: IEEE Conference on Computer Vision and Pattern Recognition, pp. 1–8 (2014)
24. Blanz, V., Vetter, T.: Face recognition based on fitting a 3d morphable model. IEEE Trans. Pattern Anal. Mach. Intell. **25**(9), 1063–1074 (2003)

Enhanced Sequence Matching for Action Recognition from 3D Skeletal Data

Hyun-Joo Jung and Ki-Sang Hong(✉)

Image Information Processing Lab, Department of Electrical Engineering, POSTECH, San 31 Hyojadong, Pohang, South Korea
{hyunjoo,hongks}@postech.ac.kr

Abstract. Human action recognition using 3D skeletal data has become popular topic with the emergence of the cost-effective depth sensors, such as Microsoft Kinect. However, noisy joint position and speed variation between actors make action recognition from 3D joint positions difficult. To address these problems, this paper proposes a novel framework, called Enhanced Sequence Matching (ESM), to align and compare action sequences. Inspired by DNA sequence alignment method used in bioinformatics, we model the new scoring function to measure the similarity between two action sequences with noise. We construct action sequence from a set of elementary Moving Poses (eMP) built from affinity propagation. By using affinity propagation, eMP set is built automatically, in other words, it determines the number of eMPs itself. The proposed framework outperforms the state-of-the-art on UTKinect action dataset and MSRC-12 gesture dataset and achieves comparable performance to the state-of-the-art on MSR action 3D dataset. Moreover, experimental results show that our method is very intuitive and robust to noise and temporal variation.

1 Introduction

Human action recognition has been an important area in computer vision due to its wide range of applications such as surveillance systems, human-computer interactions, and video analysis. While many existing recognition approaches achieve good results, recognizing human action from the RGB video still remains a challenging problem because it cannot fully capture the 3D human motion and is highly sensitive to illumination change or background clutter.

The recent introduction of the cost-effective depth sensors alleviates these problems. Specifically, 3D human skeletal data extracted from depth video enriches the motion information and is insensitive to the illumination change or background clutter. Estimating the skeletal joint positions from a single depth image [1] stimulates a renewed interest in skeleton-based action recognition.

In skeleton-based approaches, human action is considered as a *temporal evolution* of joint configurations and the position of each joint is considered as function of time. Therefore, modeling joint configurations and temporal evolution of actions are important tasks. However, estimated joint positions often

D. Cremers et al. (Eds.): ACCV 2014, Part V, LNCS 9007, pp. 226–240, 2015.
DOI: 10.1007/978-3-319-16814-2_15

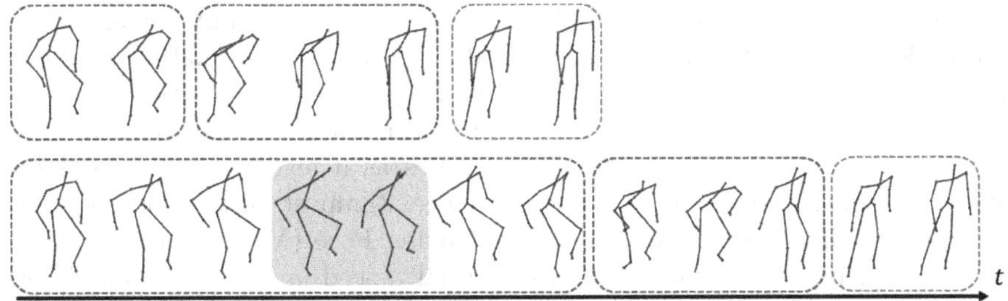

Fig. 1. Two example action sequences in the *stand up* action class of UTKinect action dataset. In both sequences, same-colored dashed box represents the same phase of the action and orange-colored box indicates that the noisy joint positions exist (in the left arm). As we can see, there are severe action speed variation and noisy poses even though both actors perform the same action (Color figure online).

have flipped noise in short-duration (usually less than 1 s) because of the noisy property of depth data. Moreover, modeling temporal evolution of actions with this unstable joint positions is a difficult task. Figure 1 shows an example of two action sequences in the same action class but have different action speed and noisy joint positions.

In this paper, to address these problems, we propose a new framework for human action recognition with 3D skeletal data which is called Enhanced Sequence Matching (ESM). Inspired by DNA sequence alignment approach used in bioinformatics [2–5], we construct action sequence from a set of elementary Moving Poses (eMPs) and match two sequences using a new scoring function. In DNA sequence alignment, if two sequences of DNA share a common ancestor, mismatches can be interpreted as point mutations and gaps as indels. Likewise, we consider human actions as a sequence of eMPs and assume that if two action sequences come from the same action class, mismatching eMPs in short-duration can be considered as a noise and should not influence the recognition result. To deal with such short-duration mismatch (mutation or gap in DNA sequence), we apply the *affine gap penalty* to our scoring function. Moreover, we construct the set of eMPs automatically by using affinity propagation [6]. Experimental results show the effectiveness of our approach, achieving the best results on UTKinect dataset and MSRC-12 gesture dataset and comparable results to the state-of-the-art on MSR action 3D dataset.

This paper is organized as follows. Section 2 reviews the related work. Our action recognition framework, elementary Moving Pose construction and Enhanced Sequence Matching (ESM), is explained in Sect. 3. Section 4 shows experimental results. Conclusion is in Sect. 5.

2 Related Work

In this section, we briefly review various skeleton-based human action recognition approaches and modeling temporal evolution of human actions.

Human action recognition using 3D skeletal data has been an active area of research for the past few years. Wang et al. [7] select an informative subset of joints as an actionlet and classifies actions using ensemble of actionlet. Their actionlet is robust to noise occurring in uninformative joints and to intra-class variation. Xia et al. [8] represent human poses as a histogram of joint locations in spherical coordinate for view-invariance. Zanfir et al. [9] propose a new descriptor for 3D skeletal data named as Moving Pose (MP) descriptor which includes both pose information and differential (speed and acceleration) information. MP descriptor is invariant to scale change and absolute speed of actions. Wang et al. [10] group the joints into five body parts and uses data mining to obtain a spatial-temporal configurations of human actions. As the first step, they improve the method that estimates human joint locations to reduce errors that comes from wrongly estimated joint positions. Luo et al. [11] construct a dictionary of poses with group sparsity and geometry constraints. By adding these constraints, learned dictionary is robust to noise and large intra-class variations. As we can see, most of skeleton-based action recognition approaches mainly focus on dealing with noise and intra-class variation such as action speed change. Our method also considers the noise and speed variation by transforming an action sequence into refined action sequence and using a novel sequence matching method.

There have been many approaches for modeling temporal evolution of actions. The simplest method is using temporal pyramid [7,11]. Luo et al. [11] divide an action sequence into 3 levels with each level containing 1, 2, 4 segments. Then histograms of sparse coefficients are generated from each segment by max pooling and concatenated to form the representation of the action sequence. Wang et al. [7] use Fourier temporal pyramid as a representation of temporal structure. For each segment at each pyramid level, they apply short time Fourier transform, obtain Fourier coefficients, and utilize its low-frequency coefficients as features. Temporal pyramid approach is easy to use and can be combined with various classification schemes such as variant of Support Vector Machine (SVM) [12,13]. However, it only works properly when the action sequence is well segmented.

Another methods employ generative model [14,15]. Hidden Markov Model (HMM) [8,16–18] and Conditional Random Field (CRF) [19–21] are popular models for this approach. These methods attempt to model the generative process of actions and perform learning and inference for recognizing actions. It produces effective representation of action because it exploits the structural information of actions but learning generative model with limited amount of training data is prone to overfit.

The most similar model to our approach is temporal warping [22–25]. Dynamic Time Warping (DTW) is the most popular model for temporal warping. Veeraraghavan and Roy-chowdhury [22] compute a nominal activity trajectory for each action category using DTW. Müller and Röder [23] use DTW for matching the 3D joint positions to a motion template. Wang and Wu [25] unify DTW and SVM using Maximum Margin Temporal Warping (MMTW). The fundamental purpose of DTW is to align action sequences and to find the best warping path between two sequences. Because it focuses on measuring similarity between

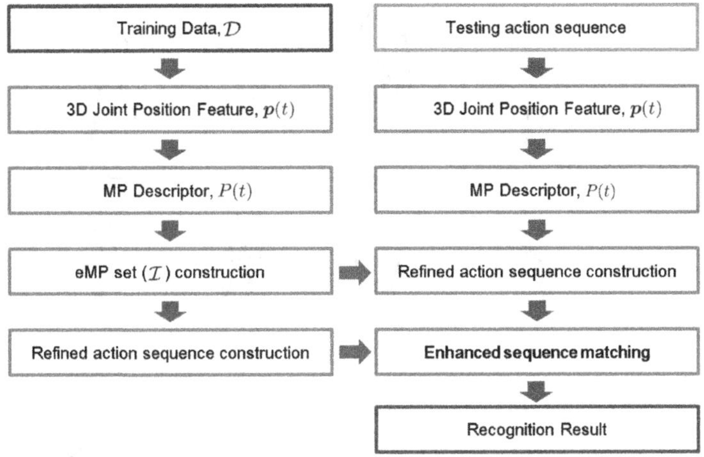

Fig. 2. Flow chart of the proposed system.

individual elements, it suffers severely from noisy elements in the sequence which occurs frequently in the skeletal data.

Our method mainly focus on matching sequences including noisy elements for the classification rather than finding optimal warping path. Therefore our method considers matching with the *gap* rather than matching with the noisy element in comparing sequences. Figure 2 shows the entire system of our method.

3 Proposed Method

3.1 Feature Extraction

We use Moving Pose (MP) descriptor [9] as a feature of each frame. The position of joint j at frame t is defined by $p^j(t) = (p^j_x(t), p^j_y(t), p^j_z(t))$, where $j \in \{1, ..., J\}$ and J is the number of joints. At frame t, the human pose $\boldsymbol{p}(t)$ is represented as

$$\boldsymbol{p}(t) = \{p^j(t) | j \in \{1, ..., J\}\} \in \mathbb{R}^{J \times 3}, \tag{1}$$

namely, the concatenation of all joints' positions.

We normalize $\boldsymbol{p}(t)$ like [9]. First we compute the expected length of skeleton limbs from the training data, and modify each joint's location so that all subjects have the same limb length. After that, we subtract the position of hip center from each joint position in order that the human pose is invariant to locations.

Before computing the MP descriptor, we apply the 5-tap 1D Gaussian filter ($\sigma = 1$) to each coordinate of the normalized pose along the temporal axis. Given the normalized and filtered pose $\tilde{\boldsymbol{p}}(t)$, the MP descriptor $P(t)$ is defined as

$$P(t) = (\tilde{\boldsymbol{p}}(t), \alpha\tilde{\boldsymbol{p}}'(t), \beta\tilde{\boldsymbol{p}}''(t)) \in \mathbb{R}^{J \times 3 \times 3}, \tag{2}$$

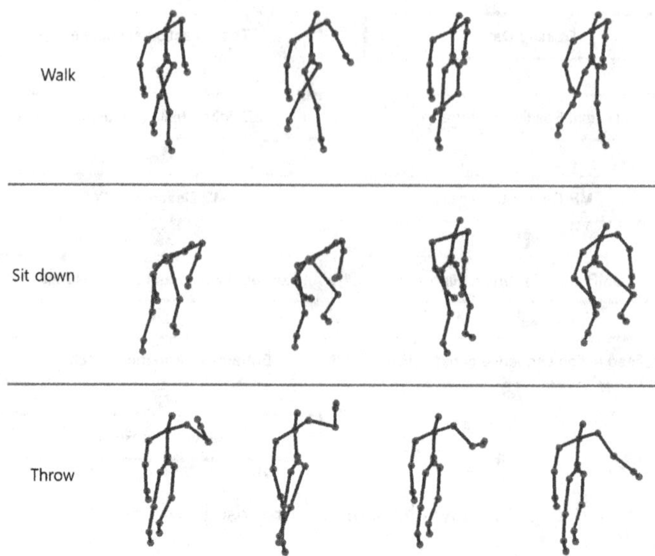

Fig. 3. Example of elementary Moving Poses of *Walk, Sit down, and Throw* action classes in the UTKinect action dataset. Note that we only plot the positional part of MP descriptor not the two derivatives.

where $\tilde{\boldsymbol{p}}'(t) = \tilde{\boldsymbol{p}}(t+1) - \tilde{\boldsymbol{p}}(t-1)$ and $\tilde{\boldsymbol{p}}''(t) = \tilde{\boldsymbol{p}}(t+2) + \tilde{\boldsymbol{p}}(t-2) - 2\tilde{\boldsymbol{p}}(t)$ are the first and second order derivatives of $\tilde{\boldsymbol{p}}(t)$ respectively. $\tilde{\boldsymbol{p}}'(t)$ and $\tilde{\boldsymbol{p}}''(t)$ are normalized so that they have unit-norm. α and β are the parameters that weight the relative importance of the two derivatives. The MP descriptor is a good feature for action classification because it captures both the static pose information and the joint kinematics at a given time.

3.2 Elementary Moving Pose (eMP)

We denote the training dataset by $\mathcal{D} = \{(X_1, Y_1), (X_2, Y_2), ..., (X_N, Y_N)\}$ where $X_n = \{P_n(t)|t = 1, ..., T_n\}$ is the n-th action sequence and T_n is its total frame number. $Y_n \in \mathcal{Y}$ is the action category label of n-th action sequence and $\mathcal{Y}$ is the set of action categories in the training dataset $\mathcal{D}$.

Let the set of entire MP descriptors in $\mathcal{D}$ is $\mathcal{P} = \{P_i|i = 1, ..., N_{\mathcal{D}}\}$ and its corresponding action category label set is $\{y_i|i = 1, ..., N_{\mathcal{D}}\}$ where $N_{\mathcal{D}} = \sum_{n=1}^{N} T_n$ is the total number of MP descriptors in the training set $\mathcal{D}$. We compute the class-confidence value $V(P_i)$ of P_i which is defined as

$$V(P_i) = \frac{\kappa_{y_i}}{\kappa}, \tag{3}$$

where κ is the number of nearest MP descriptors which is defined by user and κ_{y_i} is the number of MP descriptors that have the same action category label as P_i [9]. Large class-confidence value $V(P_i)$ means that P_i strongly belongs to its class y_i and consequently P_i has discriminative power. By thresholding class-confidence value, we exclude MP descriptors that have low discriminative power. Then the candidate of eMP is defined as

$$\tilde{\mathcal{P}} = \{P_i | V(P_i) > \tau(y_i)\}, \tag{4}$$

where the $\tau(y_i)$ is a class-specific threshold.

To construct the eMP set, we use affinity propagation [6] which clusters features by selecting representative features as exemplars (cluster centers). The input of affinity propagation is a $N_{\tilde{\mathcal{P}}} \times N_{\tilde{\mathcal{P}}}$ affinity matrix S, where $N_{\tilde{\mathcal{P}}}$ is the number of MP descriptors in $\tilde{\mathcal{P}}$. S is defined as

$$S(i,k) = -\|P_i - P_k\|^2, \qquad \forall i \neq k \tag{5}$$

$$S(k,k) = V(P_k) - \nu, \tag{6}$$

where ν is a parameter which controls the number of exemplars. Each off-diagonal element of S encodes affinity between two MP descriptors and the k-th diagonal elements give *preference* for choosing the k-th MP descriptor as an exemplar. Equation (6) means that the MP descriptor with large class confidence value is more likely to be chosen as an exemplar. Then, the selected MP descriptors have both representativeness as well as the discriminative power.

After the matrix S is computed, then the affinity propagation method iteratively updates the responsibility $r(i,k)$ and availability $a(i,k)$ of all pairs of data [6]. The output of affinity propagation is a set of exemplars $\mathcal{E}$ denoted by

$$\mathcal{E} = \{P_i | r(i,i) > 0\}, \tag{7}$$

where $r(i,i)$ is the self-responsibility of P_i. The main advantage of affinity propagation is that we do not need to specify the number of exemplars and we can assign the potential for selecting as an exemplar to each P_i. We call each exemplar as an *elementary Moving Pose* (eMP). Figure 3 shows the example of constructed eMP. As we can see, the constructed eMP is representative of each action class and discriminative between different action classes.

Then we can rewrite $\mathcal{E}$ as

$$\mathcal{I} = \{I(m) | m = 1, ..., N_{\mathcal{I}}\}, \tag{8}$$

where $I(m)$ is the m-th eMP(exemplar) and $N_{\mathcal{I}}$ is the number of eMPs. In the next subsection, we transform the action sequence into *refined* action sequence using $\mathcal{I}$.

3.3 Refined Action Sequence

Given an action sequence $X = \{P(t) | t = 1, ..., T\}$, we can transform X into *refined* action sequence R_X using $\mathcal{I}$. For each frame t, the distances between $P(t)$ and $I(m)$ $(m = 1, ..., N_{\mathcal{I}})$ are computed and the closest eMP is matched to the $P(t)$. We denote the index of matched eMP as

$$M(P(t)) = \min_m \|P(t) - I(m)\|^2. \tag{9}$$

If the closest distance is larger than a pre-defined threshold ρ, then we consider $P(t)$ as a noisy frame because there is no similar eMP in the learned eMP set $\mathcal{I}$. In this case, we exclude the matched eMP from the refined action sequence.

$$M(P(t)) = 0, \qquad \text{if } \|P(t) - I(m)\|^2 > \rho, \forall m \in \{1, ..., N_{\mathcal{I}}\}. \tag{10}$$

Then the refined action sequence of X is represented as $\tilde{R}_X$.

$$\tilde{R}_X = \{M(P(t)) | M(P(t)) \neq 0, t = 1..., T\}. \tag{11}$$

To make the refined action sequence compact, if the same eMP is matched continuously, then we merge those frames into one element. Then the final refined action sequence becomes

$$R_X = \mathcal{U}(\tilde{R}_X), \tag{12}$$

where the function $\mathcal{U}(\cdot)$ merges the continuous same value into one value. For example, $\mathcal{U}(\{5, 5, 5, 1, 7, 8, 8\}) = \{5, 1, 7, 8\}$.

3.4 Enhanced Sequence Matching (ESM)

Before explaining ESM, we mention about the DTW and traditional sequence alignment (SA) method.

Given the two action sequences X_1 and X_2, the cost of DTW is computed as

$$F_{DTW}(i, j) = D(P_1(i), P_2(j)) + \min \begin{cases} F_{DTW}(i-1, j-1) \\ F_{DTW}(i-1, j) \\ F_{DTW}(i, j-1) \end{cases}, \tag{13}$$

where $P_1(i)$ and $P_2(j)$ are MP descriptors of X_1 at frame i and X_2 at frame j respectively. $D(P_1(i), P_2(j))$ is a matching cost and the Euclidean distance is used in general. Even though DTW is very effective method for aligning two sequences, the matching cost always increase except that $P_1(i)$ and $P_2(j)$ are same. In other words, when noisy MP exists in the sequence, the cost will grow rapidly because the matching cost with noisy MP is usually large. It would degrade the classification performance.

SA [3,4] used in bioinformatics computes the alignment score as

$$F_{SA}(i, j) = \max \begin{cases} F_{SA}(i-1, j-1) + H(R_{X1}[i], R_{X2}[j]) \\ F_{SA}(i-1, j) - \zeta \\ F_{SA}(i, j-1) - \zeta \end{cases}, \tag{14}$$

where ζ is a gap penalty parameter and $R_{X1}[i]$ and $R_{X2}[j]$ are the i-th element of refined action sequence R_{X1} and j-th element of R_{X2} respectively. $H(R_{X1}[i], R_{X2}[j])$ is the matching score written as

$$H(R_{X1}[i], R_{X2}[j]) = \begin{cases} \omega & \text{if } R_{X1}[i] = R_{X2}[j] \\ \delta & \text{if } R_{X1}[i] \neq R_{X2}[j] \end{cases}, \tag{15}$$

where the parameter $\omega > 0$ is a matching reward and $\delta < 0$ is a mismatching cost. As we can see in Eq. (14), SA considers matching each element in a sequence with both an element in another sequence and gap. However, SA gives the same matching score or mismatching cost regardless of similarity between $I(R_{X1}[i])$ and $I(R_{X2}[j])$. SA also gives the same gap penalty without regard to the length of matching with gap.

Our proposed method, named as Enhanced Sequence Matching (ESM), computes the alignment score as

$$F_{ESM}(i,j) = \max \begin{cases} F_{ESM}(i-1,j-1) + S(R_{X1}[i]), R_{X2}[j]) \\ \max_{k=0,\ldots,i-1} F_{ESM}(k,j) - \gamma(|j-k|) \\ \max_{k=0,\ldots,j-1} F_{ESM}(i,k) - \gamma(|i-k|) \end{cases}, \quad (16)$$

where $S(R_{X1}[i], R_{X2}[j])$ is a matching score and $\gamma(n)$ is an *affine gap function* [5] that enables our method to model the desired property for skeleton-based action recognition. The matching score $S(R_{X1}[i], R_{X2}[j])$ is defined as

$$S(R_{X1}[i], R_{X2}[j]) = \lambda * S_{app}(I(R_{X1}[i]), I(R_{X2}[j])) + (1-\lambda) * S_{hist}(R_{X1}[i], R_{X2}[j]), \quad (17)$$

where λ is a parameter that controls the weights of the two similarity functions. $S_{app}(I(R_{X1}[i]), I(R_{X2}[j]))$ is the appearance similarity defined as

$$S_{app}(I(R_{X1}[i]), I(R_{X2}[j])) = \phi\left(\|I(R_{X1}[i]) - I(R_{X2}[j])\|^2\right), \quad (18)$$

where $\phi(\cdot)$ is a sigmoid-like function defined as $\phi(x) = \frac{1}{x+1/2} - 1$ and the class-distribution similarity, $S_{hist}(R_{X1}[i], R_{X2}[j])$, is defined as

$$S_{hist}(R_{X1}[i], R_{X2}[j]) = \phi\left(\|h(R_{X1}[i]) - h(R_{X2}[j])\|^2\right), \quad (19)$$

where $h(R_{X1}[i])$ is the class-distribution of $R_{X1}[i]$-th eMP which is computed from the training dataset. The b-th bin of $h(R_{X1}[i])$ is defined as

$$h^b(R_{X1}[i]) = \frac{1}{N} \sum_{n:Y_n=b} \sum_{t=1}^{T_n} \delta(R_{X1}[i], R_{Xn}[t]), \quad (20)$$

where N is the number of total eMPs of refined action sequence in the training set and $\delta(m_1, m_2) = 1$ if $m_1 = m_2$ and 0 otherwise. By considering class distribution of each eMP, we can additionally give more weight to the eMP that frequently occurs in the specific action class.

The affine gap function $\gamma(n)$ is defined as

$$\gamma(n) = \max[(n-1) * \eta - \theta, 0], \quad (21)$$

where η and θ are affine-cost and gap-cost parameter respectively. By using the affine gap function, we can ignore the matching with gap up to $\theta/\eta + 1$ elements for computing matching score because this gap-matching is down to noise. But we impose a gap penalty to matching with gap more than $\theta/\eta + 1$ elements since this

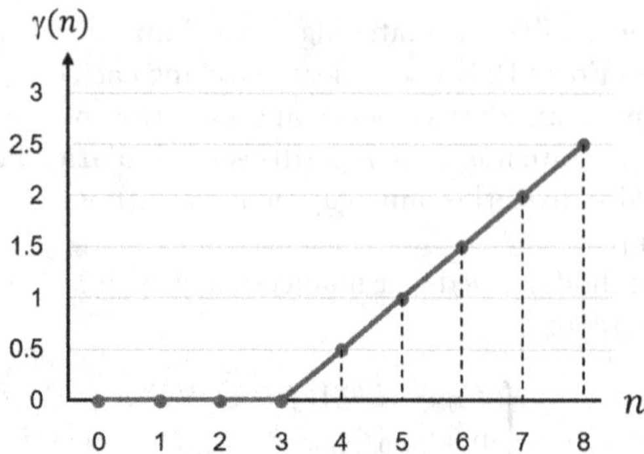

Fig. 4. Example of affine gap function when $\eta = \frac{1}{2}$ and $\theta = 1$. In this case, as we can see, we ignore the matching with gap up to 3 elements.

gap-matching is thought to be caused by different action classes. Figure 4 shows an example of affine gap function. This property is desirable for action sequence matching with noise, especially using 3D skeleton data for action classification. Moreover, our sequence matching approach is very intuitive and natural then other temporal modeling such as temporal pyramid. In the next section, we show that the effectiveness of our framework.

4 Experimental Results

We use MSR action 3D dataset [18], UTKinect action dataset [8], and MSRC-12 gesture dataset [26] to evaluate our proposed action classification framework.

In all datasets, there are $J = 20$ joints (head, shoulder center, shoulder left/right, elbow left/right, wrist left/right, hand left/right, spine, hip center, hip left/right, knee left/right, ankle left/right, foot left/right) to represent the human pose. For MP descriptor, we set $\alpha = 0.75$ and $\beta = 0.6$ which is the same as [9]. In the following experiments, unless specified, we use $\kappa = 50$, $\lambda = 0.7$, and $\theta = 1$. ν in Eq. (6) is determined so that the average number of eMPs for each action class is around 50. For classification, we use the nearest-neighbor scheme. The matching score of two refined action sequences is defined by the maximum value of $F_{ESM}(i, j)$ in Eq. (16).

4.1 Datasets

MSR Action 3D Dataset. MSR action 3D dataset contains 20 action classes: *high arm wave, horizontal arm wave, hammer, hand catch, forward punch, high throw, draw x, draw tick, draw circle, hand clap, two hand wave, side-boxing, bend, forward kick, side kick, jogging, tennis swing, tennis serve, golf swing, pickup &throw.* Each action class is performed by 10 subjects for 2–3 times. There are 567 videos in total. In [7], they do not use 10 videos because these

Table 1. Performance comparison on MSR action 3D dataset.

Method	Accuracy (%)
Action Graph on Bag of 3D Points [18]	74.70
Histogram of 3D Joints [8]	78.97
Actionlet Ensemble [7]	88.20
Pose-based Recognition [10]	90.22
Moving Pose (MP) [9]	91.70
Maximum Margin Temporal Warping (MMTW) [25]	92.70
Enhanced Sequence Matching (ours)	**94.61**
DL-GSGC [11]	96.70

Table 2. Performance comparison on UTKinect action dataset.

Method	Accuracy (%)
Skeleton Joint Features [27]	87.90
Histogram of 3D Joints [8]	90.92
Combined features with Random Forests [27]	91.90
Enhanced Sequence Matching (ours)	**93.94**

videos contain highly erroneous positions. For fair comparison we follow the same procedure with [7]. For constructing eMPs, $\tau(\cdot)$ in Eq. (4) is determined in order that the number of candidate eMPs in each action class is around 250 and ρ in Eq. (4) is set to 1.5. As a result of elementary Moving Pose construction, $N_{\mathcal{I}} = 385$ eMPs are constructed on average. For the affine gap function, we set the affine-cost η to 0.5. We use cross-subject test where the videos for half of the subjects are used for training, and the videos of the other half of the subjects for testing.

UTKinect Action Dataset. UTKinect action dataset contains 10 action classes: *walk, sit down, stand up, pick up, carry, throw, push, pull, wave hands, clap hands.* Each action class is performed by 10 subjects for 2 times, therefore there are 200 videos in total. This dataset is more challenging than MSR action 3D dataset because each actor in the dataset performs actions in different views. For that reason, we additionally normalize the human pose invariant to viewpoint. Like [8], we define the center of human poses as hip center and rotate each joint position in order that the x-axis and the vector from the left hip center to the right hip center are parallel. For this dataset, $\tau(\cdot)$ is determined in order that the number of candidate eMPs in each action class is around 200 and as a result, $N_{\mathcal{I}} = 385$ eMPs are constructed. ρ is set to 1 and η is set to 0.2. Similar to the MSR action 3D dataset, we use cross-subject testing scheme for evaluating performance.

Table 3. Performance comparison on MSRC-12 iconic gesture dataset.

Method	Accuracy (%)
Nonlinear Markov Models [28]	90.90
Enhanced Sequence Matching (ours)	**96.76**

MSRC-12 Gesture Dataset. MSRC-12 gesture dataset includes 6 iconic and 6 metaphoric gestures performed by 30 people. There are 6,244 gesture instances in 594 videos (719,359 frames in total) in the dataset and instance separation ground-truth is also given. We use 6 iconic gestures (*crouch, put goggle, shoot pistol, throw object, change weapon, kick*) from this dataset, which amounts to 3034 instances. Because the size of this dataset is too big, we sample frames in order that the number of frames in each instance becomes maximally 12 frames. $\tau(\cdot)$ is determined so that the number of candidate eMPs in each action class is around $2,000$ and $N_{\mathcal{I}} = 328$ eMPs are constructed on average. ρ is set to 1 and the affine-cost η is set to 0.5. For performance evaluation, we employ 5-fold leave-person-out cross-validation as in [28]. Specifically, for each fold, instances from 24 subjects are used for training and instances from the remaining 6 subjects are used for testing.

4.2 Comparison with the State-of-the-Art

Table 1 shows the action classification accuracies of various algorithms on MSR action 3D dataset. Our Enhanced Sequence Matching (ESM) method achieves the accuracy of 94.61 % which is comparable to the state-of-the-art accuracy 96.70 % [11] and superior to other methods. Luo et al. [11] concentrate their attention on the class-specific dictionary learning for dealing with intra-class variation rather than the temporal evolution of action. They assume that the action video is localized well therefore they use simply the 3-level temporal pyramid to keep the temporal information of actions. On the other hand, we mainly focus on the temporal evolution of action, therefore, we can handle the weekly localized action (e.g., standing still quite a while at the start of action video or missing a part of an action at the end of video). We expect that the employment of the dictionary learned from [11] in our method instead of the eMP set would improve the performance.

Tables 2 and 3 shows the classification results on UTKinect action dataset and MSRC-12 iconic gesture dataset respectively. Our ESM method achieves the state-of-the-art accuracy of 93.94 % and 96.76 % on both datasets. Especially, in MSRC-12 iconic gesture dataset, we outperform [28] by 6 %.

4.3 Discussion

To show the effectiveness of our method in constructing refined action sequence and modeling temporal evolution, we compare our framework with the two variants of DTW.

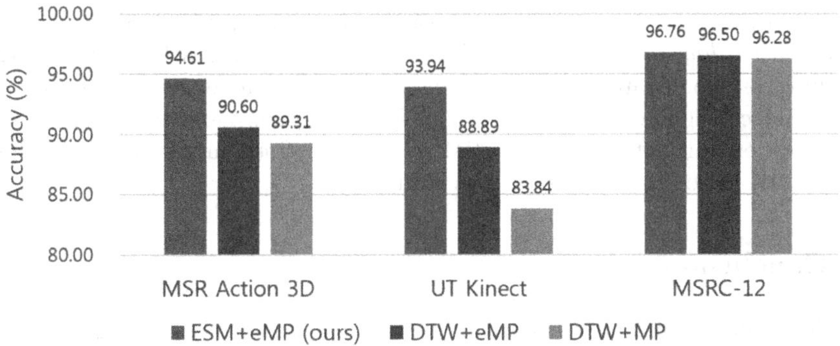

Fig. 5. Classification results of the three datasets using ESM+eMP (our method), DTW+eMP, and DTW+MP.

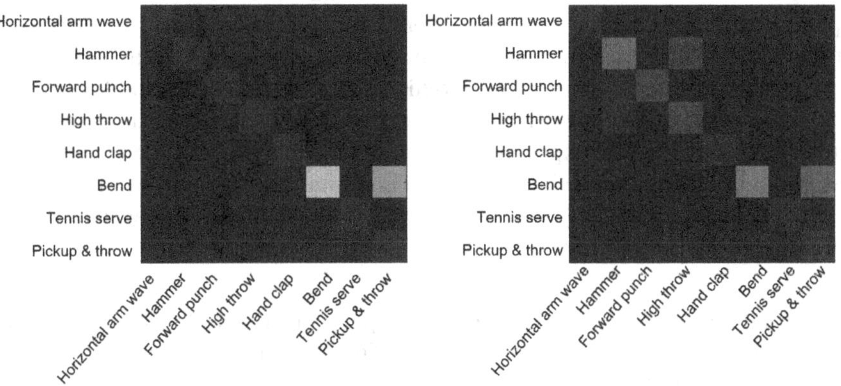

Fig. 6. Confusion matrix of MSR action 3D dataset (AS1). Result of ESM+eMP (*left*) and result of DTW+eMP (*right*).

- DTW+MP: We use the traditional DTW method with the MP descriptor as a frame-level feature. The Euclidean distance between the two MP descriptors is used for matching cost. The result of this framework is the baseline of our experiment.
- DTW+eMP: We use the traditional DTW method with the refined action sequence using eMP. The minus sign of Eq. (17) is used for the matching cost.
- ESM+eMP: This is our framework. We construct the refined action sequence using eMP and classify each sequence by scoring our Enhanced Sequence Matching(ESM) presented in Eq. (16).

Figure 5 shows the comparing result on the three datasets. Both DTW and ESM model the temporal evolution well. Comparing DTW+MP with DTW+eMP, we can see that refined action sequence is better representation for classification than frame-wise feature. Comparing ESM+eMP with DTW+eMP, the result tells us that ESM is an effective sequence matching method where the noise have potential to deteriorate performance. Example is shown in Fig. 6. Similar action classes such as *high throw* and *hammer* suffer from noise in DTW because the large matching cost would interrupt the classification between these similar actions. However, ESM can ignore the cost from the short-duration noise but penalize the long-duration mismatch so that ESM classifies actions more effectively than DTW in the case of noisy sequence matching.

5 Conclusion

In this paper, we propose a novel framework for action recognition based on 3D skeletal data. Inspired by DNA sequence alignment method used in bioinformatics, we model the new sequence matching method to measure the similarity between two action sequences. We first automatically construct the elementary Moving Pose set by using affinity propagation and then construct refined action sequence which is compact and noise-tempered representation for actions. By applying the affine gap function and similarity measure based on both feature and class-distribution to sequence matching score, our method is able to handle noise and action speed variation effectively. Our sequence matching scheme is intuitive and natural and experimental results on three benchmark datasets show that our method works well. We plan to combine part-based recognition approach with our method and to model actions using multiple sequence alignment in the future.

Acknowledgement. This work was partly supported by the National Research Foundation of Korea(NRF) grant funded by the Korea government(MEST) (No. 2011-00166669) and Samsung Electronics Co., Ltd.

References

1. Shotton, J., Fitzgibbon, A., Cook, M., Sharp, T., Finocchio, M., Moore, R., Kipman, A., Blake, A.: Real-time human pose recognition in parts from single depth images. In: CVPR, p. 3 (2011)
2. Mount, D.W.: Bioinformatics: Sequence and Genome Analysis. Cold Spring Harbor Laboratory Press, New york (2004)
3. Needleman, S.B., Wunsch, C.D.: A general method applicable to the search for similarities in the amino acid sequence of two proteins. J. Mol. Biol. **48**, 443–453 (1970)
4. Smith, T.F., Waterman, M.S.: Identification of common molecular subsequences. J. Mol. Biol. **147**, 195–197 (1981)
5. Vingron, M., Waterman, M.S.: Sequence alignment and penalty choice: review of concepts, case studies and implications. J. Mol. Biol. **235**, 1–12 (1994)
6. Frey, B.J., Dueck, D.: Clustering by passing messages between data points. Science **315**, 972–976 (2007)
7. Wang, J., Liu, Z., Wu, Y., Yuan, J.: Mining actionlet ensemble for action recognition with depth cameras. In: 2012 IEEE Conference on Computer Vision and Pattern Recognition (CVPR), pp. 1290–1297 (2012)

8. Xia, L., Chen, C.C., Aggarwal, J.: View invariant human action recognition using histograms of 3d joints. In: 2012 IEEE Computer Society Conference on Computer Vision and Pattern Recognition Workshops (CVPRW), pp. 20–27 (2012)
9. Zanfir, M., Leordeanu, M., Sminchisescu, C.: The moving pose: an efficient 3d kinematics descriptor for low-latency action recognition and detection. In: The IEEE International Conference on Computer Vision (ICCV) (2013)
10. Wang, C., Wang, Y., Yuille, A.: An approach to pose-based action recognition. In: 2013 IEEE Conference on Computer Vision and Pattern Recognition (CVPR), pp. 915–922 (2013)
11. Luo, J., Wang, W., Qi, H.: Group sparsity and geometry constrained dictionary learning for action recognition from depth maps. In: 2013 IEEE International Conference on Computer Vision (ICCV), pp. 1809–1816 (2013)
12. Yang, J., Yu, K., Gong, Y., Huang, T.: Linear spatial pyramid matching using sparse coding for image classification. In: IEEE Conference on Computer Vision and Pattern Recognition (CVPR) (2009)
13. Chapelle, O., Vapnik, V., Bousquet, O., Mukherjee, S.: Choosing multiple parameters for support vector machines. Mach. Learn. **46**, 131–159 (2002)
14. Sminchisescu, C., Kanaujia, A., Li, Z., Metaxas, D.: Conditional models for contextual human motion recognition. In: Tenth IEEE International Conference on Computer Vision, ICCV 2005, vol. 2, pp. 1808–1815 (2005)
15. Morency, L., Quattoni, A., Darrell, T.: Latent-dynamic discriminative models for continuous gesture recognition. In: IEEE Conference on Computer Vision and Pattern Recognition, CVPR 2007, pp. 1–8 (2007)
16. Lv, F., Nevatia, R.: Recognition and segmentation of 3-d human action using HMM and multi-class adaboost. In: Leonardis, A., Bischof, H., Pinz, A. (eds.) ECCV 2006, Part IV. LNCS, vol. 3954, pp. 359–372. Springer, Heidelberg (2006)
17. Li, K., Hu, J., Fu, Y.: Modeling complex temporal composition of actionlets for activity prediction. In: Fitzgibbon, A., Lazebnik, S., Perona, P., Sato, Y., Schmid, C. (eds.) ECCV 2012, Part I. LNCS, vol. 7572, pp. 286–299. Springer, Heidelberg (2012)
18. Li, W., Zhang, Z., Liu, Z.: Action recognition based on a bag of 3d points. In: 2010 IEEE Computer Society Conference on Computer Vision and Pattern Recognition Workshops (CVPRW), pp. 9–14 (2010)
19. Quattoni, A., Wang, S., Morency, L., Collins, M., Darrell, T.: Hidden conditional random fields. IEEE Trans. Pattern Anal. Mach. Intell. **29**, 1848–1852 (2007)
20. Han, L., Wu, X., Liang, W., Hou, G., Jia, Y.: Discriminative human action recognition in the learned hierarchical manifold space. Image Vis. Comput. **28**, 836–849 (2010). Best of Automatic Face and Gesture Recognition 2008
21. Wang, Y., Mori, G.: Hidden part models for human action recognition: probabilistic versus max margin. IEEE Trans. Pattern Anal. Mach. Intell. **33**, 1310–1323 (2011)
22. Veeraraghavan, A., Roy-chowdhury, A.K.: The function space of an activity. In: Proceedings of Computer Vision Pattern Recognition, pp. 959–968 (2006)
23. Müller, M., Röder, T.: Motion templates for automatic classification and retrieval of motion capture data. In: Proceedings of the 2006 ACM SIGGRAPH Eurographics Symposium on Computer Animation, SCA 2006, Aire-la-Ville, Switzerland, Switzerland, pp. 137–146. Eurographics Association (2006)
24. Yao, B.Z., Zhu, S.C.: Learning deformable action templates from cluttered videos. In: ICCV, pp. 1507–1514. IEEE (2009)
25. Wang, J., Wu, Y.: Learning maximum margin temporal warping for action recognition. In: 2013 IEEE International Conference on Computer Vision (ICCV), pp. 2688–2695 (2013)

26. Fothergill, S., Mentis, H., Kohli, P., Nowozin, S.: Instructing people for training gestural interactive systems. In: Proceedings of the SIGCHI Conference on Human Factors in Computing Systems, CHI 2012, pp. 1737–1746. ACM, New York (2012)
27. Zhu, Y., Chen, W., Guo, G.: Fusing spatiotemporal features and joints for 3d action recognition. In: 2013 IEEE Conference on Computer Vision and Pattern Recognition Workshops (CVPRW), pp. 486–491 (2013)
28. Lehrmann, A.M., Gehler, P.V., Nowozin, S.: Efficient non-linear markov models for human motion. In: IEEE Conference on Computer Vision and Pattern Recognition (CVPR), Columbus, Ohio, USA. IEEE (2014)

Multi-label Discriminative Weakly-Supervised Human Activity Recognition and Localization

Ehsan Adeli Mosabbeb[1(✉)], Ricardo Cabral[2], Fernando De la Torre[2], and Mahmood Fathy[1]

[1] Iran University of Science and Technology, Tehran, Iran
eadeli@iust.ac.ir
[2] Robotics Institute, Carnegie Mellon University, Pittsburgh, PA, USA

Abstract. Activity recognition in video has become increasingly important due to its many applications ranging from in-home elder care, surveillance, human computer interaction to automatic sports commentary. To date, most approaches to video rely on fully supervised settings that require time consuming and error prone manual labeling. Moreover, existing supervised approaches are typically tailored for classification, not detection problems (the spatial and temporal support of the action has to be detected). Recently, weakly-supervised learning (WSL) approaches were able to learn discriminative classifiers while localizing the action in space and/or time using weak labels. However, existing approaches for WSL provide coarse localization in terms of spatial regions or spatio-temporal volumes. Moreover, it is unclear how to extend current approaches to the multi-label case that is common in practical applications. This paper proposes a matrix completion approach to the problem of WSL for multi-label learning for video. Our approach localizes non-rectangular spatio-temporal discriminative regions that are inferred by clustering regions of common texture and motion features. We illustrate how our approach improves existing WSL and supervised learning techniques in three standard databases: Hollywood, UCF sports, and MSR-II.

1 Introduction

The idea of recognizing actions automatically from videos brims with potential. Solving it enables many tasks, including surveillance, human-computer interaction, patient monitoring, and automatic sports analysis. However, understanding actions in a video sequence remains a challenging problem due to several reasons: (1) there is a large variability in imaging conditions, as well as in how different people perform an action; (2) background clutter and motion blur are common; (3) data arising from video is of high dimensionality; (4) obtaining ground truth labels for every individual action in every frame of a video is cumbersome. Previous works have addressed these issues by introducing different features [1,2],

Electronic supplementary material The online version of this chapter (doi:10.1007/978-3-319-16814-2_16) contains supplementary material, which is available to authorized users.

D. Cremers et al. (Eds.): ACCV 2014, Part V, LNCS 9007, pp. 241–258, 2015.
DOI: 10.1007/978-3-319-16814-2_16

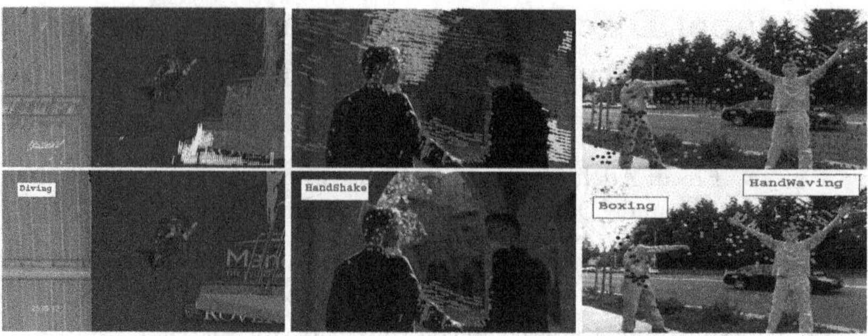

Fig. 1. Our multi-label weakly-supervised approach recognizes activities and pinpoints their spatio-temporal location on unseen videos. This figure shows results on UCF Sports, HOHA and MSR-II datasets. Top: A sample frame and the extracted spatio-temporal activity parts. Bottom: Activities recognized and localized by our method.

interest region detectors such as space-time volumes [3] or trajectories [4,5], and using different classifiers [2,6–10]. While these methods have improved recognition results, they may find correlations from background context and non-activity related regions, which result in a lack of interpretability of what is being learned. This motivates us to explore learning techniques that rely less on error-prone human annotations, and learn instead from captions describing the entire video.

In this paper, we propose a multi-label WSL approach to efficiently recognize activities and pinpoint their spatio-temporal location on unseen videos. Figure 1 shows examples of our results on different datasets. We first extract spatio-temporal activity parts throughout the video. Then, we recognize the activity/activities present in the video, along with selecting the activity parts associated with each recognized activity.

Weakly-supervised learning (WSL) approaches such as multiple instance learning (MIL) ([7–10]) have eased the problems in labeling by localizing discriminative regions while learning the classifier. Instead of class labels, MIL defines labels for positive and negative bags, each containing several instances. All instances in negative bags are negative, but there is at least one positive instance in each positive bag, and the goal is to localize the positive instances (see Fig. 2(a)). Unfortunately, the MIL paradigm has two major drawbacks: first, it is non-trivial to extend it to multi-label settings [11]; second, it typically leads to multi-pass algorithms that alternate between classification and localization. This is especially cumbersome on videos, due to the high number of degrees of freedom in voxel/cuboid search. The MIL problem gets even harder if several instances have to occur together in a bag to form a positive sample. This is the case of action recognition, since activities are typically defined by a collection of spatio-temporal parts extracted from a video [5,7,12,13]. Thus, in order to provide accurate spatio-temporal localization, activity parts cannot be labeled individually, but rather be selected coherently throughout the entire dataset.

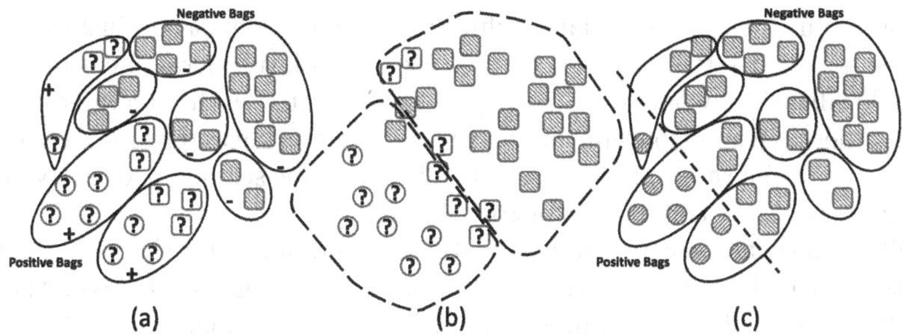

Fig. 2. (a) Multiple instance learning has positive and negative bags, and the goal is to identify positive instances in positive bags. Instead, our approach (b) clusters the instances and (c) forces the labels to agree with the clustering output and bag labels.

We explore the fact that instances from the same class usually organize themselves into clusters [14–17] and that low-rank matrix completion [18] can exploit low-rank subspaces to find relations between labels and features. Thus, we jointly cluster instances into subspaces (Fig. 2(b)) and label unknown instances consistently with the clustering, while keeping negative bag instances as negative (Fig. 2(c)). We demonstrate the effectiveness of our joint subspace clustering and classification in weakly-supervised multi-label learning for video activity recognition.

2 Related Work

Many researchers have addressed the problem of activity recognition in video sequences by using space-time interest points [1,19], dense trajectories [5] and discriminative space-time neighborhood features [20]. Some previous works have also targeted the problem of spatio-temporal action segmentation and recognition. Hoai *et al.* [21] recognized activities using a multi-class support vector machine (SVM) and infer the temporal segments with dynamic programming. Lan *et al.* [8] trained a latent SVM with a number of labeled and fully annotated videos, but each video is assigned a single label. In [22], the authors propose a weakly supervised video action classification using a similarity constrained latent SVM. Tang *et al.* [23] use a variable-duration hidden Markov model to build a model for each video. Chen *et al.* [24] construct a space-time video graph and find the subgraph that maximizes an activity classifier's score. Siva *et al.* [10] extract potential action cuboids and use genetic algorithms to select the best potential cuboids to learn a SVM for recognition. In related work, [12] introduced spatio-temporal deformable part models for activity recognition and localization.

Action localization is usually performed in the context of action detection, separate from the recognition phase (*e.g.*, [25–29]). Raptis *et al.* [7] extract spatio-temporal structures by forming clusters of trajectories. A graphical model is used to recognize a collection of these clusters as a particular action. We share with [7] the use of action parts, but they use graph search to correspond action parts and incorporate fully supervised data, while we perform subspace clustering in a weakly-supervised setting. Ma *et al.* [30] use a two level hierarchical model for activity localization, where each body part is associated with a rectangular box. They first perform a video frame hierarchical segmentation and prune a candidate segment tree. Then they extract hierarchical space-time segments for activity recognition via separate codebooks for root and parts.

Multiple-instance learning was initially proposed in [31] for the WSL problem of predicting which configurations of a pharmaceutical drug are effective. Andrews *et al.* [32] formulated a maximum margin MIL based on Support Vector Machines, where sample labels are unobserved integer variables and the margin between these is maximized directly. These MIL methods result in non-convex optimization processes and thus are heavily dependent on initialization. WSL in computer vision has been extensively studied, by generating spatio-temporal masks for objects in images and videos [33] from partially tagged Internet and YouTube videos [34]. Since labeling video by annotating every single frame is a cumbersome task, several WSL models have been developed for activity recognition and event detection in videos (*e.g.*, [8,30]). Tang *et al.* [17] propose a spatio-temporal transductive and inductive object segment annotation from weakly-tagged videos. Recently, several works have formulated the MIL and WSL problems as convex problems (*e.g.*, [35,36]). In [35] the authors have proposed a model based on calculating likelihood ratios of instances using Support Vector Regression and classifying the bags into positive and negative with a binary SVM.

Our work is most similar to [14,18]. Liu *et al.* [14] is a low-rank subspace segmentation algorithm and [18] a low-rank matrix completion (MC) framework for classification. We propose a method that intertwines these two to perform simultaneous recognition and localization in videos. In [18] each image is represented as a single column in the matrix, localization is performed in the image plane by a bounding-box exhaustive search. However, in our method each video is composed of several parts and supervision is weak and only labels entire videos. Transduction and clustering alone do not suffice, but together provide a selection coherent for all parts in the dataset. This global context means selecting parts yields space-time locations and activity labels.

3 Video Representation

In our method, each video in the dataset is treated as a collection of motion parts [5,7,12,13]. Following [5,7], videos are represented by features extracted from parts with dense motion trajectories. We perform a spatio-temporal segmentation to obtain volumetric regions that have similar visual and motion characteristics. Then, we extract trajectories using an optical flow tracker, and discard regions with little or no movement. Finally, we group trajectories with similar behavior into parts. Figure 3 illustrates this process in a sample video from the HOHA dataset. Since trajectories are asynchronous and have different lengths, we define a distance to incorporate motion similarity and spatial closeness. For two trajectories

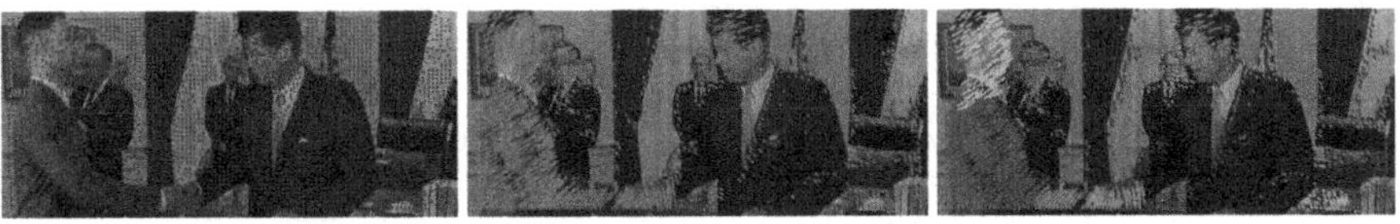

Fig. 3. Left to right: Points tracked on a frame, extracted trajectories, trajectory groups.

A and B with points $\mathbf{x_A}[t]$ and $\mathbf{x_B}[t]$, we calculate their similarity on a temporal overlap $t \in [\tau_1, \tau_2]$ as[1]

$$d(A, B) = \left(\max_{t \in [\tau_1, \tau_2]} \|\mathbf{x_A}[t] - \mathbf{x_B}[t]\|_2 \right) \times \left(\frac{\sum_{t=\tau_1}^{\tau_2} \|\dot{\mathbf{x}}_\mathbf{A}[t] - \dot{\mathbf{x}}_\mathbf{B}[t]\|_2}{(\tau_2 - \tau_1)\sigma_{[\tau_1, \tau_2]}} \right), \quad (1)$$

where $\dot{\mathbf{x}}[t] = \mathbf{x}[t] - \mathbf{x}[t-1]$ denote velocities of the trajectory points and $\sigma_{[\tau_1, \tau_2]}$ is the local optical flow variance in the interval $[\tau_1, \tau_2]$. In (1), the first term is a measure of spatial distance while the second estimates distance in motion and velocity. To group trajectories, we follow [7] and calculate the affinities between all pairs of trajectories in a video, forming an affinity matrix, calculated as $\omega(A, B) = \exp(-\eta d(A, B))$. A normalized-cut clustering is then used to group the trajectories, where a Cattell's scree test is used to determine the appropriate number of clusters.

Each trajectory group forms a part that may or may not be associated to the activities of interest. For instance, 23 parts appear in the video frame shown in Fig. 3. Each part is represented by a histogram of oriented gradients (HoG), optical flow (HoF) [1] and oriented edges in the motion boundaries (HoMB) [5]. These histograms are computed on a regular grid at three different scales. Each descriptor (HoG, HoF, HoMB) uses an independent dictionary, obtained by performing K-means on all the parts, and quantizing all descriptors to its closest ℓ_2 distance dictionary element. The concatenation of all three histograms forms the group (part) descriptor, $\mathbf{h}_k \in \mathbb{R}^n$. A video $\mathbf{V}_i$ is described by concatenating its activity parts, as $\mathbf{V}_i = [\mathbf{h}_{1i}\ \mathbf{h}_{2i}\ \ldots\ \mathbf{h}_{ki}]$.

4 Activity Recognition and Localization

In this section, we present our weakly-supervised learning algorithm for action recognition and localization in video sequences. In our problem, we have several training videos, each of which is labeled with one or more activities. However, no spatio-temporal information exists on where the activities occur. Our task is to classify whether unknown test videos contain those activities or not, and simultaneously localize them throughout the video. Our approach merges the advantages

[1] Bold capital letters denote matrices (*e.g.*, $\mathbf{D}$). All non-bold letters denote scalar variables. d_{ij} denotes the scalar in the row i and column j of $\mathbf{D}$.$\langle \mathbf{d}_1, \mathbf{d}_2 \rangle$ denotes the inner product between two vectors $\mathbf{d}_1$ and $\mathbf{d}_2$.$\|\mathbf{d}\|_2^2 = \langle \mathbf{d}, \mathbf{d} \rangle = \Sigma_i d_i^2$ denotes the squared Euclidean Norm of$\mathbf{d}$.$\|\mathbf{A}\|_*$ designates the nuclear norm (sum of singular values) of $\mathbf{A}$.

of two recently proposed low-rank models: subspace segmentation [14] clusters similar activity parts from all videos in the dataset, and a matrix completion classifier [18] determines the activity labels they belong to, such that the labeling is consistent throughout the entire dataset.

Let m be the number of different activity classes, n the dimensionality of the feature space, and N_{tr}, N_{tst} the number of training and testing parts, respectively. For the classification task, we can define a matrix $\mathbf{D_0}$ as

$$\mathbf{D_0} = \begin{bmatrix} \mathbf{D_Y} \\ \mathbf{D_X} \\ \mathbf{D_1} \end{bmatrix} = \begin{bmatrix} \mathbf{Y_{tr}} & \mathbf{Y_{tst}} \\ \mathbf{X_{tr}} & \mathbf{X_{tst}} \\ \multicolumn{2}{c}{\mathbf{1}^\top} \end{bmatrix}, \tag{2}$$

where $\mathbf{Y_{tr}} \in \mathbb{R}^{m \times N_{tr}}$ and $\mathbf{Y_{tst}} \in \mathbb{R}^{m \times N_{tst}}$ are the training and test labels and $\mathbf{X_{tr}} \in \mathbb{R}^{n \times N_{tr}}$ and $\mathbf{X_{tst}} \in \mathbb{R}^{n \times N_{tst}}$ are the training and test feature vectors, respectively. Hence, $\mathbf{D_Y}$, $\mathbf{D_X}$ and $\mathbf{D_1}$ denote the label, feature and last rows of $\mathbf{D}$, respectively. As noted by Cabral *et al.* [18], if a linear classification model holds, $\mathbf{D_0}$ is rank deficient. Therefore, classification can be posed as a matrix completion problem of filling the missing entries in $\mathbf{Y}_{tst}$ such that the nuclear norm of $\mathbf{D_0}$ (a convex approximation of its rank) is minimized. To deal with noise and outliers in the data, we can incorporate an error term $\mathbf{E^{mc}}$ in the known feature and training label entries,

$$\mathbf{D} = \mathbf{D_0} + \mathbf{E^{mc}} = \begin{bmatrix} \mathbf{Y_{tr}} & \mathbf{Y_{tst}} \\ \mathbf{X_{tr}} & \mathbf{X_{tst}} \\ \multicolumn{2}{c}{\mathbf{1}^\top} \end{bmatrix} + \begin{bmatrix} \mathbf{E_{Y_{tr}}} & \mathbf{0} \\ \multicolumn{2}{c}{\mathbf{E_X}} \\ \multicolumn{2}{c}{\mathbf{0}^\top} \end{bmatrix} \tag{3}$$

and the classification process can be posed as finding the best $\mathbf{Y_{tst}}$ and the error matrix $\mathbf{E^{mc}}$ such that the rank of $\mathbf{D}$ is minimized.

As discussed in Sect. 3, each video $\mathbf{V}_i$ is represented by the histograms of its activity parts. If labels were provided for each part in training, we could construct $\mathbf{D_0}$ by setting each column to the features corresponding to one activity part and its respective $\{0, 1\}^m$ label vector. However, in our case supervision is weak and labels are only provided for entire videos. Thus, simply labeling parts with all class labels present in the video they originate from is insufficient for obtaining correct part level classifications.

Instead, to identify the parts that comprise each activity class, we can also exploit the fact that activity parts from the same class likely cluster together. This can be formulated as a segmentation of feature vectors into low-rank subspaces, using a Low-Rank Representation (LRR) [14]. Since $\mathbf{D_X}$ contains the feature vectors for all videos in the dataset, we can cluster activity parts by computing a low-rank similarity matrix $\mathbf{Z}$, as

$$\begin{aligned} \min_{\mathbf{Z},\mathbf{E^{lrr}}} \quad & \|\mathbf{Z}\|_* + \lambda \|\mathbf{E^{lrr}}\|_{2,1}, \\ \text{subject to} \quad & \mathbf{D_X} = \mathbf{D_X Z} + \mathbf{E^{lrr}}, \end{aligned} \tag{4}$$

where $\mathbf{E^{lrr}}$ is the LRR [14] error matrix and λ is a balancing parameter between low-rank and error fit. $\mathbf{Z}$ is indicative of the similarity between each activity part in $\mathbf{D_X}$ and thus can be used as an additional cue to weak supervision for classifying which parts constitute which activities. Using the similarity matrix $\mathbf{Z}$, we can apply a clustering method such as Normalized Cuts to group similar activity parts in all train/test videos. The output of this clustering method is a $n_c \times N$ binary matrix $\mathbf{Q}$, where n_c is the number of clusters. Each row of $\mathbf{Q}$ corresponds to one cluster, with $q_{ij} = 1$ if the jth activity part belongs to the i^{th}cluster, and 0 otherwise.

Below, we show that these matrix completion classification and subspace clustering steps can be done jointly, so that labels are consistent within clusters and vice-versa.

4.1 Joint Classification and Clustering

With the matrix completion and subspace segmentation defined as above, we can simultaneously obtain a low-rank representation of the feature vector matrix $\mathbf{D_X}$, and correct and complete the labels in $\mathbf{D_Y} = [\mathbf{Y_{tr}}, \mathbf{Y_{tst}}]$. Our activity classification problem can be defined as minimizing the rank of $\mathbf{D}$ for determining the part labels, while at the same time ensuring the labels are consistent with the clustering $\mathbf{Q}$ obtained from the low-rank representation $\mathbf{Z}$ of the parts $\mathbf{D_X}$. If we define $\mathbf{\Omega_Y}$ as the set of known label entries in $\mathbf{D_0}$, this objective can be written as

$$\begin{aligned} \min \quad & \|\mathbf{D}\|_* + \gamma\|\mathbf{Z}\|_* + \lambda\|\mathbf{E_X}\|_{2,1} \\ & + \rho_1 \sum_{i,j \in \mathbf{D_Y}} c_y(d_{ij}, q_{kj}) + \rho_2 \sum_{i,j \in \mathbf{\Omega_Y}} c_y(d_{ij}, d_{0ij}) \\ \text{subject to} \quad & \mathbf{D} = \mathbf{D_0} + \mathbf{E}^{\mathbf{mc}}, \mathbf{D_1} = \mathbf{1}^\top, \mathbf{D_X} = \mathbf{D_X}\mathbf{Z} + \mathbf{E_X}, \end{aligned} \tag{5}$$

where $c_y(a, b) = \log(1 + \exp(-(2b - 1)(a - b)))$ is a logistic loss function that penalizes entries of different classes. γ, λ, ρ_1, ρ_2 are positive trade-off parameters. k is the most similar cluster to label i, calculated as $k = \mathrm{argmin}_{k=1}^{nc} \sum_j c_y(d_{ij}, q_{kj})$.

With the objective in (5), the first term seeks a low-rank $\mathbf{D}$ matrix so that labels can be expressed as a linear combination of features. The second establishes a low-rank representation $\mathbf{Z}$ for subspace clustering. The third term controls the level of noise in the clustering. The fourth term nudges the labels in $\mathbf{D_Y}$ the direction suggested by the clustering $\mathbf{Q}$ and the fifth term regularizes changes on known training labels $\mathbf{Y_{tr}}$ in the matrix completion. Therefore, we are seeking to achieve a consensus between the clustering and classification outputs. The intersection of these two tasks is incorporated by the fourth term, where inconsistent clustering outputs and labels are penalized. The minimization process will aim towards unanimity between the two and the least label changing in $\mathbf{Y_{tr}}$. Also, notice that in the process of joint minimization, both classification and clustering tasks share the feature error matrix, resulting in less variables than used when optimizing both objectives separately.

The objective in (5) can be optimized using an Alternating Direction Method of multipliers (ADMM) [37]. When it converges, the labels in $\mathbf{Y_{tst}}$ corresponding to each activity part indicate its action label(s) and the columns with that label are the parts associated to that specific activity. The highest computational complexity step in solving (5) with an ADMM is a SVD of $\mathbf{D}$, but scalable SVD/ADMM methods are currently being researched heavily [38].

As in $\mathbf{D_Y}$, each instance is assigned a set of labels, each of which belongs to an independent activity class. This enables us to model multi-label MIL problems. Many previous works have exploring the dependence among the labels [39,40]. But when the labels are incomplete (weakly-supervised) the task is harder. As also explored in previous works [18,41], the low rank assumption of the matrix $\mathbf{D}$ resembles a linear dependence among the labels and the feature vectors. We evaluate our multi-label setting in a weakly-supervised video activity recognition and localization.

5 Experiments

To evaluate the proposed technique, we set up several experiments on various synthetic and real datasets. Since our approach performs clustering and classification simultaneously, one might conceive that we could first run clustering and then use matrix completion for obtaining the labels. Thus, as a baseline, we derive a low-rank representation [14] of matrix $\mathbf{D_X}$ and then run matrix completion while incorporating the feature error term in the matrix completion formulation (LRRMC). We also compare the performance of our method to using just matrix completion (MC) of [18] for classification as described in Sect. 4 to show that solely relying on a weakly supervised labeling for part classification does not work, and the well-known MI-SVM [32], with RBF kernel.

In each iteration of (5), we obtain the clustering $\mathbf{Q}$ using $n_c = 2m$ clusters to account for intra-class variability, and use as parameters $\gamma = 0.9$, $\rho_1 = 1.5$, $\rho_2 \in \{10^{-3}, 10^{-2}, 10^{-1}, 1\}$. For experiments on activity recognition datasets, to ensure direct comparability with state of the art methods, we follow the setup of [7] for obtaining and describing activity parts, as described in Sect. 3. Each part

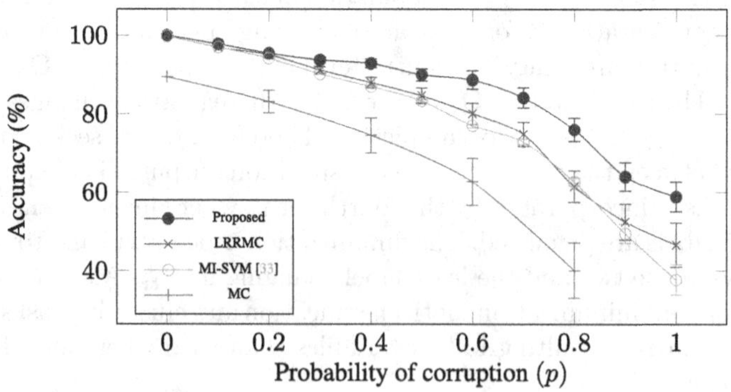

Fig. 4. Accuracy comparison according to corruption probability p on synthetic data. This figure shows the means and standard deviations for three different runs.

is represented by histogram of oriented gradients (HoG), histogram of optical flow (HoF) [1] and histogram of the oriented edges in the motion boundaries (HoMB) [5] descriptors, with 500, 500, 300 dimensions respectively.

5.1 Synthetic Data

First, in order to validate the proposed algorithm, we construct 10 independent subspaces of dimensionality 100 (as described in [14]). The first five subspaces form our desired positive classes and the second five, negative. We create 100 positive and 100 negative bags, with size 10, and sample instances from the above subspaces. Positive bags, as in MIL, are composed of uniformly distributed positive and negative instances. We corrupt each sampled instance $\mathbf{x}$ with probability p, by adding Gaussian noise with zero mean and variance $0.3\|\mathbf{x}\|$. The performance of the proposed method is compared with LRRMC, MI-SVM and matrix completion (MC) [18], as illustrated in Fig. 4 for different probabilities of corruption and noise. The performance of our method is much better when the noise level increases in the data. As mentioned in Sect. 4, MC yields worse results since it fully relies on the initial labeling, which is not accurate enough due to its weakly supervised nature. Our method performs a joint clustering and classification of the data and detects noise and outliers in both tasks collaboratively. In LRRMC these are done separately. Thus, our method deals better with noise in the data.

5.2 Action Recognition and Localization

Three popular activity recognition datasets are used: MSR-II [6], HOHA [1] and UCF sports [3] action datasets. MSR-II action dataset 2 contains 54 videos with three action categories: boxing, clapping and hand-waving. In this dataset, some of the videos contain multiple actions and some with actions even occurring at the same time. The HOHA (Hollywood1 Human Action) dataset contains 430 videos. Each video contains significant camera motion, rapid scene changes and occasionally significant clutter. Furthermore, actions in this dataset are performed in different conditions, and many actions are defined by the interactions between the subjects and/or objects. These factors make this dataset particularly challenging. The UCF sports dataset consists of 150 videos extracted from sports broadcasts. Video in this dataset contain camera motions and many different lighting and capturing conditions, as well as large displacements of most of the actions, cluttered backgrounds, and large intra-class variability.

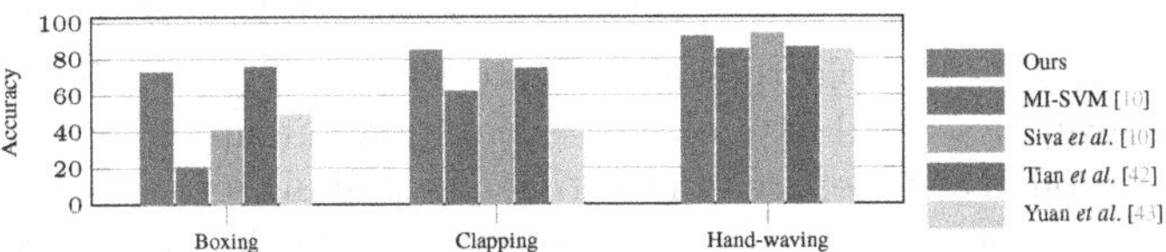

Fig. 5. Per-class recognition accuracy for MSR-II dataset.

Table 1. Recognition results on MSR-II dataset. *Cross dataset* methods are trained on KTH dataset, which only contains actions with little background motion.

Method	Supervision	Accuracy
Siva *et al.* [10]	Weak	71.2 %
MI-SVM [10]	Weak	55.8 %
Tian *et al.* [42]	Full (Cross dataset)	78.8 %
MC	Weak	41.1 %
LRRMC	Weak	54.9 %
Our Method	Weak	**83.1%**

Recognition: Tests on each of the datasets have separate experimental settings to facilitate comparisons with reference methods. We compare our recognition model with state-of-the-art models reported in the literature and with the same baselines described in the synthetic tests of Sect. 5.1. The final classification step in our model is performed via a thresholding procedure, where labels above a common threshold are selected.

MSR-II dataset- For the experiments on this dataset, a two-to-one random division of all videos in the dataset creates the training and testing sets. This dataset contains videos with multiple actions happening in the video and, in some cases, being performed at the same time, which can challenge our multi-label classification framework. Some of the videos in this dataset contain several instances of all activities. Since we expect a single instance of each activity class in the video, the videos are split such that each video contains only one instance of each activity class, but allowing for several activities from different classes. Figure 5 shows our per-class accuracy results compared to the MI-SVM model [32]. Table 1 shows the recognition accuracy results compared to state-of-the-art methods on this dataset. The supervision column shows the level of supervision used in the training phase: fully supervised methods know spatio-temporal bounding boxes of activity locations, whereas weakly-supervised methods use only the label(s).

HOHA dataset- In this experiment the test set has 211 videos with 217 labels and the training set has 219 videos with 231 labels, all manually annotated [7]. Figure 6 shows the per-class accuracy results for this dataset. This dataset is very challenging for activity recognition, due to the large amount of clutter and motion in the camera. Our approach is comparable with results from state-of-the-art methods designed specifically for this dataset, improving them by a slight margin. Table 2 gives the overall accuracy results compared to some other methods on this dataset.

UCF Sports dataset - We split this dataset into 103 training and 47 test samples, follwing the setup described in [7,8]. This separation minimizes the strong correlation of background cues between the testing and training set [7]. Some results on this dataset report leave-one-out-cross-validation (LOOCV) performance, which may take into account the similarity of the background instead of the activity itself. In this dataset the background is very similar for sports of the same kind,

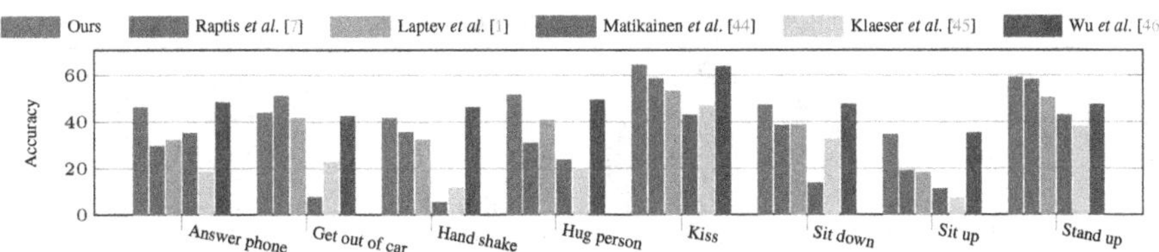

Fig. 6. Per-class recognition for HOHA dataset.

Table 2. Recognition results on HOHA dataset.

Method	Supervision	Accuracy
Klaeser *et al.* [45]	Full	27.3 %
Laptev *et al.* [1]	Full	38.4 %
Matikainen *et al.* [44]	Full	22.8 %
Raptis *et al.* [7]	Full	40.1 %
Wu *et al.* [46]	Full	47.6 %
MC	Weak	22.3 %
LRRMC	Weak	29.8 %
Our Method	Weak	**48.5%**

which affects the activity recognition rates. Figure 7 depicts the per-class classification accuracy for this dataset. As shown, our method outperforms the BoW+SVM model in almost all classes. As shown in Table 3, the overall recognition rate of our method is also competitive with the state-of-the-art. The upper part of the table compares our results with state-of-the-art methods' reported results for the same training and testing dataset split. Our method outperforms all of these works. The lower part of the table shows results from works that use LOOCV, which generally achieve better results. Our split is much harder and the difference between the results is expected. Notwithstanding a more difficult test scenario, our results are still comparable to these works.

Spatio-Temporal Localization: The second function of our method is the spatio-temporal localization of the activity in the video sequence. In order to assess spatio-temporal localization directly against reported state-of-the-art methods, we employ three metrics for assessing localization performance: (1) intersection-over-union using the selected positive parts (IOU), (2) average precision (AP) of part classification based on ground truth spatio-temporal annotations, and (3) the localization *score*, defined as in [7]. The latter is defined as the average ratio of the sets of points inside the annotated ground truth bounding box and the set of points of the selected trajectory group for each frame. If the detected activity part(s) throughout the video have at least a θ overlap with the annotated ground truth bounding box ($score \geq \theta$), the recognition/localization is considered as correct. The results are compared to the state-of-the-art methods in the

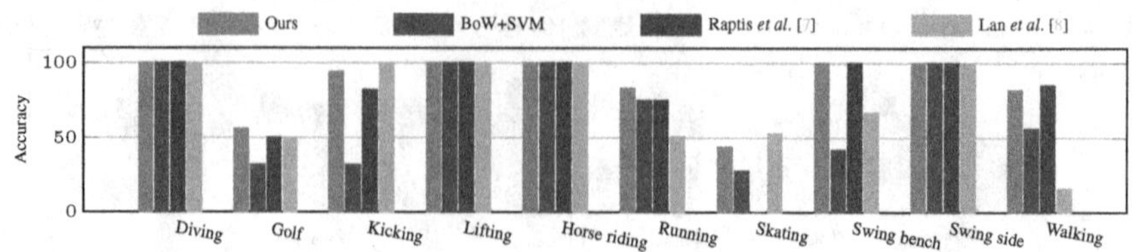

Fig. 7. Per-class recognition results for UCF Sports dataset.

Table 3. Recognition results on UCF Sports. Upper part: Results with 103:47 dataset split. Lower part: Results with LOOCV.

Method	Supervision	Accuracy
Lan *et al.* [8]	Full	73.1 %
Raptis *et al.* [7]	Full	79.4 %
Tian *et al.* [12]	Full	75.2 %
Ma *et al.* [30]	Weak	81.7 %
MC	Weak	59.8 %
LRRMC	Weak	71.2 %
Our Method	Weak	**86.9%**
Le *et al.* [47]	Full	86.5 %
Wang *et al.* [19]	Full	85.6 %
Wang *et al.* [5]	Full	88.2 %
Wang *et al.* [48]	Full	**89.1%**
Kovashka and Grauman [20]	Full	87.3 %

Table 4. Action localization AP on the MSR-II dataset. *Cross dataset* methods are trained on KTH dataset, which only contains actions with little background motion.

Method	Supervision	Clapping	Boxing	Handwaving
Siva *et al.* [10]	Full	**0.602**	0.694	0.700
Siva *et al.* [10]	Weak	0.326	0.658	0.799
Cao *et al.* [6]	Full (Cross Dataset)	0.125	0.144	0.242
Tian *et al.* [12]	Full (Cross Dataset)	0.239	0.389	0.447
Our Method	Weak	0.569	**0.724**	**0.811**

literature, using IOU, AP or localization score, where available. Tables 4, 5 and 6 show results on MSR-II, HOHA and UCF Sports datasets, respectively. Since [8] only provides localization results on a subset of frames, we also include results on this subset for comparison. The average recognition/localization accuracies for the experiments on the datasets as a function of θ are illustrated in Fig. 8. Some results are shown in Fig. 9.

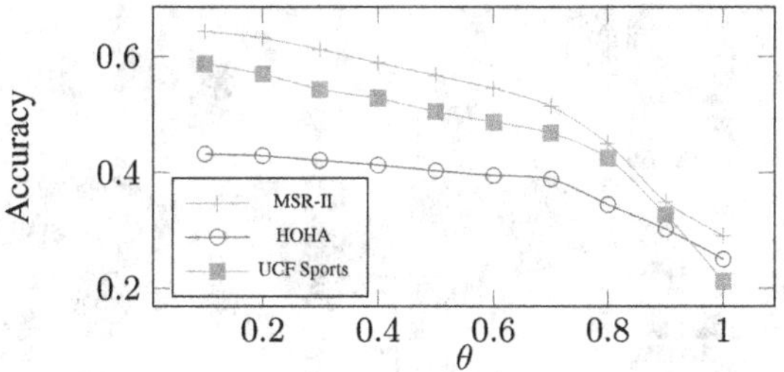

Fig. 8. Average localization accuracy as a function of the localization overlap θ.

Table 5. Localization comparisons for HOHA dataset.

Method	Supervision	Localization score		Mean IOU
		$\theta = 0.1$	$\theta = 1$	
Raptis *et al.* [7]	Full	54.3 %	**28.6 %**	–
Our Method	Weak	**56.2%**	21.0 %	**42.9%**

Table 6. Average localization IOU on the UCF Sports dataset. Note that [25] and [8] use the bounding box annotations during the training,while ours is weakly-supervised.

Action	Subset of frames				All frames			
	[25]	[8]	[30]	Ours	[25]	[8]	[30]	Ours
Diving	36.5	43.4	**46.7**	44.8	37.0	–	**44.3**	43.7
Golf	–	37.1	51.3	**53.1**	–	–	50.5	**52.3**
Kicking	–	36.8	50.6	**54.3**	–	–	48.3	**52.9**
Lifting	–	68.8	55.0	**69.0**	–	–	51.4	**63.5**
H-Ride	**68.1**	21.9	29.5	34.5	**64.0**	–	30.6	32.5
Running	**61.4**	20.1	34.3	31.2	**61.9**	–	33.1	30.1
Skating	–	13.0	40.0	**45.5**	–	–	38.5	**43.2**
Swing-B	–	32.7	54.8	**57.1**	–	–	54.3	**57.5**
Swing-S	–	16.4	19.3	**48.7**	–	–	20.6	**44.1**
Walking	–	28.3	39.5	**47.5**	–	–	39.0	**47.1**
Avg.	–	31.8	42.1	**51.3**	–	–	41.0	**46.7**

Experimental Results Discussion: Our experiments show that the proposed joint process in (5) significantly improves results, when compared to the baselines of MC and performing clustering and classification steps separately (LRRMC). We note that the multi-label nature of our method allows us to provide results for simultaneous actions on the MSR-II dataset, as seen on Fig. 9. An important note on the recognition results, is that our method performed competitively even with those specifically focused for recognition (*i.e.*, that do not perform any localization of the activity) and methods that train with fully annotated datasets. This is

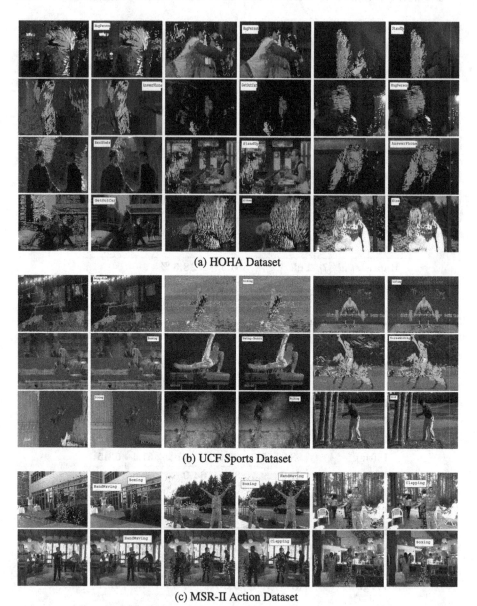

(a) HOHA Dataset

(b) UCF Sports Dataset

(c) MSR-II Action Dataset

Fig. 9. Recognition and localization results on action recognition datasets. Each result from a test video is illustrated in a pair of images, first of which is a sample frame of the video containing the action of the interest. The trajectory groups are shown on this image, each with a different color. The second image shows the selected trajectory group(s) by our algorithm. (a) results from the HOHA dataset, (b) results from the UCF Sports dataset, and (c) results from MSR-II action datset.

despite the fact that when using the whole frame or video features for recognition, we are dealing with many outliers and significant noise. Furthermore, our model extracts the exact spatio-temporal segmentation of the activity, rather than a simple bounding box, cuboid or voxel representation, as opposed to many previous works. We improve the recognition results on all datasets, and also achieve good localization scores. We believe these could be improved further if more accurate spatio-temporal annotations in the datasets were used as ground truth instead of bounding boxes.

As could be seen, our method achieved much better results compared to many state-of-the-art methods. This is basically due to two important properties of our method. Our method deals with errors and outliers in the feature vectors and the labels. As could be seen in (5) we extract the erroneous elements as well in the process of minimizing the matrix ranks. The error for both LRR and MC are incorporated simultaneously, which tend to correct one another in the process. On the other hand, our method labels the actions via transduction, which alone improves the results compared to inductive approaches. There are no separate train and test phases and our approach incorporates activity parts and information from the whole dataset when minimizing the nuclear norm and deciding on the instance classes.

6 Conclusions

In this paper, we have proposed a low-rank formulation for weakly supervised learning and have applied it to the challenging problem of activity recognition. Our approach uses a simultaneous convex matrix completion and LRR subspace clustering framework to recover the labels for the test videos and localize the spatio-temporal extent of activities throughout each video. Interactions between the activity parts are globally modeled throughout the entire dataset using the subspace clustering procedure, while the matrix completion framework labels the activities ensuring that labeling is consistent within clusters and vice-versa. Our experiments show this joint process significantly improves results, when compared to performing clustering and classification steps separately. Moreover, it attains performances comparable to state-of-the-art methods for classification and localization in all three datasets tested.

Unlike typical MIL approaches, our method to be naturally multi-label and is able to handle video sequences where several activity parts have to occur together in a bag to define an action, and actions occur simultaneously in different spatial locations.

As a direction for future work, we intend to apply and develop incremental procedures for the training and testing and exploit parallel algorithms for the SVD operations needed to optimize (5), such as in [38], in order to decrease processing time.

References

1. Laptev, I., Marszałek, M., Schmid, C., Rozenfeld, B.: Learning realistic human actions from movies. In: CVPR (2008)
2. Ryoo, M.S., Aggarwal, J.K.: Spatio-temporal relationship match: video structure comparison for recognition of complex human activities. In: ICCV (2009)
3. Rodriguez, M.D., Ahmed, J., Shah, M.: Action mach: a spatio-temporal maximum average correlation height filter for action recognition. In: CVPR (2008)
4. Sheikh, Y., Sheikh, M., Shah, M.: Exploring the space of a human action. In: ICCV (2005)
5. Wang, H., Kläser, A., Schmid, C., Cheng-Lin, L.: Action recognition by dense trajectories. In: CVPR (2011)
6. Cao, L., Liu, Z., Huang, T.S.: Cross-dataset action detection. In: CVPR (2010)
7. Raptis, M., Kokkinos, I., Soatto, S.: Discovering discriminative action parts from mid-level video representations. In: CVPR (2012)
8. Lan, T., Wang, Y., Mori, G.: Discriminative figure-centric models for joint action localization and recognition. In: ICCV (2011)
9. Nguyen, M.H., Torresani, L., De la Torre, F., Rother, C.: Weakly-supervised discriminative localization and classification: a joint learning process. In: ICCV (2009)
10. Siva, P., Xiang, T.: Weakly-supervised action detection. In: BMVC (2011)
11. Zhou, Z., Zhang, M.: Multi-instance multi-label learning with application to scene classification. In: NIPS (2006)
12. Tian, Y., Sukthankar, R., Shah, M.: Spatiotemporal deformable part models for action detection. In: CVPR (2013)
13. Wang, L., Qiao, Y., Tang, X.: Motionlets: mid-level 3D parts for human motion recognition. In: CVPR, pp. 2674–2681 (2013)
14. Liu, G., Lin, Z., Yu, Y.: Robust subspace segmentation by low-rank representation. In: ICML (2010)
15. Cheng, B., Liu, G., Wang, J., Huang, Z., Yan, S.: Multi-task low-rank affinity pursuit for image segmentation. In: ICCV (2011)
16. Elhamifar, E., Vidal, R.: Sparse subspace clustering. In: CVPR (2009)
17. Tang, K., Sukthankar, R., Yagnik, J., Fei-Fei, L.: Discriminative segment annotation in weakly labeled video. In: CVPR (2013)
18. Cabral, R.S., De la Torre, F., Costeira, J.P., Bernardino, A.: Matrix completion for multi-label image classification. In: NIPS (2011)
19. Wang, H., Ullah, M.M., Kläser, A., Laptev, I., Schmid, C.: Evaluation of local spatio-temporal features for action recognition. In: BMVC (2009)
20. Kovashka, A., Grauman, K.: Learning a hierarchy of discriminative space-time neighborhood features for human action recognition. In: CVPR (2010)
21. Hoai, M., Lan, Z., De la Torre, F.: Joint segmentation and classification of human actions in video. In: CVPR (2011)
22. Shapovalova, N., Vahdat, A., Cannons, K., Lan, T., Mori, G.: Similarity constrained latent support vector machine: an application to weakly supervised action classification. In: Fitzgibbon, A., Lazebnik, S., Perona, P., Sato, Y., Schmid, C. (eds.) ECCV 2012, Part VII. LNCS, vol. 7578, pp. 55–68. Springer, Heidelberg (2012)
23. Tang, K., Fei-Fei, L., Koller, D.: Learning latent temporal structure for complex event detection. In: CVPR (2012)
24. Chen, C.Y., Grauman, K.: Efficient Activity Detection with max-subgraph Search. In: CVPR (2012)

25. Tran, D., Yuan, J.: Max-margin structured output regression for spatio-temporal action localization. In: NIPS (2012)
26. Duchenne, O., Laptev, I., Sivic, J., Bach, F., Ponce, J.: Automatic annotation of human actions in video. In: ICCV (2009)
27. Tran, D., Yuan, J., Forsyth, D.: Video event detection: from subvolume localization to spatio-temporal path search. IEEE Trans. Pattern Anal. Mach. Intell. **36**(2), 404–416 (2014)
28. Kumar, B.G.V., Patras, I.: Supervised dictionary learning for action localization. In: FG (2013)
29. Gaidon, A., Harchaoui, Z., Schmid, C.: Temporal localization of actions with actoms. IEEE Trans. Pattern Anal. Mach. Intell. **35**, 2782–2795 (2013)
30. Ma, S., Zhang, J., Ikizler-Cinbis, N., Sclaroff, S.: Action recognition and localization by hierarchical space-time segments. In: ICCV (2013)
31. Dietterich, T.G., Lathrop, R.H., Lozano-Pérez, T.: Solving the multiple instance problem with axis-parallel rectangles. Artif. Intell. **89**, 31–71 (1997)
32. Andrews, S., Tsochantaridis, I., Hofmann, T.: Support vector machines for multiple-instance learning. In: NIPS (2003)
33. Prest, A., Leistner, C., Civera, J., Schmid, C., Ferrari, V.: Learning object class detectors from weakly annotated video. In: CVPR (2012)
34. Hartmann, G., Grundmann, M., Hoffman, J., Tsai, D., Kwatra, V., Madani, O., Vijayanarasimhan, S., Essa, I., Rehg, J., Sukthankar, R.: Weakly supervised learning of object segmentations from web-scale video. In: Fusiello, A., Murino, V., Cucchiara, R. (eds.) ECCV 2012 Ws/Demos, Part I. LNCS, vol. 7583, pp. 198–208. Springer, Heidelberg (2012)
35. Li, F., Sminchisescu, C.: Convex multiple-instance learning by estimating likelihood ratio. In: NIPS (2010)
36. Joulin, A., Bach, F.: A convex relaxation for weakly-supervised classifiers. In: ICML (2012)
37. Lin, Z., Chen, M., Wu, L., Ma, Y.: The Augmented Lagrange Multiplier Method for Exact Recovery of Corrupted Low-Rank Matrices. UIUC Technical report 2215 (2009)
38. Tron, R., Vidal, R.: Distributed computer vision algorithms through distributed averaging. In: CVPR (2011)
39. Boutell, M.R., Luo, J., Shen, X., Brown, C.M.: Learning multi-label scene classification. Pattern Recognit. **37**, 1757–1771 (2004)
40. Zhang, M.L., Zhou, Z.H.: A review on multi-label learning algorithms. IEEE Trans. Knowl. Data Eng. **26**(8), 1819–1837 (2014)
41. Goldberg, A.B., Zhu, X., Recht, B., Xu, J.M., Nowak, R.D.: Transduction with matrix completion: three birds with one stone. In: NIPS (2010)
42. Tian, Y., Cao, L., Liu, Z., Zhang, Z.: Hierarchical filtered motion for action recognition in crowded videos. IEEE Trans. Sys. Man. Cyb. Part C **42**, 313–323 (2012)
43. Yuan, J., Liu, Z., Wu, Y.: Discriminative video pattern search for efficient action detection. IEEE Trans. Pattern Anal. Mach. Intell. **33**, 1728–1743 (2011)
44. Matikainen, P., Hebert, M., Sukthankar, R.: Trajectons: action recognition through the motion analysis of tracked features. In: ICCV (2009)
45. Klaeser, A., Marszalek, M., Schmid, C.: A spatio-temporal descriptor based on 3D-gradients. In: BMVC (2008)
46. Wu, S., Oreifej, O., Shah, M.: Action recognition in videos acquired by a moving camera using motion decomposition of Lagrangian particle trajectories. In: ICCV (2011)

47. Le, Q.V., Zou, W.Y., Yeung, S.Y., Ng, A.Y.: Learning hierarchical invariant spatio-temporal features for action recognition with independent subspace analysis. In: CVPR (2011)
48. Wang, H., Kläser, A., Schmid, C., Liu, C.L.: Dense trajectories and motion boundary descriptors for action recognition. Int. J. Comput. Vis. **103**, 60–79 (2013)

Action-Gons: Action Recognition with a Discriminative Dictionary of Structured Elements with Varying Granularity

Yuwang Wang[1], Baoyuan Wang[2](✉), Yizhou Yu[3], Qionghai Dai[1], and Zhuowen Tu[4]

[1] BBNC Lab, Department of Automation, THU, Beijing, China
yw.wang2011@gmail.com, qhdai@tsinghua.edu.cn
[2] Microsoft Research, Beijing, China
baoyuanw@microsoft.com
[3] Department of Compute Science, HKU, Hong Kong, China
yizhouy@acm.org
[4] Department of CogSci, UCSD, San Diego, USA
ztu@ucsd.edu

Abstract. This paper presents "Action-Gons", a middle level representation for action recognition in videos. Actions in videos exhibit a reasonable level of regularity seen in human behavior, as well as a large degree of variation. One key property of action, compared with image scene, might be the amount of interaction among body parts, although scenes also observe structured patterns in 2D images. Here, we study high-order statistics of the interaction among regions of interest in actions and propose a mid-level representation for action recognition, inspired by the Julesz school of n-gon statistics. We propose a systematic learning process to build an over-complete dictionary of "Action-Gons". We first extract motion clusters, named as action units, then sequentially learn a pool of action-gons with different granularities modeling different degree of interactions among action units. We validate the discriminative power of our learned action-gons on three challenging video datasets and show evident advantages over the existing methods.

1 Introduction

Human action recognition has received an increasing amount of attention in the computer vision community as developing a practical action recognition system is vital for many applications ranging from mobile applications, surveillance, interactive gaming, to video annotation and retrieval. Although much progress has been made in the past few years, existing approaches are still far from being satisfactory and practical. Similar to the situation in other recognition problems, finding the right representation is still the key to deal with the challenges due to intra-class variations in viewing condition, illumination, spatial and temporal scale, and camera motion.

This work was done when Yuwang Wang was an intern at Micrsoft Research.

D. Cremers et al. (Eds.): ACCV 2014, Part V, LNCS 9007, pp. 259–274, 2015.
DOI: 10.1007/978-3-319-16814-2_17

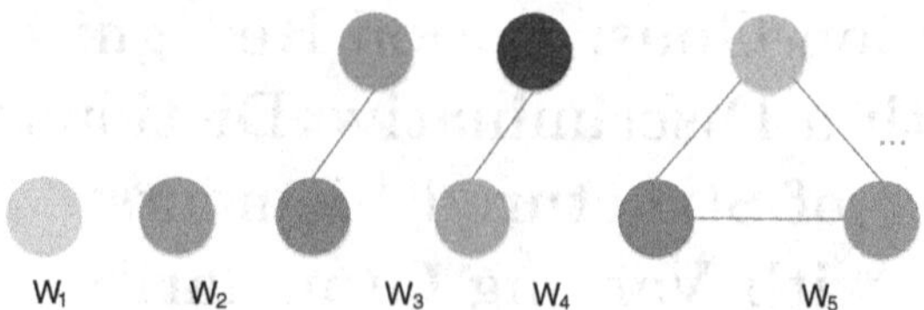

Fig. 1. Action-gons with different granularities for modeling different degrees of interaction. Action-gons shown on real images can be found in Figs. 3 and 6.

To tackle the problem of action recognition, one often designs novel low-level features [1] or applies learning techniques to mine discriminative mid-level or high-level features, as in [2,3]. Recent advances [2,4–6] show that learning mid-level action units, which are essentially spatio-temporal regions of interest, leads to large improvement in performance.

Actions in videos observe sparse, well-structured, strong temporal coherence, and dynamic interactions, which are different from objects and scenes in 2D images. First, human actions consist of coordinated movements of body parts and accessories. For example, a high jump requires precisely coordinated movements of the arms, torso and legs. It is important to model the co-occurrences and interactions among the movements of different body parts. Second, the number of interacting parts in different actions may vary. For example, the aforementioned high jump involves all body parts while certain actions, such as drinking, only involve the upper body and arms. A complex action, such as a gymnastic routine, can be decomposed spatially and temporally into a number of elementary movements, each of which may involve a different number of body parts. In addition, in the absence of 3D information, 2D videos taken from different viewpoints typically need multiple modes. Thus, we need to study statistics with respect to a variety of interactions for action analysis. In the past, not much attention has been given to explicitly characterizing the statistics of the interactions among regions of interests in actions. And there has been even little attempt to explore the graph-based dictionary with varying granularity to capture the intrinsic motion structures for action recognition.

The Julesz school of two-gon and tri-gon statistics models the intrinsic patterns of textures [7], which has rarely been studied lately in computer vision for action analysis. Our work is inspired by the n-gon statistics of Julesz. We first perform unsupervised learning to extract a set of informative motion clusters, called action units, from videos. Our focus is then to learn a dictionary of interactions among the units, named as "Action-Gons", which model co-occurring and potentially interacting regions of interest, as shown in Fig. 1. To account for varying degrees of complexity, different orders of interaction for the action units are studied. The number of co-occurring action units within an action-gon is defined as its granularity.

For the detailed pipeline of our work, we first partition the motion trajectories into canonical clusters, each of which is called an action unit; then we sequentially learn the interaction structures with varying granularities for each action class to form our proposed action-gons. Specifically, each action-gon is defined as a latent graph structure with nodes representing action units and edges representing interactions between action units. The feature vector for an action-gon includes features for the individual nodes, as well as features for the edges. Latent graphs with the same granularity for the same action class are learned simultaneously. To achieve better discriminative representation power, a classifier is eventually learned for each action-gon, which is used as an entry in the dictionary. During the recognition stage, we apply the classifier associated with every action-gon on the video and perform max pooling over the response maps to generate features for final action classification.

We validate our framework for learning action-gons on three challenging video datasets: HMDB51 [8], Youtube [9], and UCF-Sports [10]. Extensive experiments show that our approach achieves significantly improved performance over existing state-of-the-art methods, indicating the effectiveness of having a mid-level dictionary of part interactions.

In summary, this paper makes the following three contributions: (1) We propose to learn action-gons with varying granularities for action recognition, inspired by the Julesz n-gon statistics which has not been frequently studied. Each action-gon characterizes co-occurring and interacting regions of interest. (2) We introduce a principled learning method for building an informative yet discriminative dictionary of action-gons. (3) Building on top of the action-gon representation, our overall method produces significantly improved results on benchmark datasets for action recognition.

2 Related Work

Conventional video-based action recognition methods typically extract sparse (sometimes dense) spatio-temporal interest points (STIP) [11] and compute low-level appearance and motion features, followed by training a classifier on top of either the Bag-of-Words (BoW) model or the SPM feature representation. The most popular low-level features, including HOG/HOF [12], HOG3D [13], and MBH [1], indeed turn out to be very informative yet discriminative representations. Recently, to overcome the drawbacks of the traditional Bag-of-Words model, researchers [14,15] have proposed to add pairwise spatial-temporal relational features between quantized base features (i.e., HOG/HOF) to express potential interactions. A similar idea has also been employed in [16] to explore contextual features. Although those methods have been proven to be effective on certain datasets, they still lack the flexibility to adaptively infer and localize the most discriminative action parts. Therefore, they do not necessarily derive the optimal representation for characterizing natural human interactions.

Complementary to this line of effort, people have also been trying to develop better feature learning methods or models to tackle the challenges caused by differing scales, viewpoints, illumination or even occlusions. For example, action recognition by learning middle level features has recently become a popular research topic in computer vision, a variety of methods [2,4–6,17] have been

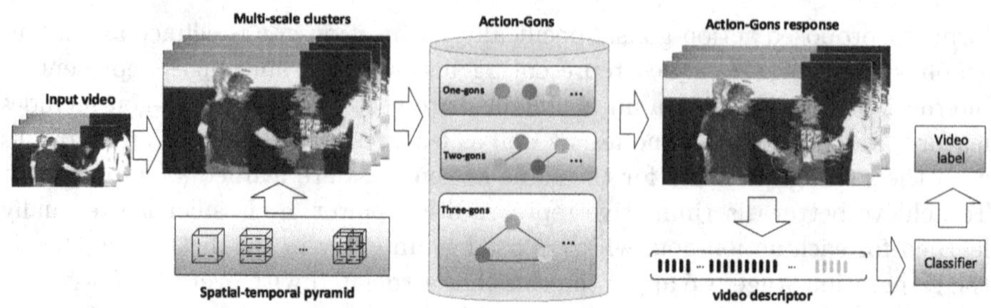

Fig. 2. Our pipeline for building the mid-level action-gon representation and training action classifiers.

proposed to learn the so-called "action parts". Such work can be roughly divided into two categories. One is based on unsupervised learning, and the other is based on supervised or weakly supervised learning.

Action Bank [3] performs action recognition by comparing a test video against a collection of manually designed action templates. Only low-level features are used during such comparison. In contrast, our work learns a mid-level representation by extracting abstract information from low-level features. Inspired by Action Bank [3], motionlets [4] adopt unsupervised learning to discover action parts. Instead of manually designing action templates, it identifies action parts with motion saliency detection and a greedy motionlet ranking method. The method in [18] also adopts unsupervised learning to learn an AND-OR grammar to build the contextual relationships for semantic video understanding, which can be regarded as one typical way of middle level feature learning.

More recently, [17] proposes to harvest middle level parts via weakly supervised learning. However, this method does not incorporate interactions among body parts, which are vital for complex human action modeling. Interactions between pairwise trajectory clusters are modeled as latent graphs in [2]. Nonetheless, it always adopts a single fixed graph structure (e.g. 3 nodes), which becomes inadequate for representing complex human actions. In comparison, this paper builds a mid-level dictionary, each word of which is defined as a graph with a potentially distinct granularity to capture one typical interaction among action units. Given a testing video, our method adaptively localizes potential interactions via optimization.

3 Action-Gon Dictionary Learning

3.1 Overview

In this section, we present a systematic approach for learning multi-granularity action-gons, each of which corresponds to a graph structure. The graph structure is a mid-level representation that models the joint occurrence and interaction among action units. In addition, to make the action-gons sufficiently diverse so that they can handle different scales, viewpoints as well as different numbers of interacting units, we study graphs with different granularities. For example, a single-node graph describes a relatively simple action unit while a two-node graph can model a higher complexity of interaction and co-occurrence. We first extract dense trajectories from each video, and then apply a multi-scale clustering method to obtain trajectory clusters that serve as action units. Given those action units, we compute action-gons with multiple granularities in separate steps through constrained optimization, and then stack these multi-granularity action-gons together into an overcomplete dictionary. Figure 2 shows an overview of our pipeline for action recognition based on action-gons. Before delving into further details, let us formally define a few terms that we frequently use in the following sections.

Terminology Definition. An action unit is defined as one trajectory cluster, which is a basic motion or shape primitive. Let V be a set of action units (graph nodes, see Fig. 1), and E be the set of edges connecting all pairs of action units. An action-gon is defined as $G = \{(V, E); h\}$, where h is a latent variable that chooses a subset of trajectory clusters to be the action-gon nodes. We define the granularity of an action-gon to be $G_{gran} = |V|$. Let us further define B_λ as a dictionary which contains a collection of action-gons with the same granularity λ, and define $B = B_1 \bigcup B_2 \bigcup ... \bigcup B_\lambda, ...$ as a larger dictionary that contains action-gons with all different granularities. To better localize such action-gons in each action video ϑ, we define a linear classifier f as a filter to localize action-gon G in ϑ, and the filter response $\rho = f(G * \vartheta)$ reflects whether G exists in ϑ. Throughout this paper, we call SPM features built on top of the descriptors constructed along with the trajectories [1] as the low-level representation (also called the first-layer in [17]), and the action-gon filter responses as the mid-level representation.

3.2 Action-Gon Modeling

Action Units. For each video, we first extract dense trajectories based on [19] (which is an improved version of [1]). Then we apply a hierarchical clustering procedure [20] to group the trajectories into a hierarchical cluster tree solely based on the trajectory geometry features, specifically, a trajectory is represented as a sequence of pixel locations in the spatio-temporal volume as follows, $(x_t, y_t; ...; x_{t+L}, y_{t+L};)$, where t is the starting frame of the trajectory and L is the number of frames along the trajectory. To increase the capability of describing actions with varying scales, we consider clusters at all different levels within the hierarchical cluster tree as potential graph nodes. A higher-level cluster occupies a larger spatial and temporal volume and overlaps with lower-level clusters. In practice, graphs built on hierarchical clusters give rise to higher recognition performance than the single-level clusters used in [2]. We name each cluster as one action unit.

For each trajectory, we extract five low-level features, including trajectory geometry, HOG, HOF, and MBH (Motion Boundary Histograms) along both x

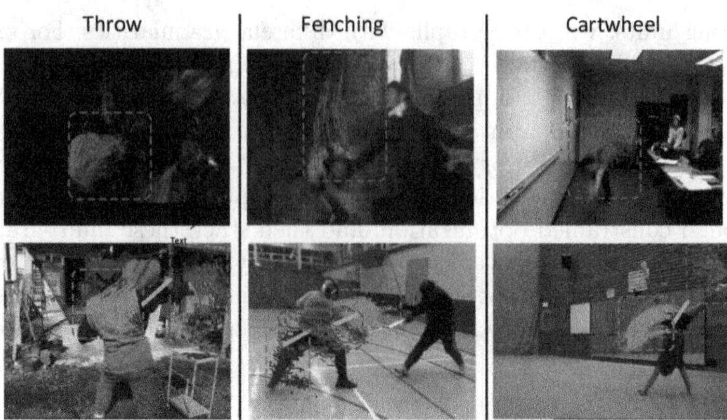

Fig. 3. Examples showing the inferred latent graphs. Note that, even for the same action class, it is still much desired to use multi-granularity graphs to tackle intra-class variations.

and y image axes [1], and build their individual dictionaries through K-means. These low-level features will be used for training and detecting action-gons. We apply localized soft assignment quantization (LSAQ) [21] to code all low-level features. Given any trajectory t_j within a cluster U_i, we use F_{t_j} to denote the concatenated codes of all low-level features along t_j, and 'max' to denote the element-wise maximum operation over a set of vectors. Then the node(trajectory cluster) feature, Γ_{U_i}, of U_i is defined as the max-pooling result over all trajectories within U_i, then

$$\Gamma_{U_i} = \max_{t_j \in U_i} F_{t_j}. \tag{1}$$

Edges and Features. The edge feature for a pair of nodes within the graph describes the relative motion and location between the nodes. We first define the edge features for a pair of trajectories t_i and t_j. Suppose a trajectory t_i spans a time interval from T_s^i to T_e^i (s, e are the frame indices). Let us denote the centroid of the trajectory as (x_m^i, y_m^i), the average image-space velocity along the trajectory as (v_x^i, v_y^i). Suppose the distribution of every type of attributes (denoted as z) follows its own Gaussian mixture model, $\mathcal{P}_z(X) = \sum_{k=1}^{N} \pi_k \mathcal{N}(X|\mu_k, \sigma_k)$. We define the features P_z for a type of attributes (z) using the probability values returned by all the Gaussian components in its own Gaussian mixture model. Let us further define $(\boldsymbol{v_1} * \boldsymbol{v_2}^T)(:)$ as the result of unfolding the outer product between $\boldsymbol{v_1}$ and $\boldsymbol{v_2}$ into a row vector. Then the feature vector for the edge between two trajectories is defined as

$$\begin{aligned} \phi(t_i, t_j) = [\ & P_T(|T_s^i - T_s^j|)^T \\ & P_x(|x_m^i - x_m^j|) * P_y(|y_m^i - y_m^j|)^T(:) \\ & P_{v_x}(|v_x^i - v_x^j|) * P_{v_y}(|v_y^i - v_y^j|)^T(:)\ ]^T. \end{aligned} \tag{2}$$

Finally, the edge feature vector, $\Phi(U_i, U_j)$, for clusters U_i and U_j is simply defined as the average feature vector of all trajectory pairs across the two clusters, namely

$$\Phi(U_i, U_j) = \frac{1}{|U_i||U_j|} \sum_{t_m \in U_i, t_n \in U_j} \phi(t_m, t_n). \tag{3}$$

Note that $P_T, P_x, P_y, P_{v_x}, P_{v_y}$ can all be estimated using the EM algorithm on a set of sampled trajectories. We empirically set N=6 to prevent overly long edge feature vectors. And it turned out to work well in all our experiments.

Latent Graph Representation. Given N candidate graph nodes within a video X, let $\mathcal{H}$ be the space of graphs defined over subsets of these candidate nodes. In this paper, every graph is a complete graph with edges connecting all possible pairs of nodes. Therefore, the configuration of a graph is uniquely determined by the nodes in the graph. Even under this assumption, there are an exponential number of graphs that can be composed by any subset of N nodes, i.e., the number of graphs with $M(M < N)$ nodes is $\binom{N}{M}$. However, only few of them have real discriminative power and can serve as mid-level action-gons. Let h be one of the graph configurations from $\mathcal{H}$. Now that we have defined the node feature as well as edge features, for a graph with fixed M nodes, we define its feature map $\psi(X, h) = [\Gamma_{U_0}, \Gamma_{U_1}, ..., \Gamma_{U_{M-1}}; \Phi(U_0, U_1), ..., \Phi(U_i, U_j), ..., \Phi(U_{M-2}, U_{M-1})]$ Once h is known, $\psi(X, h)$ can be easily established. In reality, however, h is a latent variable that should be inferred, and it is infeasible to perform exhaustive search when both M and N are large. Therefore, we need a more efficient way to infer h during both the training and classification stages, and the inference should be based on the discriminative power of h by learning a supervised classifier. Suppose we already have such a classifier $\mathbf{w}_k$ in the form of a linear SVM, then latent graph h can be inferred by the following operation,

$$h^* = \arg\max_{h \in \mathcal{H}} \mathbf{w}_k^T \psi(X, h). \tag{4}$$

The above optimization is essentially the NP-hard Quadratic Integer Programming problem, and exact inference could be computationally demanding. We therefore adopt the TRW-S method [22] to obtain an approximate solution. Figure 3 shows examples of inferred latent graphs.

3.3 Learning Multi-granularity Action-Gons

As indicated by earlier discussion and Eq. (4), we use a classifier (also called a filter) to identify the most discriminative latent graph with a predefined granularity (number of nodes) in a video or action class. However, a single classifier has limited generalization capability while actions typically have large intra-class variations due to different viewpoints and scales among other factors. Therefore, we propose to harvest intrinsic mid-level actions for every action class by training multiple latent graph configurations with a predefined granularity in that class.

The collection of classifiers for all classes are included in a mid-level dictionary, named action-gon dictionary. To learn the classifier for each action-gon, we train one-versus-all binary SVM classifiers by taking all the other classes as negative examples.

Suppose we are given a set of videos with binary class labels $S = \{(X_i, y_i)_{i=1}^n\}$, where $y_i \in \{1, -1\}$. Let $\mathcal{H}_i$ be the latent graph space defined over the trajectory clusters in X_i. To make the filters discriminative, we require each positive video X_i^+ contain at least one latent structure $h_i \in \mathcal{H}_i$ that can be identified by one of the filters $w_k, k \in \mathcal{I} = \{1, 2, ..., K\}$, while each negative video X_i^- should not contain any latent structure that can be identified by any of the classifiers. Based on these requirements, we learn the graph classifiers by solving the following optimization problem,

$$\min_{\mathbf{w}_k, \xi_i \geqslant 0, \zeta_i \geqslant 0} \frac{1}{2} \sum_{k=1}^{K} \|\mathbf{w}_k\|^2 + C_1 \sum_{i=1}^{N} \xi_i + C_2 \sum_{y_i=+1} \zeta_i \tag{5}$$

s.t.

$$\forall i = 1, 2, \cdots, n : y_i \max_{h \in \mathcal{H}_i} \max_{k \in \mathcal{I}} \mathbf{w}_k^{\mathrm{T}} \psi(X_i, h) \geqslant 1 - \xi_i,$$

$$\forall y_i = +1, k \in \mathcal{I} : \max_{h \in \mathcal{H}_i} \left[\mathbf{w}_k^{\mathrm{T}} \psi(X_i, h) - \frac{1}{K-1} \sum_{k' \neq k} \mathbf{w}_{k'}^{\mathrm{T}} \psi(X_i, h) \right] \geqslant 1 - \zeta_i,$$

$$\forall k_1, k_2 \in \mathcal{I} : \left| \sum_{y_i=+1} \frac{1}{J_i} \sum_{h \in \mathcal{H}_i} (\mathbf{w}_{k_1}^{\mathrm{T}} \psi(X_i, h) - \mathbf{w}_{k_2}^{\mathrm{T}} \psi(X_i, h)) \right| \leqslant \eta,$$

where J_i represents the number of potential graphs within the latent space $\mathcal{H}_i$. The first set of constraints enforce a multiple-instance-based margin for each bag (video) X_i; the second set of constraints try to maintain diversity among the filters, making different filters generate strong responses on different latent structures; and the last set of constraints enforce a balance among filters to avoid a trivial solution that assigns most latent structures to the same filter. Note that the above formulation can be viewed as a generalization of the learning method in [5] because we can treat a VOI (volume of interest) as a single-node graph. For more general cases, we need to infer the hidden graphs by solving an MRF labeling problem. Specifically, we use TRW-S [22] to identify graphs with maximum responses from the latent space $\mathcal{H}_i$, as shown in Eq. (4). The entire training process is solved by the Convex-Concave Cutting Plane (CCCP) algorithm [23], which alternates the following two steps, inferring latent structures with Eq. (4) and solving a structured SVM problem based on the cutting plane method.

In comparison with our simultaneous action-gon training, [2] only learns one single filter, so its learning algorithm does not impose the second and third set of constraints defined in our optimization Eq. 5. Another significant difference is that our method considers all the learned filters as codewords in a mid-level dictionary upon which a higher-level video representation is built for final classification while [2] directly takes the learned filter as the final video classifier.

Since different actions may exhibit different levels of co-occurrence and interaction among regions of interest, the number of co-occurring or interacting regions may vary. Hence, it is obviously suboptimal to use a single graph granularity across all action classes. This further inspired us to adaptively use graph configurations with different granularities during both the learning and classification stages. Ideally, our method is capable of supporting graphs with an arbitrary number of nodes. However, in practice, we restrict the granularity of an action-gon to be 1, 2 or 3 to achieve a better tradeoff between accuracy and computational cost. To build a multi-granularity dictionary, we run dictionary learning via the optimization in (5) for each supported graph granularity separately. All the filters learned from these separate runs are stacked together to form the action-gon dictionary. To the best of our knowledge, this is the first time to build a multi-granularity dictionary of structured elements.

4 Video Representation via Action-Gons

Suppose we have obtained an action-gon dictionary, which contains **g** classifiers for multi-granularity graphs. Given an input video X, we divide it into P spatiotemporal pyramid volumes as defined in [1]. We perform latent structure inference for every volume in the pyramid by taking all the trajectory clusters in the volume as input and estimating Eq. (4). This results in a confidence map, where each entry is the estimated confidence that there exists a corresponding action-gon inside the considered volume. Specifically, for the l-th volume, we obtain such a vector $F_l \in R^g$, and $F_l = [\alpha_1^l, ..., \alpha_k^l, ..., \alpha_g^l]$, where $\alpha_k^l = \max_{h \in \mathcal{H}_l} \mathbf{w}_k^T \psi(X, h)$, w_k is the k-th filter within the dictionary, and $\mathcal{H}_l$ is the latent graph space defined over the trajectory clusters in the l-th volume. The final video representation Θ_i is obtained by simply concatenating the confidence maps for all the spatio-temporal pyramid volumes. That means $\Theta_i = [F_1, F_2, \ldots, F_P]$. As most of the previous methods, i.e. [17], a linear SVM classifier built on Θ_i performs the final video category classification.

5 Experiments

In this section, we perform detailed evaluation of the discriminative power of our proposed action-gon representation on three popular and challenging action datasets: HMDB51 [8], Youtube [9] and UCF Sports [10].

5.1 Experimental Setup

For all the datasets used in our experiments, we extract refined dense trajectories as in [19] and compute low-level feature descriptors (i.e. Trajectory, HOG, HOF and MBH) with exactly the same parameters given in [1]. As we use bags of words built on top of these low-level features, we train a codebook with K-means for each type of low-level descriptors using 100,000 randomly sampled features, and set the codebook size to 4000. The parameter setting of our LSAQ coding is identical to that defined in [21] (i.e., $\beta = 10, n = 5$). We adaptively select the threshold for pruning background trajectories to make sure we can collect at least 100 clusters from each video.

For each dataset, we learn a relatively large pool of action-gons using Eq. (5). Instead of learning one set of action-gons using five concatenated low-level descriptors [1], we learn five sets of action-gons. Each set is based on one of the five descriptors. As most of previous low-level dictionary learning, at present we empirically determine the size of the action-gon dictionary. Specifically, we learn action-gons with $K = 3$ (used in Eq. (5)) different granularities (i.e., one-gon, two-gon, three-gon). This results in a large dictionary with $5 * 51 * (3 + 3 + 3) = 2295$ action-gons for the HMDB51 dataset. Likewise, we learn 1000 action-gons respectively for the Youtube and UCF Sports datasets. The problem of learning an action-gon dictionary with an optimal size requires much further investigation and, therefore, is left as future work.

Most of the other parameters in our method can take values from a relatively large range without affecting the final performance significantly. We empirically set each of them to a constant value within its working range. For example, we set $C_1 = 256$ and $C_2 = 32$ in Eq. (5) in all our experiments. We follow the same parameter settings proposed in [17] when learning final action classifiers.

Our method has been implemented primarily using Matlab except TRW-S [22][1]. We use the SVM^{struct} package[2] to perform the optimization in Eq. (5). On a modern PC, the training stage of our method spends about 24 h on the HMDB51 dataset (6776 video clips). Nevertheless, it only takes less than 5 s for our trained model to classify a test video clip.

5.2 Performance Evaluation

We first evaluate the overall performance of the action-gon representation through extensive comparisons against existing methods in the action recognition literature. For the HMDB51 dataset, we follow the default splitting rule to perform three rounds of training and testing, and report the average per-class classification accuracy. When only the mid-level action-gon representation is used, our results in the three rounds are 57.8 %, 57.8 %, and 58.4 %, respectively, resulting in an average performance of 58.0 %. As shown in Table 1, compared with other mid-level representations, action-gons have achieved significantly better results, i.e., its result is respectively 7.3 % and 15.9 % higher than those in [17] (50.7 %, the second layer performance) and [4] (42.1 %). The low-level representation in our current implementation is based on the descriptors in [19] but with one major difference, which is the replacement of fisher vectors with bag of words in LSAQ coding. Hence the average per-class classification accuracy achieved with our low-level representation is 57.0 %, which is slightly lower than the best

[1] Code is available from: http://research.microsoft.com/en-us/downloads/dad6c31e-2c04-471f-b724-ded18bf70fe3.

[2] Code is based on http://www.cs.cornell.edu/people/tj/svm_light/svm_struct.html.

Table 1. Performance of the proposed action-gon representation and comparisons with state-of-the-art methods. We report average per-class classification accuracy on the datasets. '*mid*' represents action-gons alone, '*mid + low*' represents the combination of action-gons and low-level features.

HMDB51 [8] (.%)		Youtube [9] (.%)	
Oneata et al. [24]	54.8	Le et al. [12]	75.8
Motionlet [4]	42.1	MIL-Bof [25]	80.4
Shi et al. [26]	47.6	Dense Traj. [1]	85.4
Jian et al. [27]	52.1	Brendel et al. [28]	77.8
Zhu et al. [17]	54.0	Zhu et al. [17]	89.4
Dense Traj. [19]	57.2	Oneata et al. [24]	89.0
Action-Gons	58.0	**Action-Gons**	89.7
Action-Gons+Low	**58.9**	**Action-Gons+Low**	**92.1**

Table 2. Performance comparison on the UCF-Sports dataset based on two common dataset splitting rules. Note that the middle level features facilitated by Action-Gon generates the state-of-the-art performance under both data splitting rules.

Methods	Splitting rule in [10]	Leave-one-out in [1]
Lan et al. [10]	73.1 %	n/a
Raptis et al. [2]	79.4 %	n/a
Kovashka et al. [29]	n/a	87.3 %
DenseTraj. [1]	n/a	89.1 %
Wu et al. [30]	n/a	92.5 %
ActionBank [3]	n/a	95.0 %
Action-Gons	**83.0 %**	**100 %**

performance (57.2 %) reported in [19]. Nevertheless, our proposed middle-level representation alone outperforms the high-dimensional low-level features used in [19]. In addition, when combined with our low-level features, the average performance of our method can be further elevated to 58.9 %, which indicates that our action-gon representation has a strong discrimination power complementary to low-level features, as shown in Fig. 5.

In the experiments on the UCF-Sports dataset, we apply the same setting recently proposed in [10]. As shown in Table 2, the average per-class classification accuracy achieved with our mid-level action-gon representation is 83 %, which is significantly higher than the state-of-the-art result (79.4 %) [2] among all existing work that adopts the same data splitting rule as in [10]. To fully validate the performance of action-gons, we further apply "leave-one-out" data splitting as in [1], and see that action-gons achieve a 100 % classification accuracy, which is a significant improvement over the best "leave-one-out" result reported in [1] (89.1 %). Such a large performance gain is primarily achieved with the adaptive

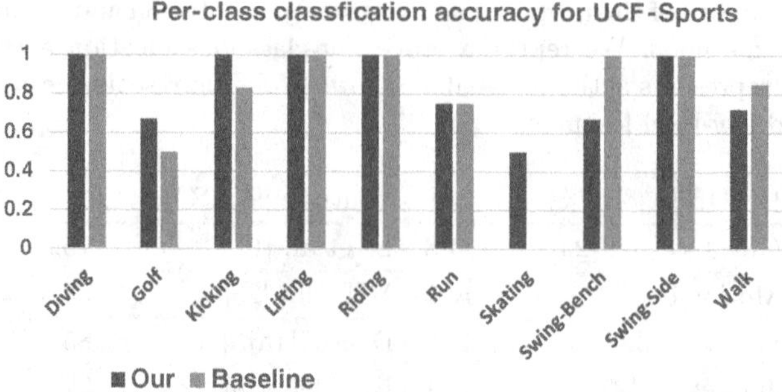

Fig. 4. Per-class classification accuracy on the UCF-Sports dataset according to the dataset splitting rule proposed in Lan et al. [10]

action unit localization ability enabled by action-gons. Refer to [10] for reasons why "leave-one-out" splitting generates better classification accuracy. Figure 4 shows the per-class classification accuracy obtained with the action-gons alone.

We have also observed advantages of using action-gons on the Youtube dataset. As shown in Table 1, by using the action-gon representation alone, we can achieve an average per-class accuracy of 89.7 %, which is superior to any existing methods that rely on low-level features alone according to [19,24]. When action-gons are combined with low-level features, the performance can be further improved to 92.1 %, indicating the two types of feature representations are complementary.

5.3 Analysis and Discussion

Analysis of Multi-granularity Action-Gons. To validate the effectiveness of multi-granularity action-gons, we compare classification performance achieved using various combinations of the action-gon dictionaries B_1, B_2 and B_3. Such combinations include any individual dictionary of the three or any group formed by two or more of these individual dictionaries, such as B_1+B_2 and $B_1+B_2+B_3$. The testing results are shown in Fig. 5, where we can see that with increasing levels of granularity, we achieve increasing classification accuracy on HMDB51. This indicates that different action-gon granularity can capture different complexity of interactions (see Fig. 3), and therefore provide complementary feature representations. Interestingly, we notice that one-gon dictionary (B_1) achieve slightly worse performance than two-gon dictionary (B_2) and three-gon dictionary (B_3) on HMDB51. However, when combined together, they can increase representation diversity and boost the overall performance.

Analysis of the Action-Gons Size. The size of Action-Gon Dictionary is actually controlled by the parameter K (used in Eq. (5)). If $K = 3$, we would have 2295 action gons. We evaluated the performances with respect to different K, take HMDB51 as an example, when $K = 1, 2, 3, 4$, their corresponding accuracy

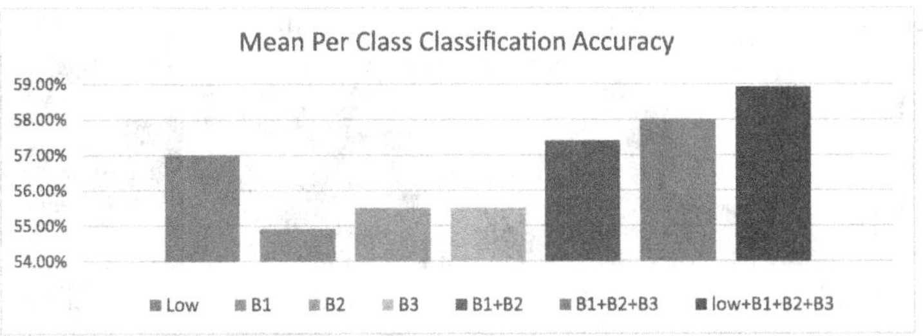

Fig. 5. Average per-class classification accuracy on HMDB51 using action-gons with increasing levels of granularity.

Table 3. Performance correlation between mid-level and low-level representations. Performance is measured on HMDB51. As ITF [19] improves over DTF [1], we found the performance of their corresponding action-gons improves as well.

	B_1	B_2	B_3	B_1, B_2	B_1, B_2, B_3
ITF [19]	54.9	55.5	55.5	57.4	58.0
DTF [1]	52.5	52.1	52.3	53.6	54.1

are 55.3 %, 57.6 %, 57.8 % and 55.8 % respectively. When K is larger, the Action-Gon based video representation would be very high dimensional, which increases the risk of over fitting. So empirically we set K = 3.

Performance Correlation with Low-Level Features. The process of learning an action-gon dictionary represents a general pipeline for building a mid-level action representation. Similar to deep learning, an action-gon learns the compositions and abstractions of low-level features. Because of this, although being complementary to low-level features, the discrimination power of action-gons is also expected to be correlated with that of the low-level features. That is, the better the low-level features, the stronger discrimination power the learned action-gons would be equipped. To demonstrate this performance correlation, we have compared the effect of the refined trajectories [19] against that of the baseline trajectories [1] on the quality of the action-gons using the HMDB51 dataset. Given the results in Table 3, we can observe that using more powerful low-level features also boosts the classification performance of the action-gons.

6 Conclusions

In this paper, we have presented a novel approach for middle level action representation and use graphs with varying granularity to serve as the mid-level dictionary which we call action-gon dictionary. Action-gons have been proven to have strong discrimination power in action classification on several popular yet challenging datasets. Extensive experiments and comparisons show that

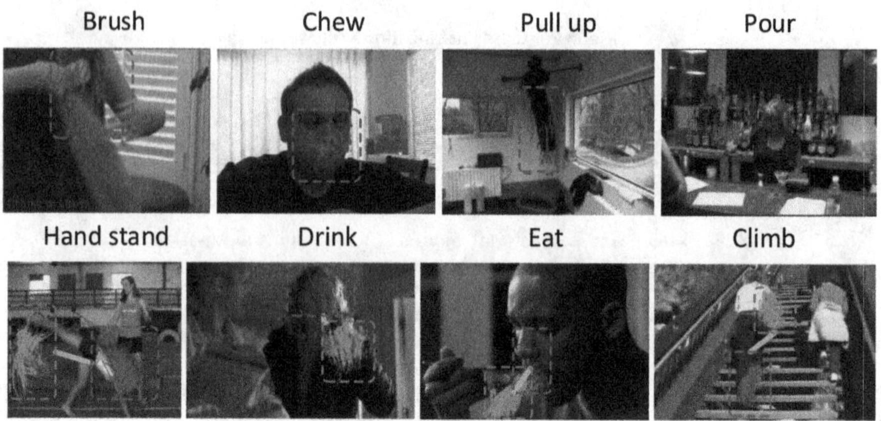

Fig. 6. Inferred action-gons for typical videos. Note that, for simple actions, we may only need a one-gon model while, for relatively complex actions, we need higher-order action-gons.

action-gons are complementary to low-level features, indicating that using more powerful low-level feature descriptors would boost the performance of action-gons at the same time. Although we have observed connections between our mid-level action-gons and other high-level representations [3], a thorough investigation on questions like "what are the optimal granularities of action-gons" and "how many action-gons should be chosen" are very much desired. In addition, it is worthwhile to explore layered representations to further improve performance correlation between action-gons and low-level features.

Acknowledge. Zhuowen Tu is supported by NSF IIS-1216528(IIS-1360566) and NSF award IIS-0844566(IIS-1360568).

References

1. Wang, H., Klser, A., Schmid, C., Liu, C.L.: Dense trajectories and motion boundary descriptors for action recognition. IJCV **103**, 60–79 (2013)
2. Raptis, M., Kokkinos, I., Soatto, S.: Discovering discriminative action parts from mid-level video representations. In: CVPR (2012)
3. Sadanand, S., Corso, J.: Action bank: a high-level representation of activity in video. In: CVPR (2012)
4. Wang, L., Qiao, Y., Tang, X.: Motionlets: mid-level 3D parts for human motion recognition. In: CVPR 2013 (2013)
5. Gaidon, A., Harchaoui, Z., Schmid, C.: Temporal localization of actions with actoms. IEEE Trans. Pattern Anal. Mach. Intell. **35**, 2782–2795 (2013)
6. Yuan, F., Xia, G.S., Sahbi, H., Prinet, V.: Mid-level features and spatio-temporal context for activity recognition. Pattern Recogn. **45**, 4182–4191 (2012)
7. Julesz, B., Gilbert, E.N., Victor, J.D.: Visual discrimination of texture with identical third-order statistics. Biol. Cybern. **31**, 137–140 (1978)

8. Kuehne, H., Jhuang, H., Garrote, E., Poggio, T., Serre, T.: HMDB: a large video database for human motion recognition. In: ICCV (2011)
9. Liu, J., Luo, J., Shah, M.: Recognizing realistic actions from videos in the wild. In: ICCV (2009)
10. Lan, T., Wang, Y., Mori, G.: Discriminative figure-centric models for joint action localization and recognition. In: 2011 IEEE International Conference on Computer Vision (ICCV), pp. 2003–2010 (2011)
11. Laptev, I.: On space-time interest points. Int. J. Comput. Vis. **64**, 107–123 (2005)
12. Le, Q., Zou, W., Yeung, S., Ng, A.: Learning hierarchical invariant spatio-temporal features for action recognition with independent subspace analysis. In: CVPR (2011)
13. Klaser, A., Marszalek, M., Schmid, C.: A spatio-temporal descriptor based on 3D gradients. In: BMVC (2008)
14. Bilinski, P., Bremond, F.: Contextual statistics of space-time ordered features for human action recognition. In: Proceedings of the 2012 IEEE Ninth International Conference on Advanced Video and Signal-Based Surveillance, AVSS 2012, pp. 228–233 (2012)
15. Matikainen, P., Hebert, M., Sukthankar, R.: Representing pairwise spatial and temporal relations for action recognition. In: Daniilidis, K., Maragos, P., Paragios, N. (eds.) ECCV 2010, Part I. LNCS, vol. 6311, pp. 508–521. Springer, Heidelberg (2010)
16. Sun, J., Wu, X., Yan, S., Cheong, L.F., Chua, T.S., Li, J.: Hierarchical spatio-temporal context modeling for action recognition. In: IEEE Conference on Computer Vision and Pattern Recognition, 2009, CVPR 2009, pp. 2004–2011 (2009)
17. Zhu, J., Wang, B., Yang, X., Zhang, W., Zhuowen, T.: Action recognition with actons. In: ICCV (2013)
18. Si, Z., Pei, M., Yao, Z., Zhu, S.C.: Unsupervised learning of event and-or grammar and semantics from video. In: ICCV (2011)
19. Wang, H., Schmid, C.: Action recognition with improved trajectories. In: International Conference on Computer Vision, Sydney, Australia (2013)
20. Tabatabaei, S.S., Coates, M., Rabbat, M.G.: Ganc: greedy agglomerative normalized cut. CoRR abs/1105.0974 (2011)
21. Liu, L., Wang, L., Liu, X.: In defense of soft-assignment coding. In: ICCV (2011)
22. Kolmogorov, V.: Convergent tree-reweighted message passing for energy minimization. IEEE Trans. Pattern Anal. Mach. Intell. **28**, 1568–1583 (2006)
23. Yuille, A., Rangarajan, A.: The concave-convex procedure (CCCP). Neural Comput. **15**, 915–936 (2003)
24. Oneata, D., Verbeek, J., Schmid, C.: Action and event recognition with fisher vectors on a compact feature set. In: IEEE Intenational Conference on Computer Vision (ICCV), Sydney, Australia (2013)
25. Michael Sapienza, F.C., Torr, P.H.: Learning discriminative space-time actions from weakly labelled videos. In: BMVC (2012)
26. Shi, F., Petriu, E., Laganiere, R.: Sampling strategies for real-time action recognition. In: CVPR 2013 (2013)
27. Jain, M., Jegou, H., Bouthemy, P.: Better exploiting motion for better action recognition. In: CVPR 2013 (2013)
28. Brendel, W., Todorovic, S.: Activities as time series of human postures. In: Daniilidis, K., Maragos, P., Paragios, N. (eds.) ECCV 2010, Part II. LNCS, vol. 6312, pp. 721–734. Springer, Heidelberg (2010)

29. Kovashka, A., Grauman, K.: Learning a hierarchy of discriminative space-time neighborhood features for human action recognition. In: 2010 IEEE Conference on Computer Vision and Pattern Recognition (CVPR), pp. 2046–2053 (2010)
30. Wu, X., Xu, D., Duan, L., Luo, J., Jia, Y.: Action recognition using multilevel features and latent structural SVM. IEEE Trans. Circ. Syst. Video Technol. **23**, 1422–1431 (2013)

Fast Inference of Contaminated Data for Real Time Object Tracking

Hao Zhu[1(✉)] and Yi Li[2]

[1] 3M Cogent Beijing R&D Center, Beijing, China
ahzhu@mmm.com
[2] NICTA and Australian National University, Canberra, Australia
yi.li@nicta.com.au

Abstract. The online object tracking is a challenging problem because any useful approach must handle various nuisances including illumination changes and occlusions. Though a lot of work focus on observation models by employing sophisticated approaches for contaminated data, they commonly assume that the samples for updating observation model are uncorrupted or can be restored in updating. For instance, in particle filter based approaches every particle has to be restored for each frame, which is time-consuming and unstable. In this paper, we propose a novel scheme to decouple the observation model and its update in a particle filtering framework. Our efficient observation model is used to effectively select the most similar candidate from all particles only, by analyzing the principal component analysis (PCA) reconstruction with L_1 regularization. In order to handle the contaminated samples while updating observation model, we adopt on an online robust PCA during the update of observation model. Our qualitative and quantitative evaluations on challenging dataset demonstrate that the proposed scheme is competitive to several sophisticated state of the art methods, and it is much faster.

1 Introduction

Visual tracking has been an active topic in computer vision because it is widely used in many applications such as surveillance, robotics, human computer interaction, vehicle tracking, and even medical imaging. In spite of great progress in last two decades, visual tracking is still an extremely challenging topic because in the real scenes visual tracker has to face different situations (e.g. sophisticated object shape or complex motion, illumination changes and occlusions).

The current methods of visual tracking can be categorized into generative or discriminative ones. The methods based on generative models aim at finding the most similar region as the target from a lot of candidates, while the methods based on the discriminative models are modeling the tracking problem as a classification problem, which build classifiers for distinguishing the target from the surrounding region of backgrounds. In this paper, we mainly focus on the visual tracking based on generative models.

D. Cremers et al. (Eds.): ACCV 2014, Part V, LNCS 9007, pp. 275–289, 2015.
DOI: 10.1007/978-3-319-16814-2_18

Among the trackers based on generative methods, the linear representation is widely employed in many trackers because it is capable of maintaining holistic appearance information and casting generative models (i.e. Gaussian model) as linear regression. These methods often adopt a dictionary (e.g., a set of basis vectors from a subspace or a series of templates) to represent the tracked target. A given candidate sample is linearly represented by the dictionary, and the representation coefficient and reconstruction error are computed, from which the corresponding likelihood (the similarity to the expected target) is determined.

Ross et al. proposed an incremental visual tracking (IVT) method [1] which employs a low dimensional PCA subspace to represent the tracked target and thus assumes that the error is Gaussian distributed with small variances (i.e., small and dense noise). Technically it is equivalent to the ordinary least squares solution under the assumption that the dictionary atoms are orthogonal, and the representation of the tracked target is capable of obtaining by inner product operator. Furthermore, the reconstruction error is also easy to compute. Thus, the IVT is a potential method for real time applications. While the IVT method is able to handle appearance changes caused by illumination variation and pose variation, it is not robust to some challenging environments (e.g. partial occlusion and background clutter) due to the following two reasons. Firstly, the ordinary least squares method has been shown to be sensitive to outliers due to the formulation is equivalent to Maximum Likelihood Estimate(MLE) under Gaussian models. Secondly, the IVT method directly uses new observations to update the observation model without any intervention such as detecting outliers and processing them accordingly.

Recently, sparse representation has been successfully employed in classification problems in computer vision. Wright et al. [2] reported sparse representation for face recognition (FR). Such a sparse representation classifier (SRC) firstly codes the query face image over the dictionary sparsely, and then makes the classification by checking which class yields the least coding error. This scheme presents an impressive performance in FR due to the robustness to different situations (e.g. face expression, illumination changes and occlusion).

Inspired by SRC, many L_1 trackers represent a candidate target by a sparse linear combination of the templates in a dictionary. Benefitting from sparsity penalty (i.e. L_0 norm and L_1 norm), these methods demonstrated robustness in various tracking environments. However, sparsity penalty is a non-differential function. Therefore these SRC based trackers are quite computationally expensive. In the classical L_1 tracker [3], L_1 minimization problems need to be solved by the interior point method [4] for each frame during the tracking process. This process is very time-consuming not only because L_1 minimization is computationally expensive but also the trivial templates significantly extend the size of the dictionary. The optimized solution proposed in [5] reduces the number of particles by a minimal error bounding strategy. Though this strategy is able to save 80 % computation. It is still far away from real time applications. Furthermore, the L_1 based trackers commonly select down-sampling particles as templates due to computational burdens [6], which significantly reduces the tracking accuracy.

Aforementioned L_1 based trackers only concern with the robust representation for observing data and employing raw inputs as "templates", which may be corrupted or contaminated. These methods ignore that corrupted templates will have significant influences on the observation model because the templates in the dictionary came from raw observations. Unlike the methods that try to solve these two problems by using sophisticated appearance models and better mechanisms of updating model, in this paper we ask two different yet essential questions. (1) Is it necessary to use sophisticated observation methods to handle corrupted data, such as partial occlusion situation? For example, it is very computationally expensive if we have to restore hundreds of particles in each frame) but only need one of them to update the observation model. (2) Is there an efficient and effective way to update the observation model, without occlusion detection in the appearance model?

In this paper, we propose to overcome the disadvantage of subspace representation by proposing an robust appearance model to deal with heavy occlusion effectively. We chose the observation model in the IVT to our model, because IVT performs remarkably more efficient than L_1 tracker in handling higher resolution image observations. During the model update, we propose to use robust online dictionary learning based method, such as those methods based on Huber loss function (Wang and Yeung [7]). which remedy the problem of corrupted samples by obtaining more robust templates. Several experiments on challenging video sequences validate that the proposed algorithm is efficient and effective for object-tracking problem.

2 Related Work

To facilitate the comparison between different methods, we briefly review the particle filter models for visual tracking and trackers based on linear representation. And then some classical trackers based on linear representation (e.g. IVT and L1 Tracker) are also reviewed briefly.

2.1 Particle Filter Tracking

In the framework of particle filtering, the problem of object tracking can be considered as a sequential Bayesian inference. Given a set of observed images $Y_t = [y_1, y_2, ..., y_t]$ at the t-th frame, the hidden state variable x_t

$$p(x_t|Y_{1:t}) \propto p(y_t|x_t) \int p(x_t|x_{t-1})p(x_{t-1}|Y_{t-1})dx_{t-1} \tag{1}$$

where $p(x_t|x_{t-1})$ is the dynamic model between two sequential states, and $p(y_t|x_t)$ denotes observation model that estimates the likelihood of observing y_t at state x_t. The optimal state of all observing targets is obtained by the maximum a posteriori estimation over N samples at time t by

$$\widehat{x_t} = \arg\max_{x_t^i} p(y_t^i|x_t^i)p(x_t^i|x_{t-1}), i = 1, 2, ... \tag{2}$$

where x_t^i denotes the i-th sample of the state x_t, and y_t^i indicates the image patch estimated by x_t^i.

Dynamic Model. The affine warp model is used to model the target motion between two sequential frames. There are six parameter of the affine transformation used to model $p(x_t|x_{t-1})$. Let $x_t = [x_1, x_2, x_3, x_4, x_5, x_6]$, which denote shift in x, y translation, rotation, scale, and shear. Usually, the each dimension of $p(x_t|x_{t-1})$ is modeled by an independent Gaussian distribution (i.e. $p(x_t|x_{t-1}) = N(x_t; x_{t-1}, \Psi)$, where Ψ is a diagonal covariance matrix).

Observation Model Based on Linear Representation. The global appearance of an object under different conditions (e.g. illumination and viewpoint change) is considered to lie approximately in a low dimensional space. Assume the target variable y is given by a deterministic function $f(T, a)$ with additive Gaussian noise as the following equation:

$$y = Ta + \epsilon \tag{3}$$

where tracking result $y \in R^d$ approximately lies in the linear span of T and is the zero mean, we denote the templates set as $T = [t_1, ..., t_n] \in R^{d \times n}(d >> n)$, containing n target templates such that each template $t_i \in R^d$ and $a = [a_1, a_2, ..., a_n]^T \in R^n$ is called a target coefficient vector. ϵ is the zero mean Gaussian random noisy term. Therefore, the observeration model is able to be extend to the following formulation:

$$p(y_t^i|x_t^i) = N(\epsilon; 0, I) \tag{4}$$

where I is a diagonal covariance matrix and ϵ is the residual of linear representation. Due to the $p(x_t|x_{t-1})$ drawing N particles from the previous the particle of target and then resetting their weights to $1/n$, thus the Eq. 2 become the ordinary least square problem $||y - Ta||_2^2$.

2.2 Incremental Subspace Learning

As a classical method, the incremental tracking method [1] uses online PCA to update templates which can efficiently handle the problem that appearance change caused by in-plane rotation, scale, illumination variation and pose change. However, because of the intrinsic character of the representation based on PCA subspace, the IVT method is sensitive to partial occlusion, especially large occlusion. In PCA scheme, the underlying assumption is that the noisy term ϵ in Eq. 3 is Gaussian distributed with small variance. It is still a ordinary least square problem. Because of the orthogonality of bases T, the representation a can be estimated by $a = T^T Y$. And the noisy term $||\epsilon||_2^2 = \left\|Y - TT^T Y\right\|_2^2$.

Commonly, the noisy energy is very small because the PCA will hold the most variance after transforming input into a subspace. However, when the input is partly occluded by other objects, the IVT method would be failed in different conditions with partial occlusions which are non-Gaussian. Additionally, the IVT directly uses a new observation without any intervention for corruptions. As a result, it makes the observation model degraded in the situation with partial situation.

2.3 Sparsity Regularization Based Tracker

Sparse representation has recently been extensively studied and applied in pattern recognition and computer vision, one of most successful applications is the sparse representation classification (SRC) in the face recognition problem [2]. In spite of existing different situations with various occlusion patterns, it always works well. Inspired by the SRC, Mei et al. [3] propose an algorithm by defining the tracking problem as finding the patch with minimum reconstruction error by sparse representation and handling occlusion with trivial templates by:

$$\min_{c} \frac{1}{2} \|y - Bc\|_2^2 + \lambda \|c\|_1 \;\; s.t. \; c \geq 0, \; B = [T \; I \; -I], \; c = [a \; e] \tag{5}$$

where y denotes an observer sample, T represents a sub dictionary of target templates, I indicates identity matrix as trivial template for error representation, a indicates the corresponding coefficient to target templates and the e is the coefficients of trivial templates. Commonly, only a few templates are necessary, whereas a lot of trivial templates are also needed. Therefore, the implementation make the dictionary too big to efficiently solve.

The Eq. 5 is able to obtain robust coefficients from the corrupted observation. In order to build a more robust model for object tracking, [7,8] propose an efficient and effective method to estimate different components from residual ϵ. They assume that the ϵ is a combination of Gaussian and Laplacian Distribution. Thus, they use huber loss function to replace least square function in the sparse representation or the ordinary least square problem.

$$f(x) = \begin{cases} x^2/2, & |x| \leq \lambda \\ \lambda|x| - \lambda^2/2, & (otherwise) \end{cases} \tag{6}$$

3 The Proposed Method

Many aforementioned methods employ the detection of pixel level outliers to solve the problem of degrading models. However, it is not an efficient and effective way to solve the problem of updating model. In this paper, we seek a different scheme which exploits a method without any prior about pixel level outliers, and update the observation model based on corrupted observations. Thus we only need a simple model which is good enough to estimate likelihood of particles.

3.1 Motivation

The Huber loss function is an efficient method to estimate different components from residual ϵ for building a more robust model. It assume that the ϵ is a combination of Gaussian and Laplacian distribution and decompose ϵ into $\mathbf{e} + \mathbf{s}$ iteratively. The relationship can be formulated as the following extend version of Eq. 3:

$$y = Ta + \epsilon, s.t. \; \epsilon = \mathbf{e} + \mathbf{s} \tag{7}$$

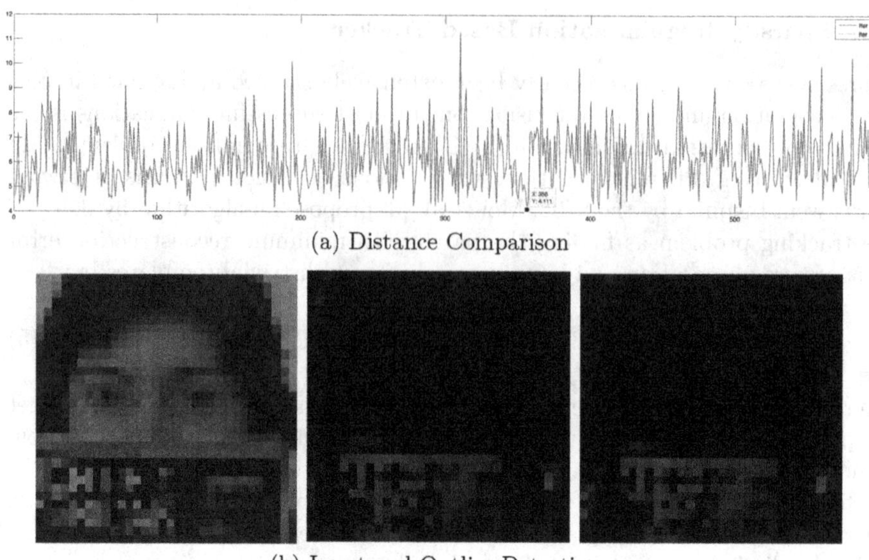

(a) Distance Comparison

(b) Input and Outlier Detection

Fig. 1. Comparison between results with different iteration numbers

where $\mathbf{e} = [e_1, ..., e_n]$ is Gaussian noisy and $\mathbf{s} = [s_1, ..., s_n]$ is sparse noisy followed Laplacian distribution. Thus, the ordinary least square problem using huber loss function [8] is equivalent to:

$$E = \min_{a,s} ||y - Ta - \mathbf{s}||_2^2 + \lambda ||\mathbf{s}||_1 \tag{8}$$

To estimate the $\mathbf{e}$ and $\mathbf{s}$, the Eq. 8 needs to repeat two steps: detecting outlier pixels and then solving ordinary least square function without the influence of outlier pixels. Commonly, the function needs to repeat these two steps many times in order to obtain convergence. This method is capable of detecting pixel level outliers but really expensive in time.

However, in the repeated processes, the cost function (Eq. 8) update is usually very small. Figure 1(a) shows a comparison between the cost value E after Iteration 1 and Iteration 8 for 600 particles. It is difficult to distinguish the difference between both lines. It is obvious to find that the tracking target is the 356-th particle because it has the lowest E. The 356-th particle and the outlier maps with different iteration numbers are shown in Fig. 1(b). It is obvious that the two outlier maps have very similar pattern, where the only difference is small.

Based on this fact, we argue that it is not necessary to use such a sophisticated method like the Huber loss function to exactly calculate which noisy of pixels are Gaussian or Laplacian distribution. For the sake of saving computation, we do not estimate these two different components accurately. According to the prior knowledge, the tiny ϵ is typically Gaussian distribution while the large

ϵ is Laplacian distribution. Therefore, we can further simplify an assumption that ***the ϵ is Gaussian distribution below a threshold, otherwise is Laplacian distribution***.

3.2 Observation Model

An image observation y_t^i can be represented by a subspace of the target object spanned by T if no occlusion occurs. Thus, many approaches use the reconstructed residual of each observed image patch to measure the observation likelihood by minimizing $||y^i - Ta^i||_2^2$:

$$p(\mathbf{y^i}|\mathbf{x^i}) = \exp(-\left\|\mathbf{y^i} - \mathbf{Ta^i}\right\|_2^2) \tag{9}$$

where we assume the y^i is centring. However, the Eq. 9 do not consider the impact introduced by complex noisy. It is necessary to account for partial occlusion in an appearance model. In [8], authors assume that a centered image observation can be represented by a linear combination of the PCA basis vectors and trivial templates. If partial occlusion occurs, the most likely image patch can be represented as a linear combination of PCA basis vectors and very few number of trivial templates (as illustrated by Fig. 1(b)). Thus, the precise localization of the tracked target can be benefited by penalizing the sparsity of trivial coefficients. But the problem of sparsity penalty is very computational expensive (i.e. Eq. 8).

We will propose the method to discriminate the type of noisy term using a threshold. As shown in Fig. 1(b), this scheme may be not perfect for pixel-wise occlusion, but it is good enough for the appearance model like Eq. 8. Specifically, we define a mask indicator M and a penalty vector W to point out Gaussian and Laplacian parts roughly:

$$m_i = \begin{cases} 1, \ |\epsilon_i| \le \lambda \\ 0, \ (otherwise) \end{cases} \tag{10}$$

where m_i is a element of $M = [m_1, m_2, ..., m_n]$, which is a vector that indicates Gaussian elements of e. The λ is a threshold constant in all experiments of this paper.

$$w_i = \begin{cases} |\epsilon_i| - \lambda, \ |\epsilon_i| > \lambda \\ 0, \qquad\quad (otherwise) \end{cases} \tag{11}$$

where w_i is a element of $W = [w_1, w_2, ..., w_n]$, which is a vector that indicates Laplacian elements of s. Equation 11 is related to the soft-threshold function using subgradient (i.e. $sgn(x)(abs(x) - \lambda)$) for solving L_1 regularization problem [9].

$$p(\mathbf{y^i}|\mathbf{x^i}) = \exp(-\left\|M^i \odot (Y^i - Ta^i)\right\|_2^2 - \beta\left\|W^i\right\|_1) \tag{12}$$

where $\odot$ is the Hadamard product (element-wise product), and β is a penalty term. The first term accounts for reconstruction errors of the unoccluded proportion of the target object, and the second term indicates the impact of occluded part of the target object.

3.3 Update of Observation Model

Due to the least square loss function used, PCA is very sensitive to corrupted and contaminated observations. Even a few such outliers enable the quality of PCA output to be degraded. Unfortunately, for the tracking problem, outlier observations are frequent. In [10], researchers propose an online PCA method for outliers. The mechanism of probabilistic admission and rejection for new samples endows this method with the ability to be robust to the outliers. Technically, the method, in wild conditions, can be resistant to 50 % breakdown point. However, this method cannot be employed in tracking problems directly. There are mainly two problems: ignoring the estimation of the mean vector and storing a full covariance matrix. The former is necessary for updating the appearance model. The latter one makes the method has to store a 1024×1024 covariance matrix and perform Eigen-decomposition on it while we have 32×32 patches as observations. It is not a small storage and computational burden for real time trackers.

By combining the conventional incremental subspace learning method and the mechanism of probabilistic admission and rejection, we propose a robust incremental subspace learning in this paper. Nevertheless, we do not select the normalization of the data point by L_2-norm to estimate admissible probability and to update eigenvectors and eigenvalues, as same as [10]. We define the $\frac{\Sigma_{j=1}^{D}\hat{y}_{ij}^2}{\Sigma_{j=1}^{K}|U_j\hat{y}_i|^2}$ as a measure to estimate acceptable probability. Once a new sample is accepted, it would be process by conventional incremental subspace learning as the same in [1]. Such a method has a theoretical performance guarantee under the noisy case. For instance, in [10] the strategy works well even in the situation of 30 % outlier fraction in the experiment, while the online PCA fails in the situation of 5 % outlier fraction.

Algorithm 1. Robust Incremental Subspace Learning

Input: Data Sequence $[y_1, ..., y_b] \in R^{D\times b}$,buffer size b, eigenvectors $U \in R^{D\times K}$, eigenvalues $\Sigma \in R^{D\times D}$ and the mean vector $I \in R^D$.
Output: updated eigenvectors U', eigenvalues Σ' and the mean vector I'.
Initialization: 1) y' = []

repeat
a) Centering the data point as $\hat{y}_i = y_i - I$;
b) Estimating the energy of data point as $e_i = \Sigma_{j=1}^{D}\hat{y}_{ij}^2$
c) Calulate the variance of y_i along the direction eigenvectors U: $\theta_i = \Sigma_{j=1}^{K}|U_j\hat{y}_i|^2$
d) Accept y_i with probability θ_i/e_i
e) If y_i is accepted, $y' = [y'\ \hat{y}_i]$

until $i > b$
2) Perform incremental subspace learning [1] on y' and obtain new eigenvectors U', eigenvalues Σ' and the mean vector I'.

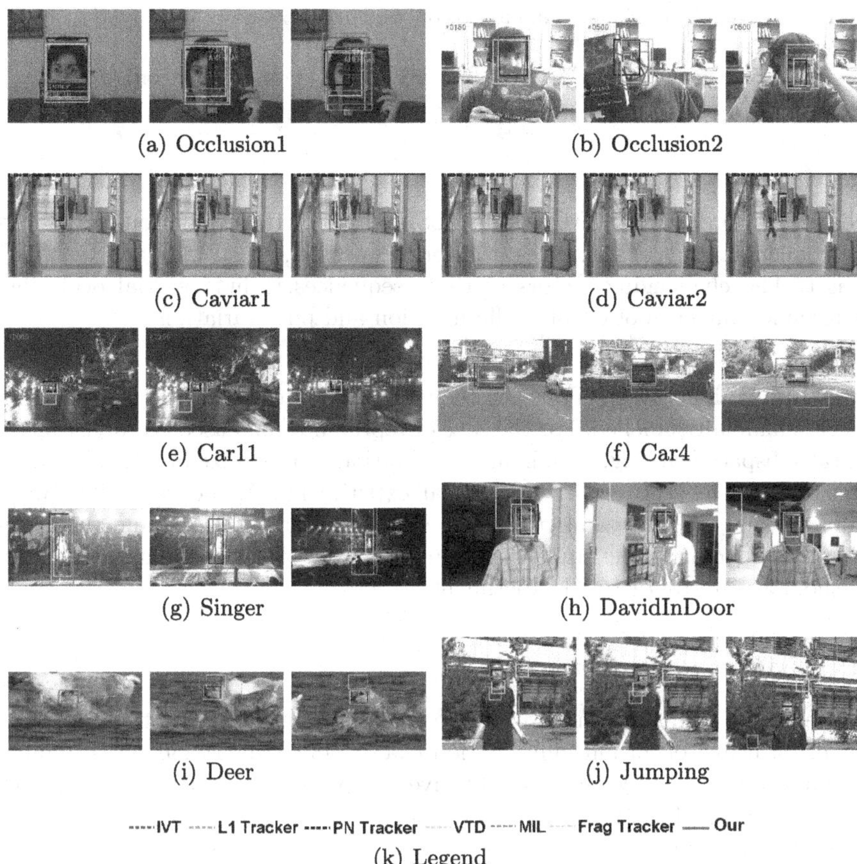

Fig. 2. Sample tracking results on ten challenging image sequences. This figure demonstrates the results of the IVT, L1 tracker, PN Tracker, VTD, MIL, Frag Tracker and the proposed method.

4 Experiments

Speed. The proposed method is implemented in both MATLAB and C. The MATLAB versions runs at 10 fps on an Air-Mac with Core i5 1.86 GHZ CPU and 4 GB memory, and the C version runs at 25–30 fps on Xeon E5305 CPU and 16 GB memory (Table 1). Please note that, our C version is single thread, and other comparison methods are usually on multi-thread (Matlab's default matrix operation option).

Dataset. We evaluate the proposed tracker against ten state-of-the-art algorithms qualitatively and quantitatively, using the source codes provided by the authors for fair comparisons, including the IVT [1], FragTrack (FT) [11], MILTrack [12], VTD [13], PN [14], TLD [15], APGL1 [6], ASLSA [16], MTT [17],

Table 1. Comparison of computational costs

Method	L1APG	ONNDL	OSPT	ASLS	Ours (C Version)
FPS	14.5	1.4	4.7	1.3	25

ONNDL [7], OSPT [8], SCM [18], and LSAT [19]. In the evaluation, we use fifteen challenging image sequences from prior works [1,3,12,13,20] and CAVIAR dataset. The challenging factors of these sequences include partial occlusion, background clutter, motion blur, illumination and pose variation.

Experimental Setting. For each sequence, the initial location of the target object is manually labelled. For the sake of representation based on robust incremental subspace learning, each image observation is normalized to 32×32 pixels patch and 16 eigenvectors are selected in all experiments. As the trade-off between computational efficiency and effectiveness, 600 particles are used and the incremental subspace learning updates parameters every 5 frames. The noisy term threshold λ is set to 0.1 to all experiments.

4.1 Qualitative Evaluation

All the sequence images in our experiment are simulating situations of three categories: heavy occlusion, illumination change and fast motion. With limited space available, we only give a qualitative comparison as shown in Fig. 2 with some key frames of ten sequences.

For the situation under heavy occlusions, such as *Occlusion*1 sequence that the face is occluded by a magazine significantly [11], our approach, FragTrack and L1 methods perform better as shown in Fig. 2(a) due to taking partial occlusion into account. Before the magazine covers the face, all trackers do a fine job. However, after that many of them only track the face inaccurately. In *Occlusion*2 sequence that simulates a more complex situation by appearing occlusion and in-plane rotation at the same time. As shown in Fig. 2(b), although all tracker work well in the partial occlusion at about frame 150. They fail in the situation combining in-plane rotation and partial occlusion at about frame 500. *Carviar*1 and *Caviar*2 are surveillance videos which are challenging as they contain scale change, partial occlusion and similar target. The L1 and IVT trackers drift away from the target at frame 225 in Fig. 2(d) or fail totally at frame 125 in Fig. 2(c) after it is occluded by a similar object. Our method is succeeded in solving the challenges.

For the situation under illumination change, such as *Car*4 in which the illumination changes abruptly due to the shallow of entrance and exit of a tunnel. All tracker work well before the car enters the tunnel at about frame 160 in the Fig. 2(f). However, after that only our method and IVT can track the car accurately and others track the target with drift or miss the target totally. In *Car*11 sequences in where the road environment is very dark with background

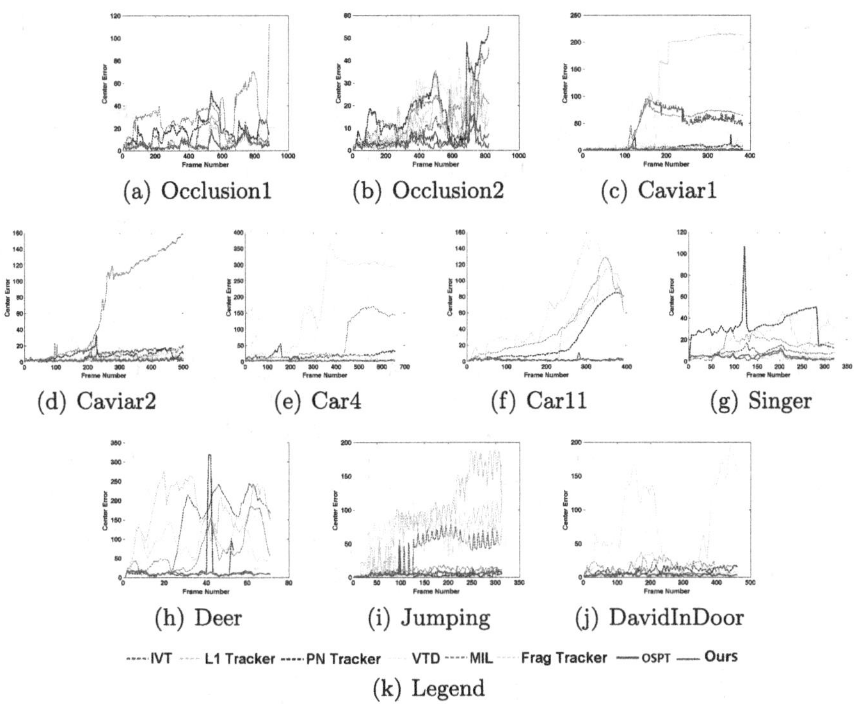

Fig. 3. Quantitative Comparison between the average center error among different methods in 10 datasets

light, we notice the IVT approach and the proposed method perform better than the other methods whereas the other methods drift away when the abrupt illumination change occurs (e.g. frame 200 in Fig. 2(e)) or when the similar objects are close to the target (e.g. frame 300 in Fig. 2(e)). In *DavidIndoor* sequence, recorded in an indoor environment, we need to track a moving face with illumination, scale and out-plane rotation changes. Most methods drift from frame 160 in Fig. 2(h) because of out-plane rotation. But some of them can recover this after several frames. In *Singer* sequence, complicated illumination changes make the tracking task more difficult. Our tracker is able to track the target more precisely than others as shown in Fig. 2(g).

For the fast motion situation, such as *Deer* sequence in which the target is a running deer with rapid changes in appearance, our method and VTD method work better than other methods. In *Jumping* sequence, the trackers have to face the challenge of appearance change caused by motion blur. The MIL, PN tracker and the proposed method can track the target even the target become blurred.

4.2 Quantitative Evaluation

There are two different evaluation for our quantitative evaluation: the difference between the predicated and the ground truth center locations, and the overlap

Table 2. Average center location error. The best three results are shown in red, blue and green fonts seperatively.

Sequence	FT	IVT	ONNDL	VTD	TLD	APGL1	MTT	LSAT	SCM	ASLAS	OSPT	Ours
Occlusion1	5.6	9.2	5.0	11.1	17.6	6.8	14.1	5.3	3.2	10.8	4.7	5.3
Occlusion2	15.5	10.2	8.6	10.4	18.6	6.3	9.2	58.6	4.8	3.7	4	3.5
Caviar1	5.7	45.2	3.2	3.9	5.6	50.1	20.9	1.8	0.9	1.4	1.7	1.4
Caviar2	5.6	8.6	4.4	4.7	8.5	63.1	65.4	45.6	2.5	62.3	2.2	2.4
Caviar3	116.1	66	63.7	58.2	44.4	68.6	67.5	55.3	2.2	2.2	45.7	3.2
DavidOut	90.5	53	53.3	61.9	173	233.4	65.5	101.7	64.1	87.5	5.8	7.9
DavidIn	148.7	3.1	6.0	49.4	13.4	10.8	13.4	6.3	3.4	3.5	3.2	3.9
Singer1	22	8.5	9.3	4.1	32.7	3.1	41.2	14.5	3.7	5.3	4.7	3.5
Car4	179.8	2.9	6.0	12.3	18.8	16.4	37.2	3.3	3.5	4.3	3	3.2
Car11	63.9	2.1	1.4	27.1	25.1	1.7	1.8	4.1	1.8	2	2.2	1.5
Deer	92.1	127.5	8.3	11.9	25.7	38.4	9.2	69.8	36.8	8	8.5	10
Football	16.7	18.2	19.6	4.1	11.8	12.4	6.5	14.1	10.4	18	33.7	7
Jumping	58.4	36.8	79.1	63	3.6	8.8	19.2	55.2	3.9	39.1	5	4.8
Owl	148	141.4	27.8	86.8	8.2	104.2	184.3	110.7	7.3	7.6	47.4	6.2
Face	48.8	69.7	29.5	141.4	22.3	148.9	127.2	16.5	125.1	95.1	24.1	12.3
Average	67.8	40.2	21.7	36.7	28.6	51.5	45.5	37.5	18.2	23.4	13.1	5

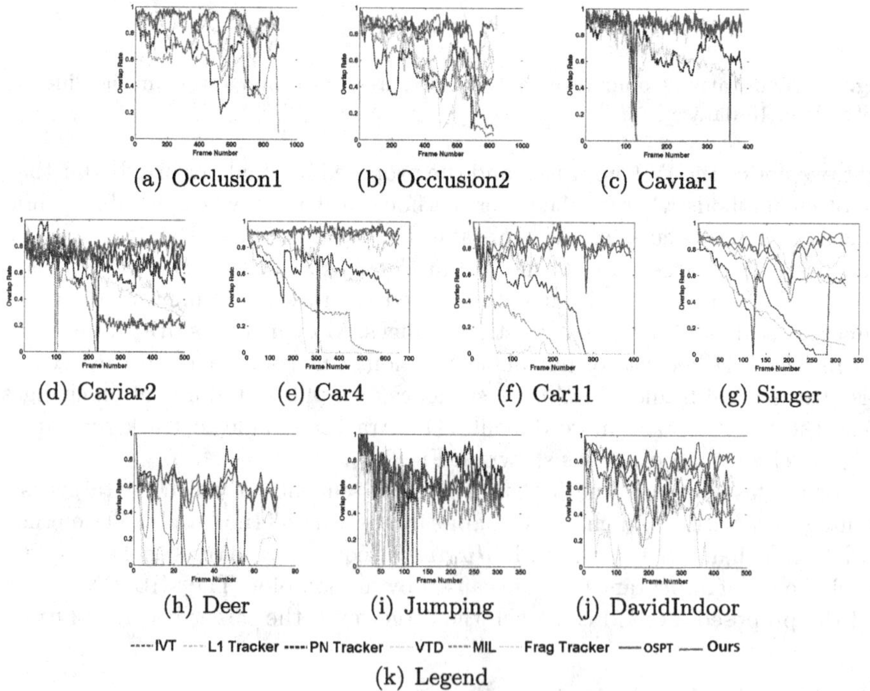

(a) Occlusion1 (b) Occlusion2 (c) Caviar1

(d) Caviar2 (e) Car4 (f) Car11 (g) Singer

(h) Deer (i) Jumping (j) DavidIndoor

(k) Legend

Fig. 4. Quantitative comparison between the overlap rates among different methods in 10 datasets

Table 3. Average overlap rate. The best three results are shown in red, blue and green fonts seperatively.

Sequence	FT	IVT	ONNDL	VTD	TLD	APGL1	MTT	LSAT	SCM	ASLAS	OSPT	Ours
Occlusion1	0.90	0.85	0.89	0.77	0.65	0.87	0.79	0.90	0.93	0.83	0.91	0.89
Occlusion2	0.60	0.59	0.54	0.59	0.49	0.70	0.72	0.33	0.82	0.81	0.84	0.82
Caviar1	0.68	0.28	0.67	0.83	0.70	0.28	0.45	0.85	0.91	0.90	0.89	0.89
Caviar2	0.56	0.45	0.46	0.67	0.66	0.32	0.33	0.28	0.81	0.35	0.71	0.80
Caviar3	0.13	0.14	0.13	0.15	0.16	0.13	0.14	0.58	0.87	0.82	0.25	0.85
DavidOut	0.39	0.52	0.71	0.42	0.16	0.05	0.42	0.36	0.46	0.45	0.77	0.74
DavidIn	0.09	0.69	0.56	0.23	0.5	0.63	0.53	0.72	0.75	0.77	0.76	0.78
Singer1	0.34	0.66	0.58	0.79	0.41	0.83	0.32	0.52	0.85	0.78	0.82	0.82
Car4	0.22	0.92	0.88	0.73	0.64	0.7	0.53	0.91	0.89	0.89	0.92	0.91
Car11	0.09	0.81	0.82	0.43	0.38	0.83	0.58	0.49	0.79	0.81	0.81	0.84
Deer	0.08	0.22	0.60	0.58	0.41	0.45	0.6	0.35	0.46	0.62	0.61	0.59
Football	0.57	0.55	0.44	0.81	0.56	0.68	0.71	0.63	0.69	0.57	0.62	0.69
Jumping	0.14	0.28	0.06	0.08	0.69	0.59	0.3	0.09	0.73	0.24	0.69	0.65
Owl	0.09	0.22	0.46	0.12	0.6	0.16	0.09	0.13	0.79	0.78	0.48	0.79
Face	0.39	0.44	0.56	0.24	0.62	0.14	0.26	0.69	0.36	0.21	0.68	0.76
Average	0.35	0.51	0.56	0.5	0.51	0.49	0.45	0.52	0.74	0.66	0.72	0.79

rate with ground truth. The results are summarized in Tables 2 and 3, respectively. The Table 2 reports the average center location errors in pixels, where the value smaller the result more accurate. Given the tracking result of each frame R_t and the corresponding ground truth R_G, the overlap rate is defined as $\frac{area(R_T \cap R_G)}{area(R_T \cup R_G)}$. Table 3 reports the average overlap rates, where the value larger the result more accurate. For each video sequence (i.e., each row), we show the best result in red, second best in blue, third best in green. We also report the central-pixel errors and the overlap rates frame-by-frame for each video sequence in Figs. 3 and 4 respectively. In terms of the overlap rate, our method is always among the best three in 13 of the 15 sequences. With respect to the central-pixel error, our method is among the best two in 13 of the 15 sequences. For the other two sequences, the gaps are quite small. We believe they can be negligible in practical applications. Looking at the overall results. Our algorithm achieves the lowest tracking errors in the most of all sequences, and archives the highest overlap rate.

5 Conclusion

In this paper, we propose a robust incremental visual tracking method which take probabilistic admission into account for observation model updating and take partial occlusion into account for object tracking. Either robust incremental subspace method or outliers detection for observations didn't introduce new computational burden. Thus they are positive to make the method be real time. Both quantitative and qualitative evaluations on challenging image sequences demonstrate that the proposed tracking method outperforms several state of the art methods. In the future work, the λ in Eq. 10 is supposed to be measured dynamically according to the real scenes.

Acknowledgement. The authors would like to thank the anonymous reviewers for constructive comments that helped in improving the quality of this manuscript and Dr. NaiYan Wang for useful discussions.

References

1. Ross, D.A., Lim, J., Lin, R.S., Yang, M.H.: Incremental learning for robust visual tracking. Int. J. Comput. Vis. **77**, 125–141 (2008)
2. Wright, J., Yang, A.Y., Ganesh, A., Sastry, S.S., Ma, Y.: Robust face recognition via sparse representation. IEEE Trans. Pattern Anal. Mach. Intell. **31**, 210–227 (2009)
3. Mei, X., Ling, H.: Robust visual tracking using 1 minimization. In: 2009 IEEE 12th International Conference on Computer Vision, pp. 1436–1443. IEEE (2009)
4. Kim, S.J., Koh, K., Lustig, M., Boyd, S., Gorinevsky, D.: An interior-point method for large-scale l1-regularized least squares. IEEE J. Sel. Top. Sign. Process. **1**, 606–617 (2007)
5. Mei, X., Ling, H., Wu, Y., Blasch, E., Bai, L.: Minimum error bounded efficient 1 tracker with occlusion detection. In: 2011 IEEE Conference on Computer Vision and Pattern Recognition (CVPR), pp. 1257–1264. IEEE (2011)
6. Bao, C., Wu, Y., Ling, H., Ji, H.: Real time robust l1 tracker using accelerated proximal gradient approach. In: IEEE Conference on Computer Vision and Pattern Recognition (CVPR), pp. 1830–1837. IEEE (2012)
7. Wang, N., Wang, J., Yeung, D.Y.: Online robust non-negative dictionary learning for visual tracking. In: 2013 IEEE International Conference on Computer Vision (ICCV), pp. 657–664 (2013)
8. Wang, D., Lu, H., Yang, M.H.: Online object tracking with sparse prototypes. IEEE Trans. Image Process. **22**, 314–325 (2013)
9. Bach, F., Jenatton, R., Mairal, J., Obozinski, G.: Optimization with sparsity-inducing penalties. Found. Trends® Mach. Learn. **4**, 1–106 (2012)
10. Feng, J., Xu, H., Mannor, S., Yan, S.: Online PCA for contaminated data. In: Advances in Neural Information Processing Systems, pp. 764–772 (2013)
11. Adam, A., Rivlin, E., Shimshoni, I.: Robust fragments-based tracking using the integral histogram. In: 2006 IEEE Computer Society Conference on Computer Vision and Pattern Recognition, Vol. 1, pp. 798–805. IEEE (2006)
12. Babenko, B., Yang, M.H., Belongie, S.: Visual tracking with online multiple instance learning. In: IEEE Conference on Computer Vision and Pattern Recognition, 2009, CVPR 2009. pp. 983–990. IEEE (2009)
13. Kwon, J., Lee, K.M.: Visual tracking decomposition. In: 2010 IEEE Conference on Computer Vision and Pattern Recognition (CVPR), pp. 1269–1276. IEEE (2010)
14. Kalal, Z., Matas, J., Mikolajczyk, K.: Pn learning: Bootstrapping binary classifiers by structural constraints. In: 2010 IEEE Conference on Computer Vision and Pattern Recognition (CVPR), pp. 49–56. IEEE (2010)
15. Kalal, Z., Mikolajczyk, K., Matas, J.: Tracking-learning-detection. IEEE Trans. Pattern Anal. Mach. Intell. **34**, 1409–1422 (2012)

16. Jia, X., Lu, H., Yang, M.H.: Visual tracking via adaptive structural local sparse appearance model. In: 2012 IEEE Conference on Computer Vision and Pattern Recognition (CVPR), pp. 1822–1829. IEEE (2012)
17. Zhang, T., Ghanem, B., Liu, S., Ahuja, N.: Robust visual tracking via multi-task sparse learning. In: 2012 IEEE Conference on Computer Vision and Pattern Recognition (CVPR), pp. 2042–2049. IEEE (2012)
18. Zhong, W., Lu, H., Yang, M.H.: Robust object tracking via sparsity-based collaborative model. In: 2012 IEEE Conference on Computer Vision and Pattern Recognition (CVPR), pp. 1838–1845. IEEE (2012)
19. Liu, B., Huang, J., Yang, L., Kulikowsk, C.: Robust tracking using local sparse appearance model and k-selection. In: 2011 IEEE Conference on Computer Vision and Pattern Recognition (CVPR), pp. 1313–1320. IEEE (2011)
20. Wu, Y., Ling, H., Yu, J., Li, F., Mei, X., Cheng, E.: Blurred target tracking by blur-driven tracker. In: 2011 IEEE International Conference on Computer Vision (ICCV), pp. 1100–1107. IEEE (2011)

Data Mining for Action Recognition

Andrew Gilbert(✉) and Richard Bowden

Centre for Vision Speech and Signal Processing (CVSSP),
University of Surrey, Guildford GU2 7XH, UK
a.gilbert@surrey.ac.uk

Abstract. In recent years, dense trajectories have shown to be an efficient representation for action recognition and have achieved state-of-the-art results on a variety of increasingly difficult datasets. However, while the features have greatly improved the recognition scores, the training process and machine learning used hasn't in general deviated from the object recognition based SVM approach. This is despite the increase in quantity and complexity of the features used. This paper improves the performance of action recognition through two data mining techniques, APriori association rule mining and Contrast Set Mining. These techniques are ideally suited to action recognition and in particular, dense trajectory features as they can utilise the large amounts of data, to identify far shorter discriminative subsets of features called rules. Experimental results on one of the most challenging datasets, Hollywood2 outperforms the current state-of-the-art.

1 Introduction

Action recognition has been a popular area of research within the computer vision and machine learning communities for a number of years. This is partly due to the huge number of applications that would benefit, given the ability to automatically recognise actions within natural videos. Driving this research has often been the ease of dataset availability, from the earliest Weizmann [1] and KTH [2] datasets, to the current state of the art, the more realistic and difficult HMDB51 [3] and Hollywood2 [4] datasets. These later datasets pose significant challenges to action recognition, for example, background clutter, fast irregular motion, occlusion and viewpoint changes. The identification of an action class is related to many other unsolved high-level visual problems, such as human pose estimation, interaction with objects, and scene context. Furthermore, determining the temporal extent of an action is much more subjective than for a static object and the size of video datasets are considerably higher than those consisting of static images.

Initially, to solve the action recognition problem, the image recognition framework was generalised to videos. This included the extension of many classical image features; 3D-SIFT [5], extended SURF [6] and HOG3D [7], Space Time Interest Points (STIPs) [8], and more recently dense trajectories [9]. Similarly the classification pipelines applied to single frame image recognition were and

D. Cremers et al. (Eds.): ACCV 2014, Part V, LNCS 9007, pp. 290–303, 2015.
DOI: 10.1007/978-3-319-16814-2_19

still are applied to action recognition. This means the extensive use of SVMs [2], boosting [10] and Multiple Instance Learning (MIL) [11]. While these approaches can provide excellent results for object recognition, it might not be optimal to directly transfer into the temporal domain, for action recognition, without compromise.

We propose standard learning approaches by data mining techniques which are especially suited for use with densely sampled features. We argue that due to the fact that these dense features are over complete compared to the final solution, mining can efficiently identify the small subset of distinctive and descriptive features that provide the greatest description of the data. In this work we propose the use of Contrast Set Mining as it is able to provide improved results over APriori association rule mining with a lower computational cost.

The rest of the paper is organized as follows. In Sect. 2, we introduce related work in action recognition and data mining. While in Sect. 3, we detail the APriori and Contrast Set Mining methods. The experimental setup and evaluation protocols are explained in Sect. 4 and experimental results in Sect. 5.

2 Related Work

Related to this work, there are two main areas of relevant work within the computer vision community; action recognition and data mining. The action recognition field is an active area, including research on the features used [5–7] and methods for spatially and temporal encoding features [12–15]. As the datasets have become more realistic, additional modelling of the videos has become a recent important area of research. For example using Optical flow, Uemura [16] estimates the dominant camera motion, while Park [17] performs simple optical flow based camera stabilisation to remove both the camera and object motion. Similarly Wang [9] uses the optical flow in conjunction with SURF features to compensate for the camera motion. While Hoai [18] performed segmentation on the actions to increase accuracy before classification. The context of the video can also provide information [4,19], learning relationships between objects in the scene and the scene itself to provide additional cues. In addition, the encoding of the features has been improved by moving away from the standard bag of words towards fisher vector encoding as employed by Oneata [20]. In our work, we concentrate on the learning method, instead of the often used SVM [2] or MIL [11] frameworks, we investigate a data mining based learning technique.

Data mining is a feature selection process increasingly used in computer vision, as the efficiency benefits with increasingly large amounts of data become more marked, where the aim is to generate a higher level super set of features. Yuan [21] mined visual features to generate a high level visual lexicon for object recognition while work by Newozin [22] learnt a temporal based sequential representation of the features to encode the temporal order of features for action recognition. Within image recognition, the spatial encoding of SIFT features by Quack [13] was be learnt through APriori data mining, while the hierarchical encoding of simple corner features were mined by Gilbert [12] to perform action recognition. More recent work on negative mining to find the *non* frequently occurring rules in images [23] has shown promise in learning the differences between classes. Finally, the work by Wang [24] uses a form of APriori data mining for action recognition to efficiently evaluate their motion features called phrases, leveraging APriori's ability to efficiently mine the large feature space. This paper continues the research into data mining techniques by proposing contrast set learning for action recognition.

3 Data Mining

In order to provide scalable solutions to learning from large datasets we propose to adapt text mining techniques. APriori data mining and Contrast Set Mining ignore noise or infrequent features and instead identify frequently reoccurring unique and discriminative subsets of the data. Term Frequency Inverse Document Frequency (TF-IDF) [25] is another popular numerical statistic providing a measure of the importance of a feature (word) to a document or class compared to the rest of the data. However, contrast set mining and APriori have efficient methods to generate the key feature rules, especially contrast set mining which is designed to identify rules that provide the maximum class separation.

3.1 APriori Association Rules Mining

One of the most popular data mining approaches, originally proposed by Agrawal and SriKant [26] is APriori, its aim is to find frequently occurring sets of features or items in the form of association rules. An association rule is a relationship between a number of items that frequently occur within the data. For example, a discovered rule might be, given the items A, B and C, people who buy the items A and B are very likely to purchase item C at the same time. This can then be written as an association rule in the form $\{A, B\} \Rightarrow C$. To assess the quality of a possible association rule, two measures are computed, the support and confidence.

Support. Given transaction T, which consists of a number of encoded features or items, a, a database of all the transactions, DB, the complete feature or item vocabulary is I, where $a \subset I$. The support $s(a)$ of a specific set of items, measures the statistical significance of the proposed rule. The support is defined in Eq. 1

$$s(a) = \frac{|\{T \mid T \in DB, a \subseteq T\}|}{|DB|} \tag{1}$$

A frequently occurring set of items is defined as a set for which $s(a) \geq \sigma > 0$, for a user defined σ, or support threshold. The support threshold σ, is used to filter the large set of transaction vectors to remove the insignificant rules that rarely occur.

Finding sets of items that frequently occur is not trivial because of its combinatorial explosion. It is characterized as a level-wise complete search algorithm using anti-monotonicity of the set of items, i.e. if a set of items is not frequent, any of its supersets will also never be frequent. In order to discover the rules of frequent items, APriori first scans the database of all transactions and searches for frequent sets of items of size $k = 1$ by accumulating the count for each item and collecting those that satisfy the minimum support requirement. Then given the set of frequent items of size k and the possible rules r_k, it iterates on the following five steps and extracts all the frequent sets of items.

1. Increment k by 1.
2. Generate r_k candidates of frequent sets of items of size k, from the frequent set of items of size r_{k-1}.
3. Compute the support for each candidate of the frequent set of items of size k.
4. Remove the candidates that do not satisfy the minimum support requirements.
5. Repeat steps until no further possible candidates exist of size k.

While the support can be used to find frequent set of items, these features could occur across multiple classes or concepts and therefore would not provide discriminative information against other classes. To solve this, the evaluation of a possible rules is extended to measure a confidence of the rule.

Confidence Measure. The confidence is key for identifying the discriminative sets of items that occur in a single class, providing a measure of how discriminative a rule is. The confidence of a frequent item a with respect to a class label α is equivalent to $P(\alpha|a)$. $P(\alpha|a)$ will be large only if a occurs frequently in transactions containing the specific class label α but infrequently in the other class labels. If a occurs frequently in multiple concepts, then $P(\alpha|a)$ will remain small as the denominator in the conditional probability will be large. It is defined as

$$K(a \Rightarrow \alpha) = \frac{s(a \cap \alpha)}{s(a)} \tag{2}$$

Through the association rule generation process outlined above, each rule is measured with respect to both a minimum support and confidence threshold. The confidence threshold γ is set high at 70 %, to ensure rules related to a single class are discriminative with respect to others.

3.2 Contrast Set Mining

APriori achieves excellent performance, however, in situations with many frequent sets of item, large sets of items, or very low minimum support, it suffers from the cost of generating a huge number of candidate sets and scanning the database repeatedly to check candidate items. The simple pruning strategy means that in the worst case it may be necessary to generate 2^{20} candidate items to obtain frequent sets of items of size $k = 20$. To reduce this figure, higher support thresholds can be used, but, this limits the search space of the approach

Table 1. Supermarket Purchases

Burger	Chips	Foie Gras	Wine	Purpose
1	1	0	0	Family meal
1	1	0	0	Family meal
0	0	1	1	Anniversary
1	1	0	0	Family meal

possibly missing significant rules. Instead, Contrast Set Mining [27,28] is based on sub sampling the transactions multiple times. It aims to identify the meaningful differences between separate classes by reverse engineering the key predictors that identify each class. To illustrate the key principle behind Contrast Set Mining, the example in Table 1 shows 4 people's supermarket transactions. The goal would be to learn that people who bought burgers and chips were *having* a family meal. APriori Association rule mining from the section above would learn that people who buy burgers and chips are *likely* to have a family meal. However Contrast Set Mining would identify that the main *difference* or *contrast* between people shopping for a family meal, compared to an anniversary, is that people buying for a family meal buy burgers and chips and *don't* buy Foie Gras and Wine. This distinction is useful for larger datasets or ones with low inter class variation, as it focuses on the discriminate information and not just the frequent. Therefore instead of modelling all the data, it identifies rules that can provide the most impact or change on the dataset and this generally results in a simple set of rules for each class that are both distinctive and descriptive. To measure the quality of possible rules, two concepts; *lift* and *support* are examined.

Lift. The *lift* of a rule is a measure of how the class distribution of the training data shifts in response to the use of the rule compared to the baseline class distribution. It will seek the smallest set of rules that induce the largest shifts. Given a set of transactions, T, which contain a number items a. The transactions will be labelled with a specific class α from the training data $\{T_1, T_2, ...\} \longrightarrow \alpha_1$ etc., where $C = \{\alpha_1, \alpha_2, ..., \alpha_A\}$. Within the transaction database, the frequency of the transactions attributed to a specific class is given by $\{F_1, F_2, ..., F_C\}$ and is used as a normalisation factor. The overall aim is to identify the short subsets of items or rules r that provide the greatest improvement in the overall class distribution. To achieve this, the frequency of the rule r occurring within each class α is computed f^r_α. Ideally the rule will have a high frequency of occurrence in the positive class and low occurrence elsewhere and this will provide maximal lift. The lift is defined as

$$lift(r) = \sum_{\alpha=0}^{C} \frac{f^r_\alpha}{U_\alpha F_\alpha} \tag{3}$$

where C denotes the set of class labels, and U_α is a class weight, where

$$U_\alpha = \begin{cases} 1 & \alpha = Positive \\ 0.1 & otherwise \end{cases} \tag{4}$$

If the lift is greater than 1, the rule is improving the input or baseline distribution of the classes, i.e. the rule is more frequent in the positive class and less so in the negative classes. Ideally the rule will have a large lift, and this can achieved by making it more specific. However, the more specific the rule is, the greater the amount of the data it filters out. This can cause over fitting, causing the unwelcome property of the rule only occurring in a very small selection of the positive examples. Therefore an additional measure related to the frequency of the rule within the data is computed.

Minimum Best Support. It is problematic to rely on the lift of a rule alone, incorrect or noisy items within the data, may results in an overfitted rule set. Such an overfitted rule may have a high lift score, but will not accurately reflect the positive data. In order to avoid overfitting, the approach uses a threshold called *minimum best support*, to reject rules below the minimum support. This is the percentage of transactions supporting the rule, it is the ratio of the frequency of occurrence of the rule within the positive class, with respect to the frequency of the occurrence of the rule in the rest of the dataset as shown in Eq. 5

$$support(r) = \frac{f^r_{\alpha_p}}{\sum_{i=0}^{C} f^r_i} where\ i \neq \alpha_p \tag{5}$$

where α_p is the positive class label.

The lift and support assesses the effectiveness of a rule, but the possible candidate rules need to be generated. A naive approach would test all possible subset item combinations in a similar fashion to the APriori rule generation. However, this is wasteful and increasingly infeasible as the complexity of data increases. Therefore we use a weighted random sampling strategy to combine the best single rules together and reduce training time.

Rule Formation. To learn the class rules, initially a random subset of individual features are selected, and the lift is calculated for each. These lift scores are then sorted and converted into a cumulative probability distribution as shown in Fig. 1. Contrast Set Mining then randomly selects K concatenations of the features, up to a maximum rule size M, generally $M = 5$ to reduce the unnecessary formation of rules that will have too low support. The use of the Cumulative Probability distribution to weight the rule formation, means that single features with a low lift are unlikely to be selected, as if the rule has a low lift it will be ignored. The K concatenations of the rules are then scored and ranked with respect to their lift and support and the process is repeated with a new random subset of individual features. If there are no changes in the top X rules after a defined number of rounds, it terminates and returns the top X rules. Contrast Set Mining is run independently for each class of the training data, to produce a set of rules for each class $M(\alpha) = \{m(\alpha)_1, m(\alpha)_2, ...m(\alpha)_A\}$.

4 Experimental Setup

In this section, we introduce the features and dataset used and the training process.

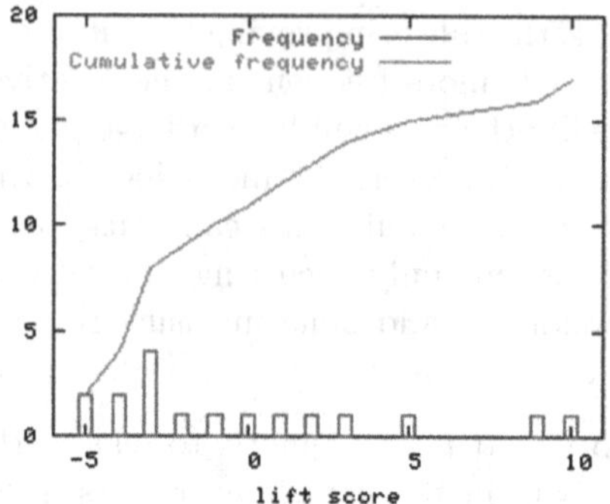

Fig. 1. Cumulative Probability distribution of single attribute lifts

4.1 Features and Dataset

For this work we test the approach on what is generally considered to be one of the most challenging but well supported action recognition datasets, Hollywood2 [4]. Hollywood2 was collected from 69 different Hollywood movies and includes 12 action classes. It contains 1,707 videos split into a training set (823 videos) and a test set (884 videos). Importantly the training and test videos come from different movies. To measure the performance, mean average precision (mAP) over all classes, as in [4] is used, with examples of the videos shown in Fig. 2.

The features extracted are based on dense trajectory features [9], the feature points on each frame are tracked by median filtering a dense optical flow field. To avoid drift, the trajectories are limited to 15 frames. In addition, feature trajectories that are static are ignored as they provide no motion information. For each trajectory, we compute and concatenate several descriptors; the Trajectory, HOG, HOF and MBH. The Trajectory descriptor is a concatenation of normalized displacement vectors. While the other descriptors are computed

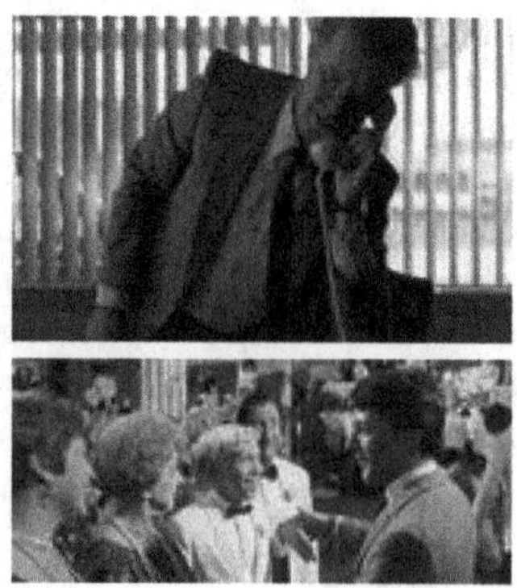

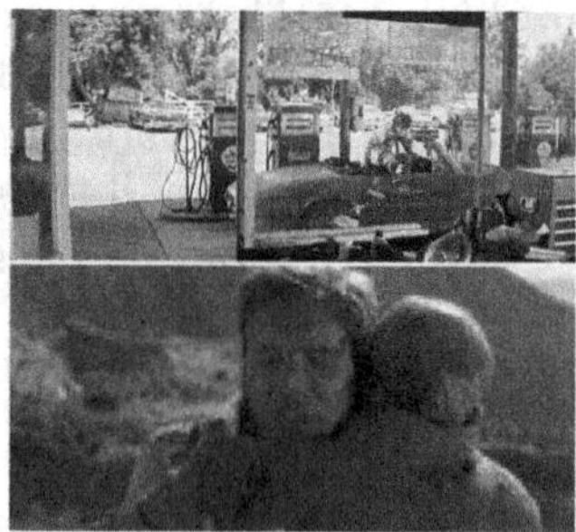

Fig. 2. Examples from the *hollywood2* dataset [4]

in the space-time volume aligned with the trajectory. HOG captures the static appearance information and is based on the orientation of image gradients. While both HOF and MBH measure motion information, and are based on optical flow. HOF directly quantizes the orientation of flow vectors, while MBH splits the optical flow into horizontal and vertical components, and quantizes the derivatives of each component. The final dimensions of the descriptors are 30 for Trajectory, 96 for HOG, 108 for HOF and 192 for MBH, giving a base feature size of 426. We then train a 4000 element codebook using 100,000 randomly sampled feature descriptors with k-means.

4.2 Training

Given the 4000 element codebook, all the trajectories detected within a given video are assigned to their closest neighbour and this results in a frequency count of specific codebook detections for a video. These frequency counts are then symbolised to allow the application of mining.

Given a feature or item vocabulary containing $|\mathbf{I}|$ items or features, where $\mathbf{I} = \{A, B, C\}$, and T_i is a transaction vector of the codebook frequency response of the input, i, with two example input transactions, $\mathbf{T}_1 = \{3, 0, 1\}$ $\mathbf{T}_2 = \{1, 3, 2\}$.

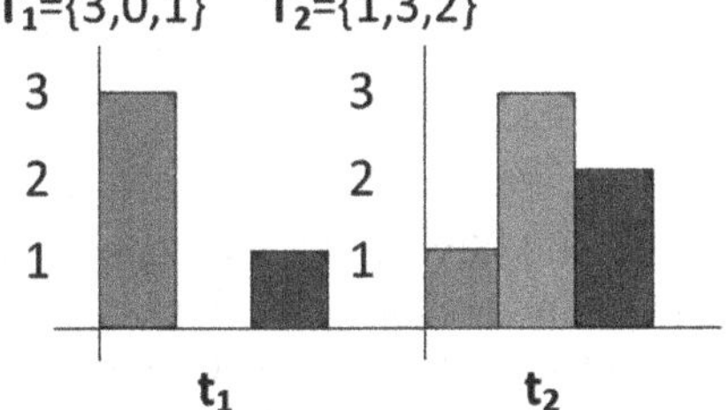

Fig. 3. The symbolisation of the codebook detections

As shown in Fig. 3, in order to convert the feature frequency response into unique symbols for data mining, the frequency of each element in $\mathbf{T}_i$ is used to form the same number of new but unique symbols as the value of the frequency. Therefore, in the example above, the transactions become, $\mathbf{T}_1^{'} = \{A1, A2, A3, C1\}$ $\mathbf{T}_2^{'} = \{A1, B1, B2, B3, C1, C2\}$.

In order to classify test videos, the rules for each class need to be mined through the two data mining techniques we propose. For each video, the codebook frequency response is symbolised into a transaction vector, and appended with the relevant class label α, and this is repeated for each video, to form a database of transactions, to be used as the input to the data mining. Generally there is between 10,500 and 20,100 unique items in each transaction each representing a video sequence, many of these items repeating both inter and intra class. Then, for each class the database is mined with respect to the class, to produce a set of rules for each class $M(\alpha) = \{m(\alpha)_1, m(\alpha)_2, ...m(\alpha)_A\}$.

4.3 Classification

Both data mining techniques generally produce concise rules for each class label, therefore the top rules can be formatted into class specific lookup tables for classification. To classify, the codebook response of a test video is found and symbolised to form a test transaction and each rule in the lookup table is compared to the transaction. The response score of the classifier R for a test transaction T_i with respect to a specific class label α is given by

$$R(T_i, \alpha) = \frac{1}{A} \sum_{j=0}^{M(\alpha)_A} \frac{1}{|M(\alpha)_j|} m(T_i, M(\alpha)_j) \tag{6}$$

where

$$m(T_i, M(\alpha)_j) = \begin{cases} 1 & T_i \in M(\alpha)_j \\ 0 & otherwise \end{cases} \tag{7}$$

This response score is computed over all class labels, and the maximum response taken as the classification label.

5 Experimental Results

In the results section, initially we compare the stability of the user specified support threshold used in the mining techniques, and computational cost. This is followed by a comparison of the approaches to the current state of the art.

5.1 Stability of Thresholds

Within both APriori and Contrast Set Mining, the support value is used to filter out rules that don't represent the data class. Table 2 shows how the mAP and training computation time on the Hollywood2 dataset varies for a range of specified support values.

It can be seen that in general, the performance for the APriori is dependent on the support value threshold specified, this is because, as the support value is increased more of the data is filtered out and, the quality of the rules is reduced. This is why the training time decreases from over 15 hours to 3 hours between the support value of 0.01 and 0.3. In comparison, in Contrast Set Mining both the performance and training time is more constant. This is due to the weighted random sampling technique used to form the rules, which means it is far less dependent on the value of the minimum support.

Table 2. Comparison of the performance of APriori and contrast set mining with varied support thresholds

Support value	APriori		Contrast sets	
	mAP (%)	Train time (mins)	mAP (%)	Train time (mins)
0.01	65.1	940	65.2	120
0.05	65.1	495	65.2	125
0.1	60.1	475	65.4	129
0.2	39.7	260	65.5	127
0.3	22.1	190	62.4	135

5.2 Evaluation of Action Learning Framework

In order to compare the use of the APriori and Contrast Set Mining with other current state-of-the-art approaches, the standard train and test subsets of the Hollywood2 dataset as provided by [4] was used. For the APriori mining, the support value was set as $\sigma = 0.1$, as this provide the highest results, when using the training data. While for the Contrast Set Mining, $\sigma = 0.2$. The results are presented in Table 3.

Table 3. Comparison of the Active learning on the of hollywood2 dataset

Approach	mAP (%)
Mathe [29]	61.0
Jain [30]	62.5
Wang Baseline [24]	60.1
Wang [24]	64.3
APriori Association Rule Mining	65.1
Contrast Set Mining	65.4

The results show that the use of a data mining technique to classify action recognition is able to improve on current Sate-of-the-art by around 1 % compared to the most recent results reported in the literature [24]. An illustration of the compact nature of the mined rules can be seen in Fig. 4, it shows the location of the matched Contrast Set Mining features for successfully classified video.

The baseline result by Wang [9], is interesting as it is using the same features and a standard SVM classifier to give a performance of 60.1 %, but with additional processing to remove camera motion and to learn a human detector was able to boost their baseline performance by around 4 % to 64.3 %. These processing techniques could be added to our approach and therefore further improve the performance. The Contrast Set Mining is able to exceed the high performance of the APriori, but with a significant reduced training time, taking only 2 h to

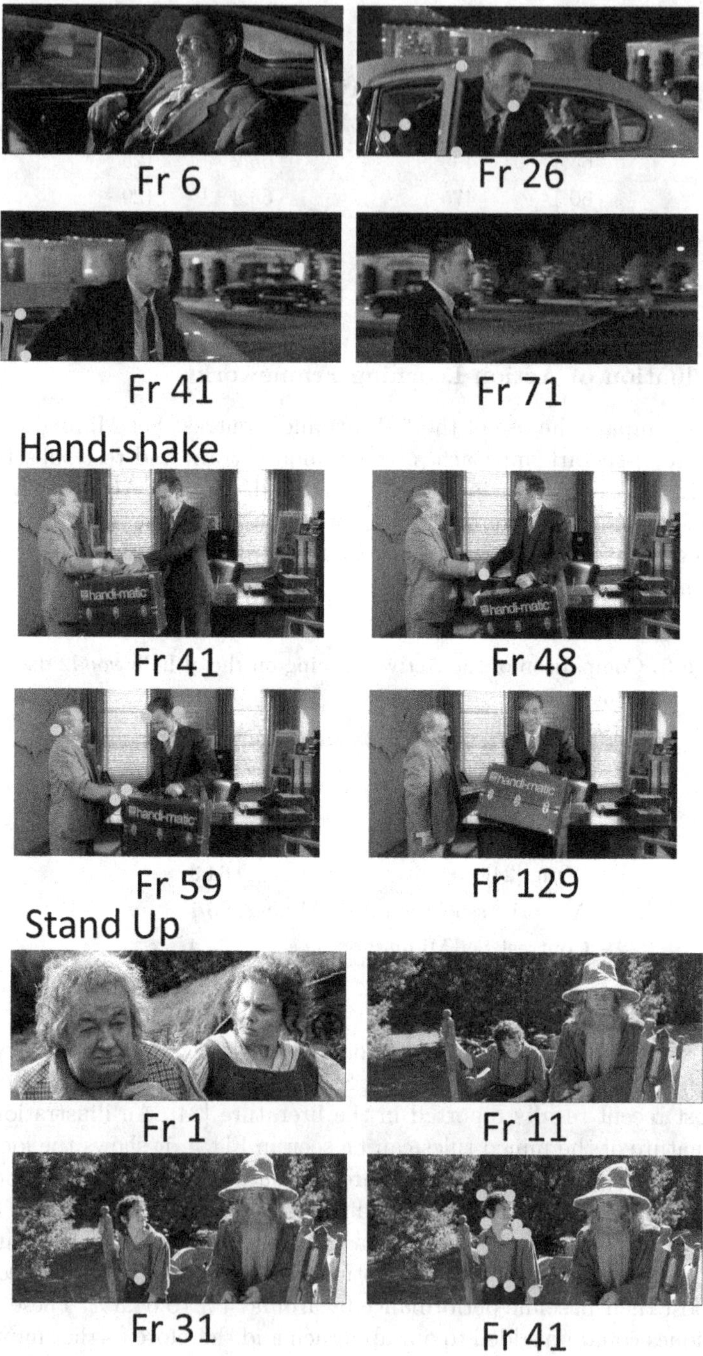

Fig. 4. Successfully classified feature locations in hollwyood2 videos

train, compared to the 8 for the APriori. Furthermore as shown previously in Table 2, the performance of the Contrast set Mining is not affected by the change in a support value of the learnt rules. An additional feature related to the rules, that is unusual compared to many other state-of-the-art approaches in the field of action recognition, is the size of the rules that are learnt. Typically the mined rules are short, the rules mined using APriori had a median length of 7 items, while in the case of Contrast Sets Mining they are at most a combination of 5 individual codebook elements. They have been identified within the mining process to provide the greatest contrast against the other classes. The compact learnt model allows for fast test time operation as well, as at run time, both data mining approaches are fast, requiring around 15 min to classify all 884 test videos, excluding the dense trajectory feature extraction.

Figure 4, shows where discriminative features fire for each class. The end coordinate of the trajectories are shown. They are generally sparse, and the mining has identified the features of the highest contrast with respect to other classes. In summary, what the rules capture are the combinations of features important to a class. If you were to treat each rule as a single classifier, this would form a very weak classifier that always fires for a certain combination of visual words. However, they often fire at points within the video sequence that are most indicative of the action, for example on the hand shake itself for the action *Hand Shake*, or the car door for the action *Get out of Car*. This high localization of the features, could be extended in future to segment the action within a longer video sequence.

6 Conclusions

This paper is able to improve on the standard dense trajectory features and SVM learning pipeline, through the inclusion of an improved training technique. We demonstrate that through using Contrast Set Mining, performance can be significantly improved on the state-of-the-art. The use of a weighted randomly sampling strategy allows for a reduction in training time and a stabilisation of the user defined minimum support thresholds. An evaluation on the current state-of-the-art action recognition dataset, Hollywood2, demonstrates the approaches effectiveness.

Acknowledgement. This work was supported by the EPSRC grant "Learning to Recognise Dynamic Visual Content from Broadcast Footage" (EP/I011811/1).

References

1. Blank, M., Gorelick, L., Shechtman, E., Irani, M., Basri, R.: Actions as space-time shapes. In: ICCV 2005, pp. 1395–1402 (2005)
2. Schuldt, C., Laptev, I., Caputo, B.: Recognizing human actions: a local SVM approach. In: ICPR 2004, pp. 32–36 (2004)

3. Kuehne, H., Jhuang, H., Garrote, E., Poggio, T., Serre, T.: HMDB: a large video database for human motion recognition. In: ICCV 2011 (2011)
4. Marszalek, M., Laptev, I., Schmid, C.: Actions in context. In: CVPR 2009 (2009)
5. Scovanner, P., Ali, S., Shah, M.: A 3-dimensional sift descriptor and its application to action recognition. In: Proceedings of MULTIMEDIA 2007, pp. 357–360 (2007)
6. Willems, G., Tuytelaars, T., Van Gool, L.: An efficient dense and scale-invariant spatio-temporal interest point detector. In: Forsyth, D., Torr, P., Zisserman, A. (eds.) ECCV 2008, Part II. LNCS, vol. 5303, pp. 650–663. Springer, Heidelberg (2008)
7. Klaser, A., Marszalek, M., Schmid, C.: A spatio-temporal descriptor based on 3D gradients. In: BMVC 2008 (2008)
8. Laptev, I., Lindeberg, T.: Space-time interest points. In: ICCV 2003, pp. 432–439 (2003)
9. Wang, H., Kläser, A., Schmid, C., Liu, C.L.: Dense trajectories and motion boundary descriptors for action recognition. Int. J. Comput. Vis. **103**, 60–79 (2013). Springer
10. Viola, P., Jones, M.: Rapid object detection using a boosted cascade of simple features. In: CVPR 2001, pp. 511–518 (2001)
11. Maron, O., Lozano-Pérez, T.: A framework for multiple-instance learning. In: Advances in Neural Information Processing Systems, pp. 570–576 (1998)
12. Gilbert, A., Illingworth, J., Bowden, R.: Action recognition using mined hierarchical compound features. IEEE Trans. Pattern Anal. Mach. Intell. **33**, 883–897 (2011)
13. Quack, T., Ferrari, V., Leibe, B., Gool, L.: Efficient mining of frequent and distinctive feature configurations. In: ICCV 2007 (2007)
14. Laptev, I., Marszalek, M., Schmid, C., Rozenfeld, B.: Learning realistic human actions from movies. In: CVPR 2008, pp. 1–8 (2008)
15. Niebles, J.C., Wang, H., Fei-Fei, L.: Unsupervised learning of human action categories using spatial-temporal words. Int. J. comput. vis. **79**, 299–318 (2008)
16. Uemura, H., Ishikawa, S., Mikolajczyk, K.: Feature tracking and motion compensation for action recognition. In: BMVC 2008 (2008)
17. Park, D., Zitnick, C.L., Ramanan, D., Dollár, P.: Exploring weak stabilization for motion feature extraction. In: CVPR 2013, pp. 2882–2889 (2013)
18. Hoai, M., Lan, Z.Z., De la Torre, F.: Joint segmentation and classification of human actions in video. In: CVPR 2011, pp. 3265–3272 (2011)
19. Han, D., Bo, L., Sminchisescu, C.: Selection and context for action recognition. In: ICCV 2009, pp. 1933–1940 (2009)
20. Oneata, D., Verbeek, J., Schmid, C.: Action and event recognition with fisher vectors on a compact feature set. In: ICCV 2013, pp. 1817–1824 (2013)
21. Yuan, J., Wu, Y., Yang, M.: Discovery of collocation patterns: from visual words to visual phrases. In: CVPR 2007, pp. 1–8 (2007)
22. Nowozin, S., Bakir, G., Tsuda, K.: Discriminative subsequence mining for action classification. In: ICCV 2007, pp. 1–8 (2007)
23. Siva, P., Russell, C., Xiang, T.: In defence of negative mining for annotating weakly labelled data. In: Fitzgibbon, A., Lazebnik, S., Perona, P., Sato, Y., Schmid, C. (eds.) ECCV 2012, Part III. LNCS, vol. 7574, pp. 594–608. Springer, Heidelberg (2012)
24. Wang, L., Qiao, Y., Tang, X.: Mining motion atoms and phrases for complex action recognition. In: ICCV 2013, pp. 2680–2687 (2013)
25. Sparck Jones, K.: A statistical interpretation of term specificity and its application in retrieval. J. Doc. **28**, 11–21 (1972)

26. Agrawal, R., Srikant, R.: Fast algorithms for mining association rules in large databases. In: Proceedings of 20th International Conference on Very Large Data Bases VLDB 1994, pp. 487–499 (1994)
27. Menzies, T., Hu, Y.: Data mining for very busy people. Computer **36**, 22–29 (2003)
28. Bay, S.D., Pazzani, M.J.: Detecting change in categorical data: Mining contrast sets. In: KDD, pp. 302–306 (1999)
29. Mathe, S., Sminchisescu, C.: Dynamic eye movement datasets and learnt saliency models for visual action recognition. In: Fitzgibbon, A., Lazebnik, S., Perona, P., Sato, Y., Schmid, C. (eds.) ECCV 2012, Part II. LNCS, vol. 7573, pp. 842–856. Springer, Heidelberg (2012)
30. Jain, M., Jégou, H., Bouthemy, P.: Better exploiting motion for better action recognition. In: CVPR 2013, pp. 2555–2562 (2013)

A Rotation-Invariant Regularization Term for Optical Flow Related Problems

Roberto P. Palomares(✉), Gloria Haro, and Coloma Ballester

DTIC, Pompeu Fabra University, 08018 Barcelona, Spain
roberto.palomares@upf.edu

Abstract. This paper proposes a new regularization term for optical flow related problems. The proposed regularizer properly handles rotation movements and it also produces good smoothness conditions on the flow field while preserving discontinuities. We also present a dual formulation of the new term that turns the minimization problem into a saddle-point problem that can be solved using a primal-dual algorithm. The performance of the new regularizer has been compared against the Total Variation (TV) in three different problems: optical flow estimation, optical flow inpainting, and optical flow completion from sparse samples. In the three situations the new regularizer improves the results obtained with the TV as a smoothing term.

1 Introduction

The optical flow problem, also called motion estimation, is a key problem in computer vision. Its aim is to recover the apparent motion field of two consecutive frames. It is a classic ill-posed problem, related to the aperture problem. Thus, additional constraints are made in order to regularize the problem and single out a solution. Horn and Schunk (HS) [1] proposed to compute the flow field as a variational problem, where the searched vector field u corresponds to the minimum of an energy functional. Their energy model has two parts: a fidelity data term imposing the brightness constancy assumption, and a regularization term. The HS model incorporates quadratic terms in both parts (regularizers and fidelity data term), so it does not allow discontinuities in the flow field. Many models, during the last thirty years, have been developed to avoid the previous problem. Several robust estimators have replaced the original quadratic norm [2], either in the data term [3] or regularization term. For the regularization term, anisotropic diffusion (image-driven) [4–7], second order smoothness assumptions [8] and isotropic diffusion as the Total Variation (TV) [9,10] have been proposed. For static scenes, the epipolar geometry can be used as a weak prior [11] or to define an over-parameterized optical flow whose parameters are regularized instead of the flow [12].

Optical flow regularization terms are also useful for motion inpainting, where the optical flow in the missing region is completed by looking for a smooth flow that matches the motion in the known region. Motion inpainting has been applied for completing the optical flow in regions of low confidence due to occlusions,

D. Cremers et al. (Eds.): ACCV 2014, Part V, LNCS 9007, pp. 304–319, 2015.
DOI: 10.1007/978-3-319-16814-2_20

transparencies, etc. [13]. It has also been used for video stabilization [14] and for video inpainting [15].

Total Variation is one of the most used regularizers due to its nice properties such as its ability to recover the image discontinuities, and the existence of efficient and robust numerical schemes with guaranteed convergence. However, it suffers from staircasing effects and does not properly handle rotations.

Our contribution in this paper is a new regularization term which is invariant to infinitesimal flow rotations and which is able to preserve discontinuities/jumps in the flow field. The proposed regularizer does not increase the energy of the functional when the flow field is a rotation movement and, moreover, it keeps some nice properties of the TV, providing a smooth flow field that preserves discontinuities. Real scenes usually contain rotation movements, sometimes at an infinitesimal level, and therefore the use of the proposed term could help to obtain accurate and realistic optical flows. It has been tested in three different optical flow related problems: motion estimation, motion inpainting, and motion reconstruction from sparse samples. In the three kinds of applications it outperforms the results obtained by the TV.

The paper is organized as follows: In Sect. 2 we give the theoretical motivation for the new regularization term. In Sect. 3 we describe a variational model for the optical flow estimation and how to minimize its energy. In Sect. 4 we provide details of the numerical implementation. Some experiments are presented in Sect. 5. Finally, in Sect. 6 we present the main conclusions.

2 Motivation for the Regularizer

Let $U : \mathcal{R}^3 \to \mathcal{R}^3$ be the velocity vector field of a fluid in $\mathcal{R}^3$. For U smooth enough, we consider a first-order Taylor approximation of U,

$$U(\boldsymbol{x} + \boldsymbol{h}) = U(\boldsymbol{x}) + J_{\boldsymbol{x}}U(\boldsymbol{x})\boldsymbol{h} + o(|\boldsymbol{h}|) \quad \text{for} \quad \boldsymbol{h} \to 0 \tag{1}$$

where $\boldsymbol{x} = (x, y, z), \boldsymbol{h} = (h_1, h_2, h_3)$ and $J_{\boldsymbol{x}}U(\boldsymbol{x})$ is the Jacobian matrix at the point $\boldsymbol{x}$. For $\boldsymbol{h}$ small enough, let us approximate

$$U(\boldsymbol{x} + \boldsymbol{h}) \approx U(\boldsymbol{x}) + J_{\boldsymbol{x}}U(\boldsymbol{x})\boldsymbol{h}. \tag{2}$$

The first term at the right-hand side of the above equation represents a translation. The second term provides information on the rotation and deformation movement (scaling and shearing). A matrix can be decomposed in two parts, the symmetric and the antisymmetric part. In our case, let us denote by $D = \frac{1}{2}\left(J_{\boldsymbol{x}}U(\boldsymbol{x}) + J_{\boldsymbol{x}}U(\boldsymbol{x})^T\right)$ the symmetric part of $J_{\boldsymbol{x}}U(\boldsymbol{x})$ and by $C = \frac{1}{2}\left(J_{\boldsymbol{x}}U(\boldsymbol{x}) - J_{\boldsymbol{x}}U(\boldsymbol{x})^T\right)$ the antisymmetric one. The symmetric part measures the area change ratio (divergence) while the antisymmetric part describes the infinitesimal rotation of the vector field (curl) [16]. It is easy to see that the previous argument is valid for $\mathcal{R}^2$. With this idea in mind, we propose to use as a motion regularizer a measure that does not penalize infinitesimal rotations and, as we will see, still produces good smoothness conditions and is able to preserve discontinuities/jumps in the flow field.

We propose the following regularization term

$$E_{D_u}(u) \equiv \int_\Omega \left\| \frac{1}{2}\left(Du + Du^T\right) \right\|_F dx \tag{3}$$

where, for smooth functions, $Du = \begin{pmatrix} u_{1x} & u_{1y} \\ u_{2x} & u_{2y} \end{pmatrix}$, being $u = (u_1, u_2) : \Omega \to R^2$ the optical flow; $||.||_F$ denotes the Frobenius norm. Let us recall that the Frobenius norm can be defined as $\|A\|_F = \langle A, A\rangle_F^{1/2}$, where $\langle A, B\rangle_F = \text{Trace}(A^t B)$.

For $u \in \mathcal{L}^1(\Omega, \mathcal{R}^2)$, $E_{D_u}(u)$ can be defined by its dual representation as

$$E_{D_u}(u) = \sup_{\|\xi\|_F \leq 1} \int_\Omega \langle u_1, \text{div}\,(\xi_{11}, \xi_{12})\rangle + \langle u_2, \text{div}\,(\xi_{12}, \xi_{22})\rangle dx, \tag{4}$$

where the supremum is taken over all $\xi \in C_c^1(\Omega; Sym(R^{2\times 2}))$ s.t. pointwise $\|\xi(x)\|_F \leq 1$. We can restrict ξ to be a symmetric matrix due to the following Lemma.

Lemma 1. *If ξ and C are symmetric and antisymmetric 2×2 matrices, respectively, then $\langle C, \xi\rangle_F = 0$.*

For u, smooth enough, (4) can be writen as

$$E_{D_u}(u) = \sup_{\|\xi\|_F \leq 1} \int_\Omega \langle \frac{1}{2}\left(Du + Du^T\right), \xi\rangle_F \, dx. \tag{5}$$

The proposed regularization term is related to the symmetric part of the following term based on the Frobenius norm which, for u smooth enough and using dual variables, can be written as

$$\int_\Omega \|Du\|_F \, dx = \sup_{\|\xi\|_F \leq 1} \int_\Omega \langle Du, \xi\rangle_F dx, \tag{6}$$

with $\xi \in C_c^1(\Omega; R^{2\times 2})$. This term has been called $\text{TV}_{\ell^2}(u)$ in the paper [17].

Let us remark that, if u is a rotation flow such as $u(x_1, x_2) = (-x_2, x_1)$, then $E_{D_u}(u)$ vanishes. Moreover, as in [17], for a translation of an object in a static background, our term handles different directions of translation equally. In a different context to ours, the authors in [18] use the idea of regularizing the symmetric part of the deformation.

3 Optical Flow Functional

In this section we present the proposed model to estimate the optical flow, and how to minimize its energy.

3.1 The Model

To show the benefits of our term, we build up from a well-known optical flow model [10] that uses TV as the regularization term and an L^1 data term

$$\min_u \int_\Omega \left(|\nabla u_1| + |\nabla u_2| + \lambda \left|I_1(x+u) - I_0\right|\right) dx, \tag{7}$$

where I_0, I_1 are two consecutive frames and $u = (u_1, u_2)$ is the estimated optical flow between them.

We replace the Total Variation as regularizing term by the new flow-rotation-invariant-regularizer defined by (3). Then, in order to compute the optical flow $u = (u_1, u_2)$ between two consecutive frames I_0 and I_1 of a video sequence, we propose to minimize the following energy

$$\int_\Omega \left\| \frac{1}{2}\left(Du + Du^T\right) \right\|_F dx + \lambda \int_\Omega |I_1(x+u) - I_0(x)| dx. \tag{8}$$

The use of L^1 type-norm measures has proven a good performance in front of L^2 norms. Unfortunately, it increases the difficulty when minimizing the functional due to its non differentiability. We introduce an auxiliar variable v representing the optical flow, as in [10], and we penalize its deviation from u. Thus, we minimize the energy

$$\int_\Omega \left\| \frac{1}{2}\left(Du + Du^T\right) \right\|_F dx + \lambda \int_\Omega |I_1(x+v) - I_0(x)| dx + \frac{1}{2\theta} \int_\Omega (u-v)^2 dx \tag{9}$$

with respect to u and v.

Notice that by minimizing this energy we do not impose regularization of the skew symmetric part of the Jacobian. Indeed, given any function f of Bounded Variation, the symmetric part of the Jacobian of the deformation $(f(x_2), -f(x_1))$ vanishes. Therefore, in order to prevent an irregular behavior of this part of the flow field, one can add to the functional, e.g., an additional classical TV term. In any case, the experiments show that the proposed term alone keeps some nice properties of the TV providing a smooth flow field that preserves discontinuities.

This energy can be minimized by an alternating minimization procedure. On the other hand, to minimize (9) with respect to v, we linearize $I_1(x+v)$ around a given optical flow map u_0 using first order Taylor approximation. Therefore, the expression in the fidelity data term can be approximated by

$$\rho(v) := I_1(x+u_0) + \langle \nabla I_1(x+u_0), (v-u_0) \rangle - I_0(x). \tag{10}$$

Then, our functional (8) becomes

$$\int_\Omega \left\| \frac{1}{2}\left(Du + Du^T\right) \right\|_F dx + \lambda \int_\Omega |\rho(v)| dx + \frac{1}{2\theta} \int_\Omega (u-v)^2 dx. \tag{11}$$

3.2 Minimizing the Energy

The energy (11) can be minimized by alternating steps updating either u or v in every iteration. The minimization procedure is

1. For v fixed, minimize (11) with respect to u.
   Chambolle and Pock proposed a primal-dual algorithm to minimize the ROF model [19]. It is based on a dual formulation of the TV [20]. Following the ideas of [19], we reformulate the optical flow model as a min-max problem incorporating dual variables. Then, our minimization problem (11) can be solved as a saddle-point problem. For v fixed, we solve

$$\min_{u} \max_{\xi} \int_{\Omega} \langle \frac{1}{2}\left(Du + Du^T\right), \xi \rangle dx + \int_{\Omega} \frac{1}{2\theta} (u - v)^2 \, dx \tag{12}$$

   where the dual variables are $\xi = \begin{pmatrix} \xi_{11} & \xi_{12} \\ \xi_{12} & \xi_{22} \end{pmatrix}$ and satisfy $||\xi||_F \leq 1$. Let us notice that, using previous Lemma 1, we can restrict ξ to be a symmetric matrix.

Proposition 1. *The solution of (12) is given by the following iterative scheme*

$$\xi_{11}^{n+1} = \frac{\xi_{11}^n + \tau \overline{u}_{1x}^n}{\max(1, ||\xi||_2)} \tag{13}$$

$$\xi_{22}^{n+1} = \frac{\xi_{22}^n + \tau \overline{u}_{2y}^n}{\max(1, ||\xi||_2)} \tag{14}$$

$$\xi_{12}^{n+1} = \frac{\xi_{12}^n + \frac{\tau}{2}\left(\overline{u}_{1y}^n + \overline{u}_{2x}^n\right)}{\max(1, ||\xi||_2)} \tag{15}$$

$$u_1^{n+1} = u_1^n - \sigma\left(\frac{(u_1^n - v_1)}{\theta} - div\left(\xi_{11}^n, \xi_{12}^n\right)\right) \tag{16}$$

$$u_2^{n+1} = u_2^n - \sigma\left(\frac{(u_2^n - v_2)}{\theta} - div\left(\xi_{12}^n, \xi_{22}^n\right)\right) \tag{17}$$

$$\overline{u}_1^{n+1} = 2u_1^{n+1} - u_1^n \tag{18}$$

$$\overline{u}_2^{n+1} = 2u_2^{n+1} - u_2^n \tag{19}$$

where u is the primal variable and ξ is the dual variable.

2. For u fixed, minimize with respect to v the following functional

$$\int_{\Omega} \lambda|\rho(v)| + \int_{\Omega} \frac{1}{2\theta}(u - v)^2 \, dx. \tag{20}$$

   Since (20) does not depend on spatial derivatives on v, a simple thresholding step gives us an explicit solution [10].

Proposition 2. *The minimum of (20) with respect to v is*

$$v = u + \begin{cases} \lambda\theta\nabla I_1 & \text{if } \rho(u) < -\lambda\theta|\nabla I_1|^2 \\ -\lambda\theta\nabla I_1 & \text{if } \rho(u) > \lambda\theta|\nabla I_1|^2 \\ -\rho(u)\frac{\nabla I_1}{|\nabla I_1|^2} & \text{if } |\rho(u)| \leq \lambda\theta|\nabla I_1|^2 \end{cases} \tag{21}$$

The whole minimization algorithm is presented in Algorithm 1.

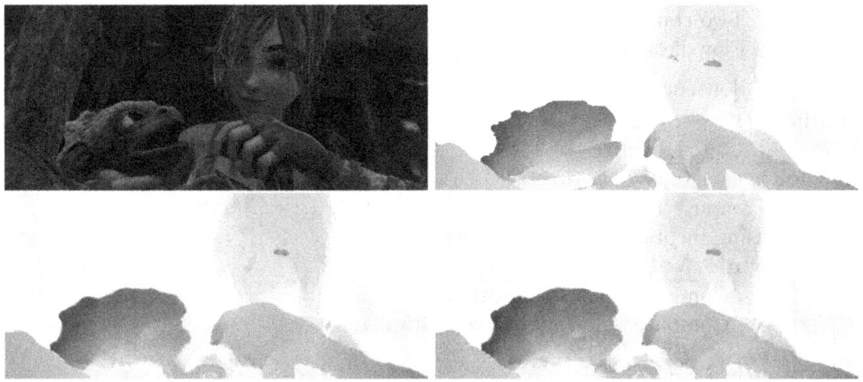

Fig. 1. Results on the MPI Sintel training set "Bandage-2" (clean version). From top to bottom and from left to right: (**a**) First frame, (**b**) optical flow ground truth, (**c**) estimated optical flow using the TV-L^1 method, (**d**) estimated optical flow using an L^1 data term and the proposed regularizer.

4 Implementation

The minimization of (11) to estimate the optical flow is embedded into a coarse-to-fine multi-level approach in order to be able to deal with large motion fields. The numerical algorithm is summarized in Algorithm 1. The image gradient is computed using a five-point stencil as in [5]. Image warpings use bicubic interpolation. Our code is written in C. To do a fair comparison against the TV-L^1 optical flow model of [10], we took the implementation of [21], which is also written in C, and changed their numerical scheme by a primal-dual approach as in our case. The algorithm parameters are initialised with the same default settings. Both time-steps are set to $\tau = \sigma = 0.125$ to ensure the convergence. As stopping criterion both optical flow methods use the infinite-norm between two consecutive values of u with a threshold of 0.01. The coupling parameter θ is equal to 0.3. Input images have been normalized between $[0, 1]$. The fidelity data term weight λ is set to 40. Let us remark that the parameters value have been fixed to ensure a good performance for all the sequences of the Middlebury Dataset. All the experiments use the previous parameters even if the images come from another database.

5 Experiments

In this section we provide two sets of experiments. The first one is designed to verify the good performance of the new regularization term over different types of movements. The second one shows the properties of the presented term to recover rotation movements. We use both real and synthetic images, and two databases: the Middlebury flow benchmark [22] and some images from the MPI Sintel Flow Dataset [23].

Input : Two consecutive frames I_1, I_2
Output: Flow field $\mathbf{u}$

Compute down-scaled images I_1^s, I_2^s for $s = 1, \ldots, N_{\text{scales}}$;
Initialize $\mathbf{u}^{N_{\text{scales}}} = \xi^{N_{\text{scales}}} = \mathbf{v}^{N_{\text{scales}}} = 0$;
for $s \leftarrow N_{\text{scales}}$ to 1 **do**
  for $w \leftarrow 1$ to N_{warps} **do**
    Compute $I_1^s(x + v_0(x))$, $I_1^{sx}(x + v_0(x))$, $I_1^{sy}(x + v_0(x))$;
    using bicubic interpolation;
    while $n < N_{\max}$ or $tol < error$ **do**
      Compute v via Proposition 2;
      Compute ξ and u via Proposition 1;
    end
  end
end

Algorithm 1. Coarse-to-fine multi-level approach to compute optical flow.

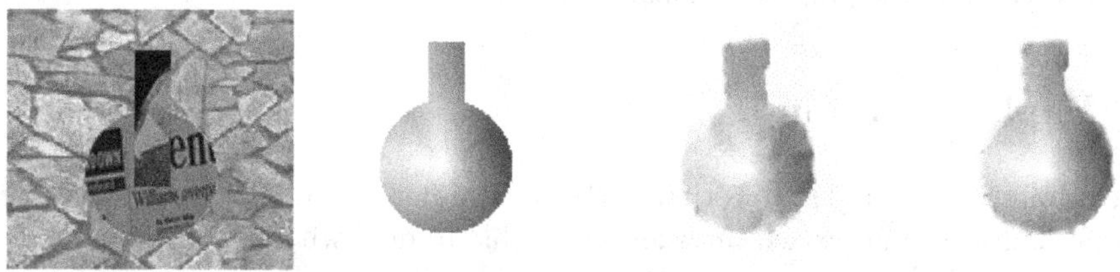

Fig. 2. Results for a pure rotation movement (3 degree anti-clockwise). *From left to right:* (**a**) First frame. (**b**) Optical flow ground truth. (**c**) Estimated optical flow using the TV regularizer. (**d**) Estimated optical flow using the proposed regularizer.

5.1 Global Accuracy

In this section we compute the optical flow from a set of images from standard datasets.

Middlebury DataSet - It contains a training set where ground truth is available. We use it to verify the accuracy of our regularization term against the well-established TV term. In order to compare our regularizer to other high-order regularization methods, we have implemented TGV_2 (see [24]). The parameters α_0 and α_1 have been chosen to ensure a good performance for all the sequences of the Middelbury Dataset. Table 1 shows how our method improves the optical flow maps for almost all the images by measuring the Average Angular Error (AEE) and Average End-point Error (EPE).

MPI Sintel Flow DataSet - MPI Sintel dataset has 23 training sequences. For every frame, there are two different images, "clean" and "final". The difference is that the second set adds complexity to the first one by incorporating atmospheric effects, depth of field blur, motion blur, color correction and other details. We evaluate the frames 32–38 from the training set "Bandage-2"

Table 1. Error measures in the Middlebury dataset with public ground truth flow.

Middlebury	Dim.	Hyd.	Rub.	Gro2	Gro3	Urb2	Urb3	Ven
EPE-TV	0.1537	0.2286	0.1916	0.1496	0.6808	0.3709	0.6034	0.3563
EPE-TGV	0.1405	0.2913	0.1868	0.1471	0.6255	0.3832	0.5639	0.3263
EPE-Ours	0.1393	0.2598	0.1716	0.1438	0.6113	0.3518	0.4815	0.3595
AAE-TV	2.8458°	2.6528°	6.0472°	2.2356°	6.5780°	2.9230°	5.3784°	5.9934°
AAE-TGV	2.6014°	3.3339°	6.0431°	2.1670°	6.0920°	3.0723°	5.4091°	5.2621°
AAE-Ours	2.5336°	3.0934°	5.6276°	2.1302°	5.9385°	2.7349°	4.7173°	6.1516°

Table 2. Global error measures in images of the sequence Bandage-2 from MPI. The first and second set of results correspond, respectively, to the "clean" and "final" frames.

$Bandage - 2$	I-32	I-33	I-34	I-35	I-36	I-37	I-38
EPE-TV	0.3012	0.2635	0.2281	0.1969	0.1819	0.1831	0.1744
EPE-Ours	0.2875	0.2528	0.2200	0.1871	0.1738	0.1744	0.1646
AAE-TV	4.1854°	4.3195°	4.4798°	4.6716°	4.5370°	4.5531°	4.4934°
AAE-Ours	3.9796°	4.0286°	4.2245°	4.3852°	4.3138°	4.3766°	4.2783°
EPE-TV	0.4871	0.4125	0.3514	0.3081	0.2788	0.2538	0.2304
EPE-Ours	0.4793	0.3833	0.3380	0.2999	0.2723	0.2464	0.2208
AAE-TV	6.7334°	6.6018°	6.7360°	6.9075°	6.6736°	6.3551°	6.0901°
AAE-Ours	6.5131°	6.0037°	6.4608°	6.5416°	6.5060°	6.1108°	5.8036°

Table 3. Local error measures in images of Bandage-2 from MPI dataset. The first and second set of results correspond, respectively, to the clean and final frames.

$Bandage - 2$	I-32	I-33	I-34	I-35	I-36	I-37	I-38
EPE-TV	0.6651	0.5622	0.4984	0.4209	0.4026	0.4326	0.4052
EPE-Ours	0.6095	0.5213	0.4651	0.3847	0.3631	0.3936	0.3693
AAE-TV	5.4301°	5.6568°	6.1474°	6.4521°	6.7121°	6.8091°	6.6867°
AAE-Ours	5.1992°	5.4078°	5.9587°	6.1164°	6.2567°	6.4884°	6.3163°
EPE-TV	0.9592	0.7842	0.7031	0.6330	0.5383	0.5389	0.4877
EPE-Ours	0.9661	0.7426	0.6839	0.6086	0.5209	0.5157	0.4575
AAE-TV	8.3658°	8.9096°	9.5192°	10.0930°	9.1798°	8.8827°	8.1718°
AAE-Ours	8.6947°	8.7647°	9.6918°	9.8830°	9.1128°	8.6662°	7.8128°

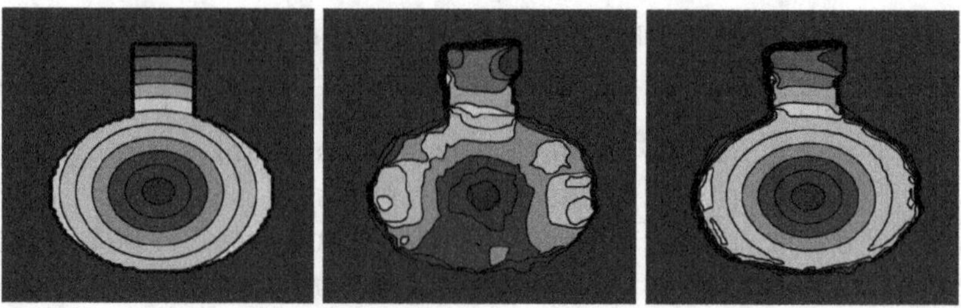

Fig. 3. Color representation of the level sets of the L^2 norm of the optical flow estimations shown in Fig. 2. *From left to right:* (**a**) ground truth, (**b**), TV regularizer, and (**c**) proposed regularized.

(see Fig. 1). We have chosen this sequence because the dragon's movement is almost a pure rotation. The quantitative results are in Table 2.

5.2 Rotation Movements

Our regularizer shows good performance in general movements, but it is specifically designed to appropriately handle rotation movements. This section contains several experiments to demonstrate the performance of our term against the TV when dealing with rotation movements in two different types of applications: motion estimation and motion inpainting. It is easy to observe how in all the figures the rotation movements look more realistic with the new regularizer and present smoother transitions as well.

Optical Flow Estimation - The following results compare the optical flow estimated by the TV$-L^1$ model [10] against the estimation obtained by solving the functional (11), i.e. an L^1 data term plus our proposed optical flow regularizer.

First, we evaluate our optical flow algorithm on a synthetic pair of images. The purpose of this synthetic sequence is to test the robustness to rotation movements. Figure 2 shows a pure anti-clockwise rotation of 3 degrees. In contrast to the TV-L^1 model, our method does not present piecewise constant zones and it is more accurate. Table 4 shows the Average Angular Error (AEE) and Average End-point Error (EPE) for both methods (TV-L^1 and our approach). Figure 3 shows a color representation of the L^2 norm of the optical flow and some of its level lines. The level lines of the ground truth flow are circles since the movement is a pure rotation. The level lines of the intensity of the estimated optical flow with the proposed regularizer are much closer to circles than the ones obtained from the flow estimated with the TV regularizer.

For the two databases with ground truth, MPI and Middlebury, we evaluate some regions that contain almost a pure rotation. The column "Local" of Table 5 shows the local errors for the RubberWhale sequence and Table 3 shows the local errors around the dragon's head in the MPI sequence. Figure 4 shows how in the

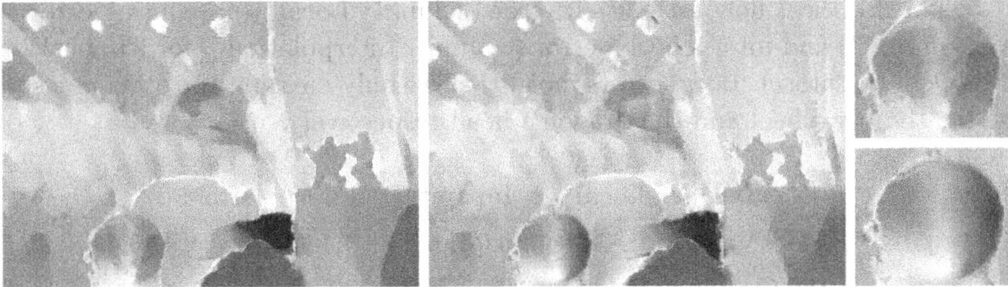

Fig. 4. Army sequence from the Middlebury dataset with a rotation movement. *From left to right* (**a**) Optical flow estimated with the TV regularizer. (**b**) Optical flow estimated with the proposed regularizer (**c**) Details of the estimations using the TV (top) and the proposed regularizer (bottom).

Army sequence the rotation movement obtained with our regularizer is more realistic than the one obtained with the TV. Figure 5 shows how our method better recovers the contour of the dragon's head and it is possible to observe little details as the eyes or the mouth.

In Fig. 7 we present another real example which consists of a video sequence of a double windmill captured by a camera with difficult light conditions. Each windmill rotates in opposite directions as is shown in the first row of Fig. 7. The last two rows of the Fig. 7 show the difference between the smooth transition of our term (third row), which agrees with the almost radially symmetric movement of a windmill, as opposite to the piecewise constant zones that appear due to the TV term (second row). Figure 6 shows this effect: it displays a color representation of the L^2 norm of the optical flow at each point and some of its level lines. Being a rotation movement, the level lines of the motion intensity should be circles, as in the synthetic example shown in Fig. 3. As seen in Fig. 6, the level lines of the optical flow norm obtained with our regularizer are closer to circles than the ones obtained with the TV, meaning that our regularization term recovers the rotation movement in a more realistic way than the TV.

Table 4. Error measures for the synthetic images in Fig. 2 of a pure rotation.

Pure Rotation	Synthetic
EPE-TV	0.0204
EPE-Ours	0.0122
AAE-TV	0.7108°
AAE-Ours	0.4351°

Optical Flow Inpainting and Interpolation from Sparse Samples - We have designed two proof of concept experiments to illustrate that the proposed regularization term is able to properly recover rotation movements. In particular,

Table 5. Local optical flow estimation error (column "Local"), inpainting error (column "Inpainting") and interpolation error (column "Interpolation") for RubberWhale, from Middlebury dataset. Local errors mean that we only measure the error in a square around the the toy wheel and the dragon's head respectively.

RubberWhale	Local	Inpainting	Interpolation
EPE-TV	0.8571	0.0611	0.4669
EPE-Ours	0.4374	0.0559	0.3088
AAE-TV	11.4892°	1.8610°	8.4497°
AAE-Ours	5.9242°	1.8118°	6.9612°

we show how it performs in reconstructing missing optical flow data and compare it to the TV. Two different cases of missing data have been addressed: data missing in a hole (we denote it as *optical flow inpainting*), and data missing along the whole image with the exception from some sparse locations (*optical flow interpolation from sparse samples*). In both cases we complete the missing data by a diffusion of the known values. The resulting diffusion depends on the smoothness term used in the minimization problem for recovering the data.

If we use the proposed regularizer, the minimization problem is

$$\min_u \int_W \left\| \frac{1}{2}\left(Du + Du^T\right) \right\|_F dx \quad \text{with } u|_{\partial W} = u_0|_{\partial W}, \tag{22}$$

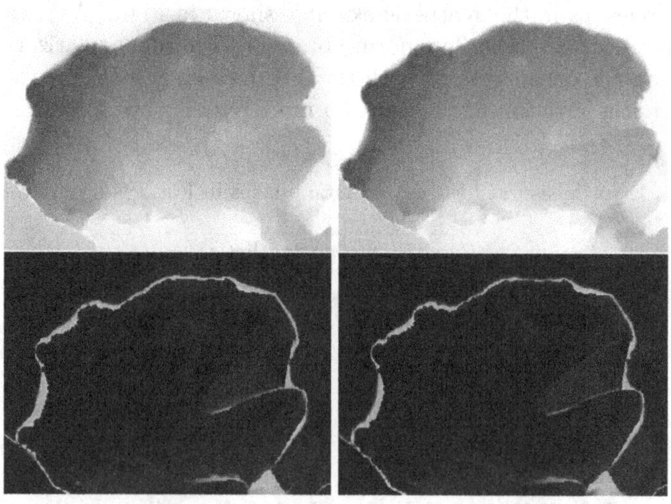

Fig. 5. Dragon's head zoom. *First row: Optical flow with an L^1 data term and* (**a**) the TV regularizer, (**b**) the proposed regularizer. *Second row: EPE.* (**c**) TV. (**d**) The proposed regularizer.

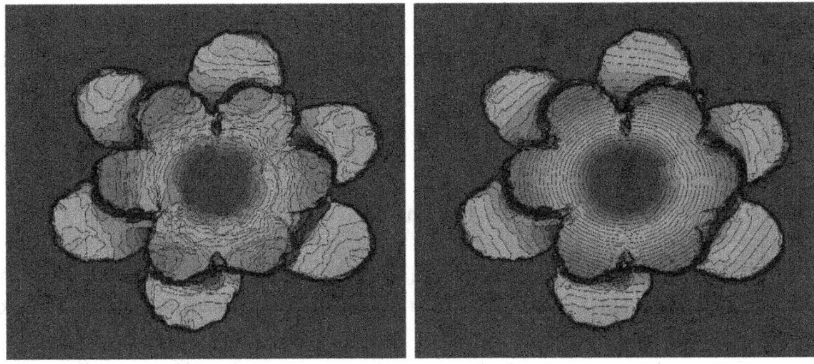

Fig. 6. Color representation of the level sets of the L^2 norm of the optical flow estimations shown in Fig. 7. *From left to right:* (**a**) TV regularizer. (**b**) The proposed regularizer (Color figure online).

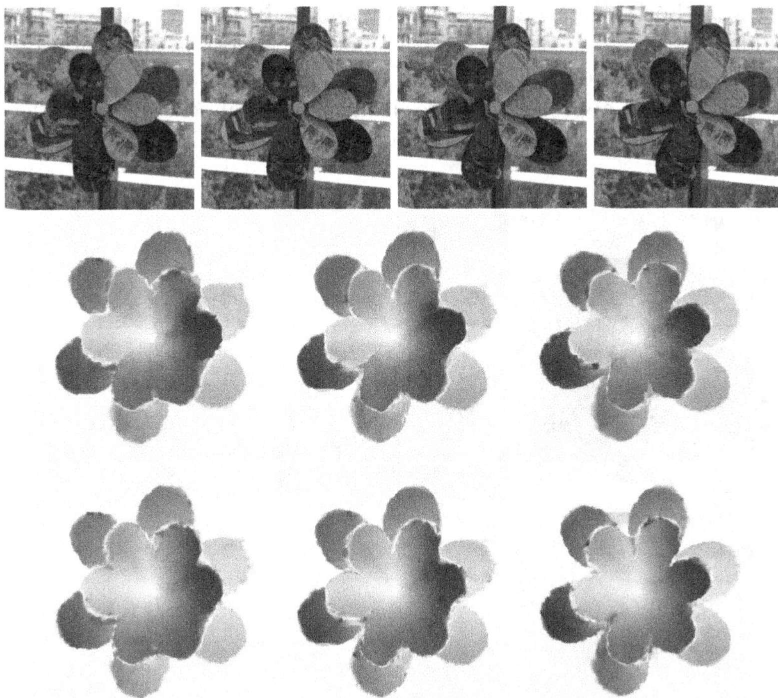

Fig. 7. Double windmill sequence. *From top to bottom:* (**a**) Original frames, (**b**) TV-L^1 optical flow and (**c**) optical flow estimated with an L^1 data term and the proposed regularizer.

where W is the missing data domain and u_0 is the known flow field in the complement of the set W. Also, the minimization problem based on the TV is

$$\min_{u} \int_{W} (|\nabla u_1| + |\nabla u_2|)\, dx \quad \text{with } u|_{\partial W} = u_0|_{\partial W}. \tag{23}$$

W is defined in the following ways for the two kind of applications:

- **Optical flow inpainting** - Squared patches are removed from the flow field (and u is initialized to zero in these regions). The motion in the known regions, u_0, is the optical flow ground truth. Regions where the ground truth is unknown also form part of the inpainting domain W, together with the squared patches.
- **Optical flow interpolation from sparse samples** - We remove the optical flow values in the 95 % of the pixels (uniformly distributed along the image). Therefore, W is made of this 95 % of pixels. Again, u_0 is defined from the optical flow ground truth.

For testing both regularization terms we use the RubberWhale sequence from the Middelbury dataset [22] because it contains almost a pure rotation. For both cases of missing data we solve the minimization problems (22) and (23) using a primal-dual approach. The resulting numerical scheme for (22) is the one explained in Proposition 1 without the terms depending on the parameter θ

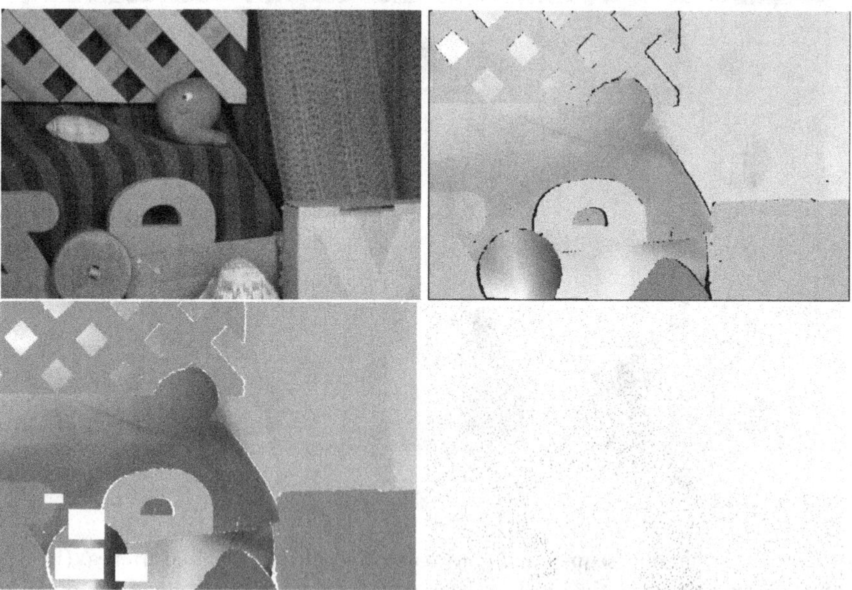

Fig. 8. RubberWhale sequence from the Middlebury dataset with a rotation movement. *First row:* (**a**) First frame. (**b**) Ground Truth. *Second row:* (**c**) Inpainting mask (in white). (**d**) Missing optical flow (white pixels) and known values at sparse locations.

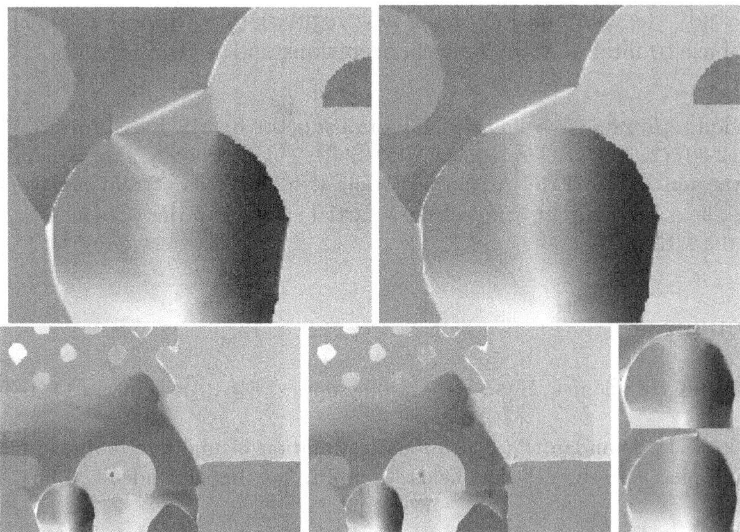

Fig. 9. Optical flow reconstruction in missing regions. *First row (from left to right):* Inpainting results. (**a**) TV regularizer. (**b**) Proposed regularizer. *Second row (from left to right):* Interpolation from sparse samples (**c**) TV regularizer. (**d**) Proposed regularizer. (**e**) Details, TV regularizer (top) and the proposed regularizer (bottom).

and with a final step that sets the boundary conditions (known optical flow in ∂W). Figures 8, 9 and Table 5 refer to this experiment. The last row of Fig. 8 shows the regions where the optical flow is missing for both kind of applications. Figure 9 shows the reconstructions obtained with the two regularizers in both experiments. Table 5 shows the quantitative results, showing that the optical flow completion based on the proposed regularizer presents a lower reconstruction error than the one based on the TV.

6 Conclusion

We have proposed a new regularization term for optical flow models with the properties of invariance to infinitesimal rotations and the ability to preserve discontinuities/jumps in the flow field. The proposed regularizer has been tested in three different kind of problems related to the optical flow: motion estimation, motion inpainting, and motion interpolation from sparse samples. For the optical flow estimation we combine it with an L^1 data fidelity term, as in [10], and the proposed variational problem is solved using a dual formulation. The numerical experiments show that the proposed regularization term combined with an L^1 data term improves the TV-L^1 model for motion estimation. For the other two problems, optical flow reconstruction in two different cases of missing regions, we show that the missing information is better recovered with a functional based on the proposed regularizer, compared to the TV regularizer. As future work we plan to study the combination of the new regularizer with more advanced data terms robust to illumination changes, occlusions and fast movements.

Acknowledgement. We acknowledge partial support by MICINN project, reference MTM2012-30772, by GRC reference 2009 SGR 773 funded by the Generalitat de Catalunya, and by the ERC Advanced Grant INPAINTING (Grant agreement no.: 319899). The second author acknowledges partial support to the Ramón y Cajal program of the MINECO.

References

1. Horn, B.K.P., Schunck, B.G.: Determining optical flow. Artif. Intell. **17**(1–3), 185–203 (1981)
2. Black, M.J., Anandan, P.: The robust estimation of multiple motions: parametric and piecewise-smooth flow fields. Comput. Vis. Image Underst. **63**(1), 75–104 (1996)
3. Zimmer, H., Bruhn, A., Weickert, J.: Optic flow in harmony. Int. J. Comput. Vis. **93**(3), 368–388 (2011)
4. Nagel, H.H., Enkelmann, W.: An Investigation of smoothness constraints for the estimation of displacement vector fields from image sequences. IEEE Trans. Pattern Anal. Mach. Intell. **8**(5), 565–593 (1986)
5. Wedel, A., Cremers D., Pock, T., Bischof, H.: Structure-and motion-adaptative regularization for high accuracy optic flow. In: IEEE 12th International Conference on Computer Vision, pp. 1663–1668 (2009)
6. Werlberger, M., Trobin, W., Pock, T., Wedel, A., Cremers, D., Bischof, H.: Anisotropic Huber-L1 optical flow. In: Proceedings of the British Machine Vision Conference (2009)
7. Weickert, J., Schnörr, C.: A theoretical framework for convex regularizers in PDE-based computation of image motion. Int. J. Comput. Vis. **45**(3), 245–264 (2001)
8. Trobin, W., Pock, T., Cremers, D., Bischof, H.: An unbiased second-order prior for high-accuracy motion estimation. In: Rigoll, G. (ed.) DAGM 2008. LNCS, vol. 5096, pp. 396–405. Springer, Heidelberg (2008)
9. Rudin, L.I., Osher, S., Fatemi, E.: Nonlinear total variation based noise removal algorithms. J. Phys. D Appl. Phys. **60**, 259–268 (1992)
10. Zach, C., Pock, T., Bischof, H.: A duality based approach for realtime TV-L1 optical flow. In: Hamprecht, F.A., Schnörr, C., Jähne, B. (eds.) DAGM 2007. LNCS, vol. 4713, pp. 214–223. Springer, Heidelberg (2007)
11. Wedel, A., Pock, T., Braun, J., Franke, U., Cremers, D.: Duality TV-L1 flow with fundamental matrix prior. In: 23rd International Conference Image and Vision Computing, pp. 1–6, New Zealand (2008)
12. Rosman, G., Shem-Tov, S., Bitton, D., Nir, T., Adiv, G., Kimmel, R., Feuer, A., Bruckstein, A.M.: Over-parameterized optical flow using a stereoscopic constraint. In: Bruckstein, A.M., ter Haar Romeny, B.M., Bronstein, A.M., Bronstein, M.M. (eds.) SSVM 2011. LNCS, vol. 6667, pp. 761–772. Springer, Heidelberg (2012)
13. Kondermann, C., Kondermann, D., Garbe, C.S.: Postprocessing of optical flows via surface measures and motion inpainting. In: Rigoll, G. (ed.) DAGM 2008. LNCS, vol. 5096, pp. 355–364. Springer, Heidelberg (2008)

14. Matsushita, Y., Ofek, E., Ge, W., Tang, X., Shum, H.-Y.: Full-frame video stabilization with motion inpainting. IEEE Trans. Pattern Anal. Mach. Intell. **28**(7), 1150–1163 (2006)
15. Shiratori, T, Matsushita, Y.: Video completion by motion field transfer. In: IEEE Computer Society Conference on Computer Vision and Pattern Recognition, pp. 411–418 (2006)
16. Chorin, A.J., Marsden, J.E.: A Mathematical Introduction to Fluid Mechanics: Texts in Applied Mathematics. Springer, New York (1990)
17. Strekalovskiy, E., Chambolle, A., Cremers, D.: Convex relaxation of vectorial problems with coupled regularization. SIAM J. Imaging Sci. **7**, 294–336 (2014)
18. Berkels, B., Rätz, A., Rumpf, M., Voigt, A.: Extracting Grain boundaries and macroscopic deformations from images on atomic scale. J. Sci. Comput. **35**(1), 1–23 (2007)
19. Chambolle, A., Pock, T.: A first-order primal-dual algorithm for convex problems with applications to imaging. J. Math. Imaging Vis. **40**(1), 120–145 (2011)
20. Chambolle, A.: An algorithm for total variation minimization and applications. J. Math. Imaging Vis. **20**, 89–97 (2004)
21. Sánchez Pérez, J., Meinhardt-Llopis, E., Facciolo, G.: TV-L1 Optical Flow Estimation. Image Processing On Line (IPOL), pp. 137–150 (2013)
22. Baker, S., Scharstein, D., Lewis, J.P., Roth, S., Black, M.J., Szeliski, R.: A database and evaluation methodology for optical flow. Int. J. Comput. Vis. **92**, 1–31 (2010)
23. Butler, D.J., Wulff, J., Stanley, G.B., Black, M.J.: A naturalistic open source movie for optical flow evaluation. In: Fitzgibbon, A., Lazebnik, S., Perona, P., Sato, Y., Schmid, C. (eds.) ECCV 2012, Part VI. LNCS, vol. 7577, pp. 611–625. Springer, Heidelberg (2012)
24. Bredies, K.: Recovering piecewise smooth multichannel images by minimization of convex functionals with total generalized variation penalty. In: Bruhn, A., Pock, T., Tai, X.-C. (eds.) Efficient Algorithms for Global Optimization Methods in Computer Vision. LNCS, vol. 8293, pp. 44–77. Springer, Heidelberg (2014)

Landmark-Based Inductive Model for Robust Discriminative Tracking

Yuwei Wu(✉), Mingtao Pei, Min Yang, Yang He, and Yunde Jia

Beijing Laboratory of Intelligent Information Technology,
School of Computer Science, Beijing Institute of Technology,
Beijing 10081, People's Republic of China
wuyuwei@bit.edu.cn
http://iitlab.bit.edu.cn/mcislab/~wuyuwei/

Abstract. The appearance of an object could be continuously changing during tracking, thereby being not independent identically distributed. A good discriminative tracker often needs a large number of training samples to fit the underlying data distribution, which is impractical for visual tracking. In this paper, we present a new discriminative tracker via the landmark-based inductive model (Lim) that is non-parametric and makes no specific assumption about the sample distribution. With an undirected graph representation of samples, the Lim locally approximates the soft label of each sample by a linear combination of labels on its nearby landmarks. It is able to effectively propagate a limited amount of initial labels to a large amount of unlabeled samples. To this end, we introduce a local landmarks approximation method to compute the cross-similarity matrix between the whole data and landmarks. And a soft label prediction function incorporating the graph Laplacian regularizer is used to diffuse the known labels to all the unlabeled vertices in the graph, which explicitly considers the local geometrical structure of all samples. Tracking is then carried out within a Bayesian inference framework where the soft label prediction value is used to construct the observation model. Both qualitative and quantitative evaluations on 65 challenging image sequences including the benchmark dataset and other public sequences demonstrate that the proposed algorithm outperforms the state-of-the-art methods.

1 Introduction

An appearance model is one of the most critical prerequisites for successful visual tracking. Designing an effective appearance model is still a challenging task due to appearance variations caused by background clutter, object deformation, partial occlusions, and illumination changes, *etc.* Numerous tracking algorithms have been proposed to address this issue [1], and existing tracking algorithms can be roughly categorized as either generative [2–7] or discriminative [8–15] approaches. Generative methods build an object representation, and then search for the region most similar to the object. However, generative models do not take into account background information. Discriminative methods train an online

D. Cremers et al. (Eds.): ACCV 2014, Part V, LNCS 9007, pp. 320–335, 2015.
DOI: 10.1007/978-3-319-16814-2_21

binary classifier to adaptively separate the object from the background, which are more robust against appearance variations of an object. In this paper, we focus on the discriminative tracking method.

In visual tracking applications, the samples obtained by the tracker are drawn from an unknown underlying data distribution. The appearance of an object could be continuously changing and thus it is impossible to be independent and identically distributed (*i.i.d*). A good discriminative tracker often needs a large number of labeled samples to adequately fit the real data distribution [16]. This is because if the dimensionality of the data is large compared to the number of the samples, then many statistical learning methods predict overfitting due to the "curse of dimensionality". However, precisely labeled samples only come from the first frame during tracking, *i.e.*, the number of labeled samples is very small. To acquire more labeled samples, in most existing discriminative tracking approaches, the current tracking result is used to extract positive samples and the surrounding regions are used to extract negative samples. Once the tracker location is not precise, the assigned labels may be noisy. Over time the accumulation of errors can degrade the classifier and cause drift. This situation makes us wonder: *with a very small number of labeled samples, whether we can design a new discriminative tracker which makes no specific assumption about the sample distribution.*

In this paper, we take full advantage of the geometric structure of the data and thus present a new discriminative tracking approach with the landmark-based inductive model (Lim). The Lim locally approximates the soft label of each sample by a linear combination of labels on its nearby landmarks. It is able to effectively propagate a limited amount of initial labels to a large amount of unlabeled samples, matching the needs of discriminative trackers. Under the graph representation of samples, the local landmarks approximation is employed to design a sparse and nonnegative adjacency matrix characterizing relationship among all samples. Based on the Nesterov's gradient projection algorithm, an efficient numerical algorithm is developed to solve the problem of the local landmarks approximation with guaranteed quadratic convergence. Furthermore, the object function of the label prediction provides a promising paradigm for modeling the geometrical structures of samples via Laplacian regularizer. Preserving the local manifold structure of samples can make our tracker have more discriminating power to handle appearance changes.

Specifically, the proposed method treats both labeled and unlabeled samples as vertices in a graph and builds edges which are weighted by the affinities (similarities) between the corresponding sample pairs. For each new frame, candidates predicted by the particle filter are considered as unlabeled samples and utilized to constitute a new graph representation together with the collected samples stored in the sample pool. A small number of landmarks obtained from the entire sample space enable nonparametric regression that calculates the soft label of each sample as a locally weighted average of labels on landmarks. Tracking is carried out within a Bayesian inference framework where the soft label prediction value is used to construct the observation model. A candidate with the highest classification score is considered as the tracking result. To alleviate the drift problem, once the tracked object is located, the labels of the newly collected samples are assigned according to the classification score of the current tracking results, in which no self-labeling is involved. The proposed tracker adapts to drastic appearance variations, as validated in our experiments.

1.1 Related Work

Discriminative tracking has received wide attention for its adaptive ability to handle appearance changes. The essential component of discriminative trackers is the classifier updating. Straightforward appearance update with newly obtained results could result in incorrectly labeled training samples and degrade the models gradually with drifts. Grabner *et al.* [9] employed an online semi-supervised learning framework to train a classifier which is less susceptible to drift but not adaptive enough to handle fast appearance changes. Babenko *et al.* [11] integrated multiple instance learning (MIL) into online boosting algorithm to alleviate the drift problem. In the MIL tracking, the classifier is updated with positive and negative bags rather than individual labeled examples. Kalal *et al.* [13] developed a semi-supervised learning approach (*i.e.*, P-N learning) to train a binary classifier with structured unlabeled data. Zhang and Maaten [17] developed a structure-preserving object tracker that learns spatial constraints between objects using an online structured SVM algorithm to improve the performance of single-object or multi-object tracking. Wu *et al.* [18] addressed visual tracking by learning a suitable metric matrix in the feature space of local sparse codes to effectively capture appearance variations.

Different from the schemes of the classifier updating in [9,11,13,18], in which candidates are not used to train the classifier, and therefore the class labels of them are assigned by the previous classifier. In our tracker, for each new frame, candidates are considered as unlabeled samples and utilized to constitute a new graph representation to update the current classifier. Explicitly taking into account the local manifold structure of labeled and unlabeled samples, we introduce a soft label propagation method defined over the graph, which has more discriminating power. In addition, once the tracked object is located, the discriminative appearance models are online updated in the manner of both supervised and unsupervised which makes our tracker more stable and adaptive to appearance changes. More details are discussed in Sect. 3.

Recently, researchers utilize the graph-based discriminative learning to construct the object appearance model for visual tracking. With the 2nd-order tensor representation, Gao *et al.* [19] designed two graphs for characterizing the intrinsic local geometrical structure of the tensor space. Based on the least square support vector machine, Li *et al.* [20] exploited a hypergraph propagation method to capture the contextual information on samples, which further improves the tracking accuracy. Kumar and Vleeschouwer [21] constructed a number of distinct graphs (*i.e.*, spatiotemporal, appearance and exclusion) to capture the spatio-temporal and the appearance information. Then, they formulated the multi-object tracking as a consistent labeling problem in the associated graphs.

Our method differs from [19,20] both in the graph construction and the label propagation method. Methods in [19,20] construct the graph representation using kNN whose computational cost is expensive. In contrast, employing local landmarks approximation, we design a new form of the adjacency matrix characterizing relationship between all samples. The total time complexity scales linearly with the number of samples. More importantly, our method is an inductive model which can be used to infer the labels of unseen data (*i.e.*, candidates). Only a few samples are selected and used to learn a new discriminative model. The label of each sample can be interpreted as the weighted combination of the labels on landmarks. Graph Laplacian is incorporated into the object function of inductive learning as a regularizer to preserve the local geometrical structure of samples.

2 Landmark-Based Inductive Model

2.1 Problem Description

Suppose that we have l labeled samples $\{(\boldsymbol{x}_i, \boldsymbol{y}_i)\}_{i=1}^{l}$ and u unlabeled samples $\{\boldsymbol{x}_i\}_{i=l+1}^{l+u}$, where $\boldsymbol{x}_i \in \mathbb{R}^d$, and $\boldsymbol{y}_i \in \mathbb{R}^c$ is the label vector. Denote $\boldsymbol{X} = \{x_1, x_2, \cdots, x_n\} \in \mathbb{R}^{d \times n}$ and $\boldsymbol{Y}_l = \{\boldsymbol{y}_1, \boldsymbol{y}_2, \cdots, \boldsymbol{y}_l\} \in \mathbb{R}^{l \times c}$, where $n = l + u$. If $\boldsymbol{x}_i$ belongs to the kth class ($1 \leq k \leq c$), the kth entry in $\boldsymbol{y}_i$ is 1 and all the other entries are 0's. In this paper, the data $\boldsymbol{X}$ is represented by the undirected graph $\mathcal{G} = \{\boldsymbol{X}, \boldsymbol{E}\}$, where the set of vertices is $\boldsymbol{X} = \{\boldsymbol{x}_i\}$ and the set of edges is $\boldsymbol{E} = \{e_{ij}\}$, where e_{ij} denotes the similarity between $\boldsymbol{x}_i$ and $\boldsymbol{x}_j$. Define a soft label prediction (*i.e.*, classification) function $f : \mathbb{R}^d \rightarrow \mathbb{R}^c$. A crucial component of our method is the estimation of a weighted graph $\mathcal{G}$ from $\boldsymbol{X}$. Then, the soft label of any sample can be inferred using $\mathcal{G}$ and known labels Y_l.

The time complexity of traditional graph-based semi-supervised learning methods is usually $O(n^3)$ with respect to the data size n, because $n \times n$ kernel matrix (*e.g.*, multiplication or inverse) is calculated in inferring the label prediction. Full-size label prediction is infeasible when n is large, the work of [22] inspired us to exploit the idea of landmark samples. To accomplish the soft label prediction, we employ an economical and practical prediction function expressed as

$$f(\boldsymbol{x}) = \sum_{k=1}^{m} K(\boldsymbol{x}, \boldsymbol{d}_k)\boldsymbol{a}_k. \tag{1}$$

The idea of this formulation is that the label of each sample can be interpreted as the locally weighted average of variables $\boldsymbol{a}_k$'s defined on m landmarks [22,23]. As a trade-off between computational efficiency and effectiveness, in this paper, k-means algorithm is used to select the centers as the set of landmarks $\boldsymbol{D} = \{\boldsymbol{d}_k\}_{k=1}^{m} \in \mathbb{R}^{d \times m}$.

Equation (1) is deemed as a inductive model, because it can diffuse the label of landmarks to all unlabeled samples, as discussed in Sect. 2.4. The above model can be written in a matrix form

$$\boldsymbol{f} = \boldsymbol{H}\boldsymbol{A}, \tag{2}$$

where $\boldsymbol{f} = [f(\boldsymbol{x}_1), f(\boldsymbol{x}_2), \cdots, f(\boldsymbol{x}_n)]^\top \in \mathbb{R}^{n\times c}$ is the landmark-based label prediction function on all samples. $\boldsymbol{A} = [f(\boldsymbol{d}_1), f(\boldsymbol{d}_2), \cdots, f(\boldsymbol{d}_m)]^\top = [\boldsymbol{A}_1, \boldsymbol{A}_2, \cdots, \boldsymbol{A}_c] \in \mathbb{R}^{m\times c}$ denotes the label of landmarks $\boldsymbol{d}_k$'s. $\boldsymbol{H} \in \mathbb{R}^{n\times m}$ is the cross-similarity matrix between the whole data $\boldsymbol{X}$ and landmarks $\boldsymbol{d}_k$,

$$\boldsymbol{H}_{ik} = K(\boldsymbol{x}_i, \boldsymbol{d}_k) > 0, 1 \le i \le n, 1 \le k \le m.$$

In what follows, we will elaborate how to effectively solve $\boldsymbol{A}$ and $\boldsymbol{H}$.

2.2 Solving Optimal $\boldsymbol{H}$

Typically, we may employ Gaussian kernel or Epanechnikov quadratic kernel to compute $\boldsymbol{H}$. However, how to choose appropriate kernel bandwidths is difficult. Instead of adopting the predefined kernel, we learn an optimal $\boldsymbol{H}$ by considering the geometric structure information between labeled and unlabeled samples. We reconstruct $\boldsymbol{x}_i$ as a combination of its s closest landmarks in the feature space. In this work, we set $s = 10$. Similar to locality-constrained linear coding (LLC) [24], a local landmarks approximation method is proposed to optimize the coefficient vector $\boldsymbol{h}_i \in \mathbb{R}^s$:

$$\begin{aligned} \min_{\boldsymbol{h}_i \in \mathbb{R}^s} g(\boldsymbol{h}_i) &= \frac{1}{2}\left\| \boldsymbol{x}_i - \sum_{j=1}^{s} \boldsymbol{d}_j \boldsymbol{h}_i \right\|^2, \\ s.t. \quad \boldsymbol{1}^\top \boldsymbol{h}_i &= 1, \ \boldsymbol{h}_i \ge 0 \end{aligned} \tag{3}$$

where s entries of the vector $\boldsymbol{h}_i$ correspond to s coefficients contributed by s nearest landmarks. The constraint $\boldsymbol{1}^\top \boldsymbol{h}_i = 1$ follows the shift-invariant requirements. The main difference between LLC and our method is that we incorporate inequality constraints (*i.e.*, non-negative constraints) into the object function as we require the similarity measure to be a positive value. Therefore we need to develop a different optimization algorithm to solve Eq. (3). In this section, Nesterov's gradient projection (NGP) method [25], a first-order optimization procedure, is employed to solve the constrained optimization problem Eq. (3). A key step of NGP is how to efficiently project a vector $\boldsymbol{h}_i$ onto the corresponding constraint set C.

Denote $\mathcal{Q}_{\beta,\boldsymbol{v}}(\boldsymbol{h}_i) = g(\boldsymbol{v}) + \nabla g(\boldsymbol{v})^\top (\boldsymbol{h}_i - \boldsymbol{v}) + \frac{\beta}{2}\|\boldsymbol{h}_i - \boldsymbol{v}\|_2^2$, as the first-order Taylor expansion of $g(\boldsymbol{h}_i)$ at $\boldsymbol{v}$ with the squared Euclidean distance between $\boldsymbol{h}_i$ and $\boldsymbol{v}$ as a regularization term. Here $\nabla g(\boldsymbol{v})$ is the gradient of $g(\boldsymbol{h}_i)$ at $\boldsymbol{v}$. We can easily obtain

$$\min_{\boldsymbol{h}_i \in C} \mathcal{Q}_{\beta,\boldsymbol{v}}(\boldsymbol{h}_i) = \Pi_C\Big(\boldsymbol{v} - \frac{1}{\beta}\nabla g(\boldsymbol{v})\Big), \tag{4}$$

where $\Pi_C(\boldsymbol{v}) = \min_{\boldsymbol{v}' \in C} \|\boldsymbol{v} - \boldsymbol{v}'\|_2^2$ is the Euclidean projection of $\boldsymbol{v}$ onto C [26]. The projection operator $\Pi_C(\cdot)$ has been implemented efficiently in $O(s \log s)$.

From Eq. (4), the solution of Eq. (3) can be obtained by generating a sequence $\{\boldsymbol{h}_i^{(t)}\}$ at $\boldsymbol{v}^{(t)} = \boldsymbol{h}_i^{(t)} + \alpha_t(\boldsymbol{h}_i^{(t)} - \boldsymbol{h}_i^{(t-1)})$, *i.e.*,

$$\boldsymbol{h}_i^{(t+1)} = \Pi_C\Big(\boldsymbol{v}^{(t)} - \frac{1}{\beta_t}\nabla g(\boldsymbol{v}^{(t)})\Big) = \min_{\boldsymbol{h}_i \in C} \mathcal{Q}_{\beta_t,\boldsymbol{v}^{(t)}}(\boldsymbol{h}_i). \tag{5}$$

In NGP, choosing proper parameters β_t and α_t is also significant for the convergence property. Similar to [25], we set $\alpha_t = (\delta_{t-1} - 1)/\delta_t$ with $\delta_t = \big(1 + \sqrt{1 + 4\delta_{t-1}^2}\big)/2$, $\delta_0 = 0$ and $\delta_1 = 1$. β_t is selected by finding the smallest nonnegative integer j such that $g(\boldsymbol{h}_i) \leq \mathcal{Q}_{\beta_t, \boldsymbol{v}^{(t)}}(\boldsymbol{h}_i)$ with $\beta_t = 2^j \beta_{t-1}$.

After getting the optimal weight vector $\boldsymbol{h}_i$, we set $\boldsymbol{H}_{ij'} = \boldsymbol{h}_i$, where j' is the indices corresponding to the s nearest landmarks and the cardinality $|j'| = s$. For the rest entries of $\boldsymbol{H}_i$, we set 0's. Apparently, $\boldsymbol{H}_{ij} = 0$ when landmark $\boldsymbol{d}_j$ is far away from $\boldsymbol{x}_i$ and $\boldsymbol{H}_{ij} \neq 0$ is only for the s closest landmarks of $\boldsymbol{x}_i$. In contrast to weights defined by kernel function (*e.g.*, Gaussian kernel), the local landmarks approximation method is able to provides optimized and sparser weights, as validated in our experiments.

2.3 Solving Label Prediction Matrix $\boldsymbol{A}$

Note that the adjacency matrix $\boldsymbol{W} \in \mathbb{R}^{n \times n}$ between all samples encountered in practice usually have low numerical-rank compared with the matrix size [27]. We consider *whether we can construct a nonnegative and empirically sparse graph adjacency matrix* $\boldsymbol{W}$ *with the nonnegative and sparse* $\boldsymbol{H} \in \mathbb{R}^{n \times m}$ *introduced in Sect.* 2.2. Intuitively, we can design the adjacency matrix $\boldsymbol{W}$ to be a low-rank form

$$\boldsymbol{W} = \boldsymbol{H}\boldsymbol{H}^\top, \tag{6}$$

where the inner product is regarded as the metric to measure the adjacent weight between samples. Equation (6) implies that if two samples are correlative (*i.e.*, $\boldsymbol{W}_{ij} > 0$), they share at least one landmark, otherwise $\boldsymbol{W}_{ij} = 0$. $\boldsymbol{W}$ defined in Eq. (6) naturally preserves some good properties (*e.g.*, sparseness and nonnegativeness).

To compute the label prediction matrix $\boldsymbol{A}$, we exploit the following optimization framework [22]:

$$\min L(\boldsymbol{f}_l, \boldsymbol{y}_l) + \eta \|\boldsymbol{f}\|_{\mathcal{G}}. \tag{7}$$

Here $L(\cdot,\cdot)$ is an empirical loss function, which requires that the prediction $\boldsymbol{f}$ should be consistent with the known class labels. η is a positive regularization parameter. $\boldsymbol{f}_l \in \mathbb{R}^{l \times c}$ is the sub-matrix corresponding to the labeled samples in $\boldsymbol{f} \in \mathbb{R}^{n \times c}$. Discriminative models take tracking as a binary classification task to separate the object from its surrounding background. In this case, $c = 2$. $\|f\|_{\mathcal{G}} = tr(\boldsymbol{f}^\top \boldsymbol{L} \boldsymbol{f})$ enforces the smoothness of $\boldsymbol{f}$ with regard to the manifold structure of the graph, where $\boldsymbol{L} \in \mathbb{R}^{n \times n}$ is the graph-based regularization matrix. Usually $\boldsymbol{L} = \boldsymbol{\Sigma} - \boldsymbol{W}$, where $\boldsymbol{\Sigma} = diag(\boldsymbol{W}\mathbf{1})$ is the vertex degree matrix of $\mathcal{G}$.

With the design of $\boldsymbol{W}$, Laplacian graph regularization can be approximated as

$$\boldsymbol{f}^\top \boldsymbol{L} \boldsymbol{f} = \boldsymbol{f}^\top (diag(\boldsymbol{H}\boldsymbol{H}^\top \mathbf{1}) - \boldsymbol{H}\boldsymbol{H}^\top)\boldsymbol{f}, \tag{8}$$

where nonnegative $\boldsymbol{W}$ guarantees the positive semi-definite (PSD) property of $\boldsymbol{L}$. Keeping PSD $\boldsymbol{L}$ is important to ensure that the graph regularizer $\boldsymbol{f}^\top \boldsymbol{L} \boldsymbol{f}$ is convex.

By plugging $\boldsymbol{f} = \boldsymbol{HA}$ into Eq. (7) and choosing the loss function $L(\cdot,\cdot)$ as the $L2$-norm, the convex differentiable object function for solving label prediction matrix $\boldsymbol{A}$ can be formulated as

$$\min_{\boldsymbol{A}} \mathcal{L}(\boldsymbol{A}) = \frac{\eta}{2} tr((\boldsymbol{HA})^\top \boldsymbol{L}(\boldsymbol{HA})) + \|\boldsymbol{H}_l \boldsymbol{A} - \boldsymbol{Y}_l\|_F^2. \tag{9}$$

Here, $\boldsymbol{H}_l \in \mathbb{R}^{l \times m}$ is the rows in $\boldsymbol{H}$ that corresponds to the labeled samples, and $\boldsymbol{L}$ is defined in Eq. (8). By setting the derivative w.r.t. $\boldsymbol{A}$ to zero, we easily obtain the globally optimal solution to Eq. (9):

$$\boldsymbol{A}^* = \left(\boldsymbol{H}_l^\top \boldsymbol{H}_l + \eta \boldsymbol{H}^\top \boldsymbol{L} \boldsymbol{H}\right)^{-1} \boldsymbol{H}_l^\top \boldsymbol{Y}_l. \tag{10}$$

2.4 Soft Label Propagation

Through applying the inductive model Eq. (2), we are able to predict the soft label for any sample $\boldsymbol{x}_i$ (unlabeled training samples or novel test samples) as

$$\widehat{f}(\boldsymbol{x}_i) = \max_{k \in \{1,2\}} \frac{\boldsymbol{H}(\boldsymbol{x}_i)\, \boldsymbol{A}_k}{\boldsymbol{1}^\top \boldsymbol{H} \boldsymbol{A}_k}, \tag{11}$$

where $\{\boldsymbol{A}_k\}_{k=1}^c \in \mathbb{R}^{m \times 1}$ is the column vector of $\boldsymbol{A}$, and $\boldsymbol{H}(\boldsymbol{x}_i) \in \mathbb{R}^{1 \times m}$ represents the weight between $\boldsymbol{x}$ and landmarks $\boldsymbol{d}_k$'s. Specifically, if $\boldsymbol{x}_i$ belongs to unlabeled training samples, $\boldsymbol{H}(\boldsymbol{x}_i) = \boldsymbol{H}_i$ where $\boldsymbol{H}_i$ denotes the i-th row of $\boldsymbol{H}$, $i = l+1, \cdots, n$. If $\boldsymbol{x}_i$ is a novel test sample, we need to compute the vector $\boldsymbol{H}_i$ as $\boldsymbol{H}(\boldsymbol{x}_i)$ described in Sect. 2.2, then update $\boldsymbol{H} \in \mathbb{R}^{(n+1) \times m}$, *i.e.*, $\boldsymbol{H} \leftarrow [\boldsymbol{H}; \boldsymbol{H}_i]$. After deriving the soft label prediction (*i.e.*, classification) of each sample, the classification score can be utilized as the similarity measure for tracking. In the next section, we will elaborate the application of the proposed landmark-based inductive model in tracking.

3 Lim Tracker

In our tracking framework, the object is represented by five different image patches inside the object region. These five image patches correspond to the five parts of an object, respectively, as exemplified in Fig. 1. Therefore, image patches corresponding to the certain part of all samples are able to construct a sub-sample set $\boldsymbol{X}^{(\tau)}$, $\tau = 1, 2, \cdots, 5$. Each sub-sample set $\boldsymbol{X}^{(\tau)}$ is used to train a single classifier $\boldsymbol{f}^{(\tau)}$ using the inductive model predefined in Eq. (2). The final tracking result can be determined by the sum of the classification scores of the five image patches inside the object region:

$$SC = \sum_{\tau=1}^{5} \omega_\tau \boldsymbol{f}^{(\tau)}, \tag{12}$$

where ω_τ is the weight of τ-th image patch ($\sum_{\tau=1}^5 \omega_\tau = 1$ and $\omega_\tau = 0.2$ in the experiments). This part-based scheme could potentially alleviate the drift caused by partial occlusions.

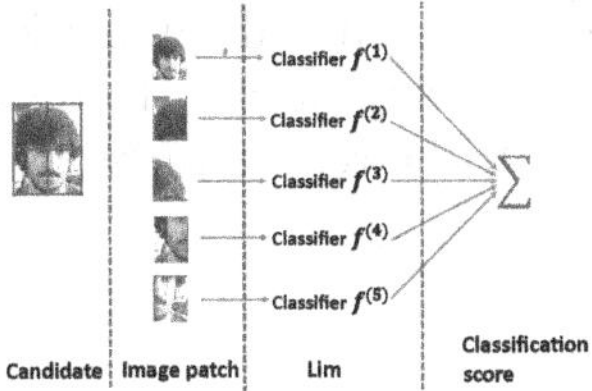

Fig. 1. Object representation using five different image patches. The candidate is normalized to the same size (24×24 in our experiment), each image patch is with 12×12.

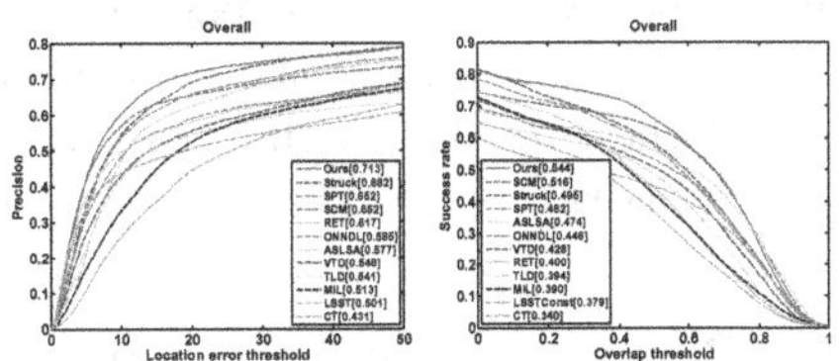

Fig. 2. Overall performance comparisons of precision plot and success rate. The performance score for each tracker is shown in the legend (best viewed on high-resolution display)

To initialize the classifier in the first frame, we draw positive and negative samples around the target location. Suppose the target is labeled manually, perturbation (e.g., shifting 1 or 2 pixels) around the object is performed for collecting N_p positive samples $\boldsymbol{X}_{N_p}$. Similarly, N_n negative samples $\boldsymbol{X}_{N_n}$ are collected far away from the located object (e.g., within an annular region a few pixels away from the object). $\boldsymbol{X}_1 = \boldsymbol{X}_{N_p} \bigcup \boldsymbol{X}_{N_n}$ is the initialized labeled sample set. K-means algorithm is exploited to select the centers as the set of landmarks $\boldsymbol{D}$. Using labeled samples and landmarks, we can train a prior classifier via the Lim.

For each new frame, candidates predicted by the particle filter are considered as unlabeled samples $\widehat{\boldsymbol{X}}$. According to Eq. (11), we can get the classification score of each candidate. A candidate with higher classification score indicates that it is more likely to be generated from the target class. The most likely candidate is considered as the tracking result for this frame. Then, perturbation (*i.e.*, the same scheme in the first frame) around the tracking result is performed for collecting sample set $\boldsymbol{X}_C$. If the classification score of the located object is higher than the predefined threshold ϵ (*i.e.*, the current tracking result is reliable), samples in $\boldsymbol{X}_C$ are regarded as labeled ones, otherwise regarded as unlabeled ones. That is, samples are collected in the manner of both supervised and unsupervised, and thus the stability and adaptivity in tracking objects of changing appearance are preserved.

3.1 Update the Classifier

We construct a *sample pool* $\boldsymbol{X}_P$ and a *sample buffer pool* $\boldsymbol{X}'$. We only keep T collected sample set $\boldsymbol{X}_C$ to constitute the sample buffer pool. Every T frames, $\boldsymbol{X}'$ is utilized to update $\boldsymbol{X}_P$. After updating the sample pool, we will leave $\boldsymbol{X}'$ blank and then reconfigure it. In our experiment, we set the sample pool capacity as $\Theta(\boldsymbol{X}_P)$ which denotes the number of samples in the sample pool. If the total number of samples in the sample pool is larger than $\Theta(\boldsymbol{X}_P)$, samples in $\boldsymbol{X}_P$ will be randomly replaced with $\boldsymbol{X}'$. To reduce the risk of visual drift, we always retain the samples $\boldsymbol{X}_1$ obtained from the first frame in the sample pool. In other words, $\boldsymbol{X}_P = [\boldsymbol{X}_1; \boldsymbol{X}']$. Similarly, landmarks also should be updated using the sample pool every T frames. Specifically, we first implement k-means in the current sample pool $\boldsymbol{X}_P$ to obtain a new landmarks set. Then, the updated landmarks set is gained by carrying out the k-means algorithm again using the new landmarks set and the previous landmarks set, which is able to better characterize the samples distribution.

3.2 Bayesian State Inference

Object tracking can be considered as a Bayesian inference task in a Markov model with hidden state variables. Given the observation set of the object $\mathcal{O}_{1:t} = \{\boldsymbol{o}_1, \boldsymbol{o}_2, \cdots, \boldsymbol{o}_t\}$, the optimal state $\boldsymbol{s}_t$ of the tracked object is obtained by the maximum a posteriori estimation $p(\boldsymbol{s}_t^i | \mathcal{O}_{1:t})$, where $\boldsymbol{s}_t^i$ indicates the state of the i-th sample. The posterior probability $p(\boldsymbol{s}_t | \mathcal{O}_{1:t})$ is formulated by Bayes theorem as $p(\boldsymbol{s}_t | \mathcal{O}_{1:t}) \propto p(\boldsymbol{o}_t | \boldsymbol{s}_t) \int p(\boldsymbol{s}_t | \boldsymbol{s}_{t-1}) p(\boldsymbol{s}_{t-1} | \mathcal{O}_{1:t-1})\ d\boldsymbol{s}_{t-1}$. This inference is governed by the dynamic model $p(\boldsymbol{s}_t | \boldsymbol{s}_{t-1})$ which models the temporal correlation of the tracking results in consecutive frames, and by the observation model $p(\boldsymbol{o}_t | \boldsymbol{s}_t)$ which estimates the likelihood of observing $\boldsymbol{o}_t$ at state $\boldsymbol{s}_t$.

We apply an affine image warp to model the object motion between two consecutive frames. The state transition distribution $p(\boldsymbol{s}_t | \boldsymbol{s}_{t-1})$ is modeled by Brownian motion, *i.e.*, $p(\boldsymbol{s}_t | \boldsymbol{s}_{t-1}) = \mathcal{N}(\boldsymbol{s}_t; \boldsymbol{s}_{t-1}, \sum)$, where $\sum$ is a diagonal covariance matrix whose diagonal elements are the corresponding variances of respective parameters. The observation model $p(\boldsymbol{o}_t | \boldsymbol{s}_t)$ is defined as

$$p(\boldsymbol{o}_t | \boldsymbol{s}_t) \propto SC_t, \tag{13}$$

where $SC_t = \widehat{f}(\boldsymbol{x}^{(t)})$ is the classification score at time t based on Eq. (11).

4 Experiments

We run our tracker on 65 challenging image sequences including the benchmark dataset [28] and 14 public sequences widely used in recent literatures. The total number of frames on the 65 sequences is more than 30000. We evaluate the proposed tracker against 11 state-of-the-art tracking algorithms including ONNDL [29], RET [30], CT [31], VTD [4], MIL [11], SCM [32], Struck [12], TLD [13], ASLSA [2], LSST [3] and SPT [14]. For fair comparisons, the source codes are provided by the benchmark with the same parameters except ONNDL, RET, LSST and SPT whose parameters of the particle filter are set as same as our tracker. As discussed in [28], we also annotate the attributes of 14 public sequences used in our paper. The proposed approach was implemented in MATLAB on a Intel Core2 2.5 GHz processor with 4GB RAM. Our tracker is about 2 frame/sec for all experiments. No code optimization is performed. The MATLAB source code and experimental results of 12 trackers are available at http://iitlab.bit.edu.cn/mcislab/~wuyuwei/.

4.1 Experimental Setup

Note that we fix the parameters of our tracker for all sequences to demonstrate its robustness and stability. The number of particles is 400 and the state transition matrix is $[8, 8, 0.01, 0, 0.005, 0]$ in the particle filter. We resize the object image to 24×24 pixels. Gray scale information and HOG feature are extracted from each object region. In the first frame, $N_p = 20$ positive samples and $N_n = 100$ negative samples are used to initialize the classifier. The regularization parameter expressed in Eq. (10) is set to $\eta = 0.02$. The predefined threshold of classification score ϵ is set as 0.3. Given the object location at current frame, if $SC \geq \epsilon$, 2 positive samples and 50 negative samples are used for the supervised learning. If $SC < \epsilon$, the tracking result is treated as the unreliable one and 100 unlabeled sample are utilized for the unsupervised learning. The sample pool capacity $\Theta(\boldsymbol{X}_P)$ is set to 310, in which the number of positive, negative and unlabeled samples are 50, 160 and 100, respectively. The number of landmarks is set to 30 empirically. As a trade-off between computational efficiency and effectiveness, the landmarks set $\boldsymbol{D}$ is updated every $T = 10$ frames.

4.2 Quantitative Comparisons

Evaluation Criteria. To measure the tracking performance, the *precision plot* [11] is adopted to measure the overall tracking performance. It shows the percentage of frames whose estimated location is within the given threshold distance of the ground truth. More accurate trackers have higher precision at lower thresholds. If a tracker loses the object, it is difficult to reach a higher precision.

The tracking overlap rate is also used for quantitative comparisons. It is defined by $score = \frac{area(ROI_T \bigcap ROI_G)}{area(ROI_T \bigcup ROI_G)}$, where ROI_T is the tracking bounding box and ROI_G is the ground truth. This can be used to evaluate the *success rate* of any tracking approach. The tracking result is considered as a success when the *score* is greater than the given threshold t_s. However, it may not be fair or representative for tracker evaluation using one success rate value at a specific threshold (*e.g.*, $t_s = 0.5$). Therefore, we count the number of successful frames at the thresholds varied from 0 to 1 and plot the *success rate* curve for our tracker and the compared trackers. The area under curve (AUC) of each success rate plot is employed to rank the tracking algorithms. More robust trackers have higher success rate at higher thresholds.

Overall Performance. The overall performance for 12 trackers is summarized by the precision plot and success rate on 65 sequence, as shown in Fig. 2. For precision plots, we use the results at error threshold of 20 for ranking these 12 trackers. The AUC score for each tracker is shown in the legend. In success rate, our tracker is 2.8 % above the SCM, and outperforms the Struck by 3.1 % in precision plot. SCM, ASLSA and LSST trackers also perform well in success rate, which suggests sparse representations are effective models to account for appearance change, especially for occlusion. Overall, our tracker outperforms

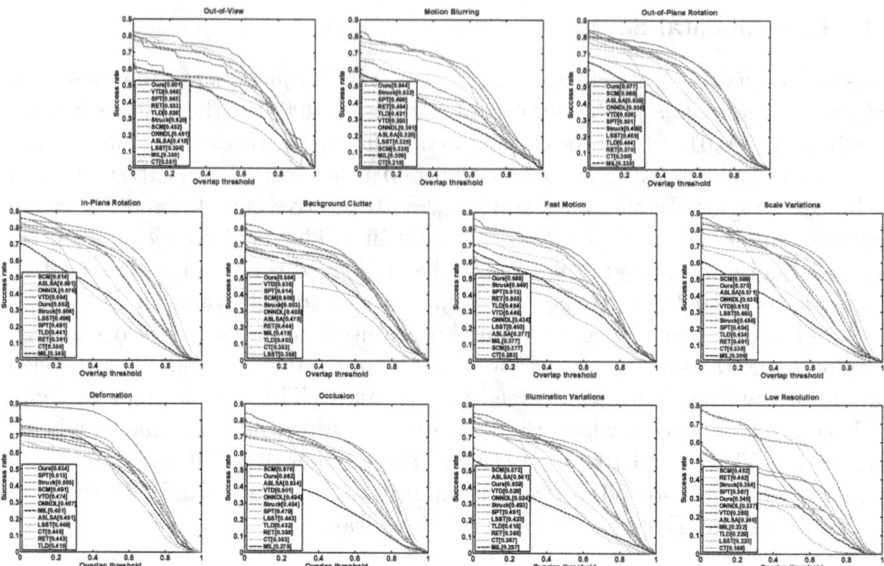

Fig. 3. Attribute-based performance analysis in success rate. The performance score of each tracker is shown in the legend (best viewed on high-resolution display)

other 11 trackers both in precision plot and success rate. Good performance of our method can be attributed to the fact that the classifier generalizes well on the new data from a limited number of training samples. That is, our method has excellent generalization ability. In addition, the local manifold structure of samples makes the classifier have more discriminating power.

Attribute-Based Performance. Apart from summarizing the performance on the whole sequences, we also construct 11 subsets corresponding to different attributes to report specific challenging conditions. Figure 3 shows the attribute-based performance analysis in success rate. Attributes OCC, IPR, OPR and SV occur more frequently than others on 65 sequences. Due to space limitations, in the following we mainly analyze the success rate and precision plot for these four attributes mentioned above and use other attributes as auxiliary.

On the OCC subset, SCM, ASLSA, LSST and our method get better results than others. The results suggest that local image representations are more effective than holistic templates in dealing with occlusions. On the SV subset, we see that trackers with affine motion models (*e.g.*, our method, SCM, ASLSA and LSST) are able to cope with scale variation better than others that only consider translational motion (*e.g.*, Struck and MIL). On the OPR and IPR subsets, besides our tracker, the SCM and ASLSA trackers is also able to obtain the satisfactory results. The performance of SCM and ASLSA trackers can be attributed to the efficient spare representations of local image patches. Similarly, on the FM and MB subsets, Struck, SPT, TLD and our trackers perform

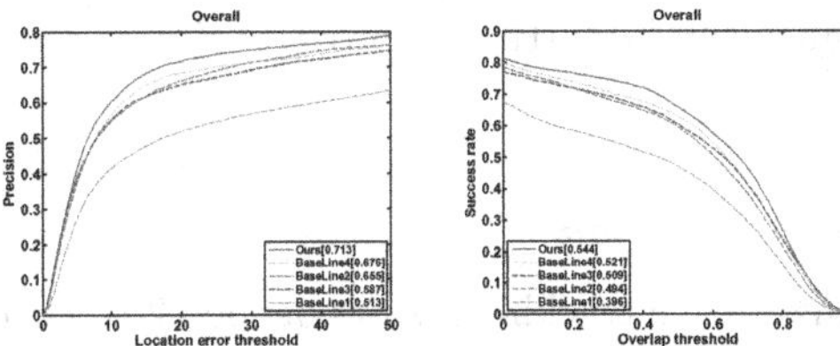

Fig. 4. The overall performance of two baseline algorithms and our method on 65 sequences is presented for comparison in terms of precision and success rate

favorably against other methods, which implies a good online learning algorithm facilitates trackers by updating the classifiers to adapt to appearance changes of the object.

Effectiveness of the Optimal $\boldsymbol{H}$. To evaluate the contribution of the optimal $\boldsymbol{H}$ described in Sect. 2.2 to the overall performance of our tracker, we compute the Nadaraya-Watson kernel regression [33] for comparison. It assigns weights smoothly with $\boldsymbol{H}_{ik} = \frac{K_\sigma(\boldsymbol{x}_i, \boldsymbol{d}_k)}{\sum_{j=1}^{m} K_\sigma(\boldsymbol{x}_i, \boldsymbol{d}_j)}, 1 \le i \le n, 1 \le j \le m$. Two kernel functions are exploited in the Nadaraya-Watson kernel regression to measure the cross-similarity matrix between the whole data $\boldsymbol{X}$ and landmarks $\boldsymbol{d}_k$'s. We first adopt Gaussian kernel for the kernel regression and the corresponding tracking method is called as the *BaseLine1*. Epanechnikov quadratic kernel is also employed for the kernel regression, whose corresponding tracking method is referred to as the *BaseLine2* tracker. We use a more robust way to get σ which uses the nearest neighborhood size s of $\boldsymbol{x}_i$ to replace σ, *i.e.*, $\sigma(\boldsymbol{x}_i) = \|\boldsymbol{x}_i - \boldsymbol{d}_s\|^2$, where $\boldsymbol{d}_s$ is the sth closest landmarks of $\boldsymbol{x}_i$. The only difference between baseline algorithms and *Ours* is that baseline algorithms utilize the predefined kernel functions to solve cross-similarity matrix $\boldsymbol{H}$ while *Ours* takes advantage of local landmarks approximation method to optimize $\boldsymbol{H}$. The overall tracking performance of these baseline algorithms and our method on the 65 challenging sequences is presented in Fig. 4. On the whole, our method obtains more accurate tracking results than baseline algorithms.

Effectiveness of the Prediction Matrix $\boldsymbol{A}$. We design another two baseline algorithms to evaluate the effectiveness of the soft label prediction matrix $\boldsymbol{A}$ described in Sect. 2.3. In the *BaseLine3*, we do not consider the Laplacian graph regularizer in Eq. (9), *i.e.*, $\eta = 0$, and thus $\boldsymbol{A}$ becomes the least-squares solution. In the *BaseLine4*, we directly construct the adjacent matrix $\boldsymbol{W}$ using the kNN algorithm instead of $\boldsymbol{W} = \boldsymbol{H}\boldsymbol{H}^\top$. If $\boldsymbol{x}_i$ is among the k-neighbors of $\boldsymbol{x}_j$ or $\boldsymbol{x}_j$ is among the k-neighbors of $\boldsymbol{x}_i$, $\boldsymbol{W}_{ij} = 1$, otherwise, $\boldsymbol{W}_{ij} = 0$. The overall tracking performance on the benchmark is illustrated in Fig. 4. Surprisingly, even without Laplacian graph regularizer, the *BaseLine3* produces the precision score of 0.587 and the success score of 0.509, outperforming the ONNDL tracker, which implies that the success is due to the framework of the landmark-based inductive model.

The overall performance can be further improved using our scheme of solving $\boldsymbol{A}$ described in Sect. 2.3.

4.3 Qualitative Comparisons

Figure 5 shows the qualitative tracking results of the 12 trackers over nine representative video sequences. In the *dragonbaby*, *Basketball* and *Freeman4* sequences are used to evaluate whether our method is able to handle significant pose changes. The *dragonbaby*, VTD, RET, ASLSA, SPT, SCM and TLD trackers are easy to drift at the beginning of the sequence when the object turns around (*e.g.*, ♯28). The LSST tracker and our methods are able to track the object well although with some errors in some frames. SCM and ASLSA trackers do not perform well in this sequence as the drastic appearance changes due to shape information are not effectively accounted for the sparse representation. In the *Basketball* sequence, we see that SPT, CT, RET and SCM trackers are easy to drift at the beginning of the sequence (*e.g.*, ♯60). The TLD, ONNDL, Struck and MIL algorithms drift to another player as the appearance between players in the same team is very similar (*e.g.*, ♯473). VTD, ASLSA and our methods are able to track the whole sequence successfully. In the *Freeman4* sequence, all the trackers except our method perform poorly since the partial occlusions appear frequently. SMC method employs a fixed histogram intersection function to compute the similarity of histograms between the candidate and the template, thereby leading to lacking the ability to adapt to scene changes.

The *Woman*, *SUV* and *Liquor* sequences are utilized to test if our methods can tackle the occlusions. In the *Woman* sequence, the CT, SCM, MIL, VTD, TLD and ONNDL trackers fail to capture the object after the woman walks behind white car (*e.g.*, ♯127). The appearance model fuses more background interference due to an occlusion, which significantly influences the samples online update of the MIL, TLD, ASLSA and RET trackers. The LSST tracker fails gradually over time (*e.g.*, ♯380). In contrast, our method, SPT and Struck trackers

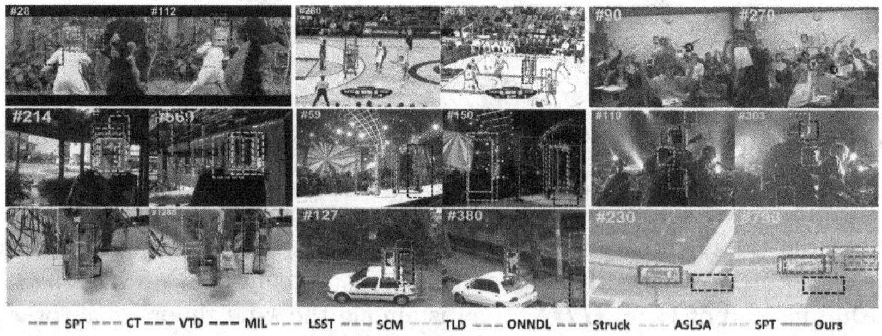

Fig. 5. Qualitative tracking results of the 12 trackers over 9 representative video sequences (*i.e.*, 'Dragonbaby", "Basketball", "Freeman4", "Trellis", "Singer2", "shaking","Liquor", "Woman" and "SUV") that are respectively aligned from left to right and from up to down (best viewed on high-resolution display)

achieve stable performance in the entire sequence. For the *SUV* sequence, most of the trackers drift when the long-term occlusion happens. In comparisons, our tracker and SCM have relatively lower center location errors and higher success rate. Although LSST and ASLSA trackers take partial occlusion into account, the results are not satisfied. The RET and TLD trackers are also achieve the satisfying results. In the *Liquor* sequence, the object suffers from background clutter besides heavy occlusions for many times. The CT, MIL, LSST and ASLSA trackers drift first when the occlusion occurs (*e.g.*, ♯361). Although the TLD, VTD, SPT, RET and Struck trackers obtain slightly better results than SCM and ONNDL trackers, they lose the object after several occlusions. Overall, our method achieves both the lowest tracking error and the highest overlap rate.

In the *Shaking*, *Singer2* and *Trellis* sequences, the objects undergo drastic illumination changes. From the *Shaking* sequence, we see that the Struck, LSST, TLD, CT and RET trackers drift from the object quickly when the spotlight blinks suddenly (*e.g.*, ♯110). SCM, VTD, ONNDL and our trackers can successfully track the surfer throughout the sequence with relatively accurate sizes of the bounding box. SPT, MIL, and ASLSA methods are also able to track the object in this sequence but with lower success rate than our method. In the *Singer2* sequence, the contrast between the foreground and the background is very low besides illumination change. Most trackers drift away at the beginning of the sequence when the stage light changes drastically (*e.g.*, ♯59). The VTD tracker performs slightly better as the edge feature is less sensitive to illumination change. In contrast, our method succeeds in tracking the object accurately. In *Trellis* sequence, a man walks under a trellis. Suffering from large changes in environmental illumination and head pose, the CT, TLD, MIL, SPT and LSST trackers drift gradually. In contrast, RET, ONNDL, ASLSA, SCM, Struck and our trackers obtain promising results.

5 Conclusion

In this paper, we have proposed a landmark-based inductive model for tracking. The idea of our method is that the label of each sample can be interpreted as the weighted combination of labels on landmarks. Through solving the cross-similarity matrix $\boldsymbol{H}$ and the label prediction matrix $\boldsymbol{A}$, our model is able to effectively propagate the landmarks' labels to all the unlabeled candidates. The Lim tracker is able to effectively fit the underlying data distribution to handle appearance changes. A candidate with the highest classification score is considered as the tracking result. In addition, explicitly considering the local geometrical structure of the samples, the graph-based regularizer is incorporated into the lim tracker, which makes our method have better discriminating power and thus is more adaptive to handle appearance changes. Compared with 11 state-of-the-art tracking methods on 65 challenging image sequences, the Lim tracker is more robust to illumination changes, pose variations and partial occlusions, *etc.* Experimental results have demonstrated the effectiveness and robustness of the proposed tracker.

Acknowledgement. This work was supported in part by the Natural Science Foundation of China (NSFC) under grant No. 61203291, the 973 Program of China under grant No. 2012CB720000, the Specialized Research Fund for the Doctoral Program of Higher Education of China under grant No.20121101120029, and the Specialized Fund for Joint Building Program of Beijing Municipal Education Commission.

References

1. Li, X., Hu, W., Shen, C., Zhang, Z., Dick, A., Hengel, A.V.D.: A survey of appearance models in visual object tracking. ACM Trans. Intell. Syst. Technol. (TIST) **4**, 58 (2013)
2. Jia, X., Lu, H., Yang, M.: Visual tracking via adaptive structural local sparse appearance model. In: Proceedings of IEEE Conference on Computer Vision and Pattern Recognition, pp.1822–1829 (2012)
3. Wang, D., Lu, H., Yang, M.H.: Least soft-thresold squares tracking. In: Proceedingsof IEEE Conference on Computer Vision and Pattern Recognition, pp. 2371–2378 (2013)
4. Kwon, J., Lee, K.: Visual tracking decomposition. In: Proceedings of IEEE Conference on Computer Vision and Pattern Recognition, pp. 1269–1276 (2010)
5. Mei, X., Ling, H.: Robust visual tracking using $\ell 1$ minimization. In: Proceedings of IEEE International Conference on Computer Vision, pp. 1–8 (2009)
6. Ross, D., Lim, J., Lin, R., Yang, M.: Incremental learning for robust visual tracking. Int. J. Comput. Vis. **77**, 125–141 (2008)
7. Wu, Y., Ma, B.: Learning distance metric for object contour tracking. Pattern Anal. Appl. **17**, 265–277 (2014)
8. Zhuang, B., Lu, H., Xiao, Z., Wang, D.: Visual tracking via discriminative sparse similarity map. IEEE Trans. Image Process. **23**, 1872–1881 (2014)
9. Grabner, H., Grabner, C., Bischof, H.: Semi-supervised on-line boosting for robust tracking. In: Forsyth, D., Torr, P., Zisserman, A. (eds.) ECCV 2008. LNCS, vol. 5302, pp. 234–247. Springer, Heidelberg (2008)
10. Yang, M., Yuan, J., Wu, Y.: Spatial selection for attentional visual tracking. In: IEEE Conference on Computer Vision and Pattern Recognition, CVPR 2007, pp. 1–8. IEEE (2007)
11. Babenko, B., Yang, M., Belongie, S.: Robust object tracking with online multiple instance learning. IEEE Trans. Pattern Anal. Mach.Intell. **33**, 1619–1632 (2011)
12. Hare, S., Saffari, A., Torr, P.H.: Struck: Structured output tracking with kernels. In: Proceedings of the IEEE International Conference on Computer Vision, pp. 263–270 (2011)
13. Kalal, Z., Mikolajczyk, K., Matas, J.: Tracking-learning-detection. IEEE Trans. Pattern Anal. Mach. Intell. **34**, 1409–1422 (2012)
14. Yao, R., Shi, Q., Shen, C., Zhang, Y., van den Hengel, A.: Part-based visual tracking with online latent structural learning. In: Proceedings of IEEE Conference on Computer Vision and Pattern Recognition, pp. 2363–2370 (2013)
15. Yang, M., Pei, M., Wu, Y., Jia, Y.: Learning online structural appearance model for robust object tracking. Sci. China Inf. Sci. **58**(3), 1–14 (2015)
16. Yu, Qian, Dinh, Thang Ba, Medioni, Gérard G.: Online tracking and reacquisition using co-trained generative and discriminative trackers. In: Forsyth, David, Torr, Philip, Zisserman, Andrew (eds.) ECCV 2008, Part II. LNCS, vol. 5303, pp. 678–691. Springer, Heidelberg (2008)

17. Zhang, L., van der Maaten, L.: Preserving structure in model-free tracking. IEEE Trans. Pattern Anal. Mach. Intell. **36**, 756–769 (2014)
18. Wu, Y., Ma, B., Yang, M., Jia, Y., Zhang, J.: Metric learning based structural appearance model for robust visual tracking. IEEE Trans. Circuits Syst. Video Technol. **24**, 865–877 (2014)
19. Gao, J., Xing, J., Hu, W., Maybank, S.: Discriminant tracking using tensor representation with semi-supervised improvement. In: Proceedings of the IEEE International Conference on Computer Vision, pp. 1569–1576 (2013)
20. Li, X., Shen, C., Dick, A.R., van den Hengel, A.: Learning compact binary codes for visual tracking. In: Proceedings of IEEE Conference on Computer Vision and Pattern Recognition, pp. 2419–2426 (2013)
21. Kumar, K., Vleeschouwer, C.: Discriminative label propagation for multi-object tracking with sporadic appearance features. In: Proceedings of the IEEE International Conference on Computer Vision, pp. 2000–2007 (2013)
22. Zhang, K., Kwok, J.T., Parvin, B.: Prototype vector machine for large scale semi-supervised learning. In: Proceedings of the 26th Annual International Conference on Machine Learning, pp. 1233–1240. ACM (2009)
23. Liu, W., Wang, J., Chang, S.F.: Robust and scalable graph-based semisupervised learning. Proc. IEEE **100**, 2624–2638 (2012)
24. Wang, J., Yang, J., Yu, K., Lv, F., Huang, T., Gong, Y.: Locality-constrained linear coding for image classification. In: Proceedings of IEEE Conference on Computer Vision and Pattern Recognition, pp. 3360–3367 IEEE (2010)
25. Nesterov, Y.: Introductory Lectures on Convex Optimization: A Basic Course. Kluwer Academic Publishers, Dordrecht (2004)
26. Duchi, J., Shalev-Shwartz, S., Singer, Y., Chandra, T.: Efficient projections onto the l1-ball for learning in high dimensions. In: Proceedings of the 25th international conference on Machine learning, pp. 272–279. ACM (2008)
27. Williams, C., Seeger, M.: Using the nyström method to speed up kernel machines. In: Advances in Neural Information Processing Systems, Citeseer (2001)
28. Wu, Y., Lim, J., Yang, M.H.: Online object tracking: a benchmark. In: Proceedings of IEEE Conference on Computer Vision and Pattern Recognition, pp. 2411–2418. IEEE (2013)
29. Wang, N., Wang, J., Yeung, D.Y.: Online robust non-negative dictionary learning for visual tracking. In: Proceedings of IEEE International Conference on Computer Vision, pp. 657–664 (2013)
30. Bai, Q., Wu, Z., Sclaroff, S., Betke, M., Monnier, C.: Randomized ensemble tracking. In: Proceedings of IEEE International Conference on Computer Vision, pp. 2040–2047 (2013)
31. Zhang, K., Zhang, L., Yang, M.-H.: Real-time compressive tracking. In: Fitzgibbon, A., Lazebnik, S., Perona, P., Sato, Y., Schmid, C. (eds.) ECCV 2012. LNCS, vol. 7574, pp. 864–877. Springer, Heidelberg (2012)
32. Zhong, W., Lu, H., Yang, M.: Robust object tracking via sparsity-based collaborative model. IEEE Trans. Image Process. **23**, 2356–2368 (2014)
33. Hastie, T., Tibshirani, R., Friedman, J.: The Elements of Statistical Learning, vol. 2. Springer, New York (2009)

Extended Co-occurrence HOG with Dense Trajectories for Fine-Grained Activity Recognition

Hirokatsu Kataoka[1,2](✉), Kiyoshi Hashimoto[2], Kenji Iwata[3], Yutaka Satoh[3], Nassir Navab[4], Slobodan Ilic[4], and Yoshimitsu Aoki[2]

[1] The University of Tokyo, Tokyo, Japan
kataoka@aoki-medialab.org
[2] Keio University, Minato, Japan
[3] National Institute of Advanced Industrial Science and Technology (AIST), Tsukuba, Japan
[4] Technische Universität München (TUM), Munich, Germany

Abstract. In this paper we propose a novel feature descriptor Extended Co-occurrence HOG (ECoHOG) and integrate it with dense point trajectories demonstrating its usefulness in fine grained activity recognition. This feature is inspired by original Co-occurrence HOG (CoHOG) that is based on histograms of occurrences of pairs of image gradients in the image. Instead relying only on pure histograms we introduce a sum of gradient magnitudes of co-occurring pairs of image gradients in the image. This results in giving the importance to the object boundaries and straightening the difference between the moving foreground and static background. We also couple ECoHOG with dense point trajectories extracted using optical flow from video sequences and demonstrate that they are extremely well suited for fine grained activity recognition. Using our feature we outperform state of the art methods in this task and provide extensive quantitative evaluation.

1 Introduction

In the past years various techniques for visual analysis of humans have been studied in the field of computer vision [1]. Human tracking, body pose estimation, activity recognition and face recognition are just some examples of analysis of humans from videos that are relevant in many real-life environments. Recently, human activity recognition has become a very active research topic and several survey papers have been published, including those by Aggarwal *et al.* [2], Moeslund *et al.* [3], and Ryoo *et al.* [4]. The number of applications is vast and they include, but are not limited to video surveillance, sports video analysis, medical science, robotics, video indexing, and games. To put these applications into practice, many activity recognition methods have been proposed in recent years to improve accuracy. Activity recognition means determining the activity of the person from a sequence of images. In case of very similar activities with the subtle

D. Cremers et al. (Eds.): ACCV 2014, Part V, LNCS 9007, pp. 336–349, 2015.
DOI: 10.1007/978-3-319-16814-2_22

differences in motion we talk about fine-grained activities. The classical recognition pipeline starts with extracting some kind of spatio temporal features and feeding them into the classifiers trained to recognize such activities. However, in case of fine-grained activities minor differences between extracted features frequently affect the classification of an activity. This makes visual distinction difficult using existing feature descriptors. For fine-grained activity recognition, Rohrbach *et al.* [5] confirmed that dense sampling of feature descriptors achieved better results than joint features based on posture information.

In this paper we propose Extended Co-occurrence HOG (ECoHOG) feature and integrate it with dense sampling and dense feature extraction approach in order to improve accuracy of fine-grained activity recognition. We rely on Co-occurrence Histograms of Oriented Gradients (CoHOG) [6] as a feature descriptor representing co-occurrence elements in an image patch. The co-occurrence feature clearly extracts an object's shape by focusing on co-occurrence of image gradients at the pairs of image pixels and in that way reduces false positives. We extend this feature by adding sum of the magnitude of the gradients as co-occurrence elements. This results in giving the importance to the object boundaries and straightening the difference between the moving foreground and static background. In addition we apply this descriptor on the dense trajectories and test it for fine grained activity recognition.

We tested influence of our ECoHOG feature coupled with dense trajectories on two fine-grained activity recognition datasets: MPII cooking activities dataset [5] and INRIA surgery dataset [7] and obtained increase of performance using only this features in contrast to the use of HOG [16], HOF (Histograms of Optical Flow) [11] and MBF (Motion Boundary Histograms) [17] used in Wang *et al.* [8,9].

2 Related Work

A large amount of activity recognition research has been undertaken in the past decade. The first noteworthy work is Space-Time Interest Points (STIPs) [10]. The STIP algorithm is an improvement of Harris corner detector for $x - y$ and time t space. STIPs are three dimensional descriptors representing motion of corner points in time. The spatio-temporal sampling and feature description framework is widely used by the activity recognition community. Klaser proposed 3D-HOG *et al.* [12], while Marszalek *et al.* [13] described feature combination using the STIP framework. Recently, Everts *et al.* proposed color STIPs with four different color spaces added to standard STIP descriptor [14].

However, up to date the best approach for activity recognition is arguably "dense trajectories" proposed by Wang *et al.* [8,9], which is a trajectory-based feature description on dense sampling feature points. Using these trajectories histograms of oriented gradients (HOG) [16], histograms of optical flow (HOF) [11], and motion boundary histograms (MBH) [17] can be acquired. Rohrbach *et al.* claimed that dense trajectories outperformed other approaches in terms of accuracy on the MPII cooking activities dataset, which is a fine-grained dataset

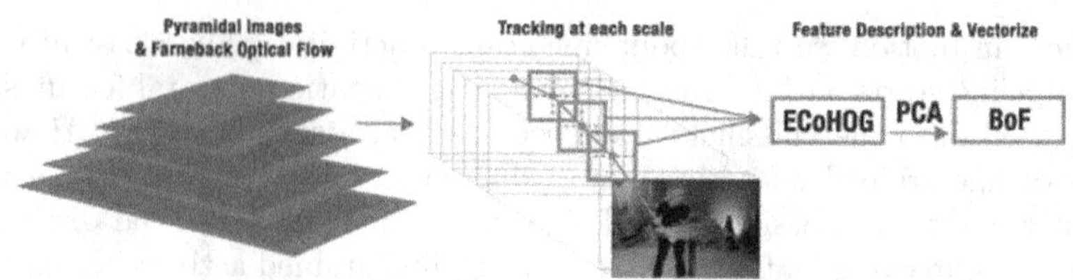

Fig. 1. Proposed framework: Pyramidal image capture and dense optical flow extraction are the same as the original dense trajectories. In feature extraction, we incorporate improved co-occurrence features (ECoHOG) in the dense trajectories. The co-occurrence vectors are reduced for effective vectorization as a bag-of-features (BoF) [23]. Finally, the co-occurrence vector is merged into other feature vectors (HOF, MBHx, MBHy, and Trajectory).

with 65 activity classes. Dense trajectories are also superior to posture-based feature descriptors on the dataset [15]. Dense sampling approaches for activity recognition have also been proposed in [18–22]) after the introduction of the first dense trajectories [8]. Raptis *et al.* implemented a middle-level trajectory yielding simple posture representation with location clustering [18]. Li *et al.* translated a feature vector into another feature vector at a different angle using the "hankelet" approach [19]. To eliminate extra-flow, Jain *et al.* applied affine matrix [20] and Peng *et al.* proposed dense optical flow capture in the motion boundary space [21]. Wang *et al.* realized improved dense trajectories [22] by adding camera motion estimation, detection-based noise canceling, and a Fisher vector [24].

Several noise elimination approaches have been considered in this field to improve recognition performance, however, feature extraction is not enough. Thus, we introduced an improved feature descriptor into dense trajectories which we call Extended Co-occurrence HOG. This feature relies on the co-occurrence of the image gradients inside an image patch described with the normalized sum of the gradient intensities of co-occurring gradients. This helped distinguishing the moving foreground from the static background while capturing a subtle differences inside the image patches of the moving human body parts.

3 Proposed Framework

In this paper, we propose an improved co-occurrence feature ECoHOG and use it for fine-grained activity recognition. ECoHOG feature represents the gradient magnitude in a co-occurring image gradients located on the image patch and emphasize the boundary between the human and the background and between the edges within the human. Figure 1 shows the proposed framework applied in the context of fine-grained activity recognition. In essence, we have implemented the original dense trajectories [9] that find trajectories and extract features on the points along the trajectories. Using this framework and the concept of dense trajectories we integrated our improved co-occurrence feature (ECoHOG) into the HOF, MBH, and trajectory vectors. Finally we performed the dimensionality reduction in order to convert the co-occurrence feature into a bag-of-features (BoF) vector [23].

The rest of the paper is organized as follows. In the next section we describe the extended co-occurrence feature descriptor and its vectorization using the BoF. In the next section we presents our experimental results using fine-grained activity datasets. Finally in the last section we conclude the paper.

4 Feature Description and Vectorization

4.1 Co-occurrence Histogram of Oriented Gradients (CoHOG)

HOG feature descriptor is calculated by computing the histogram of oriented gradients in the overlapping block inside the image patch. In practice gradient magnitude are accumulated in a corresponding orientation histogram and normalized within the block. Although the HOG can capture the rough shape of a human it often results in false positive detections in cluttered scenes when applied in tasks such as human detection. The Co-occurrence HOG (CoHOG) is designed to accumulate co-occurrences of pairs of image gradients inside the non-overlapping blocks of the image patch. Counting co-occurrences of the image gradients at different locations and in differently sized neighborhoods reduces false positives. For example, a pixel pair of the head and shoulders is described at the same time meaning that these two body parts, i.e. their edges, should always co-appear. As reported in [6] this proved to be more robust to the clutter and occlusions then standard HOG for human detection. In CoHOG eight gradient orientations are considered and co-occurrence of each orientation with each other orientation has been counted. This results in $8 \times 8 = 64$ dimensional histogram called co-occurrence matrix. In practice not only direct neighbors with offset one have been considered, but co-occurrence has also been regarded for larger offsets resulting in up to 30 co-occurrence histograms per image block. The co-occurrence histogram is computed as follows:

$$g(x, y) = \arctan \frac{f_y(x, y)}{f_x(x, y)} \tag{1}$$

$$f_x(x, y) = I(x + 1, y) - I(x - 1, y) \tag{2}$$

$$f_y(x, y) = I(x, y + 1) - I(x, y - 1) \tag{3}$$

$$C_{x,y}(i, j) = \sum_{p=1}^{n} \sum_{q=1}^{m} \begin{cases} 1, & \text{if } d(p, q) = i \text{ and } d(x + p, y + q) = j \\ 0 & \text{otherwise} \end{cases} \tag{4}$$

where $I(x, y)$ is the pixel value, $g(x, y)$ is the gradient orientation. $C(i, j)$ denotes the co-occurrence value of each element of the histogram, coordinates (p, q) depict the center of the feature extraction window, coordinates $(p + x, p + y)$ depict the position of the pixel pair in the feature extraction window, and $d(p, q)$ is one of eight the quantized gradient orientations.

The CoHOG can express the co-occurrence edge orientation acquired from two pixels and has higher accuracy than the HOG because of the co-occurrence edge representation. However, it faithfully counts all co-occurrence edges regardless of the edge magnitude. Human detection with a CoHOG results in false positives depending on the presence of an edge in a local image. Similar objects (e.g., trees and traffic signs) to a human have many elements whose histograms are similar. We believe that including the edge magnitude into the CoHoG is effective in creating a feature vector for human detection and therefore propose to extend CoHoG with magnitudes of the co-occurring gradients.

4.2 Extended Co-occurrence Histograms of Oriented Gradients (ECoHOG)

In this section, we explain the method for edge magnitude accumulation and histogram normalization, which we included in the ECoHOG. This improved feature descriptor is described below.

Accumulating Edge Magnitudes. Human shape can be described with the histograms of co-occurring gradient orientations. Here we add to it the magnitude of the image gradients which leads to improved and more robust description of the human shapes. In contrast to CoHOG, in our proposed framework we accumulate the sum of two pixel gradient magnitudes in the pairs of co-occurring pixel location inside the block of the image patch. The sum of edge magnitudes represents the accumulated gradient magnitude between two pixel edge magnitudes at different locations in the image block. In this way, for example, the difference between pedestrians and the background is more strengthened. The ECoHOG is defined as follows:

$$C_{x,y}(i,j) = \sum_{p=1}^{n}\sum_{q=1}^{m} \begin{cases} \|g_1(p,q)\| + \|g_2(p+x,q+y)\| \\ \text{if } d(p,q) = i \text{ and } d(p+x,q+y) = j \\ \\ 0 \text{ otherwise} \end{cases} \tag{5}$$

where $\|g(p,q\|$ is the gradient magnitude, and $C(i,j)$, and all the other elements are defined as in Eqs. (1)–(3).

ECoHOG describes the magnitude for each pair of co-occurring pixel gradients and in that way creates a more robust co-occurrence histogram. It efficiently expresses the boundary between human and the background and also between the different textures of the clothing of the same human. Edge magnitude representation can define a boundary depending on the strength of the edges. This feature descriptor represents not only the combination of curves and straight lines, but also performs better than the CoHOG.

Histogram Normalization. The brightness of an image changes with respect to the light sources. The feature histogram should be normalized in order to be robust for human detection under various lighting conditions. The range

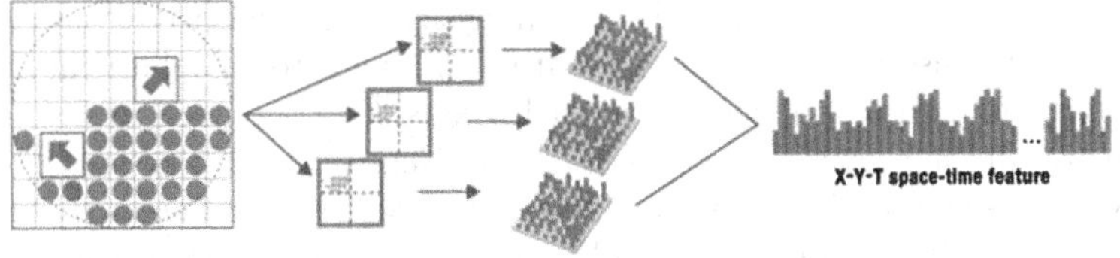

Fig. 2. Extended CoHOG in dense trajectories

of normalization is 64 dimensions, that is, the dimension of the co-occurrence histogram. The equation for normalization is given as:

$$C'_{x,y}(i,j) = \frac{C_{x,y}(i,j)}{\sum_{i'=1}^{8}\sum_{j'=1}^{8} C_{x,y}(i',j')}, \tag{6}$$

where C and C' denote histograms with and without normalization, respectively.

4.3 Extended CoHOG in Dense Trajectories

According to [9] the image is tessellated into a grid of 2×2 blocks and that small patch is tracked using optical flow in three consecutive frames. This results in dense trajectories of densely sampled image grid. In [9] propose to compute multiple features like HOG, HOF and MBH in frames along the time trajectory and concatenate into one spatio-temporal histogram resulting in (X-Y-T) space–time block as shown in Fig. 2. Instead of computing HOG, HoF and MBH we compute our ECoHOG feature and concatenate the in time. Computation of co-occurrence description seems not in real-time, however, divided blocks can be calculated in parallel. Parallel processing allows us to calculate ECoHOG nearly efficient as HOG, HOF and MBH. Depending on the size of the neighborhoods different offsets are used to collect co-occurrence of the image gradients in ECoHOG. This results into a number of histograms per image block and continuous spatio-temporal feature has huge dimension.

Dimensionality Reduction and Bag-of-Features. In order to bring it to the reasonable size and make it computationally tractable we perform PCA in order to reduce dimension of our features. A low-dimensional vector is generally easier to divide into a collection of classes, i.e. to cluster into bags of features (BoF). In related work, the CoHOG required about 35,000 dimensions for pedestrian detection [6]. However, we use a low-dimensional vector of 4000 dimensions to compose a BoF vector for activity recognition. In the experiments, we define and analyze an effective parameter for dimensionality reduction.

The BoF effectively represents a visual vector in an image [23]. An image generally consists of a large number of small patches called visual words. The BoF calculates the distribution to form feature vectors. Following the original dense trajectories, we randomly select millions of vectors from a dataset. The K-means clustering algorithm categorizes them into 4000 cluster, i.e. into

4000 visual words. The value of K is the dimension of our ECoHOG used in our experiments. We use the sum of the squared difference to calculate the nearest BoF vector f for each input feature in each frame.

So in training for each fine grained activity dense trajectories are described using ECoHOG whose dimensions are reduced using PCA and they are all clustered into 4000 visual words. In ECoHOG representation, the feature models weighting gradient magnitude and it effectively evaluate edge features in co-occurrence elements. The ECoHOG features vectorize almost the same BoF vectors if activity is in the same class. The statistical learning allows us to classify a large number of activity classes, in other words, the feature can be better approach in fine-grained activity categorization.

5 Experiments

We carried out experiments to validate influence of our ECoHOG feature in fine-grained activity recognition. In this section, we discuss the datasets, parameter selection, and comparison of the proposed approach with state-of-the-art methods. The classifier setting is based on the original dense trajectories [9].

5.1 Datasets

We used two different datasets for fine-grained categorization. Visual distinction is difficult because the categories are often subtly different in the feature space. Moreover, they are difficult to distinguish using current activity recognition approaches. The INRIA surgery dataset [7] and MPII cooking activities dataset [5] are discussed below.

INRIA Surgery Dataset [7]**.** This dataset includes four activities performed by 10 different people with occlusions; e.g., people are occluded by a table or chair (see Fig. 3). The activities include cutting, hammering, repositioning, and sitting. Each person performed the same activity twice, one for training and another for testing in this experiment.

MPII Cooking Activities Dataset [5]**.** This dataset contains 65 activities (see Table 2) performed by 12 participants. These activities can be broadly categorized into a few basic activities, such as seven ways of "cutting", five ways of "taking", and so on. In total, the dataset comprises 8 hours (881,755 frames) in 44 videos. Performance is evaluated by leave-one-person-out cross-validation.

5.2 Parameter Selection

Figure 4 shows the relationship between the parameter settings and accuracy of the co-occurrence feature. In this situation, we must set the number of dimensions for PCA and offset size in the ECoHOG. Other settings for the dense trajectories and co-occurrence feature are based on [6,9], respectively. Here we focus on the seven "cutting" activities, which represent the most fine-grained

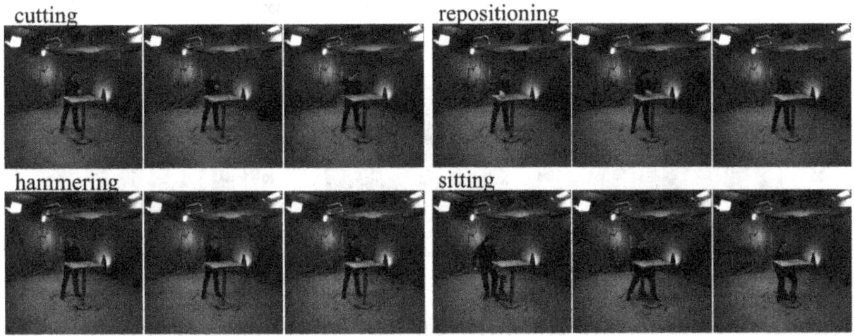

Fig. 3. INRIA surgery dataset [7], which includes four activities (cutting, hammering, repositioning, sitting).

category (Table 2 shows that activities 3 to 9 are the most confusing in terms of accurate recognition) in the MPII cooking activities dataset.

Figure 4(a) and (b) shows the number of dimensions and accuracy of the seven activities in the "cutting" category. The graph in Fig. 4(a) shows that using a feature vector with 50 dimensions achieves the highest accuracy, and therefore, detailed results for 50 to 100 dimensions are depicted in Fig. 4(b). From these results, we can judge the importance of balancing the "contribution ratio in PCA" and the "size of the feature space". As shown in Fig. 4(b), 70 is the optimal value for creating the BoF vector in the ECoHOG feature.

Figure 4(c) shows the relationship between offset (feature extraction window) size and accuracy, with 5×5 being the optimal offset in this experiment. Most edge orientation pairs are extracted with a 1.0–3.0 pixel distance in commonly used edge orientation according to this figure. It is also important to consider "pixel similarity". Since near field pixels tend to have similar features, the feature vector should be designed to capture pixel similarity. Figure 5 shows the top 50 frequently used ECoHOG elements with an offset size of 11×11. According to the figure, neighboring pixels mostly support effective feature extraction. In the rest of the experiments we used 70 dimensional features and offset length of 5×5 pixel.

5.3 Comparison of Proposed and State-of-the-Art Methods

In this section, we enumerate the experimental results on the INRIA surgery and MPII cooking activities datasets to compare the proposed approach with state-of-the-art methods. In other words, we apply the original dense trajectories, CoHOG/ECoHOG in dense trajectories, and an integrated approach (ECoHOG, HOF, MBH, Trajectory). Simple HOG is consist of any tracking method and HOG description. We track a human and extract HOG feature in a tracked bounding box.

Experiment on INRIA Surgery Dataset. Table 1 shows the classification results on the INRIA surgery dataset. The original dense trajectories [9] achieved

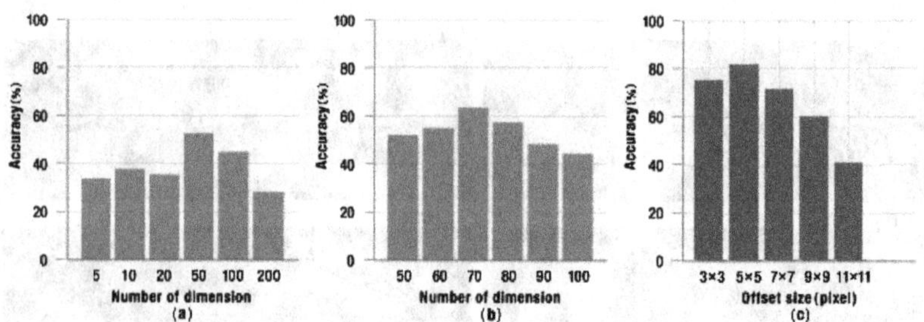

Fig. 4. Co-occurrence feature parameter settings for cutting activities (nos. 3–9 in Table 2): (a) number of dimensions for PCA; (b) detailed number of dimensions from 50 to 100 dimensions; (c) relationship between offset size and accuracy.

Table 1. Accuracy of the proposed and conventional frameworks on the INRIA surgery dataset.

Approach	Accuracy (%)
Tracking + HOG	40.16
Original Dense Trajectories (HOG, HoF, MBH, Trajectory)	93.58
CoHOG in Dense Trajectories (CoHOG)	81.05
ECoHOG in Dense Trajectories (ECoHOG)	96.36
Improved Dense Trajectories (ECoHOG, HOF, MBH, Trajectory)	97.31

93.58 % accuracy thanks to dense sampling and the use of multi-type feature descriptions, whereas our proposed approach achieved 96.36 %, applying only ECoHOG on the dense feature extraction on densely sampled trajectories. However, the integrated approach achieved a better result than the other two approaches (97.31 % accuracy). ECoHOG improves CoHOG by including edge-magnitude accumulation, which expresses co-occurrence strength. ECoHOG comprehensively evaluates edge features and effectively generates more distinguishable BoF features in an image patch. ECoHOG represents the edge-boundary, which can effectively be added to the co-occurrence feature in fine-grained categorization. Overall, ECoHOG performed 15.31 % better than CoHOG in the framework with dense trajectories, and 2.78 % better than the original dense trajectories. The integrated approach performed slightly better (0.95 %) than ECoHOG in the dense trajectories. In this context, other features, such as HOF, MBH, and Trajectory, supplement the ECoHOG feature in representing spatial and temporal image features. ECoHOG mainly represents the shape feature, while the other features capture motion features in the video sequences.

Experiment on MPII Cooking Activities Dataset. Table 2 shows the results on the MPII cooking activities dataset. The dataset contains 65 classes of cooking activities for measuring fine-grained activity recognition performance. The results for method 2, original dense trajectories, in Table 2 were taken from [5] as the baseline method. The original dense trajectories achieved 44.2 % accuracy (without pose feature combination) on the dataset using HOG, HOF, MBH, and Trajectory

Table 2. Accuracy of the proposed and conventional frameworks on the MPII cooking activities dataset. Activity tags include 1. Background activity; 2. Change temperature; 3. Cut apart; 4. Cut dice; 5. Cut; 6. Cut off ends; 7. Cut out inside; 8. Cut slices; 9. Cut strips; 10. Dry; 11. Fill water from tap; 12. Grate; 13. Lid: put on; 14. Lid: remove; 15. Mix; 16. Move from X to Y; 17. Open egg; 18. Open tin; 19. Open/close cupboard; 20. Open/close drawer; 21. Open/close fridge; 22. Open/close oven; 23. Package X; 24. Peel; 25. Plug in/out; 26. Pour; 27. Pull out; 28. Puree; 29. Put in bowl; 30. Put in pan/pot; 31. Put on bread/dough; 32. Put on cutting board; 33. Put on plate; 34. Read; 35. Remove from package; 36. Rip open; 37. Scratch off; 38. Screw closed; 39. Screw open; 40. Shake; 41. Smell; 42. Spice; 43. Spread; 44. Squeeze; 45. Stamp; 46. Stir; 47. Sprinkle; 48. Take & put in cupboard; 49. Take & put in drawer; 50. Take & put in fridge; 51. Take & put in oven; 52. Take & put in spice holder; 53. Take ingredient apart; 54. Take out of cupboard; 55. Take out of drawer; 56. Take out of oven; 57. Take out of oven; 58. Take out of spice holder; 59. Taste; 60. Throw in garbage; 61. Unroll dough; 62. Wash hands; 63. Wash objects; 64. Whisk; 65. Wipe clean.: (1) original dense trajectories [5] (**44.2 %**), (2) CoHOG in dense trajectories (**46.2 %**), (3) ECoHOG in dense trajectories (**46.6 %**), (4) combined model in dense trajectories with ECoHOG, HOF, MBH, and Trajectory (**49.1 %**). The tracking + HOG model recorded **18.2 %** on the MPII cooking activities dataset.

Activity Number	(1)	(2)	(3)	(4)	Activity Number	(1)	(2)	(3)	(4)
1	47.1	17.8	83.6	55.0	34	34.5	11.7	54.1	5.8
2	37.6	12.3	21.9	14.5	35	39.1	69.2	72.7	78.7
3	16.0	68.5	17.0	13.0	36	5.8	16.8	27.2	29.5
4	25.1	6.8	84.5	50.1	37	3.8	63.5	66.6	72.2
5	22.8	36.8	40.4	43.8	38	36.3	36.8	27.7	30.0
6	7.4	2.0	8.5	9.2	39	19.1	51.4	22.9	24.9
7	16.3	0.0	0.0	29.0	40	33.5	16.6	72.7	78.7
8	42.0	46.0	24.1	26.2	41	24.8	37.4	39.2	42.5
9	27.6	37.3	46.3	50.1	42	29.3	28.7	32.2	34.9
10	95.5	69.2	43.9	47.5	43	11.2	5.2	25.7	27.8
11	75.0	16.9	17.1	18.5	44	90.0	10.3	72.7	78.7
12	32.9	34.6	24.6	26.6	45	73.3	52.2	25.8	28.0
13	2.0	19.6	45.0	48.8	46	50.0	69.2	52.4	56.8
14	1.9	5.0	3.2	3.4	47	39.6	38.8	37.9	74.8
15	36.8	94.9	68.7	74.4	48	37.2	69.2	72.7	78.7
16	15.9	42.9	72.7	78.7	49	37.6	8.7	3.9	4.2
17	45.2	27.1	26.1	28.3	50	54.6	0.0	75.1	81.3
18	79.5	69.2	72.7	78.7	51	100	55.8	72.7	78.7
19	54.0	32.9	64.0	69.3	52	80.2	4.9	11.7	12.7
20	38.1	42.2	8.9	9.6	53	17.5	33.3	22.3	24.2
21	73.7	69.2	72.7	78.7	54	81.5	24.1	25.5	27.7
22	25.0	26.3	38.2	41.4	55	79.7	69.2	72.5	78.5

(Continued)

Table 2. *(Continued)*

Activity Number	(1)	(2)	(3)	(4)	Activity Number	(1)	(2)	(3)	(4)
23	31.9	69.2	72.7	78.7	56	73.6	48.8	27.2	29.5
24	65.2	45.6	48.3	52.4	57	83.3	45.4	27.4	29.7
25	54.7	12.0	37.1	40.2	58	67.0	42.3	50.4	54.6
26	54.2	12.5	17.1	11.9	59	18.2	30.1	2.1	22.8
27	87.5	69.2	34.2	37.1	60	84.4	4.0	42.7	46.3
28	67.1	11.5	12.9	14.0	61	100	69.2	8.3	9.0
29	18.8	69.2	72.7	78.7	62	45.9	52.0	54.4	59.0
30	15.3	29.8	12.6	13.7	63	67.1	15.1	39.7	43.0
31	42.1	18.8	5.4	5.9	64	70.0	13.9	8.8	9.6
32	7.1	9.5	72.7	78.7	65	10.6	63.1	33.4	36.2
33	11.0	36.9	45.7	49.5	**Mean**	**44.2**	**46.2**	**46.6**	**49.1**

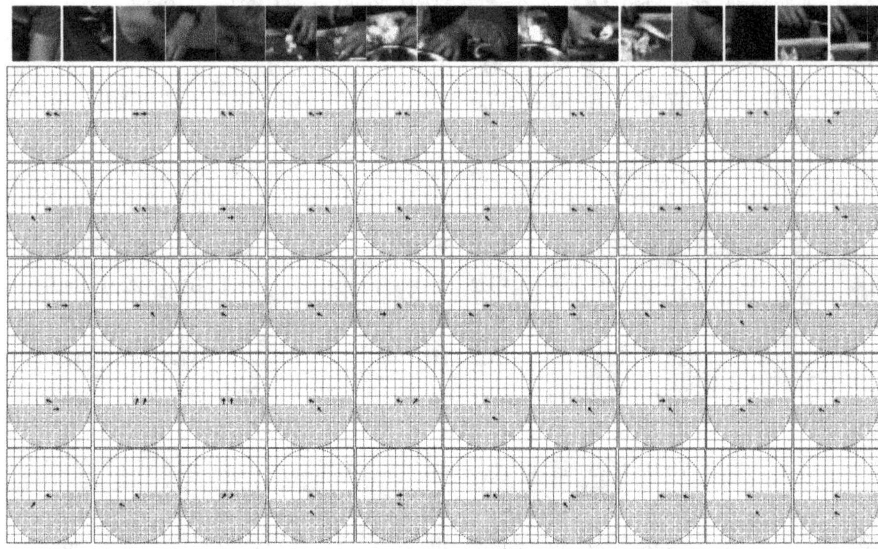

Fig. 5. (Top row) image patches on dense trajectories from MPII cooking dataset. (Remaining rows: left to right and top to bottom in decreasing order) top 50 frequently used offsets and orientations with 11 × 11 pixel offset.

features. ECoHOG in dense trajectories (method 4 in Table 2) achieved 46.6 % better accuracy than the baseline. At the same time, CoHOG in dense trajectories (method 3 in Table 2) is superior to the baseline. According to these results, the co-occurrence feature effectively represents detailed space–time shapes in fine-grained activities. The combined method (method 5 in Table 2) achieved 49.1 % better accuracy than the other approaches with all types of features (ECoHOG,

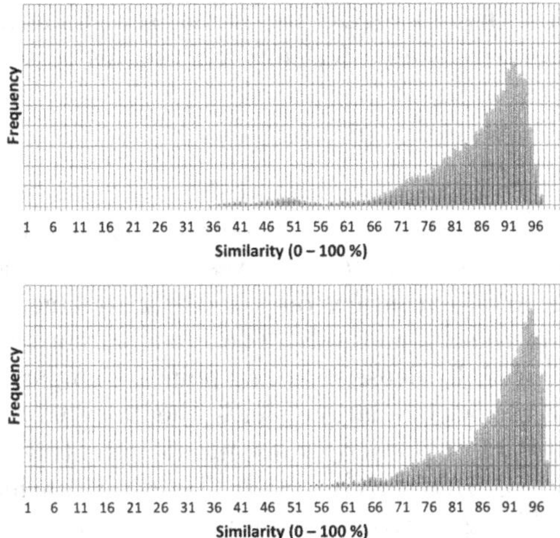

Fig. 6. Self-similarity of CoHOG (top) and ECoHOG (bottom) for 1,000 randomly chosen image patches from MPII cooking activities dataset: ${}_nC_k$ self-similarities in the graph ($n = 1000, k = 2$), the vertical axis denotes frequency and the horizontal axis gives the percentage similarity.

HOF, MBH, Trajectory). According to these results, HOF/MBH/trajectory features complementarily extract image features from the ECoHOG feature, which contains co-occurrence orientation and edge magnitude information on the edge extraction window. The co-occurrence feature mainly captures shape information; however, a detailed configuration is expressed from image patches on trajectories. On the other hand, the HOF/MBH/Trajectory features handle motion features between frames, which aid activity recognition in the fine-grained dataset. The combined approach achieves slightly better accuracy than ECoHOG in dense trajectories. In this experiment, performance of ECoHOG was 0.4 % better than CoHOG and 2.4 % better than the original dense trajectories. The combined model with ECoHOG/HOF/MBH/Trajectory features represents image features comprehensively and achieves 4.9 % better accuracy than the baseline method.

The similarity of feature histogram is directly linked to significant BoF vector. We evaluate the similarities of CoHOG and ECoHOG feature as co-occurrence representation. Figure 6 shows the histograms of self-similarity on image patches (similar to Fig. 5) from the MPII cooking activities dataset. In this case, 1,000 image patches were selected to calculate histogram similarity, giving the number of combinations ${}_nC_k, n = 1000, k = 2 (= 499500)$. We used the Bhattacharyya coefficient [25] to calculate histogram similarity:

$$S = \sum_{u=1}^{m} \sqrt{h_u^1 h_u^2} \tag{7}$$

where S is the similarity value ($0 \leq S \leq 1$), h^1 and h^2 are feature vectors normalized as $\sum_{u=1}^{m} h_u^1 = \sum_{u=1}^{m} h_u^2 = 1.0$, and m denotes the number of histogram bins. The graphs show that ECoHOG has higher self-similarity scores; that is, ECoHOG tends to evaluate similar features and creates better BoF vectors.

6 Conclusion

In this paper, we proposed an improved co-occurrence feature in dense trajectories. The proposed approach, which achieves 96.36 % accuracy on the INRIA surgery dataset and 46.6 % accuracy on the MPII cooking activities dataset, is superior to state-of-the-art methods. The co-occurrence feature represents detailed shapes on temporally dense sampling points. Comparing ECoHOG with CoHOG, the magnitude accumulation yields the boundary division between objective motion and the background by magnitude weighting. We found that an integrated approach (ECoHOG, HOF, MBH, Trajectory) achieves better accuracy 97.1 % and 49.1 %, respectively. These values are 3.73 % and 4.9 % better than the proposed approach on the INRIA surgery dataset and MPII cooking activities dataset, respectively.

We also investigated the parameter settings in the video datasets, that is, offset length and number of dimensions in PCA of the co-occurrence feature. Optimal parameter values for creating the BoF vector in the co-occurrence feature are 5×5 (pixel) offset length and 70 PCA dimensions. "Pixel similarity", which is the co-occurrence pairs are extracted from neighbor area must be considered in the offset length to adjust the dimension size. Moreover, the PCA dimension should balance the "contribution ratio in PCA" and "size of the feature space" for the BoF vector. Given the above, we experimentally chose 70 dimensions from the original 640 ECoHOG dimensions.

References

1. Moeslund, T.B., Hilton, A., Kruger, V., Sigal, L.: Visual Analysis of Humans: Looking at People. Springer, London (2011)
2. Aggarwal, J.K., Cai, Q.: Human motion analysis: a review. Comput. Vis. Image Underst. (CVIU) **73**(3), 428–440 (1999)
3. Moeslund, T.B., Hilton, A., Kruger, V.: A survey of advances in vision-based human motion capture and analysis. Comput. Vis. Image Underst. (CVIU) **104**(2), 90–126 (2006)
4. Ryoo, M.S., Aggarwal, J.K.: Human activity analysis: a review. ACM Comput. Surv. (CSUR) **43**(3), 16 (2011)
5. Rohrbach, M., Amin, S., Andriluka, M., Schiele, B.: A database for fine grained activity detection of cooking activities. In: IEEE Conference on Computer Vision and Pattern Recognition (CVPR) (2012)
6. Watanabe, T., Ito, S., Yokoi, K.: Co-occurrence histograms of oriented gradients for pedestrian detection. In: Wada, T., Huang, F., Lin, S. (eds.) PSIVT 2009. LNCS, vol. 5414, pp. 37–47. Springer, Heidelberg (2009)
7. Huang, C.-H., Boyer, E., Navab, N., Ilic, S.: Human shape and pose tracking using keyframes. In: IEEE Conference on Computer Vision and Pattern Recognition (CVPR) (2014)

8. Wang, H., Klaser, A., Schmid, C., Liu, C.L.: Action recognition by dense trajectories. In: IEEE Conference on Computer Vision and Pattern Recognition (CVPR), pp. 3169–3176 (2011)
9. Wang, H., Klaser, A., Schmid, C., Liu, C.L.: Dense trajectories and motion boundary descriptors for action recognition. Int. J. Comput. Vis. (IJCV) **103**, 60–79 (2013)
10. Laptev, I.: On space-time interest points. Int. J. Comput. Vis. (IJCV) **64**, 107–123 (2005)
11. Laptev, I., Marszalek, M., Schmid, C., Rozenfeld, B.: Learning realistic human actions from movies. In: IEEE Conference on Computer Vision and Pattern Recognition (CVPR), pp. 1–8 (2008)
12. Klaser, A., Marszalek, M., Schmid, C.: A spatio-temporal descriptor based on 3D-gradients. In: British Machine Vision Conference (BMVC) (2008)
13. Marszalek, M., Laptev, I., Schmid, C.: Actions in context. In: IEEE Conference on Computer Vision and Pattern Recognition (CVPR), pp. 2929–2936 (2009)
14. Everts, I., Gemert, J.C., Gevers, T.: Evaluation of color STIPs for human activity recognition. In: IEEE Conference on Computer Vision and Pattern Recognition (CVPR), pp. 2850–2857 (2013)
15. Zinnen, A., Blanke, U., Schiele, B.: An analysis of sensor-oriented vs. model - based activity recognition. In: IEEE International Symposium on Wearable Computers (ISWC) (2009)
16. Dalal, N., Triggs, B.: Histograms of oriented gradients for human detection. In: IEEE Conference on Computer Vision and Pattern Recognitino (CVPR), pp. 886–893 (2005)
17. Dalal, N., Triggs, B., Schmid, C.: Human detection using oriented histograms of flow and appearance. In: Leonardis, A., Bischof, H., Pinz, A. (eds.) ECCV 2006. LNCS, vol. 3952, pp. 428–441. Springer, Heidelberg (2006)
18. Raptis, M., Kokkinos, I., Soatto, S.: Discovering discriminative action parts from mid-level video representation. In: IEEE Conference on Computer Vision and Pattern Recognition (CVPR), pp. 1242–1249 (2013)
19. Li, B., Camps, O., Sznaier, M.: Cross-view activity recognition using hankelets. In: IEEE Conference on Computer Vision and Pattern Recognition (CVPR), pp. 1362–1369 (2012)
20. Jain, M., Jegou, H., Bouthemy, P.: Better exploiting motion for better action recognition. IEEE Conference on Computer Vision and Pattern Recognition (CVPR), pp. 2555–2562 (2013)
21. Peng, X., Qiao, Y., Peng, Q., Qi, X.: Exploring motion boundary based sampling and spatial temporal context descriptors for action recognition. In: British Machine Vision Conference (BMVC) (2013)
22. Wang, H., Schmid, C.: Action recognition with improved trajectories. In: International Conference on Computer Vision (ICCV), pp. 3551–3558 (2013)
23. Csurka, G., Bray, C., Dance, C., Fan, L.: Visual categorization with bags of keypoints. In: European Conference on Computer Vision (ECCV) Workshop on Statistical Learning in Computer Vision, pp. 59–74 (2004)
24. Perronnin, F., Sánchez, J., Mensink, T.: Improving the fisher kernel for large-scale image classification. In: Daniilidis, K., Maragos, P., Paragios, N. (eds.) ECCV 2010, Part IV. LNCS, vol. 6314, pp. 143–156. Springer, Heidelberg (2010)
25. Bhattacharyya, A.: On a measure of divergence between two statistical populations defined by their probability distributions. Bull. Calcutta Math. Soc. **35**, 99–109 (1943)

Motion Based Foreground Detection and Poselet Motion Features for Action Recognition

Erwin Kraft[1](✉) and Thomas Brox[2]

[1] Fraunhofer ITWM, Fraunhofer-Platz 1, Kaiserslautern, Germany
erwin.kraft@itwm.fhg.de

[2] University of Freiburg, Georges-Köhler-Allee 52, Freiburg, Germany
brox@cs.uni-freiburg.de

Abstract. For action recognition, the actor(s) and the tools they use as well as their motion are of central importance. In this paper, we propose separating foreground items of an action from the background on the basis of motion cues. As a consequence, separate descriptors can be defined for the foreground regions, while combined foreground-background descriptors still capture the context of an action. Also a low-dimensional global camera motion descriptor can be computed. Poselet activations in the foreground area indicate the actor and its pose. We propose tracking these poselets to obtain detailed motion features of the actor. Experiments on the Hollywood2 dataset show that foreground-background separation and the poselet motion features lead to consistently favorable results, both relative to the baseline and in comparison to the current state-of-the-art.

1 Introduction

All actions involve an actor and in most cases the actor must move to perform the action. Surprisingly, these facts have not been used much in the literature on action recognition. State-of-the-art works rather rely on global feature aggregation that do not make explicit use of the notion of an actor [2–6]. Exceptions are Ullah et al. [7], who run a person detector to find persons, and Prest et al. [8], who even try to detect action specific objects, such as cups and cigarettes. Wang et al. [6] also use a person detector but it is only used to improve their video stabilization method.

In static action classification, the important role of the actor is more appreciated, which is reflected by the fact that in the Pascal VOC Action Classification challenge, the bounding box of the actor is already provided [9]. In the 2012 challenge, a task was offered, where only the coarse location of the actor is provided, but there was not any submission on this task.

In this paper, we advocate focusing on foreground items of an action, which includes especially the actor. In contrast to Ullah et al. [7] and Prest et al. [8], who suggested finding the actor and other persons in the video directly with a person detector, we propose to first detect the foreground items based on motion before running poselet detectors [12] to localize the (relevant) actor(s) in these

D. Cremers et al. (Eds.): ACCV 2014, Part V, LNCS 9007, pp. 350–365, 2015.
DOI: 10.1007/978-3-319-16814-2_23

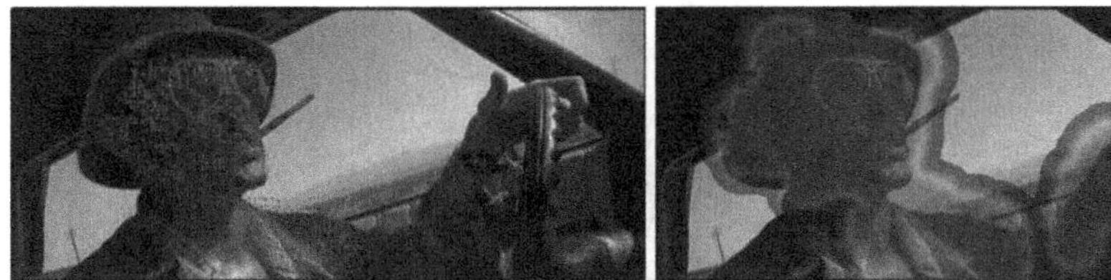

Fig. 1. Foreground scores are computed from sparse point trajectories (left). The intensities of the red pixels reflect the soft foreground scores. From these we can compute dense saliency maps (right) (Color figure online).

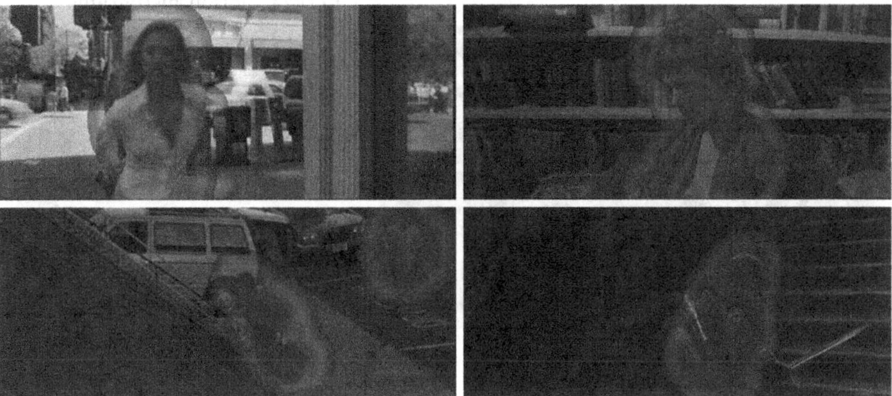

Fig. 2. Motion based foreground detection for some videos of the Hollywood2 dataset [1]. Foreground objects are marked with red pixels. Features computed specifically on the foreground help action classification (Color figure online).

foreground areas. While there has been much progress on person detectors in recent years [10–12], person detection is still error prone. Here we exploit the fact that the actor usually has to move to perform an action, i.e., motion indicates the relevance of a person detection for the action. Motion cues enable separation of moving foreground objects from the background quite reliably, as demonstrated in [13]. Admittedly, there are cases, where items of an action and even the main actor itself are static. However, such failure cases are quite rare, and they are outnumbered by those cases where current person detectors fail. Hence, compared to [7], we achieve much better performance. We also compare to [14], where an eye tracking system was used to emphasize the part of the image that humans consider most important. Although this approach uses additional supervision, we obtain higher performance with the proposed motion based saliency Fig. 1.

In the foreground we collect poselet activations for two reasons. First, poselets indicate which parts of the foreground are indeed persons. As the examples in Figs. 2 and 7 show, the foreground in an action dataset consists mostly of persons, but it can contain also a car that enters the scene and stops before a person

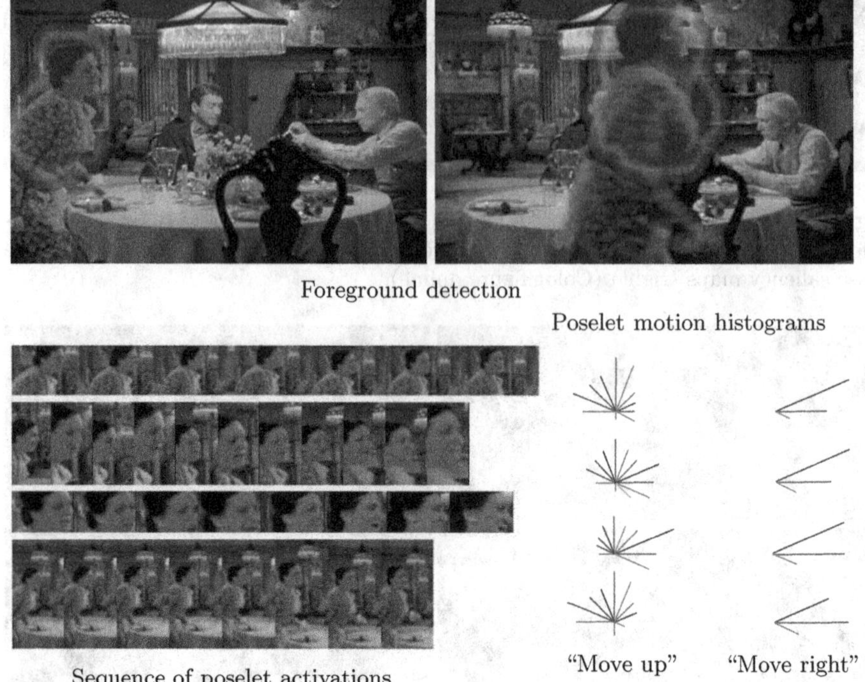

Fig. 3. Illustration of the proposed poselet motion features: we detect poselets [12] in the foreground and describe their motions over time. Thus, we encode pose information as well as the movement of specific body parts into our feature representation.

(the real actor) gets out. Second, poselets are not just person detectors but each poselet type indicates a specific body part and pose. Already static poselet activations help classify actions, as shown in [15,16]. Here we propose motion histograms accumulated for each poselet along its trajectory, which makes a strong feature on how body parts move in a particular action; see the illustration in Fig. 3.

In general, having separate foreground features is advantageous since many actions are mostly independent of the scene background. For instance, the action "Answer Phone" may occur in multiple settings: indoors, while riding a car, or outdoors in a park. In all those cases the background holds only very little information about the action class, while foreground objects (persons holding a phone) are the main indicators.

On the other hand, there *is* correlation between the action and the background. Therefore, the strategy here is to have descriptors specific to the foreground *additionally* to joint descriptors that can capture the context. The same is true for motion compensation, as used in [4–6]. While it is advantageous to define separate descriptors for motion compensated videos to be invariant to the

Table 1. Overview of all features used in our action recognition approach.

A	Trajectory aligned features from Wang et al. [3]
B	A on motion compensated trajectories
C	A only on foreground
D	B only on foreground
E	Global camera motion histogram
F	Global foreground motion histogram
G	Poselet motion features [12]

camera motion, there is much correlation between certain actions and the camera motion. Rather than the ignorance of such correlation, we advocate the separation into correlated and non-correlated descriptors. For this reason, we also propose a very low-dimensional descriptor that explicitly represents the camera motion, which is a by-product of the foreground separation. Table 1 gives an overview of the overall feature combination. We show that this leads to state-of-the-art results on the challenging Hollywood2 dataset [1].

2 Motion Based Foreground Separation

In this section we aim for separating the actor and other moving objects that may be involved in the action from the background. We assume that for action recognition the most relevant parts of an image are those that show independent motion, i.e., the segmentation comes down to a special type of motion segmentation. The foreground separation allows us to define features that are independent of the background.

Previously, [5,6] have used video stabilization by computing a global homography and subtracting it from the motion vectors. The main motivation for such motion compensation is the improved invariance of motion features to the camera motion. For this reason, we also use video stabilization when we compute motion features. However, motion compensation also allows for a rough foreground/background separation because, under good conditions, background trajectories become static. In [5,6] a simple thresholding of the motion magnitude after stabilization was used to emphasize foreground objects. In Fig. 4 we illustrate that this procedure oftentimes does not lead to a clean foreground separation.

The method we propose is based on clustering dense trajectories, which are computed using the LDOF-tracker from [17]. In contrast to [13], we are interested in exactly two clusters (foreground and background) and we model the background with a rigid 3D motion model. First, we compute a foreground score for each trajectory and then use a standard spatio-temporal minimum cut to obtain a segmentation.

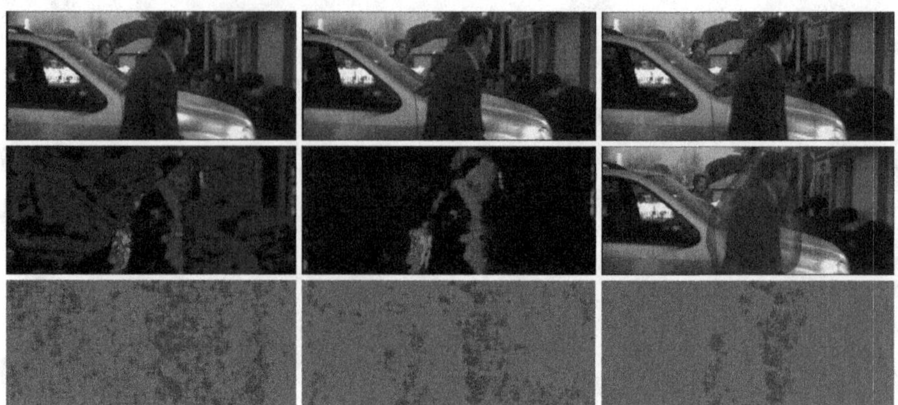

Fig. 4. Background feature pruning based on video stabilization versus foreground saliency maps. **Top row:** Sample input sequence. **Middle row, left:** Optical flow. **Middle row, center:** Optical flow after motion compensation. **Middle row, right:** Foreground saliency map computed with our approach. **Bottom row, left:** Case without camera motion compensation keeps all feature points. **Middle:** The camera motion has been compensated and features on static trajectories have been pruned [5,6]. Due to the remaining residual motion many features in the background are not pruned. **Right:** The proposed foreground saliency maps are based on a much more accurate motion model and include the long-term aspect of motion. The foreground separation is much cleaner.

2.1 Foreground Scores

Foreground scores are computed by comparing each trajectory to a background motion model that is estimated with a factorization approach [18,19]. This motion model explores the assumption that under orthogonal projections the background motion can be described by three trajectories. A projection matrix P_τ is constructed from trajectories $\mathbf{w}_i = [\mathbf{x}_{1,i}^{\mathrm{T}}, ..., \mathbf{x}_{F,i}^{\mathrm{T}}] \in \mathbb{R}^{2F}$, where $\mathbf{x}_{t,i} = (x_{t,i}, y_{t,i})^{\mathrm{T}}$ are the spatial positions of the tracked points at time t, and F is the size of a temporal window centered at time τ [19]:

$$\mathrm{P}_\tau = \mathrm{W}_3(\mathrm{W}_3^{\mathrm{T}}\mathrm{W}_3)^{-1}\mathrm{W}_3^{\mathrm{T}}. \tag{1}$$

The matrix $\mathrm{W}_3 = [\mathbf{w}_i^{\mathrm{T}}\mathbf{w}_j^{\mathrm{T}}\mathbf{w}_k^{\mathrm{T}}]$ holds the three trajectories $\mathbf{w}_i$, $\mathbf{w}_j$ and $\mathbf{w}_k$, which describe the background motion hypothesis. The likelihood that a trajectory $\mathbf{w}$ is compatible with this hypothesis is measured by the projection distance:

$$f_\tau(\mathbf{w}|\mathrm{W}_3) = \|\mathrm{P}_\tau\mathbf{w} - \mathbf{w}\|_2 \tag{2}$$

The background motion is found using RANSAC. Motion hypotheses are scored by computing the projection errors for all trajectories and selecting the 25 % quantile as a score.

Once a background model has been estimated, the projected distance of a trajectory is converted into a foreground score:

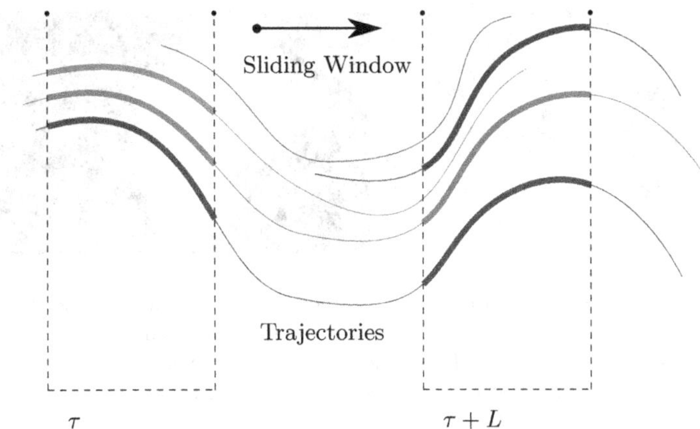

Fig. 5. Illustration of the sliding temporal window approach: only those trajectories that cover the temporal window completely are considered.

$$s_\tau(\mathbf{w}) = \exp\left(-\frac{f_\tau(\mathbf{w}|\mathrm{W}_3)}{2\sigma_0^2}\right), \tag{3}$$

where σ_0 is the average distance over all trajectories. Small s_τ indicate trajectories that do not fit to the background model. Thus we use $1-s_\tau$ as the foreground score and s_τ as the background score.

The above approach assumes that all trajectories have the same length. In practice this is not the case due to occlusion. Hence, we run the approach in sliding temporal windows of size $L = 6$. In each window we only consider those trajectories that fully cover that window; see Fig. 5. Since most of the LDOF-trajectories are much longer than the window size, they typically receive multiple scores, one from each window they cover. We assign the maximum foreground score (and equivalently the minimum background score) as the overall score for a trajectory:

$$s(\mathbf{w}) = \min_\tau s_\tau(\mathbf{w}). \tag{4}$$

2.2 Binary Segmentation and Foreground Saliency Maps

We formulate the dense, binary segmentation as independent minimum cut problems on each frame. To ensure a labeling that is smooth in time, we build the graph for a spatio-temporal volume around the frame of interest (size 5 in time) and use a 26-neighborhood to connect the pixels in the volume. The unary term is only defined for the pixels covered by a trajectory. For pixels i covered by a trajectory $\mathbf{w}$ we have costs $\theta_i(0) = (1 - l(\mathbf{w})s(\mathbf{w}))$ and $\theta_i(1) = l(\mathbf{w})s(\mathbf{w})$, where $l(\mathbf{w})$ is the length of the trajectory normalized to a range between 0 and 1. Longer trajectories are assigned a larger score to emphasize objects that are

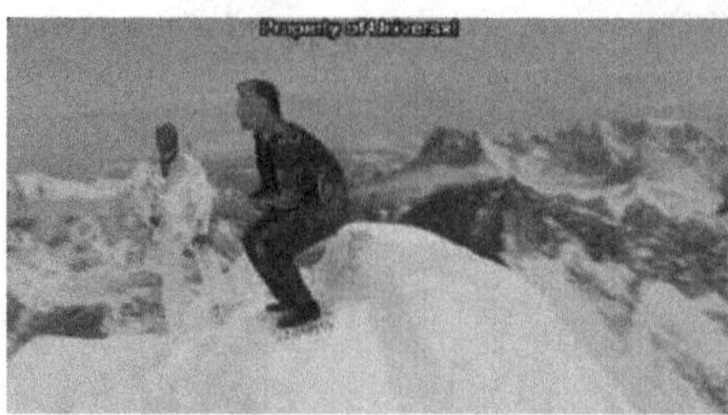

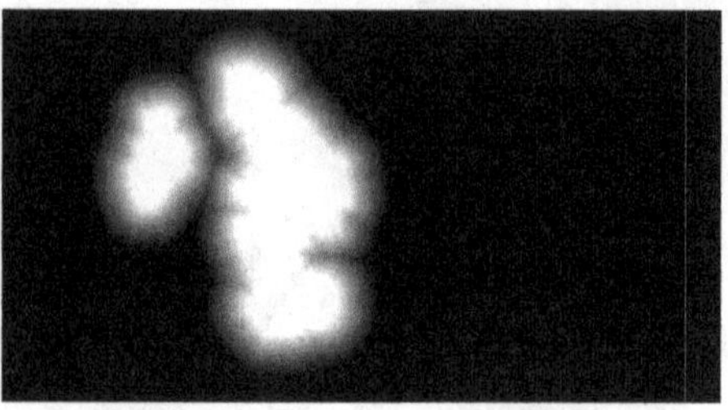

Fig. 6. Dense, binary segmentations are obtained from the sparse foreground scores (red pixels in the left image) by solving a set of minimum cut problems with the foreground scores as unary cost. The segmented image is then turned into a saliency map by applying a Euclidean distance transform (Color figure online).

visible for a longer time, since these are more likely to correspond to the actor in the shot. The energy on the binary labels X_i

$$E(X) = \sum_i \theta_i(X_i) - \kappa \sum_{i,j} \delta(X_i, X_j) \tag{5}$$

is minimized with the code from Kolmogorov [20]. δ is the 0-1 indicator function and we set $\kappa = 0.18$. This parameter was optimized using grid search on a small subset of the training set of the Hollywood2 [1] benchmark. Figure 6 shows an example of the final segmentation of the actor.

Since features in the area directly around the actor are often beneficial for action recognition, we extend the foreground region to a saliency map by applying a Euclidean distance transform; see Fig. 7.

3 Poselet Motion Features

It has been shown by Jhuang et al. [21] that high-level pose information improves action recognition performance significantly. Unfortunately, person detectors [11,12] and pose estimators [22] are not yet reliable enough to provide fine-grained information about the position of limbs and body parts on challenging action datasets. For instance, person detectors have difficulties with poses that are uncommon in static images but appear more often in videos. We experimented with the person detector from Bourdev et al. [12] on a small set of action clips and found that the detection scores decrease strongly when the pose changes from standing to sitting. This problem can be approached by tracking detections over time, i.e., scores from easy frames are propagated to more difficult ones.

Rather than relying on the functioning of a person detector, we consider the statistics of the raw poselet activations in the foreground region. Restricting the activations to the foreground ignores persons not involved in the action (as they do not move) but also false positive detections in the background; see Fig. 8. In contrast to a full person detector, the poselets also localize certain body parts

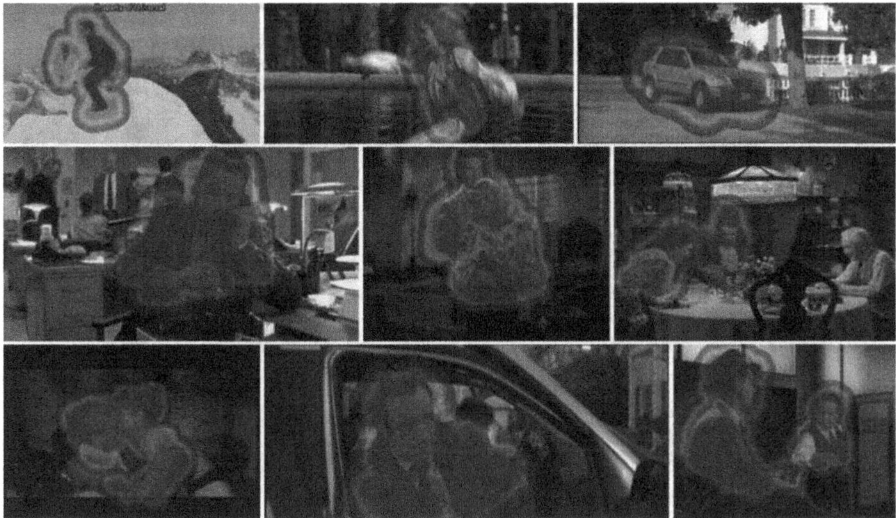

Fig. 7. Soft saliency maps generated from our foreground segmentation on some sample videos from the Hollywood2 benchmark [1]. The main actors are well covered by our saliency maps and are clearly separated from the scene background.

and their rough pose. It was demonstrated in [16] that the pose of a person can be encoded by the poselet activation vector. This may not be accurate, but still helps classify the action.

We are particularly interested in how the body parts described by the poselets move. For instance, it can be expected that the head and torso have to move upwards to perform the action "stand up" and downwards to perform the action "sit down". We extract the motion of a poselet from LDOF-trajectories [17]. For each poselet activation we consider all trajectories which are located inside the predicted bounding box. For all activations of a certain poselet we aggregate the motion vectors from an 8-frame time window in a motion histogram. A separate motion histogram is computed from stabilized and non-stabilized motion vectors. The histograms have 16 angular bins and two temporal bins. The latter allows consideration of whether a certain motion pattern appears more at the beginning or more at the end of a shot. Each motion vector votes with its magnitude for the respective bins using bilinear interpolation. The aggregation area of the temporal bins is deduced from the median length of the LDOF-trajectories. This ensures that a motion sequence will not be disrupted as it might be the case with evenly sized temporal bins. Since the video clips are in general very short, we found that a higher temporal resolution does not provide any further useful information. All motion histograms are normalized using the RootSIFT method [23]. Some poselet detections and the corresponding motion histograms are shown in Fig. 9.

We consider 150 poselets. For each we have two motion histograms (one aggregated over the stabilized and one over the non-stabilized motion vectors) and two temporal bins. Poselets that are not active in the first and/or second

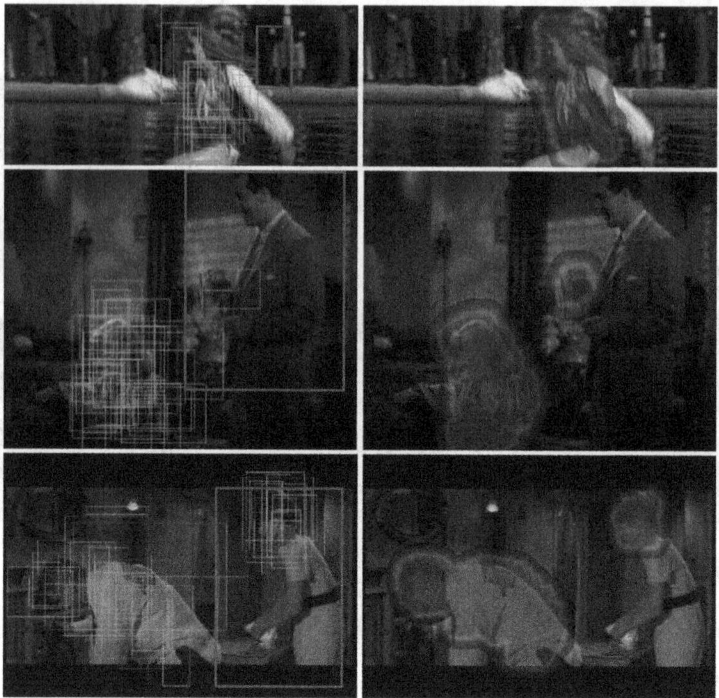

Fig. 8. Left: Poselet activations in three sample images. Green boxes show individual poselet activations [12] in the foreground region. Red boxes show the detected persons using [12]. **Right:** Foreground saliency maps. In all these examples, the main actor is missed by the person detector. Increasing the detection threshold would also lead to more false positives in the dataset. The motion based foreground saliency, on the other hand, indicates the main actor correctly in most cases. The individual poselet activations in the foreground indicate specific body parts and poses. We use the histogram over the motion of these poselets as features for classifying the action; see Fig. 9 (Color figure online).

part of a shot lead to a zero histogram. This means, the presence of a certain body part and pose is implicitly part of the overall feature vector.

4 Descriptors and Classification

With the foreground saliency maps from Sect. 2 and the poselet motion features from Sect. 3 we can define the descriptors as listed in Table 1. We build upon the local descriptors introduced by Wang et al. [3]: trajectory aligned HOG, HOF and MBH descriptors [10,24], as well as normalized trajectory shape descriptors. The descriptors can be seen as histograms that capture local image and motion structure along a trajectory path of fixed length. They are aggregated individually using the VLAD representation [25].

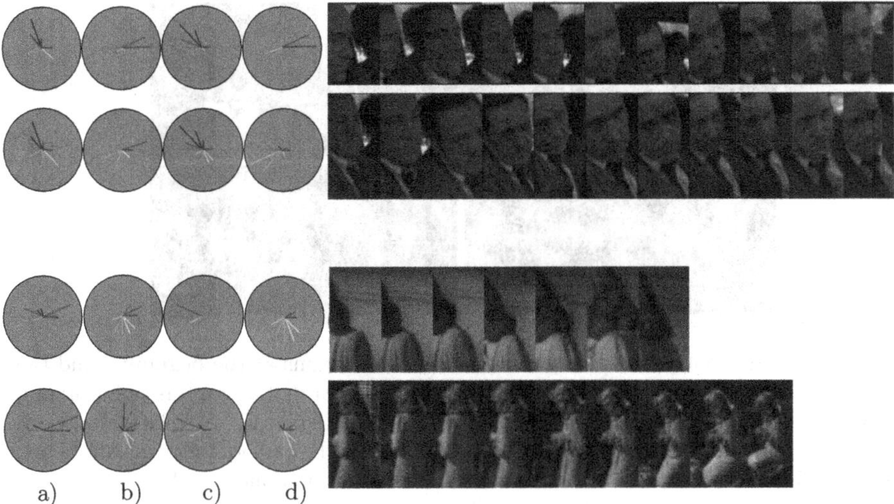

Fig. 9. Left: Poselet motion histograms for two video shots and two different poselets each. **a + b:** Histograms computed on non-stabilized motion vectors. **c + d:** Histograms computed on stabilized motion vectors. The poselet motion histograms have two temporal bins. a + c and b + d show the earlier and the later temporal bin, respectively. **Right:** Some of the activations of each of these poselets.

Based on the same methodology, we create additional VLAD features by using motion compensated trajectories similar to [5], and by using the foreground saliency maps. In the latter case, feature aggregation takes into account the saliency scores as weights. Features located in the background have very small or zero weights, which means they have hardly any influence.

We add the poselet motion features as described in Sect. 3. Moreover, we suggest using two global histograms, which encode the camera motion and the foreground motion. The camera motion histogram is aggregated over non-stabilized trajectories in the background, while the foreground motion histogram is computed from camera motion compensated trajectories in the foreground region. The histograms capture the directions of the trajectory displacements in the same way as for the poselet motion features. Each displacement vector votes with its magnitude into one of the 16 angular bins of the histogram and there are two temporal bins that cover the beginning and the end of the video clip. The global motion feature vector has a total size of 64 dimensions. An example is shown in Fig. 10.

All features are combined in the kernel function of a multi-channel SVM:

$$K(v_i, v_j) = \sum_c h(v_i^c, v_j^c), \tag{6}$$

where v_i^c and v_j^c are the individual features with respect to the c-th channel and $h(v_i^c, v_j^c)$ computes the histogram intersection between v_i^c and v_j^c. The

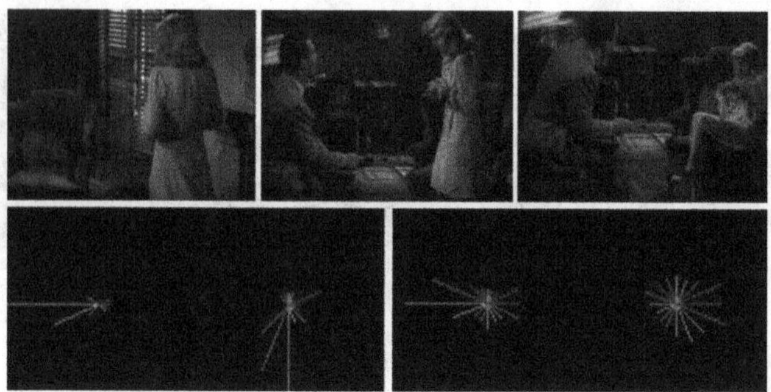

Fig. 10. Camera motion and foreground motion histograms at the beginning and the end of a video shot. Lines visualize the relative number of motion vectors pointing in a certain direction, as comprised in the histogram bins. Despite the correlation between camera motion and foreground motion, which is due to the camera following the actor, there are clear differences between foreground and background motion. This is exploited in our representation.

SVM-parameter $C = 0.001$ was selected based on cross-validation on the training set of the Hollywood2 benchmark [1].

5 Experiments

We evaluated our action recognition approach using the Hollywood2 benchmark [1]. This benchmark consists of 1707 video clips collected from 69 movies. It is divided into a training set (823 clips) and a test set (884 clips). Both sets were sampled from different movies. We increased the size of the training set by mirroring the training video clips. There are 12 action classes: stand up,

Table 2. Comparison of our results to the currently best results reported in literature.

	Hollywood2 mAP [1]
Marzałek et al. [1]	33.9 %
Gilbert et al. [26]	50.9 %
Ullah et al. [7]	55.7 %
Wang et al. [3]	58.3 %
Jiang et al. [4]	60.3 %
Vig et al. [14]	61.9 %
Jain et al. [5]	62.5 %
Oneaţă et al. [27]	63.3 %
Wang et al. [6]	64.3 %
Our method	**67.8** %

sit down, sit up, run, get out of car, hand shake, eat, drive, kiss, hug, fight and answer phone. Each action is evaluated by computing the average precision, and the mean average precision (mAP) is reported as overall result for the benchmark. The Hollywood2 benchmark can be considered as a very challenging benchmark. Many video clips contain multiple shots and show frequent and dynamic camera motion. Moreover, some of the actions have to be learned from a very small number of training samples. To show that the approach works on other datasets, we also evaluated it on the Olympic Sports dataset [28]. The performance is 77.5 % (without poselets) and 85.5 % (with poselet motion features). However, the Olympic Sports dataset [28] uses a very small test set (some actions are evaluated on only 3–4 video clips). This means that the overall score for Olympic Sports can be strongly affected based on just a few test examples. We therefore focus our detailed evaluation on the Hollywood2 benchmark where classification results depend on a significantly larger test set. A comprehensive overview of the plethora of different action recognition benchmarks can be found in [29].

Table 2 shows that our approach outperforms all other methods reported in literature so far. In particular, results are better than those of Ullah et al. [7], who used a person detector, and Vig et al. [14], who built upon saliency from an eye tracking system. A detailed analysis of the contribution of each set of features is presented in Table 3. It reveals that already the foreground saliency

Table 3. Action recognition results for the Hollywood2 benchmark [1]. We report the average precision (AP) for each action class and the mean average precision (mAP) as overall score. An overview and description of the individual features named A–G is given in Table 1.

Hollywood2 action class	Motion-stabilization B	Foreground-separation with saliency maps (A–F)	Foreground-separation with saliency maps + poselet motion (A–G)
Stand up	77.3 %	79.2 %	**81.8** %
Sit down	76.6 %	78.9 %	**80.3** %
Sit up	38.1 %	44.2 %	**50.8** %
Run	80.8 %	**85.3** %	84.9 %
Get out of car	68.1 %	**68.8** %	64.3 %
Hand shake	43.6 %	**48.4** %	46.9 %
Eat	60.2 %	66.2 %	**69.1** %
Drive car	96.3 %	**97.2** %	97.0 %
Kiss	61.6 %	68.2 %	**70.2** %
Hug	37.6 %	**46.2** %	45.8 %
Fight	**81.4** %	81.1 %	79.5 %
Answer phone	30.5 %	35.8 %	**36.0**%
mAP	62.7 %	66.6 %	**67.2** %

Table 4. Automatic selection of poselet motion features based on cross-validation: we split the Hollywood2 training set randomly into 7 subsets. For each feature set (A–F and A–G) we compute the mAP on the validation subsets and select the median as final score. An overview and description of the individual features named A–G is given in Table 1.

Hollywood2 action class	Validation score (A–F)	Validation score (A–G)	Use poselet motion	Score on test set
Stand up	64.3 %	**66.5** %	**Yes**	81.8 %
Sit down	61.7 %	**68.5** %	**Yes**	80.3 %
Sit up	25.8 %	**27.9** %	**Yes**	50.8 %
Run	**93.3** %	85.6 %	No	85.3 %
Get out of car	**30.6** %	21.8 %	No	68.8 %
Hand shake	**43.3** %	27.3 %	No	48.4 %
Eat	39.5 %	**47.3** %	**Yes**	69.1 %
Drive car	**89.1** %	88.3 %	No	97.2 %
Kiss	**67.1** %	62.7 %	No	68.2 %
Hug	**35.0** %	34.8 %	No	46.2 %
Fight	**74.7** %	70.8 %	No	81.1 %
Answer phone	**28.1** %	23.8 %	No	35.8 %
mAP				**67.8** %

maps in conjunction with the global motion histograms compare favorably to the current state-of-the-art by [6]. It also shows that separating the foreground and background based on our saliency maps leads to much better results than using just stabilized features.

The new poselet motion features increase the results even further, especially the actions stand up, sit down, sit up, eat and kiss show a strong improvement in performance while the other actions do not benefit. We assume that this is because the performance of poselet detectors is mostly limited to certain body parts, such as the head or shoulder. Some actions, e.g. hand shake, would require strong poselets on hands and arms. Also, the vast majority of the 150 poselets represents body parts seen from the front. Table 4 shows the performance of each individual action with and without poselets. By using poselets only on action classes where they improved performance on the validation set, the overall test set performance can be improved further.

5.1 Computation Times

Computation times for a $576 * 304$ video with 144 frames on a single workstation (purchased in the year 2009) are as follows: $288s$ for optical flow computation and point tracking, $47s$ for the non-stabilized features by Wang et al. [3], $127s$ including stabilization. Our contributions saliency map computation and poselet motion features require 160s and 199s, respectively. The most computationally expensive operations are: (1) LDOF computation, (2) running the poselets detector, (3) running the RANSAC part of the background subtraction, (4) video stabilization.

6 Conclusions

We have demonstrated that explicit separation of the video into foreground and background and computation of separate features has positive effects on action recognition performance. Since foreground detection with a person detector is still erroneous, we have proposed a bottom-up approach based on point trajectories. This is justified by the fact that most actions require the main actors (or the relevant parts of them) to move relative to the background. The foreground-background separation also allows us to define global, low-dimensional histograms for the camera motion and the foreground motion. To include more detailed evidence on the motion of the actor, we have proposed poselet motion features, which indicate how a certain body part in a certain pose usually moves in a certain action. These features strongly improve action recognition performance when actors are seen from a frontal view. We conclude that this is an artifact of the current poselet detectors and the poselet motion features will become even more useful as body part detectors will improve. Even now our method sets the state-of-the-art on the most challenging Hollywood2 dataset.

References

1. Marzałek, M., Laptev, I., Schmid, C.: Actions in context. In: Computer Vision and Pattern Recognition (CVPR), pp. 2929–2936 (2009)
2. Laptev, I., Lindeberg, T.: Space-time interest points. In: International Conference on Computer Vision (ICCV), pp. 432–439 (2003)
3. Wang, H., Kläser, A., Schmid, C., Liu, C.-L.: Action recognition by dense trajectories. In: Computer Vision and Pattern Recognition (CVPR), pp. 3169–3176 (2011)
4. Jiang, Y.-G., Dai, Q., Xue, X., Liu, W., Ngo, C.-W.: Trajectory-based modeling of human actions with motion reference points. In: Fitzgibbon, A., Lazebnik, S., Perona, P., Sato, Y., Schmid, C. (eds.) ECCV 2012, Part V. LNCS, vol. 7576, pp. 425–438. Springer, Heidelberg (2012)
5. Jain, M., Jégou, H. Bouthemy, P.: Better exploiting motion for better action recognition. In: Computer Vision and Pattern Recognition (CVPR), pp. 2555–2562 (2013)
6. Wang, H., Schmid, C.: Action recognition with improved trajectories. In: International Conference on Computer Vision (ICCV), pp. 3551–3558 (2013)
7. Ullah, M.M., Parizi, S.N., Laptev, I.: Improving bag-of-features action recognition with non-local cues. In: British Machine Vision Conference (BMVC), pp. 1–11 (2010)
8. Prest, A., Schmid, C., Ferrari, V.: Weakly supervised learning of interactions between humans and objects. In: Pattern Analysis and Machine Intelligence (PAMI), pp. 601–614 (2012)

9. Pascal Visual Object Challenge. http://pascallin.ecs.soton.ac.uk/challenges/VOC/
10. Dalal, N., Triggs, B.: Histograms of oriented gradients for human detection. In: Computer Vision and Pattern Recognition (CVPR), pp. 886–893 (2005)
11. Felzenszwalb, P., Girshick, R., McAllester, D., Ramanan, D.: Object detection with discriminatively trained part based models. IEEE Trans. Pattern Anal. Mach. Intell. **32**, 1627–1645 (2010)
12. Bourdev, L., Maji, S., Brox, T., Malik, J.: Detecting people using mutually consistent poselet activations. In: Daniilidis, K., Maragos, P., Paragios, N. (eds.) ECCV 2010, Part VI. LNCS, vol. 6316, pp. 168–181. Springer, Heidelberg (2010)
13. Brox, T., Malik, J.: Object segmentation by long term analysis of point trajectories. In: Daniilidis, K., Maragos, P., Paragios, N. (eds.) ECCV 2010, Part V. LNCS, vol. 6315, pp. 282–295. Springer, Heidelberg (2010)
14. Vig, E., Dorr, M., Cox, D.: Space-variant descriptor sampling for action recognition based on saliency and eye movements. In: Fitzgibbon, A., Lazebnik, S., Perona, P., Sato, Y., Schmid, C. (eds.) ECCV 2012, Part VII. LNCS, vol. 7578, pp. 84–97. Springer, Heidelberg (2012)
15. Yang, W., Wang, Y., Mori, G.: Recognizing human actions from still images with latent poses. In: Computer Vision and Pattern Recognition (CVPR), pp. 2030–2037 (2010)
16. Maji, S., Bourdev, L., Malik, J.: Action recognition from a distributed representation of pose and appearance. In: Computer Vision and Pattern Recognition (CVPR), pp. 3177–3184 (2011)
17. Sundaram, N., Brox, T., Keutzer, K.: Dense point trajectories by GPU-accelerated large displacement optical flow. In: Daniilidis, K., Maragos, P., Paragios, N. (eds.) ECCV 2010, Part I. LNCS, vol. 6311, pp. 438–451. Springer, Heidelberg (2010)
18. Tomasi, C., Kanade, T.: Shape and motion from image streams under ortography: a factorization method. Int. J. Comput. Vis. **9**, 137–154 (1992)
19. Sheikh, Y., Javed, O., Kanade, T.: Background subtraction for freely moving cameras. In: International Conference on Computer Vision (ICCV), pp. 1219–1225 (2009)
20. Kolmogorov, V., Zabih, R.: What energy functions can be minimized via graph cuts? IEEE Trans. Pattern Anal. Mach. Intell. **26**, 147–159 (2004)
21. Jhuang, H., Gall, J., Zuffi, S., Schmid, C., Black, M.J.: Towards understanding action recognition. In: International Conference on Computer Vision (ICCV), pp. 3192–3199 (2013)
22. Zuffi, S., Black, M.J.: From pictorial structures to deformable structures. In: Computer Vision and Pattern Recognition (CVPR), pp. 3546–3553 (2012)
23. Arandjelović, R., Zisserman, A.: Three things everyone should know to improve object retrieval. In: Computer Vision and Pattern Recognition (CVPR), pp. 2911–2918 (2012)
24. Dalal, N., Triggs, B., Schmid, C.: Human detection using oriented histograms of flow and appearance. In: Leonardis, A., Bischof, H., Pinz, A. (eds.) ECCV 2006. LNCS, vol. 3952, pp. 428–441. Springer, Heidelberg (2006)
25. Jégou, H., Perronnin, F., Douze, M., Sánchez, J., Pérez, P., Schmid, C.: Aggregating local image descriptors into compact codes. IEEE Trans. Pattern Anal. Mach. Intell. **34**, 1704–1716 (2012)
26. Gilbert, A., Illingworth, J., Bowden, R.: Action recognition using mined hierarchical compound features. IEEE Trans. Pattern Anal. Mach. Intell. **33**, 883–897 (2011)

27. Oneaţă, D., Verbeek, J., Schmid, C.: Action and event recognition with fisher vectors on a compact feature set. In: International Conference on Computer Vision (ICCV), pp. 1817–1824 (2013)
28. Niebles, J.C., Chen, C.-W., Fei-Fei, L.: Modeling temporal structure of decomposable motion segments for activity classification. In: Daniilidis, K., Maragos, P., Paragios, N. (eds.) ECCV 2010, Part II. LNCS, vol. 6312, pp. 392–405. Springer, Heidelberg (2010)
29. Hassner, T.: A critical review of action recognition benchmarks. In: Computer Vision and Pattern Recognition Workshops (CVPRW), pp. 245–250 (2013)

Global Motion Estimation from Relative Measurements in the Presence of Outliers

Guillaume Bourmaud[1,2(✉)], Rémi Mégret[1,2,3], Audrey Giremus[1,2], and Yannick Berthoumieu[1,2]

[1] University Bordeaux, IMS, UMR 5218, 33400 Talence, France
guillaume.bourmaud@ims-bordeaux.fr
[2] CNRS, IMS, UMR 5218, 33400 Talence, France
[3] Department of Mathematical Sciences, University of Puerto-Rico at Mayaguez, Mayaguez, USA

Abstract. This work addresses the generic problem of global motion estimation (homographies, camera poses, orientations, etc.) from relative measurements in the presence of outliers. We propose an efficient and robust framework to tackle this problem when motion parameters belong to a Lie group manifold. It exploits the graph structure of the problem as well as the geometry of the manifold. It is based on the recently proposed iterated extended Kalman filter on matrix Lie groups. Our algorithm iteratively samples a minimum spanning tree of the graph, applies Kalman filtering along this spanning tree and updates the graph structure, until convergence. The graph structure update is based on computing loop errors in the graph and applying a proposed statistical inlier test on Lie groups. This is done efficiently, taking advantage of the covariance matrix of the estimation errors produced by the filter. The proposed formalism is applied on both synthetic and real data, for a camera pose registration problem, an automatic image mosaicking problem and a partial 3D reconstruction merging problem. In these applications, the framework presented in this paper efficiently recovers the global motions while the state of the art algorithms fail due to the presence of a large proportion of outliers.

1 Introduction

This paper deals with the generic problem of estimating globally consistent motion parameters (global motions) from relative motion measurements in the presence of outliers. Such a problem occurs for instance in the context of camera pose registration [1] encountered in 3D localization, structure from motion, camera network calibration, etc. In this case, a motion or transformation is a rigid body transformation matrix. Thus, the relative measurements correspond to the rigid transformations between two cameras and the global motions we wish to estimate are the rigid transformation matrices between a reference camera and all the other cameras. For this specific application, two different kinds of outlier measurements can occur. The first kind of outliers are statistically independent

D. Cremers et al. (Eds.): ACCV 2014, Part V, LNCS 9007, pp. 366–381, 2015.
DOI: 10.1007/978-3-319-16814-2_24

from each other and arise from random failures such as RANSAC [2] failure, erroneous matches between pair of images, etc. The second kind of outliers are not independent and are due to duplicated structures in the environment [3]. For example, 3 images taken in 3 different places that are very similar match each other and thus produce 3 outlier relative motion measurements that are coherent with each other.

The generic problem considered in this work has several other applications such as multiple rotation averaging [4] (3-dimensional rotation matrices), image mosaicking [5] (3-dimensional homographies) and partial 3D reconstruction merging [6] (4-dimensional similarity transformation matrices).

All these applications can be seen as an inference problem in a pairwise factor graph (PFG) where both the vertices, i.e. the global motions, and the edges, i.e. the noisy relative motions, evolve on a matrix Lie group [7]. Indeed, a 3D rotation matrix evolves on the Lie group $SO(3)$ [7], the rigid body motion matrices correspond to the Special Euclidean Lie group $SE(3)$ [8], the homography matrices can be identified with the Special Linear Lie group $SL(3)$ [9], and the 3D similarity transformation matrices form the Lie group $Sim(3)$ [10].

In these applications, as explained above for the camera pose registration problem, the outlier measurements might not be independent and frequently outnumber the inlier measurements. As a consequence, robust optimization approaches, such as Huber norm [11], that do not explicitly exclude the outliers from the estimation process, typically fail. Without additional information, such as priors on whether a relative motion measurement is inlier or outlier, the solution forming the largest coherent set of relative motions may include dependent outliers. Consequently, the global motions are not correctly recovered.

The formalism proposed in this paper can deal with any matrix Lie group and includes the a priori information on whether a relative motion measurement is inlier or outlier as a weighted adjacency matrix (WAM) of the PFG. Consequently, it is able to tackle each of the previously mentioned applications while excluding the outliers in the relative motion measurements. It relies on the recently proposed Iterated Extended Kalman Filter on Lie Groups (LG-IEKF) [12]. Our algorithm iteratively samples a minimum spanning tree (MST) in the WAM of the PFG, applies the LG-IEKF along this MST and updates the WAM, until convergence. The WAM update is based on computing loop errors in the graph and applying a proposed statistical inlier test on Lie groups. This is performed efficiently, taking advantage of the covariance matrix of the estimation errors produced by the LG-IEKF.

The rest of the paper is organized as follows: the next section deals with related work. Section 3 introduces the formalism of Lie groups. The proposed framework is described in Sect. 4. In Sect. 5, our formalism is evaluated experimentally on several applications. Finally the conclusion is provided in Sect. 6.

2 Related Work

A large amount of work has been recently devoted to specifically dealing with multiple rotation averaging in the presence of outliers. This problem is also known as synchronization of rotations in the mathematics community and is usually tackled by minimizing a given criterion. In [13,14], spectral relaxations of the problem are proposed while [15] uses their results as initialization for a second order Riemannian trust-region algorithm to compute a local maximizer. [16] derives an algorithm that exactly estimates the global rotations when a subset of the measurements are perfect and outperforms [14]. In [17,18], two robust iterative algorithms, based on L1 and L1-L2 minimization criterion, respectively, are devised. However, the considered error functions are not convex and consequently need a good initialization such as [16] to avoid poor local minima. Finally, [19] proposes a discretization of $SO(3)$ to apply a loopy belief propagation algorithm on the resulting Markov random field.

All the previously cited approaches, assume that the outliers are statistically independent. Consequently, none of them is able to correctly recover the global motions when this assumption is violated. The works [20–22] are also relevant for the multiple rotation averaging problem. However, they are specifically tailored for $SO(3)$ and it is not straightforward to apply them to other Lie groups.

In [23], a method, that also assumes independent outliers, is derived to infer the set of outliers. The authors introduce a Bayesian framework based on collecting the loop errors in the PFG to infer outliers. Unfortunately, collecting the loop errors becomes quickly intractable and the maximum loop length is limited to 6. Consequently, many outliers cannot be detected (see [20] Fig. 4). Limiting the maximum loop length to 6 also allows them not to take into account the uncertainty induced by the length of a loop. Moreover, when the outliers are not independent, it is possible to find loops containing outliers that have a very low loop error. Thus, in this case, the method fails to infer the dependent outliers as it was shown on several examples in [3,24].

To the best of our knowledge, only one approach [3] was proposed to deal with the generic problem of global motion estimation from relative measurements in the presence of statistically dependent outliers. It is inspired by [25] which proposed a RANSAC-like algorithm to estimate the global motions. It consists in drawing spanning trees (ST) in the PFG. However, using random sampling, the number of ST to draw before finding an outlier free ST is huge. Thus, [3] proposes to sample the STs from a WAM in order to increase the chances to draw an ST without outliers. For each sampled ST, an Expectation Maximization (EM) algorithm is applied, introducing latent variables to classify the measurements as inliers or outliers. Finally, from these labels, a likelihood based on the weights of the WAM is defined and the solution of the ST which maximizes this likelihood is chosen. This approach is shown to perform very well on several small datasets. However, as we show in our experiments, it can only be applied when the number of global motions is small. Moreover, the proposed EM algorithm, although initialized with an outlier free ST, can converge to a poor local minimum (see Sect. 5).

[26] is also a relevant work dedicated to large scale problems though, as specified by the authors themselves, this method "cannot disambiguate" as well as [3]. Consequently, in the rest of the paper, this approach is not considered.

In robotics, several relevant works [27–29] dedicated to robust graph SLAM, have been published. However, they assume that an outlier free ST is given. Furthermore, neither parameter estimation on Lie group nor measurements on Lie group is addressed.

In this paper, we propose a generic approach combining a sampling approach, as in [25], the use of a WAM, as in [3], and the computation of loop errors, as in [23]. Based on these three ingredients, the recently proposed LG-IEKF [12] and a proposed statistical inlier test on Lie groups, we derive an efficient algorithm which is able to recover the global motions in the presence of statistically dependent outliers when the state of the art algorithms, previously cited, fail.

3 Preliminaries

Introduction to matrix Lie groups In this section, we briefly introduce the matrix Lie Groups for the specific purpose of transformation/motion estimation. For a detailed description of these notions the reader is referred to [7]. If G is a matrix Lie group, then $X_{ij} \in G \subset \mathbb{R}^{n \times n}$ is a transformation matrix that takes a point $x^j \in \mathbb{R}^n$ defined in the reference frame (RF) j to RF i, i.e. $x^i = X_{ij}x^j$. Two transformations $X_{ij} \in G$ and $X_{jk} \in G$ can be composed using matrix multiplication to obtain another transformation $X_{ik} = X_{ij}X_{jk} \in G$. Inverting a transformation matrix X_{ij} produces the inverse transformation, i.e. $X_{ij}^{-1} = X_{ji}$. Consequently multiplying a transformation with its inverse produces the identity matrix: $X_{ij}X_{ji} = Id_{n \times n}$. The matrix exponential exp_G and matrix logarithm log_G mappings establish a local diffeomorphism between an open neighborhood of $\mathbf{0}_{n \times n}$ in the tangent space at the identity T_eG, called the *Lie Algebra* $\mathfrak{g}$, and an open neighborhood of $Id_{n \times n}$ in G. The Lie Algebra $\mathfrak{g}$ associated to a p-dimensional matrix Lie group is a p-dimensional vector space. Hence there is a linear isomorphism between $\mathfrak{g}$ and $\mathbb{R}^p$ that we denote as follows: $[\cdot]_G^{\vee} : \mathfrak{g} \to \mathbb{R}^p$ and $[\cdot]_G^{\wedge} : \mathbb{R}^p \to \mathfrak{g}$. We also introduce the following notations: $exp_G^{\wedge}(\cdot) = exp_G\left([\cdot]_G^{\wedge}\right)$ and $log_G^{\vee}(\cdot) = [log_G(\cdot)]_G^{\vee}$. It means that a transformation $X_{jj'}$ that is "close enough" to $Id_{n \times n}$ can be parametrized as follows: $X_{jj'} = exp_G^{\wedge}(\delta_{jj'}) \in \mathbb{R}^p$. Finally, we remind the adjoint representation $Ad_G(\cdot) \subset \mathbb{R}^{p \times p}$ of G on $\mathbb{R}^p$ that enables us to transport an increment $\epsilon_{ij}^i \in \mathbb{R}^p$, that acts onto an element X_{ij} through left multiplication, into an increment $\epsilon_{ij}^j \in \mathbb{R}^p$, that acts through right multiplication:

$$exp_G^{\wedge}\left(\epsilon_{ij}^i\right) X_{ij} = X_{ij} exp_G^{\wedge}\left(Ad_G\left(X_{ij}^{-1}\right)\epsilon_{ij}^i\right) = X_{ij} exp_G^{\wedge}\left(\epsilon_{ij}^j\right) \tag{1}$$

where $\epsilon_{ij}^j = Ad_G\left(X_{ij}^{-1}\right)\epsilon_{ij}^i = Ad_G\left(X_{ji}\right)\epsilon_{ij}^i$.

Concentrated Gaussian Distribution on Lie Groups In this section, we briefly introduce the concept of concentrated Gaussian on Lie groups [30–33] as a generalization of the normal distribution to Lie group manifolds. The distribution of $X_{ij} \in G$ is called a (right) concentrated Gaussian distribution on G of "mean" μ_{ij} and "covariance" P_{ii} denoted $X_{ij} \sim \mathcal{N}_G^R(\mu_{ij}, P_{ii})$ if:

$$X_{ij} = exp_G^{\wedge}\left(\epsilon_{ij}^i\right)\mu_{ij} = \mu_{ij}exp_G^{\wedge}\left(Ad_G\left(\mu_{ij}^{-1}\right)\epsilon_{ij}^i\right) = \mu_{ij}exp_G^{\wedge}\left(\epsilon_{ij}^j\right) \quad (2)$$

where $\epsilon_{ij}^i \sim \mathcal{N}_{\mathbb{R}^p}\left(\mathbf{0}_{p\times 1}, P_{ii}\right)$, $\epsilon_{ij}^j \sim \mathcal{N}_{\mathbb{R}^p}\left(\mathbf{0}_{p\times 1}, Ad_G\left(\mu_{ij}^{-1}\right)P_{ii}Ad_G\left(\mu_{ij}^{-1}\right)^T\right)$ and $P_{ii} \subset \mathbb{R}^{p\times p}$ is a definite positive matrix. Such a distribution gives us a meaningful covariance representation. In the rest of the paper, it will allow us to quantify the uncertainty of both the global and the relative motions and thus to statistically define a threshold to reject outlier measurements.

4 Global Motion Estimation from Relative Measurements in the Presence of Outliers

In this work, we aim at estimating global motions $\{X_{iR}\}_{i=1:N}$, where each global motion $X_{iR} \in G^{'}$ is defined as the motion between a main RF R and a RF i, and $G^{'}$ is a p-dimensional matrix Lie group such as $SO(3)$, $SE(3)$, $SL(3)$, $Sim(3)$, etc. An illustration of global motions in the context of an outlier free consistent pose registration problem (Lie group $SE(3)$) is presented in Fig. 1a. First of all, we describe the case where relative motion measurements are not corrupted with outliers. Then, we treat the case of robust estimation.

4.1 Outlier Free Estimation

This section is mainly a summary of [12], however, its understanding is mandatory for the rest of the paper.

Model. We consider the case where the noises on the (inlier) relative motion measurements $\{Z_{ij}\}_{1\leq i<j\leq N}$ are mutually independent. Each $Z_{ij} \in G^{'}$ denotes a noisy relative motion between a RF j and a RF i expressed as follows:

$$Z_{ij} = exp_G^{\wedge}\left(b_{ij}^i\right)X_{iR}X_{jR}^{-1} \quad (3)$$

where $b_{ij}^i \sim \mathcal{N}_{\mathbb{R}^p}\left(\mathbf{0}_{p\times 1}, \Sigma_{ii}\right)$ is a white Gaussian noise. The problem considered can be seen as the inference in a PFG $\mathcal{G} = \{\mathcal{V}, \mathcal{E}\}$, where each vertex $\mathcal{V}_i$ corresponds to a global motion X_{iR} and each pairwise factor $\mathcal{E}_{ij}$ corresponds to a relative measurement Z_{ij} (see Fig. 1b). In this paper, $\mathcal{G}$ denotes either the PFG itself or its (weighted) adjacency matrix.

Under the concentrated Gaussian assumption, the maximum likelihood estimates of the global motions denoted $\{\mu_{iR}\}_{i=1:N}$ are then defined as:

$$\{\mu_{iR}\}_{i=1:N} = \underset{\{X_{iR}\}_{i=1:N}}{\text{argmin}}\left(\sum_{i,j}\left\|log_{G'}^{\vee}\left(Z_{ij}X_{jR}X_{iR}^{-1}\right)\right\|_{\Sigma_{ii}}^2\right) \quad (4)$$

where $\|\cdot\|_{\Sigma}^2$ stands for the squared Mahalanobis distance.

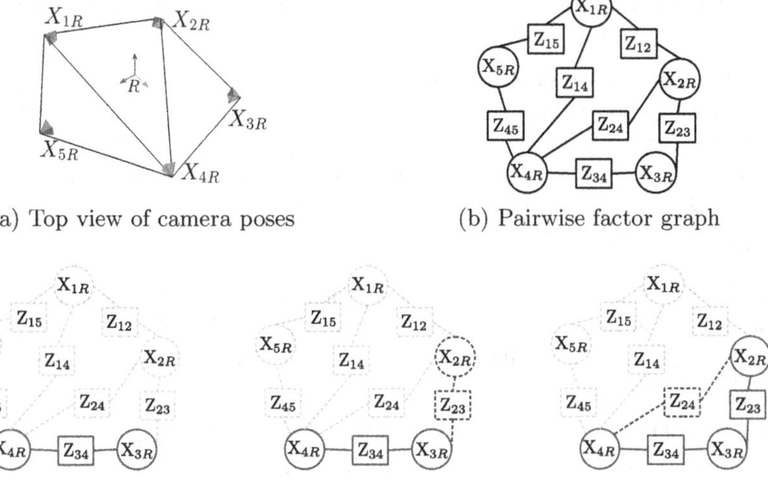

(c) Initialization (d) Propagation (e) Update

Fig. 1. Illustration of an outlier free consistent pose registration problem (Lie group $SE(3)$): (a) a cone represents a camera (global motion) and a link between two cones indicates that a relative motion measurement is available. (b)-(e) please see explanations in Sect. 4.1

Iterated Extended Kalman Filter on Matrix Lie Groups. The problem considered in (4) has several local minima and an efficient way to reach a "good" local minimum is to apply an LG-IEKF (see [12]). The idea is to draw an ST from the adjacency matrix $\mathcal{G}$ of the PFG that guides the global motion estimates at each propagation step of the filter. At each update step of the filter, the relative motions that close loops in the graph are used to refine the global motion estimates and reduce their uncertainty.

Spanning Tree $\mathcal{T}$: Let's consider an ST of the PFG $\mathcal{G} : \mathcal{T} = \{\mathcal{V}, \mathcal{E}_\mathcal{T}\}$. $\mathcal{E}_\mathcal{T} = (C^m)_{m=0:N-2}$ corresponds to a tree traversal ordered such that $C^n = Z_{i_\mathcal{T}(n) j_\mathcal{T}(n)}$ is connected to the tree built from $(C^m)_{m=0:n-1}$. The index m can be seen as a time instant and will be referred as such in the rest of the paper. The notations $i_\mathcal{T}(m)$ and $j_\mathcal{T}(m)$ indicate the referential frames i and j associated to the relative measurement C^m.

Loop Closure $\mathcal{L}$: In this context, a loop closure (LC) at time instant n is a relative measurement $Z_{ij} \notin \mathcal{E}_\mathcal{T}$ connected to the tree built from $(C^m)_{m=0:n+1}$ and not connected to the tree built from $(C^m)_{m=0:n}$. We define the ordered LCs as $\mathcal{L} = (M^m)_{m=1:N-2}$. Note that the size of M^m depends on the time instant m. Indeed, for instance, if two LC occur at time instant m, then $M^m = \left\{Z_{i_\mathcal{L}(m,1) j_\mathcal{L}(m,1)}, Z_{i_\mathcal{L}(m,2) j_\mathcal{L}(m,2)}\right\}$ is a set that contains two relative measurements. The notations $i_\mathcal{L}(m,\mathfrak{z})$ and $j_\mathcal{L}(m,\mathfrak{z})$ indicate the referential frames i and j for the $\mathfrak{z}^{th}$ LC of M^m. We introduce the following notation: $M^m_\mathfrak{z} = Z_{i_\mathcal{L}(m,\mathfrak{z}) j_\mathcal{L}(m,\mathfrak{z})}$ which means that at time instant m, the $\mathfrak{z}^{th}$ LC is a transformation from RF $j_\mathcal{L}(m,\mathfrak{z})$ to RF $i_\mathcal{L}(m,\mathfrak{z})$. From an implementation point of view, the variables $i_{\mathcal{T}}$, $j_{\mathcal{T}}$, $i_{\mathcal{L}}$ and $j_{\mathcal{L}}$ are tables of indices indicating the RFs associated to the relative transformation measurements in $\mathcal{E}_{\mathcal{T}}$ and $\mathcal{L}$.

Measurement Covariance: In the two previous paragraphs, we have introduced notations to distinguish a relative measurement $Z_{i_{\mathcal{T}}(n)j_{\mathcal{T}}(n)}$ that is part of $\mathcal{E}_{\mathcal{T}}$ from a relative measurement $Z_{i_{\mathcal{L}}(m,\mathfrak{z})j_{\mathcal{L}}(m,\mathfrak{z})}$ that is part of $\mathcal{L}$. All these measurements arise from the same generative model (3). Thus the covariance matrix of $Z_{i_{\mathcal{T}}(n)j_{\mathcal{T}}(n)}$ is noted $\Sigma_{i_{\mathcal{T}}(n)i_{\mathcal{T}}(n)}$ whereas the covariance matrix of $Z_{i_{\mathcal{L}}(m,\mathfrak{z})j_{\mathcal{L}}(m,\mathfrak{z})}$ is noted $\Sigma_{i_{\mathcal{L}}(m,\mathfrak{z})i_{\mathcal{L}}(m,\mathfrak{z})}$.

Scheduling: A scheduling is a choice of $\mathcal{E}_{\mathcal{T}}$ for a given graph $\mathcal{G}$. A possible scheduling for the graph presented Fig. 1b is: $\mathcal{E}_{\mathcal{T}} = (C^0 = Z_{34}, C^1 = Z_{23}, C^2 = Z_{45}, C^3 = Z_{14})$. It implies the following set of LC: $\mathcal{L} = (M^1 = Z_{24}, M^2 = \{\emptyset\}, M^3 = \{M_1^3, M_2^3\} = \{Z_{12}, Z_{15}\})$.

Algorithm: Once a scheduling is decided, the LG-IEKF algorithm (see [12]) can be applied to estimate both the global motions μ and the covariance of the estimation errors P. Step 1 (Initialization), 2 (Propagation) and 3 (Update) of the LG-IEKF algorithm are illustrated Figs. 1c, 1d and 1e for the scheduling previously defined.

4.2 Estimation in the Presence of Outliers

The LG-IEKF algorithm described in the previous section is not robust to outliers in the relative motion measurements all the more the noise is modeled as a concentrated Gaussian distribution on Lie groups (see (3)). In this section, we show how to perform the estimation in the presence of outliers.

Outlier Definition and Inlier Test. As previously explained, the outliers arising in the problem we consider in this paper can be statistically dependent. It is a difficult task to propose a generative model in this case. Consequently, in this work, we simply use a discriminative way to define an outlier. A relative motion measurement Z_{ij} is an outlier if and only if:

$$\left|\left|log_{G'}^{\vee}\left(Z_{ij}X_{jR}X_{iR}^{-1}\right)\right|\right|_{\Sigma_{ii}}^{2} > thresh \tag{5}$$

where *thresh* is a threshold to be defined. Note that, with this definition, a relative measurement generated using the inlier model (3) can be classified as outlier. However, if *thresh* is large enough, it is very unlikely to happen.

From the outlier definition given in (5), we propose a statistical inlier test on matrix Lie groups that will be employed in our robust estimation framework: let's assume that we have estimated the two global motions X_{iR} and X_{jR}, as well as the covariance of the estimation errors from the relative motion measurements $\{Z_{kl}\}_{(k,l)\in T}$ (T is a subset of all the measurements) without involving the relative measurement Z_{ij}, i.e. $(i,j) \notin T$. We would like to know whether Z_{ij} is an "inlier" or not w.r.t the current estimates of X_{iR} and X_{jR}. Assuming that the distribution of the two global motions X_{iR} and X_{jR} conditioned by the relative measurements $\{Z_{kl}\}_{(k,l)\in T}$ is a Gaussian distribution on Lie groups, we have:

$$X_{iR}|\{Z_{kl}\}_{(k,l)\in\mathcal{T}} = exp^{\wedge}_{G'}\left(\epsilon^i_{iR}\right)\mu_{iR} \text{ and } X_{jR}|\{Z_{kl}\}_{(k,l)\in\mathcal{T}} = exp^{\wedge}_{G'}\left(\epsilon^j_{jR}\right)\mu_{jR} \tag{6}$$

where $cov(\epsilon) = cov\left(\begin{bmatrix}\epsilon^i_{iR}\\ \epsilon^j_{jR}\end{bmatrix}\right) = \begin{bmatrix}P_{ii} & P_{ij}\\ P_{ji} & P_{jj}\end{bmatrix}$. From (3), we have the following result:

$$Z_{ij} = exp^{\wedge}_{G}\left(b^i_{ij}\right)exp^{\wedge}_{G'}\left(\epsilon^i_{iR}\right)\mu_{iR}\mu^{-1}_{jR}exp^{\wedge}_{G'}\left(-\epsilon^j_{jR}\right) \tag{7}$$

$$= exp^{\wedge}_{G}\left(b^i_{ij} + \epsilon^i_{iR} - Ad_{G'}\left(\mu_{iR}\mu^{-1}_{jR}\right)\epsilon^j_{jR} + O\left(\|\epsilon\|^2, \|b^i_{ij}\|^2\right)\right)\mu_{iR}\mu^{-1}_{jR} \tag{8}$$

Thus, neglecting second order terms, the error negative log-likelihood has the following expression:

$$err = \left\|log^{\vee}_{G'}\left(Z_{ij}\mu_{jR}\mu^{-1}_{iR}\right)\right\|^2_{Q_{err}} \tag{9}$$

where

$$Q_{err} = cov\left(\epsilon^i_{iR} - Ad_{G'}\left(\mu_{iR}\mu^{-1}_{jR}\right)\epsilon^j_{jR} + b^i_{ij}\right) \tag{10}$$

$$= \left[Id_{p\times p}\ -Ad_{G'}\left(\mu_{iR}\mu^{-1}_{jR}\right)\right]\begin{bmatrix}P_{ii} & P_{ij}\\ P_{ji} & P_{jj}\end{bmatrix}\begin{bmatrix}Id_{p\times p}\\ -Ad_{G'}\left(\mu_{iR}\mu^{-1}_{jR}\right)^T\end{bmatrix} + \Sigma_{ii} \tag{11}$$

and is distributed according to the chi-squared distribution with p degrees of freedom, i.e. $err \sim \chi^2(p)$. Consequently, one way to decide whether Z_{ij} is an inlier w.r.t the current estimates of X_{iR} and X_{jR} is to define a threshold based on the p-value of $\chi^2(p)$ [34]. Note that since we neglected second order terms, this threshold is possibly restrictive, thus in practice we take a larger threshold than the theoretical one.

Loop Voting. The robust framework that is presented in the next section is based on "loop voting". The idea of "loop voting" is simple: assuming an ST $\mathcal{E}_{\mathcal{T}} = (C^m)_{m=0:N-2}$, which probably contains outliers, has been drawn from $\mathcal{G}$, we apply the LG-IEKF algorithm. At time instant k, between Step 2 and Step 3 of this algorithm, we perform the inlier test described in Sect. 4.2 for the upcoming loop closures M^k. For simplicity let's consider the first loop closure $M^k_{i_{\mathcal{L}}(k,\mathfrak{1})j_{\mathcal{L}}(k,\mathfrak{1})}$, moreover we define $\mathfrak{m} = i_{\mathcal{L}}(k,\mathfrak{1})$ and $\mathfrak{n} = j_{\mathcal{L}}(k,\mathfrak{1})$. If the inlier test, for this loop closure, is validated, i.e $\left\|log^{\vee}_{G'}\left(Z_{\mathfrak{mn}}\mu^{k|k-1}_{\mathfrak{n}R}\left(\mu^{k|k-1}_{\mathfrak{m}R}\right)^{-1}\right)\right\|^2_{Q_{err}} < thresh$, then we found a measurement that is "coherent" with the path $\mathcal{P}$ in $\mathcal{E}_{\mathcal{T}}$ from RF $\mathfrak{m}$ to RF $\mathfrak{n}$. Thus we mark the relative motions of $\mathcal{P}$ as "checked"[1]. Note that, if $\mathcal{E}_{\mathcal{T}}$ contains dependent outliers (from duplicate structures in the scene for instance), then it is possible to close wrong loops and thus to "check" outliers. This point is discussed in the next two sections.

[1] We use the Matlab library Matgraph [35] to find the path between $\mathfrak{m}$ and $\mathfrak{n}$.

Proposed Framework. In order to perform the robust estimation of global motions from relative motions in the presence of statically dependent outliers, we proposed to combine three ideas:

- sampling Minimum Spanning Trees (MST) from a weighted adjacency matrix (WAM), as in [3,25]. The WAM contains prior information on whether a relative measurement is inlier or outlier. Without this prior information, the solution forming the largest coherent set of relative motions may include dependent outliers. However, even with a WAM, the combinatorial search of the "best" relative motions configuration is intractable. In [3], it is proposed to sample a large number of spanning trees from the WAM, to perform an optimization on each ST and to keep the best solution. Nevertheless, we show in Sect. 5 that their approach can only be applied for a small number of global motions. In order to obtain an algorithm that is applicable for larger problems, we assume that an MST of $\mathcal{G}$ does not contain dependent outliers (it may contain independent outliers). This assumption might appear restrictive, however, for image sequences for example, it is usually satisfied (see Sect. 4.2). Indeed, the image timestamps can be used to build a WAM that favors images that are close in time. In this case, an MST will not contain dependent outliers since the relative motion measurement between two consecutive images is normally either an inlier or a statistically independent outlier (in the case of a RANSAC failure for example). When timestamps are not available, one way to attribute weights to the edges is to consider "missing correspondence cue" (see [3]). Note that if there is only statistically independent outliers, our approach does not need a WAM.
- applying the LG-IEKF proposed in [12]. This algorithm achieves similar performances as compared to a Gauss-Newton (GN) approach while taking only a fraction of its computational time. It also estimates the covariance of the estimation errors which is necessary for our inlier test (see Sect. 4.2). Recovering those covariances from the solution of a GN is computationally very expensive.
- performing loop voting in order to infer the set of inliers. In [23], the maximum loop length is limited to 6 in order not to take into account the uncertainty induced by the length of a loop. On the contrary, we explicitly model this uncertainty with the LG-IEKF and derive a statistical inlier test on matrix Lie groups. Thus we are able to close long loops. Consequently, even in the case of statistically independent outliers assumed in [23], our approach outperforms the algorithm proposed in [23].

Our approach works as follows: first of all, we sample an MST from the WAM $\mathcal{G}$. Then an LG-IEKF is applied on this MST with inlier test (see Sect. 4.2) and loop voting (see Sect. 4.2) at each loop closure. If every relative motion that is part of the MST have been "checked" at least once, i.e. each relative motion in the MST is involved in at least one validated loop closure, then the global motion estimates correspond to the output of the LG-IEKF. Otherwise, the relative motions involved in the MST that have not been "checked" are upweighted (or deleted) from $\mathcal{G}$ and a new MST is drawn. The algorithm iterates

Algorithm 1. Robust approach

Inputs: $\mathcal{G}$ (weighted adjacency matrix), $\{Z_{ij}\}_{1 \leq i < j \leq N}$ (relative motions), $\{\Sigma_{ii}\}_{1 \leq i < j \leq N}$ (covariance matrices), *thresh* (p-value of $\chi^2(p)$)

Outputs: μ (global motions), P (full covariance matrix of global motions)

1. Draw an MST in $\mathcal{G}$ to get $\mathcal{E}_{\mathcal{T}} = (C^m)_{m=0:N-2}$, $\mathcal{L} = (M^m)_{m=1:N-2}$ and the tables of indices $i_{\mathcal{T}}$, $j_{\mathcal{T}}$, $i_{\mathcal{L}}$ and $j_{\mathcal{L}}$
2. Initialize[1] μ and P
   with inputs C^0, $Q_0 = \Sigma_{i_{\mathcal{T}}(0) i_{\mathcal{T}}(0)}$, $i_{\mathcal{T}}$, $j_{\mathcal{T}}$
   to get $\mu^{0|0}$ and $P^{0|0}$
3. Propagate[1] $\mu^{k-1|k-1}$ and $P^{k-1|k-1}$
   with inputs $\mu^{k-1|k-1}$, $P^{k-1|k-1}$, C^k, $Q_k = \Sigma_{i_{\mathcal{T}}(k) i_{\mathcal{T}}(k)}$, $j_{\mathcal{T}}$
   to get $\mu^{k|k-1}$ and $P^{k|k-1}$
4. Verify Loop Closures $M_{\mathfrak{z}}^k$ as explained in Sect. 4.2
   with inputs $\mu^{k-1|k-1}_{i_{\mathcal{L}}(k,\mathfrak{z})R}$, $P^{k-1|k-1}_{i_{\mathcal{L}}(k,\mathfrak{z}) i_{\mathcal{L}}(k,\mathfrak{z})}$, $\mu^{k-1|k-1}_{j_{\mathcal{L}}(k,\mathfrak{z})R}$, $P^{k-1|k-1}_{j_{\mathcal{L}}(k,\mathfrak{z}) j_{\mathcal{L}}(k,\mathfrak{z})}$, $P^{k-1|k-1}_{i_{\mathcal{L}}(k,\mathfrak{z}) j_{\mathcal{L}}(k,\mathfrak{z})}$, $M_{\mathfrak{z}}^k$, $\Sigma_{i_{\mathcal{L}}(k,\mathfrak{z}) i_{\mathcal{L}}(k,\mathfrak{z})}$, *thresh*
   (a) if $M_{\mathfrak{z}}^k$ is not validated, remove it from M^k, $i_{\mathcal{L}}$ and $j_{\mathcal{L}}$
   (b) else mark as "checked" the path in $\mathcal{E}_{\mathcal{T}}$ that led to this loop closure as explained in Sect. 4.2
5. Update[1] $\mu^{k|k-1}$ and $P^{k|k-1}$
   with inputs $\mu^{k|k-1}$, $P^{k|k-1}$, M^k, $R_k = \text{blkdiag}\left(\left\{\Sigma_{i_{\mathcal{L}}(k,\mathfrak{z}) i_{\mathcal{L}}(k,\mathfrak{z})}\right\}_{\mathfrak{z}}\right)$, $i_{\mathcal{L}}$, $j_{\mathcal{L}}$
   to get $\mu^{k|k}$ and $P^{k|k}$
6. Iterate Step 3 to Step 6 until $k = N - 2$
7. If every relative motion in $\mathcal{E}_{\mathcal{T}}$ has been "checked" at least once, return μ and P, otherwise up-weight (or remove) from $\mathcal{G}$ the relative motions involved in $\mathcal{E}_{\mathcal{T}}$ that have not been "checked" and go to 1.

[1] Further details on steps 2, 3 and 5 are provided as supplementary material.

until convergence of $\mathcal{G}$, i.e. until an MST is completely checked. The complete algorithm is summarized in Algorithm 1.

Limitations. The proposed approach may fail in several cases.

First of all, we assume that an MST of the WAM does not contain dependent outliers. If it does, depending on the graph structure, it may be possible to close loops that involve these dependent outliers. In this case, those outlier measurements are not rejected and the global motions are not correctly recovered. In practice, this limitation is not as strong as it appears. For instance, this was satisfied for all experiments shown in [3] (see the ground truth matrix of each dataset in [3]) as well those shown in this paper (see Sect. 5). Note that if there is only statistically independent outliers, our approach does not need a WAM to recover the global motions.

Secondly, if a relative motion measurement is deleted after an iteration of our algorithm, the graph might become disconnected. If it happens, it means

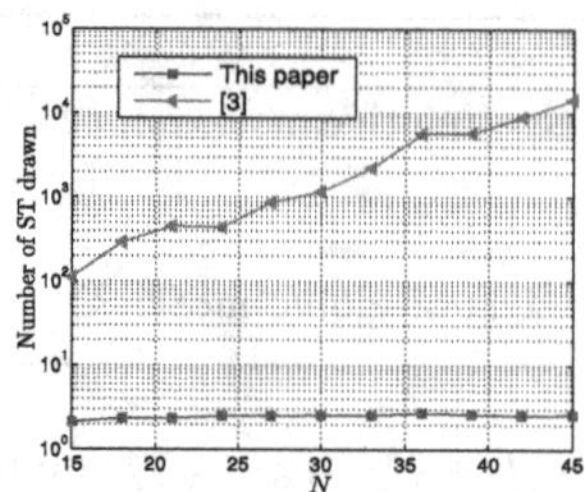

(a) Number of ST drawn to find an ST without outliers.

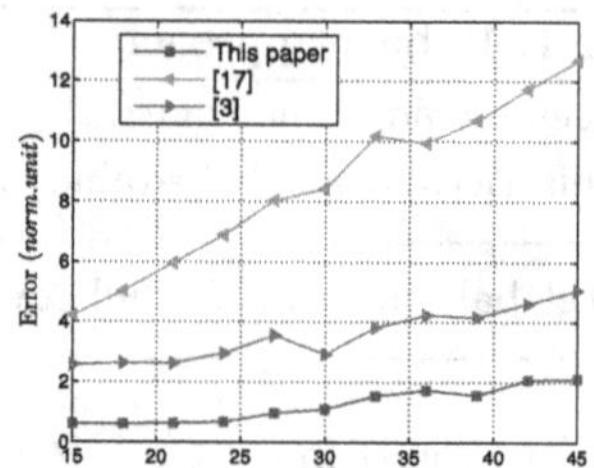

(b) Estimation error of the global motions (please see text for details)

Fig. 2. Comparison of our approach to [3,18] on a camera pose estimation problem ($\lambda = \frac{1}{10}$ and number of relative motions fixed to $5N + n$ with $n = 60$).

that there is not enough redundancy in the graph structure to correctly recover the global motions. In this case, our approach can be applied to each connected component separately.

5 Applications and Results

In this section, the proposed framework is experimentally validated both on simulated and real data.

Simulated data with independent outliers: Camera pose registration problem In this section, we compare the performance of the proposed approach to two state of the art algorithms [3] and [18] on a camera pose registration problem (Lie group $SE(3)$). [18] was developed to deal with $SO(3)$ but its extension to $SE(3)$ is straightforward. We simulate circular camera trajectories (see Fig. 3) with N cameras where each camera $X_{iR_{True}}$ has a timestamp t_i and we generate noisy relative motions as follows: first of all, a measurement can be either an inlier or an outlier. We model the probability of a measurement as $P(Z_{ij} \text{ is inlier}) = exp(-\lambda |t_i - t_j|)$ where λ is a user-chosen parameter, i.e. a

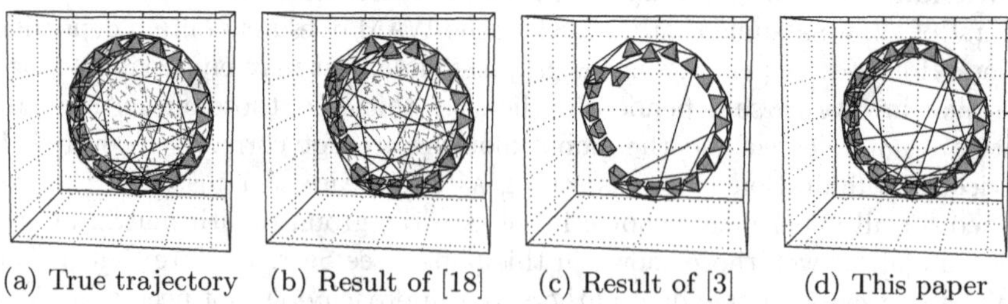

(a) True trajectory (b) Result of [18] (c) Result of [3] (d) This paper

Fig. 3. Camera Pose registration problem results, a cone represents a camera pose, a black line is an inlier measurement and a gray dashed line is an outlier

larger time difference increases the chance to produce an outlier. After having drawn the label of a measurement (inlier or outlier), we sample the measurement. The distribution of the independent outliers is modeled as a centered Gaussian distribution on Lie groups with a large covariance matrix (the large covariance is not a problem in this case since $log^{\vee}_{SE(3)}$ is defined on the whole group) while an inlier can be sampled using (3). In our implementation, we use the Lie algebra basis of $\mathfrak{se}(3)$ given in [8] and the WAM $\mathcal{G}$ is built from the absolute time differences of the camera timestamps, i.e. a low weight corresponds to a confident measurement and an infinite weight is given when a measurement is missing.

In Fig. 2a, we show that the method proposed in [3] can be applied only on very small problems. Indeed, one can see that when the number of cameras increases (N grows), it becomes quickly very difficult to draw an ST without outliers even with the help of a weighted adjacency matrix. In comparison, our approach, that iteratively updates the weighted adjacency matrix, always finds an ST without outliers in a few samplings.

In Fig. 2b, we compare our optimization method (LG-IEKF with inlier test) against the robust approach proposed in [18] and the Expectation Maximization algorithm (EM) of [3]. The three approaches are provided the same outlier free spanning tree. [3,18] are initialized by composing the relative measurements of the ST as it is proposed by the authors of those papers. In order to compare the results of each approach to the true global motions, we need to add a step to align the estimated global motions with the true global motions. For that purpose, we apply a Gauss-Newton algorithm to minimize the sum of the following error: $\left\| log_{SE(3)}\left(\mu_{iR} X_{RR_{True}} X^{-1}_{iR_{True}}\right)\right\|^2$. The error obtained, for each approach, at convergence of the Gauss-Newton is presented in Fig. 2b. We show that our method outperforms both [3,18]. Indeed, [18] is based on a robust convex L2-L1 norm to mitigate the influence of the outliers. However, because of the Lie group curvature, the complete functional is not convex. Therefore, the algorithm usually gets stuck in a poor local minimum. [3] introduces latent variables to classify the relative motions as inliers or outliers. However, the labels obtained at the initialization of the global motions are very difficult to modify. Indeed, the E-step does not take into account the estimation errors of the current global motion estimates which is negligible only when N is small. Therefore, a lot of inlier relative motion remain classified as outliers. In comparison, our approach incrementally rejects outliers, taking into account the current uncertainty of the global motions, and refines its estimates with the inliers. Consequently, the global motions are correctly recovered. An example of recovered global motions with the three different approaches is presented Fig. 3.

Real data with statistically dependent outliers: Partial 3D reconstruction merging problem. The algorithm presented in this paper is applied to a partial 3D reconstruction merging problem (Lie group $Sim(3)$). Due to the lack of space, the details and results of this experiment are provided as supplementary material.

Real data with statistically dependent outliers: Automatic planar image mosaicking problem. The algorithm presented in this paper is applied to an automatic planar image mosaicking problem. We took 53 photos of a planar scene (see Fig. 4a) with a smartphone, detected points of interest and estimated the homographies (lie group $SL(3)$) between every pair of images using a RANSAC algorithm followed by a Gauss-Newton algorithm on $SL(3)$. The covariance matrix of each relative motion is obtained by inverting the approximated Hessian matrix once the Gauss-Newton has converged. In our implementation, we use the Lie algebra basis of $\mathfrak{sl}(3)$ given in [36] and the weighted adjacency matrix is obtained from the absolute time differences from the images timestamps. In this dataset, there are 65 % of statistically dependent outliers (see Fig. 4b) due to the ambiguity of the scene (some paper sheets are almost identical). In Fig. 4, we compare the results of our approach against the EM algorithm of [3] which is initialized by composing the relative homographies of the MST obtained with our algorithm. On the one hand, once again, the proposed EM of [3] classifies a lot of inliers as outliers since the estimation errors of the global motions estimates is not taken into account during the E-step. Consequently, [3] is not able to correctly recover the global motions (see Fig. 4c). On the other hand, our approach perfectly infers the set of inliers and produces a very precise mosaic (see Fig. 4d). We could not apply [18] because $log_{SL(3)}$ is not defined on the whole group. We also tried to compare our formalism to the openCV implementation of [5], however, due to the high ambiguity of the scenes, it was not able to produce any result.

6 Discussion and Conclusion

First of all, we would like to stress 3 aspects concerning the paper:

- This work addresses the fundamental problem of robust motion averaging for any Lie group especially "mixed" groups such as $SE(3)$, $SL(3)$ or $Sim(3)$;
- It deals with cases where there are more correlated outliers than inliers. For instance, our image mosaicking dataset has 65 % of dependent outliers. Therefore, we are beyond the stage at which the independent outlier assumption starts to degrade gracefully (see comparison with [23] in [3]);
- The proposed approach significantly outperformed the two state of the art algorithms [3,18], on $SE(3)$, $SL(3)$ and $Sim(3)$.

The contributions[2] of the paper are:

- Proper handling of non-isotropic covariances on Lie groups coupled with an efficient incremental approach to avoid local minima;
- Definition of a new χ^2 inlier test that deals with "mixed" groups;
- A new tree sampling scheme aimed at significantly reducing the computational cost of the sampling scheme of [3]. This new sampling scheme allows to handle a much larger number of motions N (typically $N = 1000$). N is no longer limited by the sampling scheme but only by the memory size of the estimated covariance matrix ($6N \times 6N$ for $SE(3)$);

[2] The supplementary material and the Matlab code are available at https://sites.google.com/site/guillaumebourmaud/.

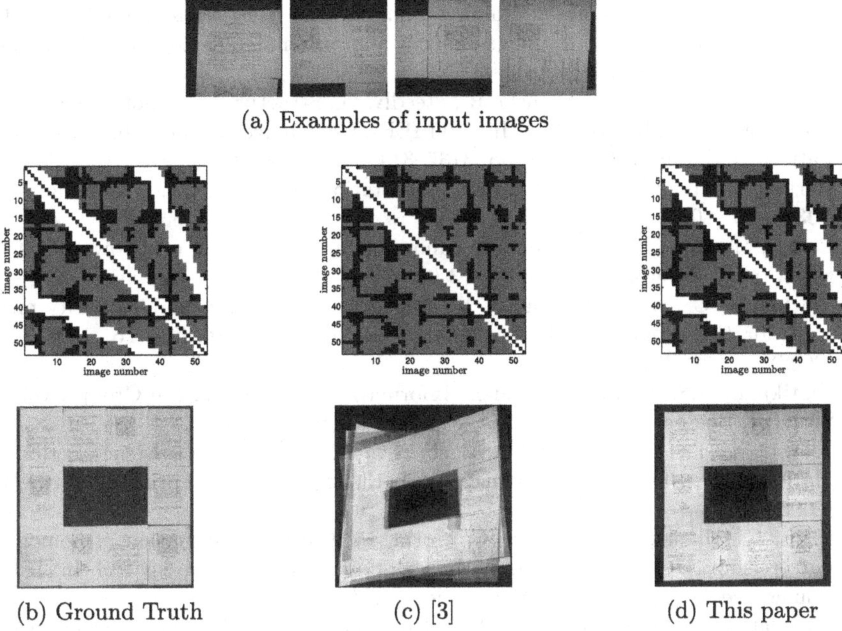

(a) Examples of input images

(b) Ground Truth (c) [3] (d) This paper

Fig. 4. Image mosaicking: in the labeling matrices a white pixel is an inlier, a black pixel corresponds to an unavailable measurement, a gray pixel corresponds to an outlier. Observe that our labeling inlier/outlier is perfect (see 4d).

The first 3 contributions of this paper could be applied inside a Structure from Motion pipeline such as [3] or [21] but this is out of the scope of the current paper and left as future work. Thus, when comparing to [3], we consider only their robust motion averaging approach and did not use their Structure from Motion datasets. Consequently, we compared neither to [21] nor to [24] (that do not solve any motion averaging problem).

In fact, our contributions concern mainly "mixed" groups which do not have robust enough solutions yet. The proposed approach is based on a generic matrix Lie group formulation, which should be usable on a wide variety of applications.

Acknowledgment. The research leading to these results has received funding from the European Community's Seventh Framework Programme (FP7/2007-2013) under grant agreement 288199 - Dem@Care. The authors would like to thank the reviewers, Moncef Hidane and Cornelia Vacar for their valuable help.

References

1. Agrawal, M.: A Lie algebraic approach for consistent pose registration for general Euclidean motion. In: IROS, pp. 1891–1897 (2006)

2. Fischler, M.A., Bolles, R.C.: Random sample consensus: a paradigm for model fitting with applications to image analysis and automated cartography. Commun. ACM **24**, 381–395 (1981)
3. Roberts, R., Sinha, S.N., Szeliski, R., Steedly, D.: Structure from motion for scenes with large duplicate structures. In: 2011 IEEE Conference on Computer Vision and Pattern Recognition (CVPR), pp. 3137–3144. IEEE (2011)
4. Hartley, R., Trumpf, J., Dai, Y., Li, H.: Rotation averaging. Int. J. Comput. Vis. **103**, 1–39 (2013)
5. Brown, M., Lowe, D.G.: Automatic panoramic image stitching using invariant features. Int. J. Comput. Vis. **74**, 59–73 (2007)
6. Wachinger, C., Wein, W., Navab, N.: Registration strategies and similarity measures for three-dimensional ultrasound mosaicing. Acad. Radiol. **15**, 1404–1415 (2008)
7. Chirikjian, G.S.: Stochastic Models, Information Theory, and Lie Groups, vol. 2. Springer, Boston (2012)
8. Selig, J.M.: Lie Groups and Lie Algebras in Robotics. NATO Science Series II: Mathematics, Physics and Chemistry, vol. 136, pp. 101–125. Springer, Dordrecht (2005)
9. Malis, E., Hamel, T., Mahony, R., Morin, P.: Dynamic estimation of homography transformations on the special linear group of visual servo control. In: IEEE Conference on Robotics and Automation (2009)
10. Strasdat, H., Davison, A., Montiel, J., Konolige, K.: Double window optimisation for constant time visual SLAM. In: IEEE International Conference on Computer Vision (ICCV) (2011)
11. Huber, P.J., et al.: Robust estimation of a location parameter. Ann. Math. Stat. **35**, 73–101 (1964)
12. Bourmaud, G., Mégret, R., Giremus, A., Berthoumieu, Y.: Global motion estimation from relative measurements using iterated extended Kalman filter on matrix Lie groups. In: ICIP 2014
13. Bandeira, A.S., Singer, A., Spielman, D.A.: A Cheeger inequality for the graph connection laplacian (2012). arXiv preprint arXiv:1204.3873
14. Singer, A., Shkolnisky, Y.: Three-dimensional structure determination from common lines in cryo-em by eigenvectors and semidefinite programming. SIAM J. Imaging Sci. **4**, 543–572 (2011)
15. Boumal, N., Singer, A., Absil, P.A.: Robust estimation of rotations from relative measurements by maximum likelihood. In: Proceedings of the 52nd Conference on Decision and Control, CDC (2013)
16. Wang, L., Singer, A.: Exact and stable recovery of rotations for robust synchronization. Inf. Infer. **2**, 145–193 (2013)
17. Hartley, R., Aftab, K., Trumpf, J.: L1 rotation averaging using the Weiszfeld algorithm. In: 2011 IEEE Conference on Computer Vision and Pattern Recognition (CVPR), pp. 3041–3048. IEEE (2011)
18. Chatterjee, A., Govindu, V.M.: Efficient and robust large-scale rotation averaging. In: ICCV (2013)
19. Crandall, D.J., Owens, A., Snavely, N., Huttenlocher, D.: Discrete-continuous optimization for large-scale structure from motion. In: CVPR, pp. 3001–3008 (2011)
20. Enqvist, O., Kahl, F., Olsson, C.: Non-sequential structure from motion. In: ICCV Workshops, pp. 264–271 (2011)
21. Jiang, N., Cui, Z., Tan, P.: A global linear method for camera pose registration. In: 2013 IEEE International Conference on Computer Vision

22. Moulon, P., Monasse, P., Marlet, R.: Global fusion of relative motions for robust, accurate and scalable structure from motion. In: 2013 IEEE International Conference on Computer Vision
23. Zach, C., Klopschitz, M., Pollefeys, M.: Disambiguating visual relations using loop constraints. In: 2010 IEEE Conference on Computer Vision and Pattern Recognition (CVPR), pp. 1426–1433. IEEE (2010)
24. Jiang, N., Tan, P., Cheong, L.F.: Seeing double without confusion: Structure-from-motion in highly ambiguous scenes. In: 2012 IEEE Conference on Computer Vision and Pattern Recognition (CVPR), pp. 1458–1465. IEEE (2012)
25. Govindu, V.M.: Robustness in motion averaging. In: Narayanan, P.J., Nayar, S.K., Shum, H.-Y. (eds.) ACCV 2006. LNCS, vol. 3852, pp. 457–466. Springer, Heidelberg (2006)
26. Wilson, K., Snavely, N.: Network principles for sfm: Disambiguating repeated structures with local context. In: 2013 IEEE International Conference on Computer Vision
27. Sunderhauf, N., Protzel, P.: Switchable constraints for robust pose graph SLAM. In: IROS (2012)
28. Latif, Y., Cadena, C., Neira, J.: Robust loop closing over time for pose graph SLAM. Int. J. Robot. Res. **32**(14), 1611–1626 (2013)
29. Olson, E., Agarwal, P.: Inference on networks of mixtures for robust robot mapping. In: RSS (2012)
30. Bourmaud, G., Mégret, R., Giremus, A., Berthoumieu, Y.: Discrete extended Kalman filter on Lie groups. In: 2013 Proceedings of the 21st European Signal Processing Conference (EUSIPCO) (2013)
31. Wang, Y., Chirikjian, G.: Error propagation on the Euclidean group with applications to manipulators kinematics. IEEE Trans. Rob. **22**, 591–602 (2006)
32. Wolfe, K., Mashner, M., Chirikjian, G.: Bayesian fusion on Lie groups. J. Algebraic Stat. **2**, 75–97 (2011)
33. Barfoot, T.D., Furgale, P.T.: Associating uncertainty with three-dimensional poses for use in estimation problems. IEEE Trans. Robot. **30**, 679–693 (2014)
34. Fisher, R.A., Yates, F., et al.: Statistical tables for biological, agricultural and medical research. Oliver & Boyd, London (1949)
35. Scheinerman, E.R.: (Matgraph: a matlab toolbox for graph theory)
36. Benhimane, S., Malis, E.: Homography-based 2d visual tracking and servoing. Int. J. Rob. Res. **26**, 661–676 (2007)

Clustering Ensemble Tracking

Guibo Zhu(✉), Jinqiao Wang, and Hanqing Lu

National Laboratory of Pattern Recognition, Institute of Automation, Chinese Academy of Sciences, Beijing 100190, China
{gbzhu,jqwang,luhq}@nlpr.ia.ac.cn

Abstract. A key problem in visual tracking is how to handle the ambiguity in decision to locate the object effectively using the target appearance model with online update. We address this problem by incorporating sequential clustering and ensemble methods into the tracking system. In this paper, clustering is used for mining the potential historical structure in the parameter space and feature space. Then we fuse multiple weak hypotheses to construct a strong ensemble learner for object tracking. Different from previous methods for updating classifier ensemble in a fixed weak classifier pool frame-to-frame, the proposed ensemble method is taking three weak hypotheses into consideration: spatial object-part view, parameter space view, and feature space view. Specially, spatial object-part view represents the object by a collection of part models that are spatially related (e.g. tree-structure). Meanwhile, analyzing the latent group structure in the parameter space and feature space is essential to take full advantage of the historical data in the tracking process. Therefore, we propose a novel ensemble algorithm that fuses object-part predictor, parameter clustered predictors and feature clustered predictors together. Furthermore, the weights of different views are updated by the relative consistency between weak predictors and final ensemble tracker. The formulation is tested in a tracking-by-detection implementation. Extensive comparing experiments on challenging video sequences demonstrate the robustness and effectiveness of the proposed method.

1 Introduction

Visual tracking has attracted significant attention due to its wide variety of applications such as terrorist detection, wearable computing and self-driving cars. Much progress has been made in the last two decades. However designing robust visual tracking methods is still an open issue. Challenges in visual tracking methods include no-rigid shape and appearance variations of the object, occlusions, illumination changes, cluttered scenes, etc. [1,2].

To solve the above problem, a popular approach is to learn a discriminative appearance model for coping with complicated appearance changes [3]. Typically, this assumes that the object/non-object discriminative information from different frames during long-term tracking is generated from a temporally homogeneous source. However this assumption may not hold in practice, as object appearance and environmental conditions vary dynamically over time.

D. Cremers et al. (Eds.): ACCV 2014, Part V, LNCS 9007, pp. 382–396, 2015.
DOI: 10.1007/978-3-319-16814-2_25

In face of challenging factors, only fitting one updating discriminative model which can satisfy all cases is unlikely to optimally distinguish an object from its background through tracking-by-detection methods [4–8]. Tracking-by-detection requires training of a classifier for detecting the object in each frame. One common approach for detector training is to use a detector ensemble framework that linearly combines the weak classifiers with different associated weights, e.g., [4,6]. A larger weight implies that the corresponding weak classifier is more discriminative and thus more useful.

Although most previous online ensemble methods originated from offline algorithms achieve many successes in online visual learning task, there are some limitations in visual tracking. As noted by Bai *et al.* [9], the common assumption was that the observed data (examples and their labels) had an unknown but stationary joint distribution. It may not apply in tracking scenarios where the appearance of an object can undergo significant changes. Due to the uncertainty in the appearance changes that may occur over time and the difficulty of estimating the non-stationary distribution of this observed data directly, they used Bayesian estimation theory to estimate a Dirichlet distribution of classifier weights. Different from their pre-defined non-stationary distribution and high computational complexity, we propose a simple and robust cumulative sum method to model how the different view predictor weights evolve so as to represent the non-stationary distribution which doesn't need to satisfy some specific distribution and is efficient.

At the same time, Grabner and Bischof [6] noted that updating the weights of online self-learning classifiers through the incoming data without annotation is difficult. Babenko *et al.* [5] treated tracking as multiple instance learning problem. Bai *et al.* [9] estimated the ensemble weights using Bayesian interpretation and ensures that the update of the ensemble weights is smooth. Yu *et al.* [10] proposed a co-training based approach to continuously label incoming data and online update a hybrid discriminative and generative model. We consider the three views of the object-part view, parameter space view and object feature space view at the same time. They are robust to different cases that object-part view covers the occlusion, discriminative parameter space view focuses the difference between the object and the background and the generative object feature space view handles the variants of the object appearance itself.

Moreover, the tracking problem has a temporal dimension which is not present in the classification methods [11] or subspace learning methods [12] by the previous works. We get temporal interval predictors through sequential clustering so as to better utilize the temporal learned structural information in parameter space and object appearance space directly.

Our method models three views of predictors whose weights ensemble with a non-stationary distribution, where their information geometry can be explored by sequential clustering methods. Our method focus on estimating the state of the object with three diverse view predictors in temporal dimension, not the independent and identically distributed variable in a fixed weak classifier pool. In summary, our contributions are as follows:

1. We first propose a clustering ensemble tracker with three diverse views of weak predictors: object-part predictor, parameter space predictor, and feature space predictor. The different views have specific properties for tracking.
2. The sequential clustering is utilized to estimate the temporal non-stationary distributions of weak structure predictor in parameter space and appearance predictor in feature space. Based on sequential clustering theory, it provides a probabilistic interpretation of which interval structured predictor of the object are more discriminative.
3. We propose a simple weighting strategy to ensemble different weak predictors based on the prediction consistency between weak predictors and final ensemble tracker.

2 Related Work

A tracking-by-detection method usually has two major components: object representation and model update. Previous methods employ various object representations [5–8, 13–15]. Our approach is most related to the methods that use structured prediction [7,8].

From the perspective of that the tracked objects are treated as labeled positive samples and the other as training samples with some structure loss, the tracking problem can be considered as supervised learning problem in each frame. Supervised learning algorithms are commonly described as performing the task of searching through a hypothesis space to find a suitable hypothesis that makes good prediction for one particular problem. Even if the hypothesis space contains hypotheses that are very well-suited for object tracking, it may be very difficult to find a good one to locate the object precisely.

"Ensemble methods" is a machine learning paradigm where multiple (homogenous/heterogenous) individual learners are trained for the same problem, e.g., neural network ensemble [16], bootstrap aggregating (bagging) [17], boosting [18], Bayesian model averaging [19,20], etc. Avidan [4], who was the first to explicitly apply ensemble methods to tracking-by-detection, extended the work of [21] by adopting the Adaboost algorithm [18] to combine a set of weak classifiers maintained with an online update strategy. Along this thread, Grabner *et al.* [6] inspired from the online boosting algorithm [22] by introducing feature selection from a pool of features for weak classifiers. Several other extensions to online boosting also existed, including the work by Banbenko *et al.* [5] who adopted Multiple Instance Learning in designing weak classifiers. In a different approach [23], Random Forests undergoed online update to grow or discard decision trees during tracking. Bai *et al.* [9] treated weight vector as a random variable and estimate a Dirichlet distribution for ensemble's weight vector. They all are a binary classifier realized by an ensemble method and don't exploit the structured data properties which can improve the tracking performance significantly, like as [7,24]. At the same time, online boosting based trackers [5,6] only considered the parameter state in current time period. Different from them, we explore the structure of parameter state in parameter space over different time periods in tracking process.

Zhong *et al.* [25] considered visual tracking in a weakly supervised learning scenario where (possibly noisy) labels but no ground truth are provided by multiple imperfect oracles (i.e., trackers). Kwon and Lee [26] proposed visual tracker sampler to track a target by searching for the appropriate trackers in each frame. They are all ensemble methods applied in visual tracking. Unlike these methods, our method is not a heterogenous method which focuses on the tracker space but an homogenous approach which there is just one tracker. Due to the trained weak trackers in historical sequences, our method is more efficient than heterogenous methods.

Our online ensemble method is most related with online bagging scheme, in the sense that we adopt random combination of weak classifiers. However, we characterize the temporal ensemble weight vector as a clustering center and evolve its distribution with sequential clustering manner. As a result, the final strong classifier is an expectation of the ensemble with respect to the weight vector, which is approximated by an average of the ensemble clustering centers. To the best of our knowledge, in the context of tracking-by-detection, we are the first to present such an online learning scheme that adopt clustering in parameter space and object appearance space to characterizes the uncertainty of a self-learning algorithm.

3 Clustering Ensemble Tracking

In this section, we introduce our tracking algorithm, clustering ensemble tracking (CET), which is a clustering ensemble based appearance model. We begin with an overview of our tracking system which includes a description of structure learning-based part models predictor. We then briefly review the concepts of sequential clustering and ensemble with temporal weak structure predictors. Finally, we give our clustering ensemble based tracking algorithm.

3.1 Overview

We illustrate the framework of our tracking system (diagram shown in Fig. 1). At each frame, our method starts with a structure predictor $h(x)$, several clustering centers based on historical weight vectors $W = \{w_1, w_2, ..w_N, ...\}$ of $h(x)$ and input data x. Our method obtains the incremental parameter cluster centers $C_p = \{C_{p,1}, ..., C_{p,M}\}$ and object appearance cluster centers $C_o = \{C_{o,1}, ..., C_{o,M}\}$ through sequential clustering method, where there is only one cluster, and then the number of clusters increases as the change of the input parameter vectors W or object feature vectors $O = \{o_1, ...o_N ...\}$. Every parameter cluster center $C_{p,i}$ and the latest parameter vector w_N are treated as the parameters of weak structure predictors $h(x)$. Meanwhile, each appearance cluster center $C_{o,i}$ evaluates the object candidates through similarity measurement. Then the output of these weak structure predictors $h(x)$ and the degree of similarity with respective weights $l = \{l_1, l_2, l_3\}$ are combined to yield the final decision where the object is. For reducing the computing complexity, the

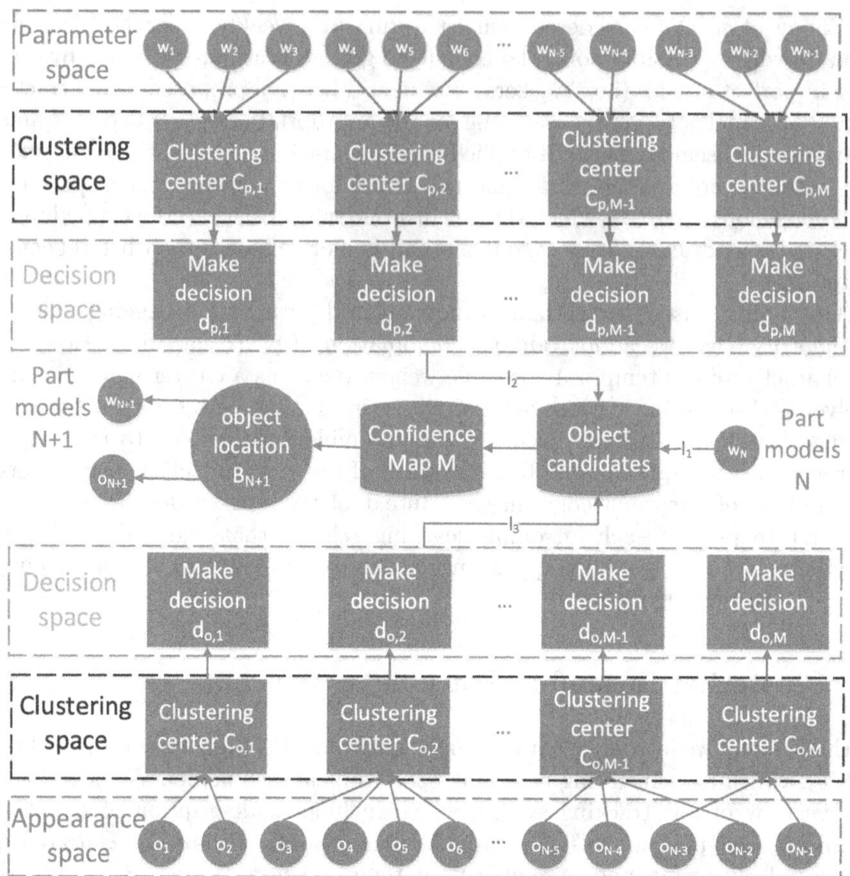

Fig. 1. Framework of the proposed clustering ensemble algorithm. W_i represents the parameter of part models in i^{th} frame. $C_{i,j}$ denotes clustering center. $d_{i,j}$ expresses the decisions related to $C_{i,j}$.

cascade method are adopted in experiments. The cascade is that using the most stable weak classifier or the latest classifier rejects most of object candidates and retains a small number of object candidates which are difficult to predict precisely by one weak classifier so that multiple weak predictors give a combined solution of higher quality than any individual solution (empirically proved by [25,26]).

3.2 Sequential Clustering

In online visual object tracking, the tracked object appearance usually changes gradually. While there are some various factors such as noise or occlusion or fast and abrupt object motion or illumination changes or variations in pose and scale, the object appearance got from the object location will changes much. Meanwhile, the weight vector trained through the changed object training samples varies with the changes of object appearance. Through updating object appearance model, the classifier can adapt the variation of the object appearance. However, model update itself is not absolutely correct without effective supervised information. For alleviating the drift problem resulted by degraded classifier update which comes from incorrectly labeled training samples, we exploit the structure of the parameter space of the trained weak trackers and the predicted object appearance space in historical temporal dimension to guarantee the accuracy of current decision by the final ensemble tracker through sequential clustering. We will introduce the sequential clustering algorithm as follows.

In basic form, parameter or weight vectors $W = \{w_1, ..., w_n\}$ are presented only once and the number of clusters $C = \{C_1, ..., C_m\}$ is not known a priori. The common approach is to define the dissimilarity $d(x_i, C_j)$ and set the threshold of dissimilarity Θ and the number of maximum clusters allowed q. The idea is to assign every newly presented vector to an existing cluster or create a new cluster for this sample, depending on the distance to the already defined clusters. In the application of online tracking, the parameter vector changes gradually so that the threshold Θ and the number q are difficult to set. Here, to avoid the setting problem above, we create a new cluster using a simple heuristic. As pseudo, the algorithm works like the following:

Algorithm 1. Sequential clustering

Init the first sample as the first cluster $C_m = \{w_1\}, m = 1$;
for each $w_i \in \{w_2, ..., w_n\}$ **do**
  find the cluster C_k such that min $d(w_i, C_k)$;
  if i mod $D == 0$ **then**
    Create a new cluster $C_m = \{w_i\}, m = m + 1$;
    Using K-means clustering algorithm to re-clustering the space of samples w, $K = m + 1$
  else
    Add the sample w_i to the nearest cluster $C_k = \{C_k, w_i\}$, while the predicted object satisfied some update condition.
  end if
end for

As can be seen the algorithm is simple but still quite efficient. Different choices for the distance function $d(w_i, C_k)$ lead to different results. We define:

$$d(w_i, C_k) = 1 - \frac{< w_i, C_{k,c} >}{||w_i||||C_{k,c}||} \tag{1}$$

where $< A, B >= \sum_{i=1}^{n} A_i \times B_i$ is the dot product of two vectors, $||A|| = \sqrt{\sum_{i=1}^{n}(A_i)^2}$, and $C_{k,c}$ is the average of all vectors in the set C_k. Due to structured time series property of online tracking, our method creates one new cluster after each D interval frames and uses K-means [27] to re-clustering. The sequential clustering is used in Sect. 3.3.

3.3 Clustering Ensemble Tracker

We adopt the bagging-like method to get the final ensemble results. Bagging predictors is a method for generating multiple versions of a predictor and using these to get an aggregated predictor. The aggregation averages over the versions when predicting a numerical outcome and does a plurality vote when predicting a class. The multiple versions are formed by making bootstrap replicates of the learning set and using these as new learning sets. Here, we use the trained structure predictor in every frame as the basic version of a predictor.

Object-Part Predictor. In our paper, similar to [24], a structured part models predictor is trained by an online manner based on the tracked object locations in previous frames. We represent the object bounding box $B_i = \{\mathbf{x}_i, w_i, h_i\}$ with center location $\mathbf{x}_i = (x_i, y_i)$, width w_i and height h_i. The HOG features extracted from image $\mathbf{I}$ that correspond to locations inside the object bounding box B_i are extracted to obtain feature vector $\Phi(\mathbf{I}; B_i)$. The part indicators $i \in V$ where $V = \{V_0, V_1, ..., V_n\}$ represents the set of object and object parts. Here, V_0 denotes the object itself. Subsequently, we define a graph $G = (V, E)$ over all objects $m \in V$ that we want to track with edges $(m, n) \in E$ between the objects. The edges in the graph model can be viewed as springs that represent spatial constraints between the tracked objects. Next, we define the score of a configuration $S = \{P_1, ..., P_{|V|}\}$ of multiple tracked parts as the sum of two terms: (1) an appearance score that sums the similarities between the observed image features and the classifier weights for all objects and (2) a deformation score that measures how much a configuration compresses or stretches the springs between the tracked objects. Different from [8], the weak base predictor is not our focus, but just part of our method. Mathematically, the score of a configuration S_b is defined as:

$$S_b = \sum_{i \in V} \mathbf{w_i^T} \Phi(\mathbf{I}; B_i) + \lambda \sum_{(m,n) \in E} ||(\mathbf{x_m} - \mathbf{x_n}) - \mathbf{e_{mn}}||^2. \quad (2)$$

Where the parameters $\mathbf{w}_i$ represent linear weights on the HOG features for object i, $\mathbf{e}_{ij}$ is the vector that represents the length and direction of the spring between objects i and j, the set of all parameters is denoted by $\Theta = \{\mathbf{w_1}, ..., \mathbf{w_{|V|}}, \mathbf{e_1}, ..., \mathbf{e_{|E|}}\}$. We treat the parameter λ as a hyper-parameter that determines the trade-off between the appearance and deformation scores. For reducing the computing complexity, we set $m = 0$, which means only to compute the distance between the parts V_i and the root V_0 in $D(x)$. We use a passive-aggressive algorithm to perform the parameter update [24,28].

Parameter and Feature Clustered Predictor. In this paper, we redefine the goal of tracking problem as to find the best state that not only using the current trained classifier in the case where the object is easy to identify (see Fig. 2(a)),

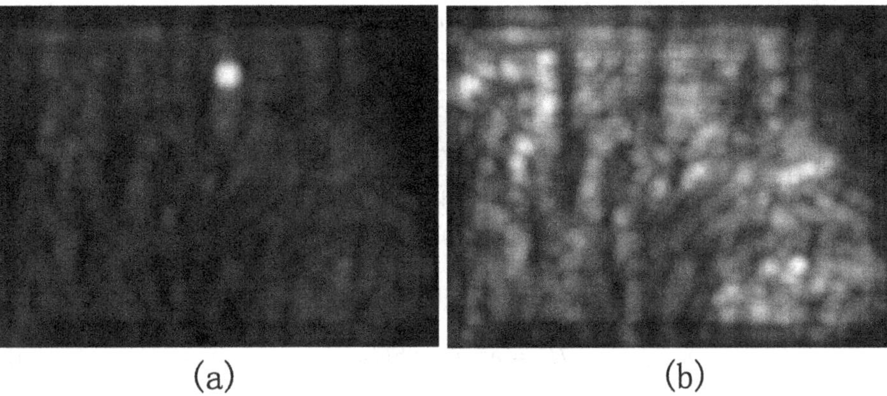

Fig. 2. Two confidence maps to decide where object is. The lighter, the more likely the object is.

but also exploiting the historical trained classifier through clustering ensemble methods in the case where the object is difficult to identify (see Fig. 2(b)). In Fig. 2(a)), the object is easy to decide because other regions' confidences are much lower than the lighter region so that the object is discriminated easier from the background. In Fig. 2(b), the background has many regions in which there are similar confidences as the object so that if the current trained classifier's decision is wrong, the tracker will drift to the background. After drift, the classifier's update will be wrong. For reducing the decision ambiguities of the object, we adopt the clustering ensemble method (see Sec. 3.2) in the historical parameter space and object appearance space and use the clustering centers to make a decision where the object is. To improve the computational efficiency and robustness, we get the extremal points in the confidence map as the object candidates. After getting the object candidates, we use the clustering centers as weak classifiers to vote the best state.

Each cluster center is treated as a sub-weak clustered predictor in ether discriminative parameter space or generative object appearance space. The score of one object candidate B_c based on the predictor in parameter space can be computed:

$$S_p(B_c) = \sum_{i=1}^{N_p} C_{p,i}^T \Phi(\mathbf{I}; B_c) \tag{3}$$

where N_p is the total number of clusters in parameter space by the end of the current frame, and $C_{p,i}$ is the representation of the ith cluster center in parameter space. The score of one object candidate using the jth predictor in object parameter space can be mathematically expressed:

$$S_o^j(B_c) = \rho(Q(B_C), C_{o,j}), \tag{4}$$

where ρ is euclidean metric function, $Q(B_C)$ is object representation directly extracted from the object candidate bounding box, $C_{o,j}$ is the jth clustering center in object feature space. In our experiment, $Q(B_C)$ is a vectorization after resizing the B_C to its quarter. The same is to extract feature in object space.

According to the Eq. (2–4), then the final object candidate's score is:

$$S = \lambda_1 S_b + \lambda_2 S_p + \lambda_3 S_o, \lambda_1 + \lambda_2 + \lambda_3 = 1, \tag{5}$$

where $\{S_b, S_p, S_o\}$ are the scores of weak part models predictor, weak parameter predictor and weak object appearance predictor and $\{\lambda_1, \lambda_2, \lambda_3\}$ are their weights respectively. How to learn the λ is introduced in next section. The final object location is inferred based on Eq. (5):

$$B^* = \arg\max_{B_c} S(B_c), \tag{6}$$

where the B_c is object bounding box candidates sampled from the search region near the previous object location.

3.4 Weight Update

Our model updates the weights of three different predictors after the decision stage in each step, not each frame which doesn't satisfy the update condition (e.g. heavily occluded), so that the model can evolve. For each step, after performing the decision, our method obtains the labels of data predicted by our strong predictor and the observation of performance of weak view predictors, that is, the prediction consistency of weak classifiers with respect to the strong classifier, likely to [9,29].

The weight distribution is dependent on the accumulative normalized central-pixel error probability. The accumulative property reflects on the cumulative sum of observation of relative reliability of each predictor. The normalized central-pixel error probability is incarnated by normalized probability directly related to the distance between the object's center and weak predictor observations' centers. Mathematically, we have

$$p(o_i^t|x^t) = \frac{1}{Z_t} exp(-(o_i^t - x^t)^2/\sigma^2), \tag{7}$$

$$Z_t = \sum_i^n p(o_i^t|x^t) \tag{8}$$

where o_i^t is the observation state center location of the ith weak predictor in step t, x^t is the predicted object's center location, Z_t is a normalization factor in each step t, and $\sigma = 25$. Each part weight is defined as:

$$\lambda_i = \frac{\sum_{t=2}^T p(o_i^t|x^t)}{\sum_{t=2}^T Z_t} \tag{9}$$

which computes relative reliability of each part predictor.

4 Experiments

For the experiments, publicly available video sequences obtained from [5,11,30,31] were utilized. Using the sequences, the proposed method (CET) was analyzed and compared with 7 state-of-the-art tracking methods: Multiple Instance Learning (MIL) [5], Visual tracking decomposition [30], Struck [7], Tracking-Learning-Detection (TLD) [32], PartTracker (PT) [33], Structure preserving object tracking (SPOT) [24], Randomized Ensemble Tracking (RET) [9]. All algorithms are compared in terms of the same initial positions in first frame in [31].

4.1 Implement Details

In all of the experiments, the parameters of our trackers are fixed. The experimental results of MIL, VTD, Struck, TLD are dependent on the public dataset where the sequences' ground truth are re-annotated by Wu *et al.* [31] and some trackers' results through the third party appraisal are attached. For fairness, we adopt the other tracker codes provided by the respective authors in their homepages. The binary code of PT is public. We just need to prepare a config file and then can get their results. The source code of SPOT is published in the website of zhang and van der Maaten [24]. There is one limitation in SPOT is that the parts' initialization for single object tracking is missing in their source code because it is mainly designed for multiple object tracking. We want to use it as our base tracker so that it is necessary to initialize the parts. For handleability and robustness, we divide the object into four parts equally and then complete the part initialization. The source code of RET is also provided by its authors. MIL and TLD use the haar-like feature [34] or LBP-like feature which is sensitive to large illumination, while Struck, VTD, PT, SPOT, RET and CET are based on edge information or HOG feature [35] that is robust to illumination and mirror misalignment. We use the given parameter in their code and get the sequences' results. In our method, one cluster is initialized newly in every $D = 100$ frames. The time complexity is mainly determined by the number of parts, the clustering computation complexity, feature extraction and the search region for deciding where object is.

4.2 Quantitative Analysis

The quantitative comparison results with several state-of-the-art trackers and our tracker (CET) are shown in Fig. 3 and Table 1. We follow the same evaluation protocol proposed in [31]. Overall, our method outperforms them consistently in the view of overall performance (see Fig. 3). In addition, Fig. 4 shows the comparison on different subsets such as occlusion and illumination subsets. The quantitative results are shown in Table 1. From the table, CET achieves the competitive performances well against the other state-of-the-art algorithms on all tested sequences. As summarized in Table 1, our method (CET) most accurately tracked the targets in terms of the center location error and the success rate, even though there are several types of appearance changes.

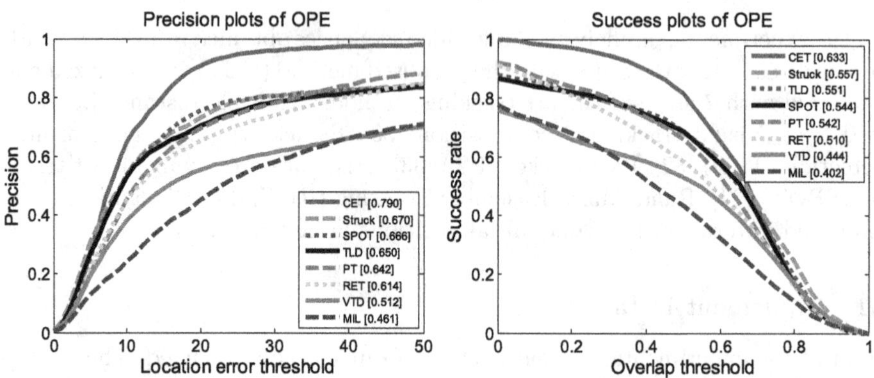

Fig. 3. Plots of overall performance comparison for the 22 videos in the benchmark [31]. The proposed method ("CET") obtain better performance in terms of precision (left) and success (right) plot

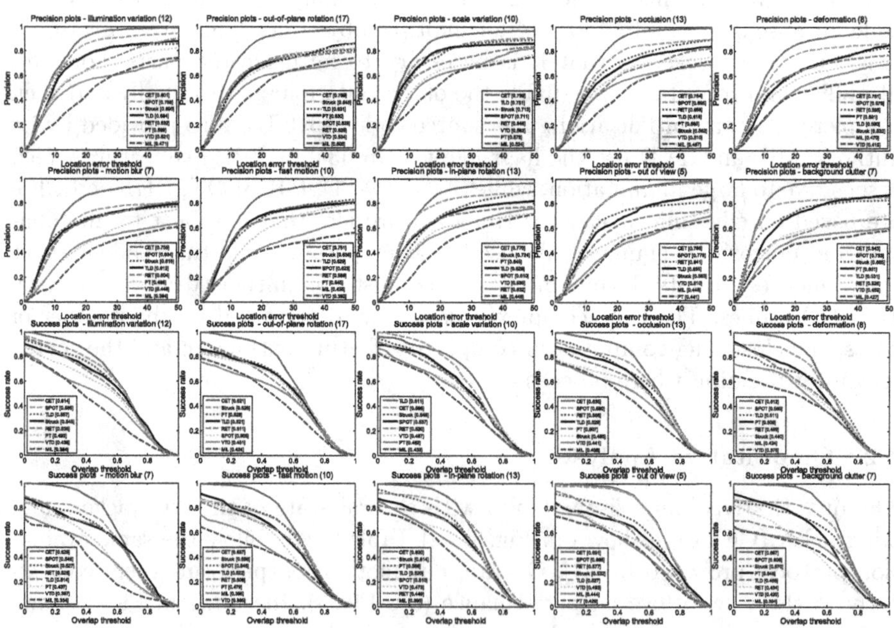

Fig. 4. Several comparisons in different subsets divided based on main variation of the object to be tracked. The details of the subsets refer to [31]. The proposed method ("CET") obtains better or comparable performance in all the subsets

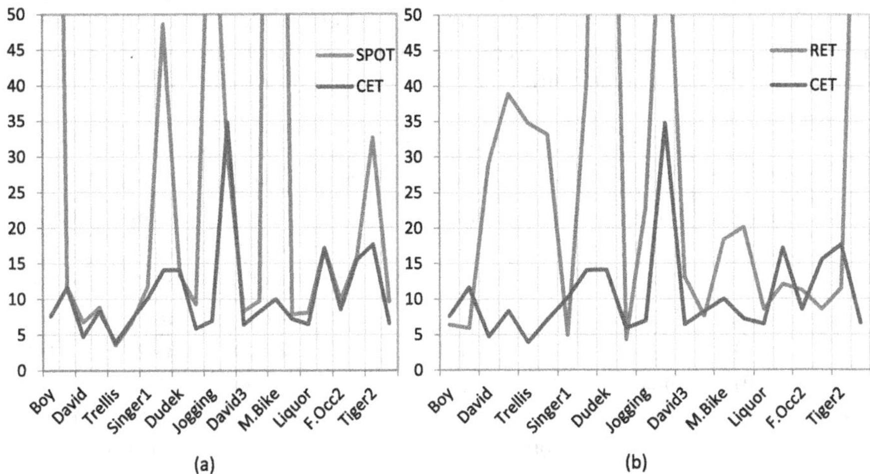

Fig. 5. Center location errors comparing CET with SPOT and RET. (a) represents the comparison between CET and its base tracker SPOT; (b) denotes the comparison between CET and the latest state-of-the-art ensemble tracker RET

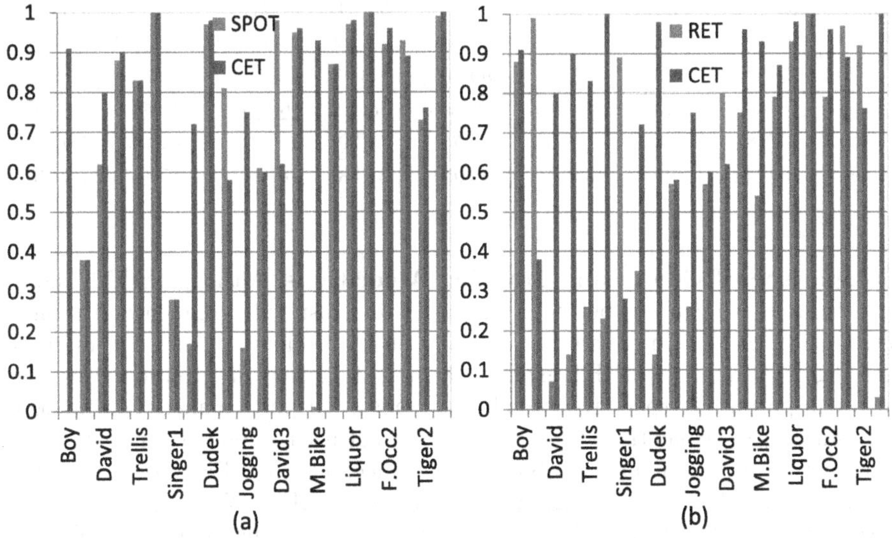

Fig. 6. Success rate based on overlap rate comparing CET with SPOT and RET. (a) represents the comparison between CET and its base tracker SPOT; (b) denotes the comparison between CET and the latest state-of-the-art ensemble tracker RET

Table 1. Comparison of tracking results. The numbers indicate the average center location errors in pixels. The bold, underlined, and italic represent the best, the second, and the third best, respectively. Other numbers in () indicate the percent of successfully tracked frames, where tracking is success when the overlap ratio between the predicted bounding box A_p and ground truth bounding box A_g is over than 0.5: $\frac{A_p \cap A_g}{A_p \cup A_g} > 0.5$

	TLD [32]	MIL [5]	VTD [30]	Struck [7]	PT [33]	SPOT [24]	RET [9]	CET
Boy	5(94)	13(39)	8(79)	**4(98)**	8(78)	238(0.3)	*6(88)*	8(*91*)
Car4	13(79)	51(28)	37(35)	*9(40)*	8(*40*)	12(38)	**6(99)**	12(38)
David	**5(97)**	24(16)	12(68)	10(57)	47(71)	*7(62)*	29(7)	**5**(80)
Sylv	7(93)	12(74)	20(80)	**6**(93)	**6(95)**	9(88)	39(14)	*8(90)*
Fish	31(47)	72(24)	32(50)	7(78)	*8*(80)	**4(83)**	35(26)	**4(83)**
Trellis	7(*96*)	27(23)	17(64)	**3(100)**	6(**100**)	7(**100**)	33(23)	7(**100**)
Singer1	*8*(**99**)	16(28)	**4**(*43*)	15(30)	31(22)	12(28)	5(89)	10(28)
Coke	25(29)	70(3)	69(14)	**12(94)**	*15(71)*	49(17)	40(35)	14(72)
Dudek	18(84)	18(86)	**10(100)**	12(98)	15(94)	*13(97)*	140(14)	14(98)
Couple	**3(100)**	35(67)	104(8)	11(54)	21(36)	9(81)	4(57)	*6(58)*
Jogging	**7(97)**	95(23)	83(22)	62(23)	**7**(88)	75(16)	23(26)	**7**(*75*)
F.Face	41(57)	63(54)	46(*71*)	23(67)	**22(86)**	*31*(61)	75(57)	35(60)
David3	208(10)	30(68)	67(48)	107(34)	7(89)	*8*(**98**)	13(*80*)	**6**(62)
Suv	13(*84*)	82(13)	57(55)	50(58)	35(53)	*10*(95)	**8**(7)	8(**96**)
M.Bike	216(26)	73(58)	*10*(**100**)	**9(86)**	**9(100)**	198(1)	18(54)	10(93)
Lem	*16*(59)	171(17)	79(49)	38(*64*)	136(45)	8(**87**)	20(79)	**7(87)**
Liquor	38(58)	142(20)	60(58)	91(41)	95(34)	8(97)	*9(93)*	**7(98)**
F.Occ1	27(83)	37(62)	20(93)	*19*(100)	17(100)	17(100)	**12(100)**	17(**100**)
F.Occ2	12(83)	20(68)	8(99)	**6(100)**	**6(100)**	10(92)	11(79)	9(*96*)
Tiger1	50(46)	37(37)	107(12)	129(18)	33(49)	16(93)	**9(97)**	16(*89*)
Tiger2	37(18)	30(36)	41(17)	*22(65)*	48(29)	33(73)	**12(92)**	18(76)
Deer	31(*73*)	101(13)	135(4)	**5(100)**	24(38)	*10*(99)	97(3)	7(**100**)

Comparison of Competing Tracking Algorithms. Although SPOT is our base tracker, we can get better performance in most video sequences through introducing the hidden clustering information by sequential clustering method (see Figs. 5(a) and 6(a)). RET exploits the non-stationary distribution of weight vector in parameter space to ensemble and get good performance. Our tracker CET adopts the sequential clustering method to utilize the hidden non-stationary distribution of parameter and object appearance. Through Figs. 5(b) and 6(b), we also get the better performance comparing with RET. We compare the proposed tracking algorithm with nine state-of-the-art tracking algorithms, Table 1 summarises the average center location error performance and success rate of the compared tracking algorithms over the 22 sequences. From the experimental results, we see that our tracking algorithm obtains the best performance on ten sequences in the terms of the center location error or the success rate, seven sequences the second best, four sequences the third best. Figure 4 shows that our method can handle occlusion, illumination and out-of-view well. The robustness of our CET tracker lies in the object-part structure which are discriminatively trained online to account for the variations, the historical hidden structure information in parameter space of base tracker and in the object appearance space of the historical predicted object.

5 Conclusion

In this paper, we deal with the tracking problem about decision ambiguities by fusing object-part predictor, parameter clustered predictor and feature clustered predictor together. Object-part predictor exploits the structure between object and its parts which is effective to object deformative appearance changes. Parameter clustered predictor utilizes temporal hidden group structure in object parameter space in some extent. Feature clustered predictor guarantees the object from the distracters in parameter space and get the better performance. Then we propose a tracker, clustering ensemble tracking (CET), based on structure learning and sequential clustering framework to avoid the drifting problem. Extensive experiments show that our algorithm is robust to occlusion, illumination and out-of-view because different predictors have different properties. The accuracy of CET is superior or competitive to several state-of-the-art tracking algorithms in a more effective way.

Acknowledgement. This work was supported by 863 Program (2014AA015104), and National Natural Science Foundation of China (61273034 and 61332016).

References

1. Yilmaz, A., Javed, O., Shah, M.: Object tracking: a survey. CSUR **38**, 13 (2006)
2. Smeulders, A.W.M., Chu, D.M., Cucchiara, R., Calderara, S., Dehghan, A., Shah, M.: Visual tracking: an experimental survey. IEEE-TPAMI **99**, 1 (2013)
3. Li, X., Hu, W., Shen, C., Zhang, Z., Dick, A., Hengel, A.: A survey of appearance models in visual object tracking. IEEE-TIST **4**, 1–58 (2013)
4. Avidan, S.: Ensemble tracking. IEEE-TPAMI **29**, 261–271 (2007)
5. Babenko, B., Yang, M.H., Belongie, S.: Visual tracking with online multiple instance learning. In: CVPR, pp. 983–990. IEEE (2009)
6. Grabner, H., Bischof, H.: On-line boosting and vision. In: 2006 IEEE Computer Society Conference on Computer Vision and Pattern Recognition, vol. 1, pp. 260–267. IEEE (2006)
7. Hare, S., Saffari, A., Torr, P.: Struck: structured output tracking with kernels. In: ICCV, pp. 263–270. IEEE (2011)
8. Zhang, L., van der Maaten, L.: Structure preserving object tracking. In: CVPR, pp. 1838–1845. IEEE (2013)
9. Bai, Q., Wu, Z., Sclaroff, S., Betke, M., Monnier, C.: Randomized ensemble tracking. In: ICCV. IEEE (2013)
10. Yu, Q., Dinh, T.B., Medioni, G.G.: Online tracking and reacquisition using co-trained generative and discriminative trackers. In: Forsyth, D., Torr, P., Zisserman, A. (eds.) ECCV 2008, Part II. LNCS, vol. 5303, pp. 678–691. Springer, Heidelberg (2008)

11. Ross, D., Lim, J., Lin, R., Yang, M.H.: Incremental learning for robust visual tracking. IJCV **77**, 125–141 (2008)
12. Mei, X., Ling, H.: Robust visual tracking and vehicle classification via sparse representation. IEEE-TPAMI **33**, 2259–2272 (2011)
13. Adam, A., Rivlin, E., Shimshoni, I.: Robust fragments-based tracking using the integral histogram. In: CVPR, vol. 1, pp. 798–805. IEEE (2006)
14. Zhang, T., Ghanem, B., Liu, S., Ahuja, N.: Robust visual tracking via multi-task sparse learning. In: CVPR, pp. 2042–2049. IEEE (2012)
15. Zhang, K., Zhang, L., Yang, M.-H.: Real-time compressive tracking. In: Fitzgibbon, A., Lazebnik, S., Perona, P., Sato, Y., Schmid, C. (eds.) ECCV 2012, Part III. LNCS, vol. 7574, pp. 864–877. Springer, Heidelberg (2012)
16. Hansen, L.K., Salamon, P.: Neural network ensembles. IEEE-TPAMI **12**, 993–1001 (1990)
17. Breiman, L.: Bagging predictors. Mach. Learn. **24**, 123–140 (1997)
18. Freund, Y., Schapire, R.E.: A decision-theoretic generalization of on-line learning and an application to boosting. J. Comput. Syst. Sci. **55**, 119–139 (1997)
19. Jennifer, A., David, M., Adrian, E., Chris, T.: Bayesian model averaging: a tutorial. Stat. Sci. **14**, 382–417 (1999)
20. Hong, S., Kwak, S., Han, B.: Orderless tracking through model-averaged posterior estimation. In: ICCV. IEEE (2013)
21. Avidan, S.: Support vector tracking. IEEE-TPAMI **26**, 1064–1072 (2004)
22. Oza, N.C.: Online bagging and boosting. In: 2005 IEEE International Conference on Systems, Man and Cybernetics, vol. 3, pp. 2340–2345. IEEE (2005)
23. Saffari, A., Leistner, C., Santner, J., Godec, M., Bischof, H.: On-line random forests. In: ICCVW, pp. 1393–1400. IEEE (2009)
24. Zhang, L., van der Maaten, L.: Preserving structure in model-free tracking. IEEE-TPAMI **36**, 756–769 (2014)
25. Zhong, B., Yao, H., Chen, S., Ji, R., Ji, X., Yuan, X., Liu, S., Gao, W.: Visual tracking via weakly supervised learning from multiple imperfect oracles. In: CVPR, pp. 1323–1330. IEEE (2010)
26. Kwon, J., Lee, K.: Tracking by sampling and integrating multiple trackers. IEEE-TPAMI **PP**, 1 (2013)
27. MacQueen, J., et al.: Some methods for classification and analysis of multivariate observations. In: Proceedings of the Fifth Berkeley Symposium on Mathematical Statistics and Probability, California, USA, vol. 1, pp. 281–297 (1967)
28. Crammer, K., Dekel, O., Keshet, J., Shalev-Shwartz, S., Singer, Y.: Online passive-aggressive algorithms. JMLR **7**, 551–585 (2006)
29. Wang, N., Yeung, D.: Ensemble-based tracking: aggregating crowdsourced structured time series data. In: ICML. JMLR. org (2014)
30. Kwon, J., Lee, K.M.: Visual tracking decomposition. In: CVPR, pp. 1269–1276. IEEE (2010)
31. Wu, Y., Lim, J., Yang, M.H.: Online object tracking: a benchmark. In: CVPR, pp. 2411–2418. IEEE (2013)
32. Kalal, Z., Mikolajczyk, K., Matas, J.: Tracking-learning-detection. IEEE-TPAMI **34**, 1409–1422 (2012)
33. Yao, R., Shi, Q., Shen, C., Zhang, Y., van den Hengel, A.: Part-based visual tracking with online latent structural learning. In: CVPR (2013)
34. Paul, V., Michael, J.: Rapid object detection using a boosted cascade of simple features. In: CVPR, vol. 1, pp. I–511. IEEE (2001)
35. Dalal, N., Triggs, B.: Histograms of oriented gradients for human detection. In: CVPR, vol. 1, pp. 886–893. IEEE (2005)

Query Based Adaptive Re-ranking for Person Re-identification

Andy Jinhua Ma(✉) and Ping Li

Department of Statistics, Department of Computer Science,
Rutgers University, Piscataway, NJ 08854, USA
jma@stat.rutgers.edu

Abstract. Existing algorithms for person re-identification hardly model query variations across non-overlapping cameras. In this paper, we propose a query based adaptive re-ranking method to address this important issue. In our work, negative image pairs can be easily generated for each query under non-overlapping cameras. To infer query variations across cameras, nearest neighbors of the query positive match under two camera views are approximated and selected from positive matches in the training set. Locality preserving projections (LPP) are employed to ensure that each feature vector under one camera shares similar neighborhood structure with the corresponding positive match. Using existing re-identification algorithms as base score function, the optimal adaptive model is learnt by least-square regression with manifold regularization. Experimental results show that the proposed method can improve the ranking performance and outperforms other adaptive methods.

1 Introduction

The task of person re-identification is to re-identify a person when she/he disappears from the field of view of a camera and appears in another. The problem is very challenging due to non-trivial variations of viewpoint, illumination condition, human pose, etc. Existing methods solve these challenges by extracting features robust to these variations [1–10] or using label information to train discriminative models [11–17]. Since there are limited labeled images for each person and the query person who needs to be re-identified is usually not contained in the training set, most discriminative methods [11–16] assume all individuals share an unified model for identification. Based on this assumption, these methods generate matched (positive) and unmatched (negative) image pairs by limited person labels to train a score function. However, the learnt generic model may not be optimal for each query image, and consequently the re-identification performance is often not satisfactory.

To learn a matching function specific to each query image, Liu *et al.* [18] proposed an unsupervised approach to on-the-fly feature importance mining by person appearance attributes for re-identification. Based on manifold ranking, the score of the probe image is propagated to the gallery for performance improvement in [19]. Given the assumption that the transition time across cameras is available

D. Cremers et al. (Eds.): ACCV 2014, Part V, LNCS 9007, pp. 397–412, 2015.
DOI: 10.1007/978-3-319-16814-2_26

to prune the candidate set, Li *et al.* [20] proposed to learn an adaptive metric by selecting and re-weighting the training data according to the query and pruned candidates. Using a different approach, in [21], feature vectors of a query-gallery image pair were first projected to a locally aligned space and then matched by specific local metrics. For post-rank optimization, weak negatives and strong negatives are manually selected from the gallery set to train an adaptive classification function for each query image in [22]. It was shown that the selected weak negatives and strong negatives can help improve the re-identification performance remarkably, but the process of manual labeling is still costly, especially when the number of query images becomes large.

In this paper, we propose a novel re-ranking method without using manually labeled information for the query data. Although negative image pairs can be easily generated for each query under non-overlapping cameras, it is more difficult and important to infer the query based positive information across cameras. To model query variations, positive image pairs in the training set are selected as nearest neighbors of the query positive match under two cameras. Since the query match is unknown, such nearest neighbors cannot be computed directly. Thus, we propose to approximate the neighborhood of the query match by employing Locality Preserving Projections (LPP) [23] to ensure that each image under the camera of the query shares the same neighborhood with the corresponding positive image pair across two cameras. Based on the available negative and estimated positive information for the query, the optimal adaptive re-ranking model is learnt by least-square regression with manifold regularization for the smoothness of the decision function.

Our contributions are summarized as follows:

1. We propose a novel query variation inference method to select nearest neighbors of the query match under two cameras based on images under one camera. Positive image pairs under two cameras in the training set are used to construct the adjacency graph for the training images under the camera of the query. A locality preserving mapping is learnt to preserve the neighborhood structure, so that nearest neighbors of the query match can be determined by the query image. Thus, query variations across cameras can be modeled by the positive image pairs in the training set corresponding to nearest neighbors of the query image.
2. We develop a new **Q**uery based **A**daptive **Re**-**R**anking (QARR) algorithm to improve the ranking performance of existing re-identification methods. Given a (generic) base score function, we learn a regression based adaptive re-ranking model by negative image pairs generated under non-overlapping cameras and the query match estimated by modeling query variations. To ensure the smoothness of the adaptive score function over the query-gallery image pairs, a manifold regularization term is incorporated in the objective function to learn the optimal QARR model.

We will first briefly review related work in Sect. 2. Then we elaborate on our proposed method in Sect. 3. Experimental results are given in Sect. 4. Finally, Sect. 5 concludes the paper.

2 Related Work

In [24] proposed a descriptive and discriminative classification model for person re-identification. Given a specific query, all the images are ranked by appearance features of region covariance descriptors. After that, a human operator is assigned to check whether the searched person has a high rank. If not, a discriminative model is learnt for re-ranking under the assumption that there are multiple frames for the query under a camera. While it was shown that this query based re-ranking model could achieve better results than the generic models, the method did not model query variations across non-overlapping cameras.

Besides person re-identification, many adaptive re-ranking algorithms [25–29] have been developed for image retrieval. Most of these methods [25–28] first rank a query image by key word features and then re-rank the text-based search results by adaptive visual similarity measure. For content-based image retrieval [29], initial ranked lists are first determined by comparing the similarities between visual features and then images are re-ranked based on the similarities of their ranked lists as contextual information. While these methods are designed for image retrieval, they do not take advantage of the special characteristics in person re-identification under non-overlapping cameras.

Domain adaptation [30] is one of the research areas related to this paper. If we consider the training data as the source domain, the query image and the gallery set as the target domain, domain adaptation techniques can be employed to learn an adaptive classification model. Without any label information in the target domain, the unsupervised domain adaptation methods [31,32] aim at aligning the marginal distributions under the assumption that the conditional probabilities are equal with each other in the source and target domain. Since the equal conditional probability assumption may not be valid, adaptive learning methods [33,34] make use of a small amount of labeled data in the target domain to improve the recognition performance. Nevertheless, such label information is not available in query based learning for person re-identification, hence existing adaptive learning methods cannot be applied directly.

3 Proposed Method

We consider the re-identification task for images from a pair of cameras a and b. Denote feature vectors of images under cameras a and b as $\boldsymbol{x}_i^a$ and $\boldsymbol{x}_j^b$, respectively. As indicated in [15], the absolute difference space exhibits certain advantages over the common difference space. Hence we use the Absolute Difference Vector (ADV) $\boldsymbol{z}_{ij}$ as feature representation for each image pair:

$$\boldsymbol{z}_{ij} = (|\boldsymbol{x}_i^a(1) - \boldsymbol{x}_j^b(1)|, \cdots, |\boldsymbol{x}_i^a(d) - \boldsymbol{x}_j^b(d)|, \cdots, |\boldsymbol{x}_i^a(D) - \boldsymbol{x}_j^b(D)|)^T \quad (1)$$

where $\boldsymbol{x}(d)$ is the d-th element of feature vector $\boldsymbol{x}$ and D is the dimension of $\boldsymbol{x}$. Let the training data be $\boldsymbol{x}_i^a$ under camera a and $\boldsymbol{x}_j^b$ under camera b. With corresponding person labels y_i^a and y_j^b for training, positive and negative ADVs can be generated and denoted by z_{ij}^{+} for $y_i^a = y_j^b$ and z_{mn}^{-} for $y_m^a \neq y_n^b$, respectively. Without loss of generality, suppose the query image come from camera a with feature vector x_q^a. Let feature vector for gallery image g under camera b be x_g^b. Since the same person cannot be presented at the same instant under different non-overlapping cameras a and b, negative ADVs z_{qg^-} can be obtained for each x_q^a. Therefore, the key problem is to infer information about the positive ADV z_{qg^+} for query variation modeling across cameras. In Sect. 3.1, we present a query variations inference method. Based on the inferred information for query variations, an adaptive re-ranking model is reported in Sect. 3.2.

3.1 Cross-Cameras Query Variation Inference

Let the person image in the gallery set sharing the same identity with x_q^a be $x_{g^+}^b$. The corresponding positive ADV for the query is z_{qg^+}. With the positive ADVs z_{ij}^+ in the training set, we propose to select some z_{ij}^+ such that the distance between z_{ij}^+ and z_{qg^+} is small. According to (1), the l_1 distance between two ADVs z_{ij}^+ and z_{qg^+} is given by the following equation:

$$\|z_{qg^+} - z_{ij}^+\| = \sum_{d=1}^{D} \Big| |x_q^a(d) - x_{g^+}^b(d)| - |x_i^a(d) - x_j^b(d)| \Big| \tag{2}$$

If $(x_q^a(d) - x_{g^+}^b(d))(x_i^a(d) - x_j^b(d)) < 0$, then the element-wise difference on the right hand side of (2) becomes

$$\begin{aligned} &\Big| |x_q^a(d) - x_{g^+}^b(d)| - |x_i^a(d) - x_j^b(d)| \Big| \\ =&|(x_q^a(d) + x_i^a(d)) - (x_{g^+}^b(d) + x_j^b(d))| \end{aligned} \tag{3}$$

Since the variations between non-overlapping cameras a and b can be large, the right hand side of (3) is a large number. In this case, we cannot obtain positive ADVs z_{ij}^+ from the training data, which are close to the positive ADV z_{qg^+} for the query. This implies that, in order to have small distance between z_{ij}^+ and z_{qg^+}, it is necessary to have $(x_q^a(d) - x_{g^+}^b(d))(x_i^a(d) - x_j^b(d)) \geq 0$, which means

$$\begin{aligned} &\Big| |x_q^a(d) - x_{g^+}^b(d)| - |x_i^a(d) - x_j^b(d)| \Big| \\ =&|(x_q^a(d) - x_i^a(d)) + (x_j^b(d) - x_{g^+}^b(d))| \\ \leq&|x_q^a(d) - x_i^a(d)| + |x_j^b(d) - x_{g^+}^b(d)| \end{aligned} \tag{4}$$

According to (4), we have an upper bound for $\|z_{qg^+} - z_{ij}^+\|$, i.e.

$$\|z_{qg^+} - z_{ij}^+\| \leq \|x_q^a - x_i^a\| + \|x_j^b - x_{g^+}^b\| \tag{5}$$

By (5), it is reasonable to see that if x_i^a is close to x_q^a and x_j^b close to $x_{g^+}^b$ for $y_i^a = y_j^b$, the distance between z_{ij}^+ in the training set and z_{qg^+} for the query is small. Therefore, we can obtain the information about the positive ADV $\boldsymbol{z}_{qg^+}$ by the intersection of the neighborhood of $\boldsymbol{x}_q^a$ and the one of $\boldsymbol{x}_{g^+}^b$.

Although the feature vector $\boldsymbol{x}_{g^+}^b$ under camera b corresponding to the query under camera a is unknown, we can select the corresponding positive ADVs from the training data by the feature vector of the query $\boldsymbol{x}_q^a$. Since $\boldsymbol{x}_q^a$ and $\boldsymbol{x}_{g^+}^b$ are feature vectors for the same person under different camera views, they must be related and it is reasonable to assume that $\boldsymbol{x}_{g^+}^b$ can be obtained by a mapping Φ on $\boldsymbol{x}_q^a$, i.e., $\boldsymbol{x}_{g^+}^b = \Phi(\boldsymbol{x}_q^a)$. Although we may not be able to determine such Φ due to limited size of available training data, we make use of this assumption as follows. Applying Φ on $\boldsymbol{x}_i^a$ for $y_i^a = y_j^b$, we get $\boldsymbol{x}_j^b = \Phi(\boldsymbol{x}_i^a)$. Therefore, the second term on the right hand side of (5) becomes

$$\|\boldsymbol{x}_j^b - \boldsymbol{x}_{g^+}^b\| = \|\Phi(\boldsymbol{x}_i^a) - \Phi(\boldsymbol{x}_q^a)\| \tag{6}$$

If Φ is a continuously differentiable function, the right hand side of (6) is bounded by the following equation according to mean value theorem [35],

$$\|\Phi(\boldsymbol{x}_i^a) - \Phi(\boldsymbol{x}_q^a)\| \leq \|\boldsymbol{J}(\Phi)\|\|\boldsymbol{x}_i^a - \boldsymbol{x}_q^a\| \tag{7}$$

where $\boldsymbol{J}$ denotes the Jacobian matrix of all first-order partial derivatives of mapping function Φ. With (6) (7), the inequality (5) becomes

$$\|\boldsymbol{z}_{qg^+} - \boldsymbol{z}_{ij}^+\| \leq (1 + \|\boldsymbol{J}(\Phi)\|)\|\boldsymbol{x}_q^a - \boldsymbol{x}_i^a\| \tag{8}$$

Therefore, if $\boldsymbol{x}_i^a$ is a neighbor of $\boldsymbol{x}_q^a$, the positive ADV $\boldsymbol{z}_{ij}^+$ in the training set is a neighbor of $\boldsymbol{z}_{qg^+}$ for the query. This means the neighborhood of the positive ADV $\boldsymbol{z}_{qg^+}$ can be determined by the neighborhood of the feature vector $\boldsymbol{x}_q^a$.

According to (8), the upper bound of the distance between two ADVs can be determined by the distance between two feature vectors $\boldsymbol{x}_q^a$ and $\boldsymbol{x}_i^a$ under the same camera. Thus, we propose to construct the neighborhood of the query image pair by the neighborhood of the query image. Although it is plausible to directly select the nearest neighbors of the query image, we need to consider that the neighborhood structures are different in the image pair and image spaces. Thus, we propose to employ Locality Preserving Projections (LPP) [23] to align such differences by learning a projection matrix P.

For each feature vector $\boldsymbol{x}_i^a$ under camera a in the training set, we compute the corresponding positive ADV as

$$\boldsymbol{z}_i^+ = \frac{1}{N_i^+} \sum_{y_j^b = y_i^a} \boldsymbol{z}_{ij}^+ \tag{9}$$

where N_i^+ is the number of positive matches for $\boldsymbol{x}_i^a$. To construct the weight matrix A, k nearest neighbors are selected for each positive ADV $\boldsymbol{z}_i^+$. Then, the simple-minded weighting scheme is employed to determine the weight between $\boldsymbol{z}_i^+$ and $\boldsymbol{z}_{i'}^+$. In other words, if $\boldsymbol{z}_i^+$ is in the neighborhood of $\boldsymbol{z}_{i'}^+$, or $\boldsymbol{z}_{i'}^+$ is in the neighborhood of $\boldsymbol{z}_i^+$, $A_{ii'} = 1$; otherwise, $A_{ii'} = 0$. Thus, the neighborhood information for the positive ADVs $\boldsymbol{z}_i^+$ is enclosed in the weight matrix A.

Algorithm 1. Cross-Camera Query Variation Inference

Input: Feature vectors $\boldsymbol{x}_i^a$ under camera a and positive ADVs $\boldsymbol{z}_{ij}^+$ in the training set, query feature vector $\boldsymbol{x}_q^a$, projection dimension p, neighborhood parameters k for LPP and k_q for query based positive ADV;

1: Compute positive ADV $\boldsymbol{z}_i^+$ by (9) for each $\boldsymbol{x}_i^a$;

2: Construct k nearest neighbors for each $\boldsymbol{z}_i^+$ to obtain weight matrix A;

3: Solve optimization problem (10) to obtain projection P with dimension p;

4: Compute the distances between the projected feature vector $P^T\boldsymbol{x}_q^a$ for the query and the projected feature vectors $P^T\boldsymbol{x}_i^a$ for the training data;

5: Select k_q nearest neighbors $P^T\boldsymbol{x}_{i_1}^+, \cdots, P^T\boldsymbol{x}_{i_{k_q}}^+$ of $P^T\boldsymbol{x}_q^a$;

6: Calculate the estimation $\tilde{\boldsymbol{z}}_{qg^+}$ for the query positive ADV by (11);

Output: Estimated query positive ADV $\tilde{\boldsymbol{z}}_{qg^+}$.

We would like to learn a projection matrix such that the indexes of the neighbors of $\boldsymbol{x}_i^a$ are nearly the same as those of $\boldsymbol{z}_i^+$. We use A to define the objective function for feature vectors $\boldsymbol{x}_i^a$ as follows,

$$\min_{\boldsymbol{e},\ \text{s.t.}\ \sum_{i,i'} A_{ii'}(\boldsymbol{e}^T\boldsymbol{x}_i^a)^2=1} \sum_{i,i'} A_{ii'}(\boldsymbol{e}^T\boldsymbol{x}_i^a - \boldsymbol{e}^T\boldsymbol{x}_{i'}^a)^2 \tag{10}$$

where $\boldsymbol{e}$ denotes the column vector in P. The optimization problem (10) can be solved by calculating the eigenvectors and eigenvalues for the generalized eigenvalue problem. The projection matrix P is obtained by the eigenvectors corresponding to the first p eigenvalues (details can be referred to [23]).

Based on the above analysis, we infer the cross-camera query variations by selecting k_q nearest neighbors $P^T\boldsymbol{x}_{i_1}^+, \cdots, P^T\boldsymbol{x}_{i_{k_q}}^+$ of $P^T\boldsymbol{x}_q^a$ from the training data. The corresponding positive ADVs $\boldsymbol{z}_{i_1}^+, \cdots, \boldsymbol{z}_{i_{k_q}}^+$ in the training set are used to represent $\boldsymbol{z}_{qg^+}$ for the query. Since the assumption that $\boldsymbol{x}_j^b = \Phi(\boldsymbol{x}_i^a)$ may not be satisfied for all the selected positive ADVs $\boldsymbol{z}_{i_1}^+, \cdots, \boldsymbol{z}_{i_{k_q}}^+$, we compute the mean of them for the estimation of $\boldsymbol{z}_{qg^+}$, i.e.,

$$\tilde{\boldsymbol{z}}_{qg^+} = \frac{1}{k_q}(\boldsymbol{z}_{i_1}^+ + \cdots + \boldsymbol{z}_{i_{k_q}}^+) \tag{11}$$

Algorithm 1 lists the procedure for cross-camera query variation inference.

3.2 Adaptive Regression with Graph Propagation for Re-ranking

Given a (generic) base score function f for feature vectors $\boldsymbol{x}_q^a$ of the query and $\boldsymbol{x}_g^b$ of the gallery image, we learn an adaptive function f_q specific to the query. Inspired by adaptive learning methods [33,34] for domain adaptation, we define

$$f_q(\boldsymbol{x}_q^a, \boldsymbol{x}_g^b) = \theta f(\boldsymbol{x}_q^a, \boldsymbol{x}_g^b) + \boldsymbol{w}^T\boldsymbol{z}_{qg} \tag{12}$$

where $\boldsymbol{z}_{qg}$ denote the ADV between feature vectors $\boldsymbol{x}_q^a$ of the query and $\boldsymbol{x}_g^b$ of a gallery image as defined in (1), θ is a positive parameter to measure the importance of the base score function f and $\boldsymbol{w}$ is the perturbation weight vector adapted for the query.

With the estimated query positive ADV $\tilde{\boldsymbol{z}}_{qg^+}$ and negative ADVs $\boldsymbol{z}_{qg^-}$ generated under non-overlapping cameras, we formulate the objective function in a least-square regression framework. Since the score of the positive image pair must be larger than the negative ones, we set $f_q(\boldsymbol{x}_q^a, \boldsymbol{x}_{g^+}^b) - f_q(\boldsymbol{x}_q^a, \boldsymbol{x}_{g^-}^b) \approx 1$. This way, we can formulate the following optimization problem:

$$\min_{\theta, \boldsymbol{w}} \frac{1}{N_q^-} \sum_{g^-} [\boldsymbol{w}^T(\tilde{\boldsymbol{z}}_{qg^+} - \boldsymbol{z}_{qg^-}) + \theta(\tilde{s}_{qg^+} - s_{qg^-}) - 1]^2 + \lambda \boldsymbol{w}^T \boldsymbol{w} + \mu\theta^2 \tag{13}$$

where $\tilde{s}_{qg^+} = \frac{1}{k_q}\sum_{t=1}^{k_q} \frac{1}{N_i^+} \sum_{y_j^b = y_{i_t}^a} f(\boldsymbol{x}_{i_t}^a, \boldsymbol{x}_j^b)$, $s_{qg^-} = f(\boldsymbol{x}_q^a, \boldsymbol{x}_{g^-}^b)$, N_q^- is the number of negative image pairs for the query, λ and μ are positive parameters for the regularization terms of $\boldsymbol{w}$ and θ, respectively. To solve the optimization problem (13), we convert it to a matrix form as,

$$\begin{aligned} &\min_{\bar{\boldsymbol{w}}} \bar{\boldsymbol{w}}^T M \bar{\boldsymbol{w}} - 2\bar{\boldsymbol{w}}^T \boldsymbol{m} + \bar{\boldsymbol{w}}^T M_r \bar{\boldsymbol{w}} \\ &\bar{\boldsymbol{w}} = \begin{pmatrix} \boldsymbol{w} \\ \theta \end{pmatrix}, M = \frac{1}{N_{q-}} \sum_{g^-} \begin{pmatrix} \tilde{\boldsymbol{z}}_{qg^+} - \boldsymbol{z}_{qg^-} \\ \tilde{s}_{qg^+} - s_{qg^-} \end{pmatrix} \begin{pmatrix} \tilde{\boldsymbol{z}}_{qg^+} - \boldsymbol{z}_{qg^-} \\ \tilde{s}_{qg^+} - s_{qg^-} \end{pmatrix}^T, \\ &\boldsymbol{m} = \frac{1}{N_{q-}} \sum_{g^-} \begin{pmatrix} \tilde{\boldsymbol{z}}_{qg^+} - \boldsymbol{z}_{qg^-} \\ \tilde{s}_{qg^+} - s_{qg^-} \end{pmatrix}, M_r = \begin{pmatrix} \lambda I & \boldsymbol{0} \\ \boldsymbol{0} & \mu \end{pmatrix} \end{aligned} \tag{14}$$

where I is the unit matrix with the same dimension as $\boldsymbol{w}$.

Note that, if two ADVs $\boldsymbol{z}_{qg}$ and $\boldsymbol{z}_{qg'}$ are close to each other, they must have similar matching scores. Thus, we employ manifold regularization [36] in our adaptive re-ranking method. A weight matrix A_q is constructed for the ADVs $\boldsymbol{z}_{q1}, \cdots, \boldsymbol{z}_{qN_G}, \boldsymbol{z}_{q(N_G+1)}$, where N_G is the number of images in the gallery set and $\boldsymbol{z}_{q(N_G+1)} = \tilde{\boldsymbol{z}}_{qg^+}$. For each query-gallery ADV $\boldsymbol{z}_{qg}$, k_m nearest neighbors are selected and the weights are determined by the simple-minded weighting scheme to avoid parameter selection in heat kernel as described in the previous section. Then, the manifold based regularization term for the continuity of the query score function f_q is given as follows,

$$\frac{1}{(N_G+1)^2} \sum_{g=1}^{N_G+1} \sum_{g'=1}^{N_G+1} A_{qgg'}[(\boldsymbol{w}^T \boldsymbol{z}_{qg} + \theta s_{qg}) - (\boldsymbol{w}^T \boldsymbol{z}_{qg'} + \theta s_{qg'})]^2 \tag{15}$$

where $s_{q(N_G+1)} = \tilde{s}_{qg^+}$. Denote the column concatenation of $\boldsymbol{z}_{qg}$ and s_{qg} by $\bar{\boldsymbol{z}}_{qg}$, and $Z_q = (\bar{\boldsymbol{z}}_{q1}, \cdots, \bar{\boldsymbol{z}}_{q(N_G+1)})$, respectively. Adding the regularization term (15) (in matrix form) into (14), the optimization problem becomes

$$\begin{aligned} &\min_{\bar{\boldsymbol{w}}} \bar{\boldsymbol{w}}^T M \bar{\boldsymbol{w}} - 2\bar{\boldsymbol{w}}^T \boldsymbol{m} + \bar{\boldsymbol{w}}^T M_r \bar{\boldsymbol{w}} + \bar{\boldsymbol{w}}^T Z_q L_q Z_q^T \bar{\boldsymbol{w}}, \\ &\text{s.t. } L_q = \frac{\eta(D_q - A_q)}{(N_G+1)^2} \end{aligned} \tag{16}$$

Algorithm 2. Training Query Score Function

Input: ADVs $\boldsymbol{z}_{qg}$ for query-gallery image pairs, estimated query positive ADV $\tilde{\boldsymbol{z}}_{qg^+}$, negative ADVs $\boldsymbol{z}_{qg^-}$ under non-overlapping cameras, base scores $\tilde{s}_{qg^+}, s_{q1}, \cdots, s_{qN_G}$, parameters λ, μ, η, k_m;

1: Compute $M, M_r, \boldsymbol{m}$ by (14);

2: Construct k_m nearest neighbors for each $\boldsymbol{z}_{qg}$ to obtain weight matrix A_q;

3: Calculate the normalized Laplacian matrix L_q by (16);

4: Obtained the optimal augmented weight vector $\bar{\boldsymbol{w}}^*$ by (17);

Output: Optimal weights $\boldsymbol{w}^*$ and θ^* for the query score function f_q.

where η is a positive parameter for the manifold based regularization term and D_q is a diagonal matrix with diagonal element $D_{qgg} = \sum_{g'} A_{qgg'}$. The optimization problem (16) can be solved by setting the first derivative of the objective function to zero. The solution is given by

$$\bar{\boldsymbol{w}}^* = (M + M_r + Z_q L_q Z_q^T)^{-1} \boldsymbol{m} \tag{17}$$

According to the definition of $\bar{\boldsymbol{w}}$ in (14), the optimal $\boldsymbol{w}^*$ and θ^* can be obtained to determine the query score function defined in (12).

Algorithm 2 summarizes the algorithmic procedure for training the Query based Adaptive Re-Ranking (QARR) model.

4 Experiments

We first introduce the datasets and settings for experiments. Then we present the results on query variation inference across cameras in Sect. 4.2. Based on the inferred query variations, we demonstrate that our method can improve the ranking performance for person re-identification in Sect. 4.3. Finally, we compare our method with existing adaptive re-identification algorithms in Sect. 4.4.

4.1 Datasets and Settings

Two publicly available datasets, namely VIPeR[1] [37] and CUHK[2] [21], are used for experiments. Example images in these two datasets are shown in Figs. 1 and 2, respectively. VIPeR is a re-identification dataset containing 632 person image pairs captured by two cameras outdoor. In this dataset, 632 image pairs are randomly separated into half for training and the other half for testing. CUHK dataset contains five pairs of camera views. Under each camera view, there are two images for each person. Following the single shot setting in [21], images from camera pair one with 971 persons are used for experiments. For this dataset, 971 persons are randomly split into 485 for training and 486 for testing. For the testing data in

[1] http://soe.ucsc.edu/~dgray/VIPeR.v1.0.zip.

[2] http://www.ee.cuhk.edu.hk/~xgwang/CUHK_identification.html.

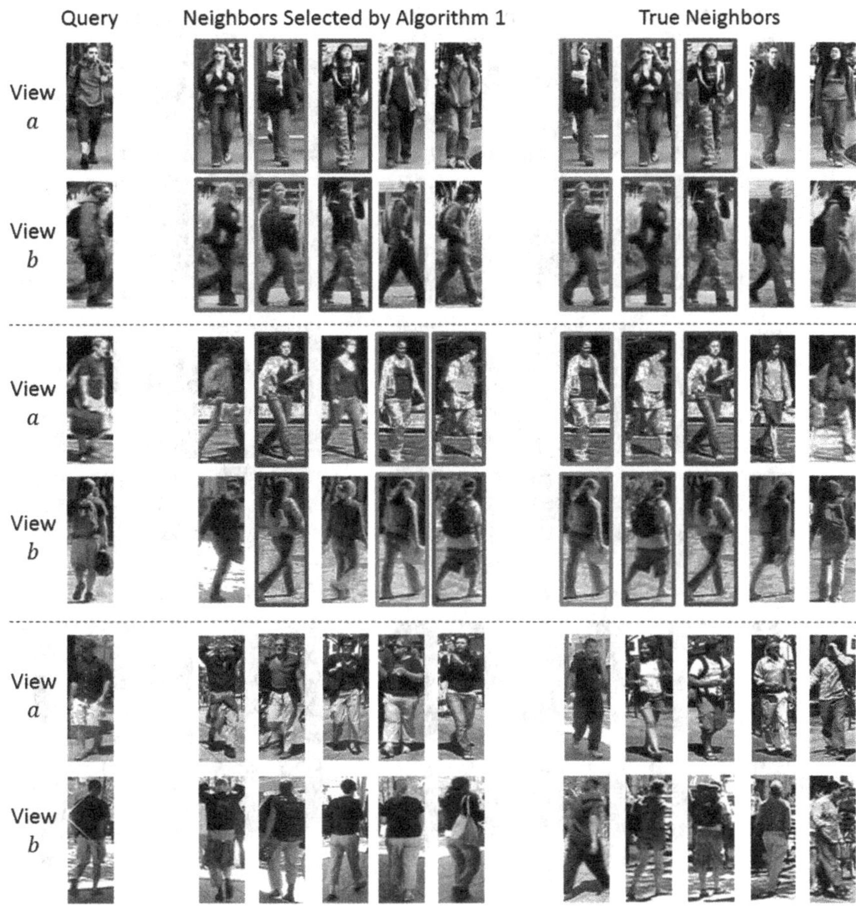

Fig. 1. Examples of $k_q = 5$ nearest neighbors obtained by Algorithm 1 on VIPeR [37] dataset (better viewed in color) (Color figure online).

VIPeR or CUHK, the evaluation is performed by searching the 316 or 486 persons in one camera view from another view. Ten negative image pairs are randomly generated for each query image. These experiments were performed ten times and the average results are reported. For feature representation, we follow [11,12,15] and divide a person image into 6 horizontal stripes and compute the RGB, YCbCr, HSV color features and two types of texture features extracted by Schmid and Gabor filters on each stripe.

In our experiments, we implemented three state-of-the-art algorithms, namely Ranking Support Vector Machines (RSVM) [12], Relaxed Pairwise Metric Learning (RPML) [14] and Relative Distance Comparison (RDC) [15], and use each as the base score function. The parameter C in RSVM is empirically set as 1, while the PCA dimension in RPML is set as 80 for robust performance. To avoid singular matrix problem, we perform PCA with dimension 80 before learning the projection matrix P in our method. The parameters for neighborhood construction are set as

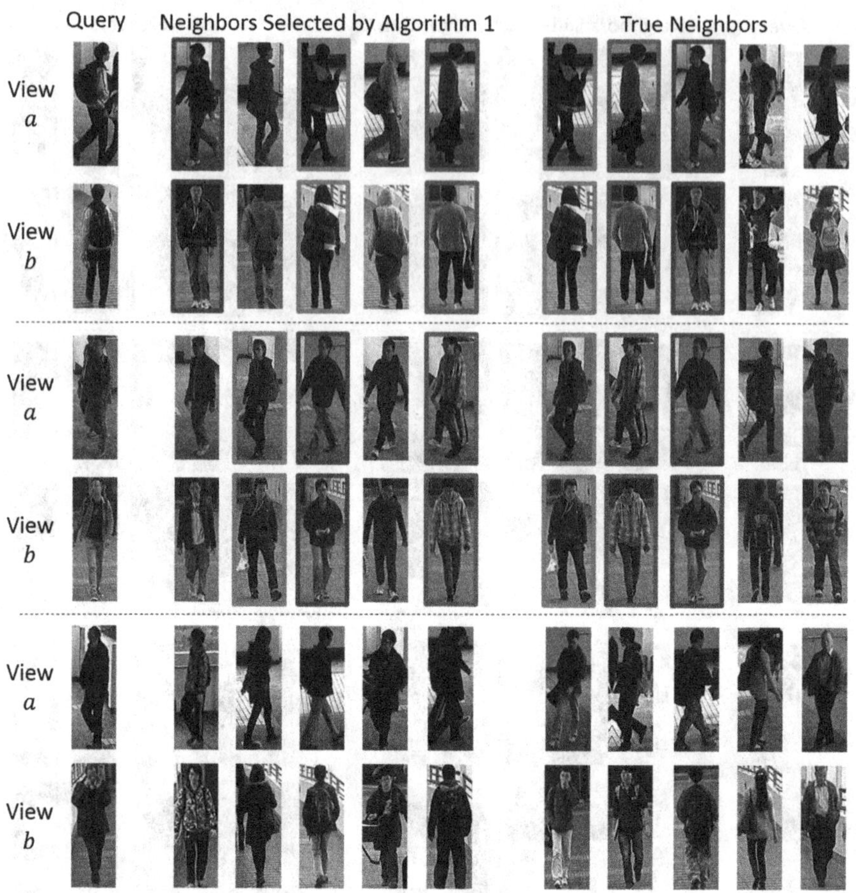

Fig. 2. Examples of $k_q = 5$ nearest neighbors obtained by Algorithm 1 on CUHK [21] dataset (better viewed in color) (Color figure online).

$k = k_q = k_m = 5$. For the regularization parameters, if λ is too large, the norm of the adaptive weight $\boldsymbol{w}$ will be very small. In this case, the query score function f_q will be very close to the base score function f. On the other hand, if λ is too small, the norm of $\boldsymbol{w}$ will be very large, which implies the model could be over-fitted and the base score function hardly affects the decision for the query. Similar analysis can be applied to parameter μ for the weight of the base score function. Thus, we empirically set $\lambda = 10^{-2}$ and $\mu = 10^{-3}$. Since η is the parameter to measure the importance of the manifold based regularization term, we set it with a larger number as $\eta = 10^{-1}$.

4.2 Results on Cross-Camera Query Variation Inference

In this section, we first evaluate whether the proposed cross-camera query variation inference method can discover the true neighborhood of the positive ADV

$\boldsymbol{z}_{qg^+}$. For evaluation, $k_q = 5$ nearest neighbors of $\boldsymbol{z}_{qg^+}$ are selected from the positive ADVs in the training set as ground truth. We calculate the intersection ratio given by the number of elements in the intersection set of the true neighborhood and the one constructed by Algorithm 1 divided by $k_q = 5$. The intersection ratios averaged over all the query images are 59.18 % on VIPeR dataset and 58.89 % on CUHK dataset, respectively. This means that on average nearly 3 out of 5 nearest neighbors are correctly detected by Algorithm 1 for the query positive ADV $\boldsymbol{z}_{qg^+}$. Since the majority of the detected nearest neighbors are in the true neighborhood of $\boldsymbol{z}_{qg^+}$, the inferred query variations can help improve the re-identification performance across cameras.

To visualize the query based positive inference results, we show the true nearest neighbors and the ones selected by Algorithm 1 for three query images under camera a in Fig. 1 for VIPeR and Fig. 2 for CUHK dataset. The image pairs in the intersection of the nearest neighbor sets are marked in the same color. From the first to the fourth rows in Figs. 1 and 2, we can see that 3 nearest neighbors selected by Algorithm 1 are in the true neighborhood of the query match, which is approximately equal to the average intersection ratios. Since we do not know which nearest neighbors are correctly selected, we compute the mean of them by (11) to reduce the error caused by incorrect selection. It is also possible that the intersection of the selected nearest neighbors and the true ones is an empty set as illustrated in the last two rows in Figs. 1 and 2. Although the order of the positive image pairs in the training set computed by Algorithm 1 may not be the same as the true one, the selected image pairs still look similar to the query ones, e.g., similar jackets, pants, and/or pose under the same camera. Therefore, the selected positive ADVs can still help improve the ranking performance, which will be shown in the following subsection.

4.3 Results on Query Based Adaptive Re-ranking

The CMC curves of the proposed Query based Adaptive Re-Ranking (QARR) method are compared with those of RSVM, RPML and RDC in Fig. 3(a)–(c) on VIPeR and Fig. 4(a)–(c) on CUHK dataset. From these figures, we can see that our method outperform RSVM, RPML and RDC on both datasets by learning a score function specific to the query. Results in Fig. 3 show that the rank one accuracy of our method using RSVM, RPML or RDC as the base score function is over 5 % higher than that without adaptive learning on VIPeR dataset. Interestingly, although the RPML should be a better score function compared with RSVM and RDC on these two datasets, our method can still achieve higher matching accuracies with different numbers of top ranks based on it. In other words, regardless of the base score function, our adaptive learning method can improve the re-identification performance robustly.

Note that the proposed method implicitly assumes that there are positive image pairs in the training set which are similar to the query positive match. When the number of training image pairs increases, this assumption will more

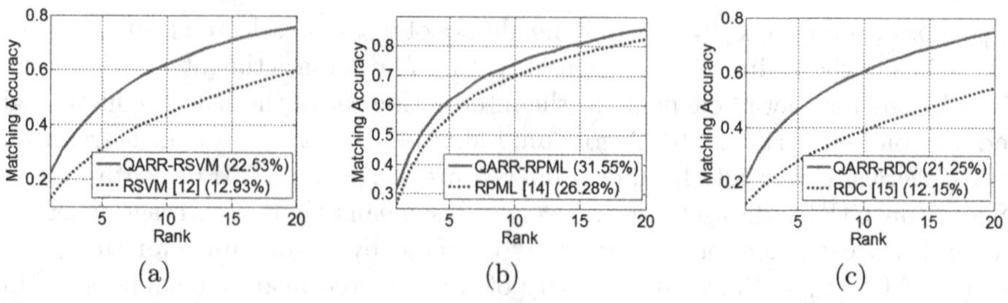

Fig. 3. CMC curves of our method using (a) RSVM [12], (b) RPML [14] or (c) RDC [15] as base score function on VIPeR [37] dataset with 316 image pairs for training.

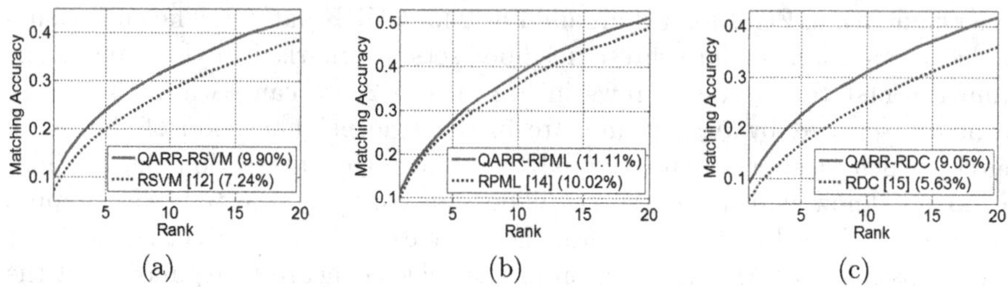

Fig. 4. CMC curves of our method using (a) RSVM [12], (b) RPML [14] or (c) RDC [15] as base score function on CUHK [21] dataset with 485 image pairs for training.

easily satisfied and we should observe better improvement of the ranking performance. To verify this argument, we increase the number of persons for training from 316 to 500 on VIPeR and 485 to 700 on CUHK dataset. The CMC curves on VIPeR dataset in Fig. 5 show that the rank one accuracy improvement by our method is increased from 9.60 % to 14.70 % using base score function RSVM, from 5.27 % to 6.06 % using RPML and from 9.10 % to 15.94 % using RDC. Similar statistics can be observed on CUHK dataset in Fig. 6. These results confirm that our method can achieve better improvement with more training data.

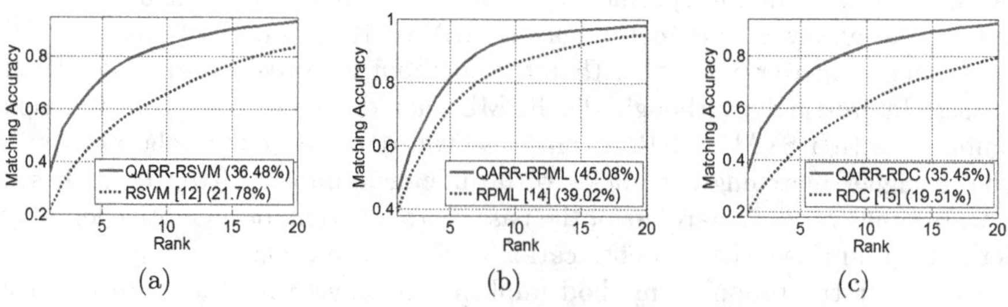

Fig. 5. CMC curves of our method using (a) RSVM [12], (b) RPML [14] or (c) RDC [15] as base score function on VIPeR [37] dataset with 500 image pairs for training.

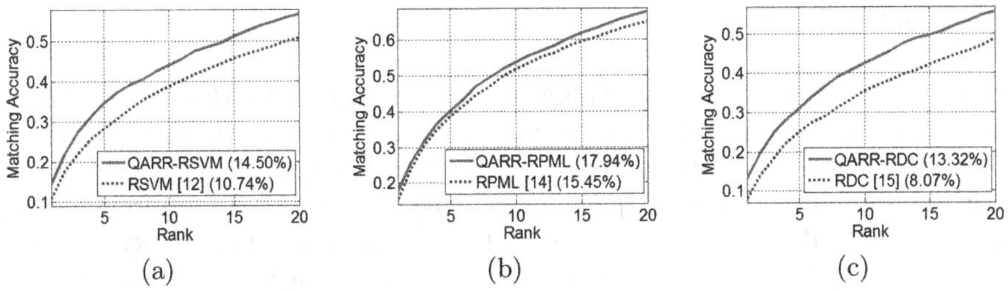

Fig. 6. CMC curves of our method using (a) RSVM [12], (b) RPML [14] or (c) RDC [15] as base score function on CUHK [21] dataset with 700 image pairs for training.

4.4 Comparison with Existing Adaptive Re-ranking Methods

In this section, we compare our method with other query based re-identification algorithms namely, Prototype-Specific Feature Importance (PSFI) [18], Individual-Specific Feature Importance (ISFI) [18], Manifold Ranking with Normalised graph Laplacian (MRNL) [19] and Manifold Ranking with Unnormalised iterated graph Laplacian (MRUL) [19]. The results are copied from their papers and recorded in Table 1 for comparison. It is shown in Table 1 that all the query based re-ranking methods can achieve higher matching accuracy by learning a score function specific to the query. Comparing our method with PSFI and ISFI, we can see that our method remarkably outperforms them using either RSVM or RDC as the base score function. The rank one accuracy of our method is over 6 % higher than those of the PSFI and ISFI based on RSVM and over 4 % higher than them based on RDC. Furthermore, our method can also outperforms the manifold ranking algorithms, MRNL and MRUL, by modeling the inter-camera variations specific to the probe image.

Table 1. Top rank matching accuracy (%) on VIPeR

Method \ Rank	1	5	10	15	20
QARR-RSVM	**22.53**	**47.59**	**62.20**	**70.85**	**75.82**
MRNL-RSVM [19]	19.27	42.41	55.00	63.86	70.06
MRUL-RSVM [19]	19.34	42.47	55.51	64.11	70.44
PSFI-RSVM [18]	15.76	38.70	51.36	n/a	66.84
ISFI-RSVM [18]	16.46	38.76	51.36	n/a	67.18
RSVM [12]	12.93	31.46	43.91	53.05	59.64
QARR-RDC	**21.15**	**46.46**	**60.47**	**68.94**	**74.84**
MRNL-RSVM [19]	19.37	42.78	54.78	63.77	69.62
MRUL-RSVM [19]	18.45	41.74	53.67	62.72	69.27
PSFI-RDC [18]	16.99	38.10	52.37	n/a	66.84
ISFI-RDC [18]	17.12	38.96	52.94	n/a	67.34
RDC [15]	12.15	27.78	38.94	47.36	54.46

5 Conclusions

In this paper, we have developed a Query based Adaptive Re-Ranking (QARR) method to learn a discriminative model specific to the query data. Negative image pairs can be generated for the query under non-overlapping cameras, while positive information about the query across cameras is inferred by approximating the neighborhood of the query positive match. By analyzing the distance between two positive ADVs, we show that such neighborhood can be determined by the nearest neighbors of the query feature vector. Locality Preserving Projection (LPP) [23] is employed to ensure the similarity of the neighborhood structures between the ADV space and feature vector space under the camera of the query. Given a base score function, a regression based adaptive re-ranking model is learnt by propagating the negative and estimated positive information about the query match to all the query-gallery image pairs.

Experimental results show that the majority of the nearest neighbors selected by our method are in the true neighborhood of the query positive match. Thus, the QARR method can improve the ranking performance of existing re-identification methods by using the positive matching information of the query across cameras. Compared with other adaptive methods for person re-identification, our method achieves the best results on VIPeR dataset.

Acknowledgement. The work is supported in part by ONR-N00014-13-1-0764, NSF-III-1360971, AFOSR-FA9550-13-1-0137, and NSF-Bigdata-1419210.

References

1. Farenzena, M., Bazzani, L., Perina, A., Murino, V., Cristani, M.: Person re-identification by symmetry-driven accumulation of local features. In: CVPR (2010)
2. Bauml, M., Stiefelhagen, R.: Evaluation of local features for person re-identification in image sequences. In: AVSS (2011)
3. Cheng, D.S., Cristani, M., Stoppa, M., Bazzani, L., Murino, V.: Custom pictorial structures for re-identification. In: BMVC (2011)
4. Doretto, G., Sebastian, T., Tu, P., Rittscher, J.: Appearance-based person reidentification in camera networks: problem overview and current approaches. JAIHC **2**, 127–151 (2011)
5. Jungling, K., Arens, M.: View-invariant person re-identification with an implicit shape model. In: AVSS (2011)
6. Bazzani, L., Cristani, M., Perina, A., Murino, V.: Multiple-shot person re-identification by chromatic and epitomic analyses. Pattern Recogn. Lett. **33**, 898–903 (2012)
7. Bąk, S., Charpiat, G., Corvée, E., Brémond, F., Thonnat, M.: Learning to match appearances by correlations in a covariance metric space. In: Fitzgibbon, A., Lazebnik, S., Perona, P., Sato, Y., Schmid, C. (eds.) ECCV 2012, Part III. LNCS, vol. 7574, pp. 806–820. Springer, Heidelberg (2012)
8. Ma, B., Su, Y., Jurie, F.: Local descriptors encoded by fisher vectors for person re-identification. In: Fusiello, A., Murino, V., Cucchiara, R. (eds.) ECCV 2012 Ws/Demos, Part I. LNCS, vol. 7583, pp. 413–422. Springer, Heidelberg (2012)

9. Kviatkovsky, I., Adam, A., Rivlin, E.: Color invariants for person reidentification. TPAMI **35**, 1622–1634 (2013)
10. Xu, Y., Lin, L., Zheng, W.S., Liu, X.: Human re-identification by matching compositional template with cluster sampling. In: ICCV (2013)
11. Gray, D., Tao, H.: Viewpoint invariant pedestrian recognition with an ensemble of localized features. In: Forsyth, D., Torr, P., Zisserman, A. (eds.) ECCV 2008, Part I. LNCS, vol. 5302, pp. 262–275. Springer, Heidelberg (2008)
12. Prosser, B., Zheng, W.S., Gong, S., Xiang, T.: Person re-identification by support vector ranking. In: BMVC (2010)
13. Avraham, T., Gurvich, I., Lindenbaum, M., Markovitch, S.: Learning implicit transfer for person re-identification. In: Fusiello, A., Murino, V., Cucchiara, R. (eds.) ECCV 2012 Ws/Demos, Part I. LNCS, vol. 7583, pp. 381–390. Springer, Heidelberg (2012)
14. Hirzer, M., Roth, P.M., Köstinger, M., Bischof, H.: Relaxed pairwise learned metric for person re-identification. In: Fitzgibbon, A., Lazebnik, S., Perona, P., Sato, Y., Schmid, C. (eds.) ECCV 2012, Part VI. LNCS, vol. 7577, pp. 780–793. Springer, Heidelberg (2012)
15. Zheng, W.S., Gong, S., Xiang, T.: Reidentification by relative distance comparison. TPAMI **35**, 653–668 (2013)
16. Ma, A.J., Yuen, P.C., Li, J.: Domain transfer support vector ranking for person re-identification without target camera label information. In: ICCV (2013)
17. Zhao, R., Ouyang, W., Wang, X.: Person re-identification by salience matching. In: ICCV (2013)
18. Liu, C., Gong, S., Loy, C.C.: On-the-fly feature importance mining for person re-identification. Pattern Recogn. **47**, 1602–1615 (2014)
19. Loy, C.C., Liu, C., Gong, S.: Person re-identification by manifold ranking. In: ICIP (2013)
20. Li, W., Zhao, R., Wang, X.: Human reidentification with transferred metric learning. In: Lee, K.M., Matsushita, Y., Rehg, J.M., Hu, Z. (eds.) ACCV 2012, Part I. LNCS, vol. 7724, pp. 31–44. Springer, Heidelberg (2013)
21. Li, W., Wang, X.: Locally aligned feature transforms across views. In: CVPR (2013)
22. Liu, C., Loy, C.C., Gong, S., Wang, G.: POP: person re-identification post-rank optimisation. In: ICCV (2013)
23. He, X., Niyogi, P.: Locality preserving projections. In: NIPS (2003)
24. Hirzer, M., Beleznai, C., Roth, P.M., Bischof, H.: Person re-identification by descriptive and discriminative classification. In: Heyden, A., Kahl, F. (eds.) SCIA 2011. LNCS, vol. 6688, pp. 91–102. Springer, Heidelberg (2011)
25. Cui, J., Wen, F., Tang, X.: Real time google and live image search re-ranking. In: ACM MM (2008)
26. Zitouni, H., Sevil, S., Ozkan, D., Duygulu, P.: Re-ranking of web image search results using a graph algorithm. In: ICPR (2008)
27. Jain, V., Varma, M.: Learning to re-rank: query-dependent image re-ranking using click data. In: ACM WWW (2011)
28. Wang, X., Liu, K., Tang, X.: Query-specific visual semantic spaces for web image re-ranking. In: CVPR (2011)
29. Pedronette, D.C.G., da S Torres, R.: Image re-ranking and rank aggregation based on similarity of ranked lists. Pattern Recogn. **46**, 2350–2360 (2013)
30. Pan, S.J., Yang, Q.: A survey on transfer learning. TKDE **22**, 1345–1359 (2010)
31. Gopalan, R., Li, R., Chellappa, R.: Domain adaptation for object recognition: an unsupervised approach. In: ICCV (2011)

32. Pan, S.J., Ivor, W., Tsang, J.T.K., Yang, Q.: Domain adaptation via transfer component analysis. TNN **22**, 199–210 (2011)
33. Yang, J., Yan, R., Hauptmann, A.G.: Cross-domain video concept detection using adaptive svms. In: ACM MM (2007)
34. Duan, L., Xu, D., Tsang, I.H., Luo, J.: Visual event recognition in videos by learning from web data. TPAMI **34**, 1667–1680 (2012)
35. Rudin, W.: Principles of Mathematical Analysis. McGraw-Hill, New York (1976)
36. Belkin, M., Niyogi, P., Sindhwani, V.: Manifold regularization: a geometric framework for learning from labeled and unlabeled examples. JMLR **7**, 2399–2434 (2006)
37. Gray, D., Brennan, S., Tao, H.: Evaluating appearance models for recognition, reacquisition, and tracking. In: PETS (2007)

Improved Color Patch Similarity Measure Based Weighted Median Filter

Zhigang Tu, Coert Van Gemeren, and Remco C. Veltkamp(✉)

Department of Information and Computing Sciences, Utrecht University, Utrecht, The Netherlands
{Z.Tu,C.J.Vangemeren,R.C.Veltkamp}@uu.nl

Abstract. Median filtering the intermediate flow fields during optimization has been demonstrated to be very useful for improving the estimation accuracy. By formulating the median filtering heuristic as non-local term in the objective function, and modifying the new term to include flow and image information that according to spatial distance, color similarity as well as the occlusion state, a weighted non-local term (a practical weighted median filter) reduces errors that are produced by median filtering and better preserves motion details. However, the color similarity measure, which is the most powerful cue, can be easily perturbed by noisy pixels. To increase robustness of the weighted median filter to noise, we introduce the idea of non-local patch denoising method to compute the color similarity in terms of patch difference. Most importantly, we propose an improved color patch similarity measure (ICPSM) to modify the traditional patch manner based measure from three aspects. Comparative experimental results on different optical flow benchmarks show that our method can denoise the flow field more effectively and outperforms the state-of-the art methods, especially for heavy noise sequences.

1 Introduction

Estimation of a dense motion field between video frames plays a fundamental role in computer vision and image processing. One of the most successful techniques that address this problem is the variational optical flow method [2,3,9], and it has been widely used for various visual tasks, such as tracking, object segmentation and recognition, and super-resolution reconstruction. Since the seminal work of Horn-Schunck (HS) [1], various subsequent extensions and improvements have been proposed over the past 30 years to tackle drawbacks of the HS model, and there has been tremendous progresses, such as: pre-processing the input images with photometric invariant constraints or structure-texture decomposition technique to handle illumination changes [11], or with pre-filtering approaches (e.g. Gaussian filter [1] and Laplacian filter [3]) to reduce outliers (e.g., image noise and estimated flow errors). Penalty functions [2,4,5] are utilized to preserve motion discontinuities and increase robustness to outliers and occlusions. Additionally, occlusions can also be handled according to bilateral filters [6,7]. Large displacements can be estimated by employing traditional coarse-to-fine

D. Cremers et al. (Eds.): ACCV 2014, Part V, LNCS 9007, pp. 413–427, 2015.
DOI: 10.1007/978-3-319-16814-2_27

strategy [8] or matching techniques (e.g. sparse feature matching [9] and dense correspondence matching [10]). However, there are still outstanding problems in existing optical flow methods, such as outliers and large displacements. This paper addresses the issue of outliers removing in terms of median filtering.

In a current survey paper, in comparing various modern optimization and implementation techniques, Sun *et al.* [5] point out that applying a median filter [11,12] to intermediate flow values during incremental estimation and warping produces the most significant improvements. Median filtering is beneficial for every optical flow algorithm they tested, since it can effectively denoises the intermediate flow fields and reduces gross outliers. All in all, it can make even non-robust methods much more robust.

However, median filtering in a large neighborhood has negative effects on edges and corners. A neighborhood centered on a corner or thin structure is dominated by its surroundings, leading to oversmoothing. To improve the performance of the classic median filtering [5,11,12] formulated the median filtering heuristic as a non-local term in the objective function, and incorporated flow and image information to construct a weighted version (a practical weighted median filter). The weighted non-local term is very useful to avoid smoothing at edges and motion boundaries, and can well preserve motion details. Because pixels that belong to the same surface are given higher weight and it ensures pixels only propagate information within their same region.

Although the weighted median filter (WMF) has great advantages, it still has one serious problem. As the weight of WMF heavily depends on the color similarity between pixels, it can be easily violated by noisy pixels [13]. Consequently, improving the robustness of the color similarity measure to noise is a good way to improve the performance of the WMF.

Since Buades *et al.* [14] proposed a non-local means (NLM) method, which uses patches instead of pixels to compare photometric similarities, the non-local denoising methods [15,16] have attracted a lot of attention recently and outperforms conventional filters, leading to the patch-based non-local manner becoming the central part of many state-of-the-art algorithms [17,18]. The NLM denoises a pixel as the weighted sum of its noisy neighbors, where each weight reflects the similarity between the local patch centered at the noisy pixel (i, j) to be denoised and the patch centered at the neighbor pixel (i', j') [15]. In this way, the NLM not only compares the intensity in a single point but also the geometrical configuration in a whole neighborhood. This characteristic allows a more robust comparison than traditional neighborhood filters, and pixels with a similar intensity neighborhood to the noisy pixel will assign higher weights on average.

In this paper, we adopt the idea of the non-local patch method [17], and propose an improved color patch similarity measure (ICPSM) to compute the color measure from three aspects: (1) we introduce a patch manner to compute the color similarity and apply a non-linear median filter function to replace the general linear Gaussian function to reduce blurring; (2) we construct a replicated patch that centered at the noisy pixel (i, j) to substitute the normal patch to reject noise more effectively; (3) we calculate the smoothing parameter of the proposed ICPSM adaptively based on the noise degree of the input image to steer smoothing.

Our paper is organized as follows: Sect. 2 introduces the WMF based optical flow method. Section 3 describes our proposed improved color patch similarity measure. We describe the implementation detailed in Sect. 4. Experimental comparisons are shown in Sect. 5. A brief conclusion is given in Sect. 6.

2 Weighted Median Filter Based Optical Flow Method

Median filtering [11, 12] the intermediate flow fields during incremental estimation and warping is effective to remove outliers. However, it also over-smoothes corners, edges or thin structures. To prevent this kind of over-smoothing, Sun *et al.* [5] construct a weighted non-local term (a practical WMF). We use the WMF based variational optical flow algorithm [5] as a baseline method, and its objective function is expressed as:

$$\begin{aligned} E(\mathbf{u},\mathbf{v},\widehat{\mathbf{u}},\widehat{\mathbf{v}}) &= \sum_{i,j} \rho_D(\mathrm{I}_2(i+u_{i,j}, j+v_{i,j}) - \mathrm{I}_1(i,j)) + \lambda(\rho_S(\|\nabla\mathbf{u}\|) + \rho_S(\|\nabla\mathbf{v}\|)) \\ &+ \lambda'(\|\mathbf{u}-\widehat{\mathbf{u}}\|^2 + \|\mathbf{v}-\widehat{\mathbf{v}}\|^2) \\ &+ \sum_{i,j}\sum_{(i',j')\in N_{i,j}} w_{i,j,i',j'}(|\widehat{u}_{i,j}-\widehat{u}_{i',j'}| + |\widehat{v}_{i,j}-\widehat{v}_{i',j'}|) \end{aligned} \tag{1}$$

where $\mathbf{u}$ and $\mathbf{v}$ are the horizontal and vertical components of the optical flow field that represents the displacements between the input image pair I_1 and I_2 and, λ and λ' are the weighting parameters controlling the relative importance of each term. $\rho_S(x) = \rho_D(x) = (x^2 + \xi^2)^\alpha$ is the slightly non-convex penalty function, with $\alpha = 0.45, \xi = 0.001$. $\widehat{\mathbf{u}}$ and $\widehat{\mathbf{v}}$ are the auxiliary flow fields of $\mathbf{u}$ and $\mathbf{v}$, and approximate to them. (i', j') is the spatial position of any pixel that belongs to a neighborhood $N_{i,j}$ of pixel (i, j).

$w_{i,j,i',j'}$ is the weighting function of the last weighted non-local term, it denotes the similarity between pixel (i, j) and its neighborhood pixels. $w_{i,j,i',j'}$ gives high values to pixels belonging to the same surface, while it gives low values to pixels corresponding to corners, edges and thin structures. It is calculated according to spatial distance and color similarity between pixels, and the occlusion state:

$$w_{i,j,i',j'} \propto \exp\{-(Spa(i,j,i',j') + Col(i,j,i',j'))\}\frac{O(i',j')}{O(i,j)} \tag{2}$$

in particular, the spatial distance measure is defined as:

$$Spa(i,j,i',j') = \frac{|i-i'|^2 + |j-j'|^2}{2\sigma_S^2} \tag{3}$$

the color similarity is defined as:

$$Col(i,j,i',j') = \frac{|\mathrm{I}(i,j) - \mathrm{I}(i',j')|^2}{2\sigma_C^2} \tag{4}$$

where $\mathrm{I}(i,j)$ and $\mathrm{I}(i',j')$ are the color vectors in the CIELab space of the central pixel (i,j) and its neighborhood pixel (i',j') respectively, $\sigma_s = 7$ and $\sigma_c = 7$.

The occlusion state $O(i,j)$ is computed by considering both the flow divergence and pixel projection difference:

$$O(i,j) = \exp\{-\frac{d^2(i,j)}{2\sigma_d^2} - \frac{e^2(i,j)}{2\sigma_e^2}\} \tag{5}$$

where $\sigma_d = 0.3$ and $\sigma_e = 20$. In particular, $d(i,j)$ is the one-sided flow divergence function, defined as:

$$d(i,j) = \begin{cases} \mathrm{div}(i,j), & \mathrm{div}(i,j) < 0 \\ 0, & \text{otherwise} \end{cases} \tag{6}$$

in which the flow divergence $\mathrm{div}(i,j)$ is computed as:

$$\mathrm{div}(i,j) = \frac{\partial}{\partial x}u(i,j) + \frac{\partial}{\partial y}v(i,j) \tag{7}$$

where $\frac{\partial}{\partial x}$ and $\frac{\partial}{\partial y}$ are respectively the horizontal and vertical flow derivatives.

The pixel projection difference $e(i,j)$ is defined as:

$$e(i,j) = \mathrm{I}(i,j) - \mathrm{I}(i + u_{i,j}, j + v_{i,j}) \tag{8}$$

Among the three cues, color similarity plays a most significant role [5]. However, as Rashwan *et al.* [13] stated: the reliance on color similarity of the non-local term causes it is affected by noisy pixels, resulting in inaccurate flow vectors and blurred motion boundaries. In the next section, we will describe a patch based color similarity measure to handle the problem of WMF.

3 Improved Color Similarity Measure

We now explain how to improve the color similarity measure by integrating the non-local patch strategy. In particular, we will first introduce a general patch manner [14] based color similarity measure. Afterwards, we describe an improved replicated patch which has better performance to reject noise. Thirdly, we propose an adaptive scheme to select the smoothing parameter to control denoising.

3.1 Color Patch Similarity Measure (CPSM)

After Buades *et al.* [14] proposed an NLM algorithm, the non-local denoising methods have drawn significant attention. The primary advantage of the NLM denoising method is that they utilize patches instead of pixels to calculate intensity similarity, which makes the NLM methods more robust to pixel-based filters. According to this fact, as shown in Fig. 1, we employ the between-patch manner to replace the between-pixel way to compute the color similarity to reduce the influence of the noisy pixels:

$$PCol(i,j,i',j') = \frac{\| \mathbf{PI}(i,j) - \mathbf{PI}(i',j') \|^2}{2\sigma_{PC}^2} \tag{9}$$

where $\mathbf{PI}(i,j)$ and $\mathbf{PI}(i',j')$ denote the local image patches of size $k \times k$ (we set k = 3 in this paper) centered at pixel (i, j) and (i',j') respectively. $\|\mathbf{PI}\|$ is the Euclidean norm of patch $\mathbf{PI}$ as a point in $\mathbf{R}^{k^2}$.

3.2 Improved Color Patch Similarity Measure (ICPSM)

With the above modification, the patch difference is used to substitute the pixel difference. For example, for a noisy pixel (i, j), the modification of $PCol(i,j,i',j')$ is expressed as (a 3×3 patch):

$$\frac{\sum_{p\in P,q\in P} \| \mathrm{I}(i+p,j+q) - \mathrm{I}(i'+p,j'+q) \|^2}{2\sigma_{PC}^2} \rightarrow \frac{|\mathrm{I}(i,j) - \mathrm{I}(i',j')|^2}{2\sigma_C^2} \tag{10}$$

where $P = [-1,0,1]$. However, the traditional patch measure stills has some defects, in this paper, we improve the CPSM from following three aspects.

PColWMF. Greenberg and Kogan [19] stated that applying a non-linear median filter function rather than a linear Gaussian function can produce less blurring during denoising and make the filter more robust to noise. Based on the idea of [19], we can improve the CPSM $PCol(i,j,i',j')$ as following:

$$PCol(i,j,i',j') = \mathrm{median}(\mathrm{ID}_1, \mathrm{ID}_2, \ldots, \mathrm{ID}_5, \ldots, \mathrm{ID}_9) \tag{11}$$

the color difference $\mathrm{ID}_n (n = 1, 2, \ldots, 9)$ is computed as:

$$\mathrm{ID}_n = \frac{|\mathrm{I}(i+p,j+q) - \mathrm{I}(i'+p,j'+q)|^2}{2\sigma_{PC}^2} \tag{12}$$

where $p \in P, q \in P$. In particular, $\mathrm{ID}_1 = \frac{|\mathrm{I}(i-1,j-1)-\mathrm{I}(i'-1,j'-1)|^2}{2\sigma_{PC}^2}$, ..., $\mathrm{ID}_5 = \frac{|\mathrm{I}(i,j)-\mathrm{I}(i',j')|^2}{2\sigma_{PC}^2}$, ..., $\mathrm{ID}_9 = \frac{|\mathrm{I}(i+1,j+1)-\mathrm{I}(i'+1,j'+1)|^2}{2\sigma_{PC}^2}$.

RPColWMF. The traditional patch based color measure Eq. (9) focuses on comparing the similarity between the patch $\mathbf{PI}(i,j)$ and its neighboring patches $\mathbf{PI}(i',j')$, and the patches that belong to the same surface will be given higher weight during filtering. However, in each $\mathbf{PI}(i,j)$, the central pixel (i, j) is the most significant, and its neighborhood pixels are not so important. For example, as shown in Fig. 1(b), if one (or more) neighboring pixel of (i, j) in $\mathbf{PI}(i,j)$ is an outlier (like the red point), the correctness of the similarity between $\mathbf{PI}(i,j)$ and $\mathbf{PI}(i',j')$ is badly violated. Colors in natural images are locally consistent, one pixel has a very large chance of being similar to some of its neighbors [22]. That is to say, one non-noise pixel should be similar to some of its neighboring patches.

According to this characteristic, to overcome the above mentioned problem, we replicate the central pixel (i, j) to construct a new patch $\mathbf{RPI}(i, j)$ (see Fig. 1(c)) and compute the color similarity between the replicated patch $\mathbf{RPI}(i, j)$ and its neighboring patches $\mathbf{PI}(i', j')$, which can be expressed as $RPCol(i, j, i', j')$:

$$RPCol(i, j, i', j') = \text{median}(\text{RID}_1, \text{RID}_2, \ldots, \text{RID}_5, \ldots, \text{RID}_9) \quad (13)$$

where $\text{RID}_n = \frac{|\text{I}(i,j) - \text{I}(i'+p, j'+q)|^2}{2\sigma_{PC}^2}$, $(p \in P, q \in P)$.

This improvement ensures that if the color of a pixel (i, j) is approximate to the color of its neighboring patch $\mathbf{PI}(i', j')$, a large value will be assigned to $RPCol(i, j, i', j')$, if not, the value of $RPCol(i, j, i', j')$ is small. Clearly, this strategy is very effective to remove noisy pixels as nearly no noise can have a similar color to an image patch.

Smoothing Parameter Selection. Different from [5] which just set the color smoothing parameter $\sigma_C = 7$ fixed for all sequences, we calculate the σ_{PC} according to:

$$\sigma_{PC} = 9(1 + \log_{10}(\sigma)) \quad (14)$$

where σ is the standard deviation of the noise of the input color image I, and under a constraint $\sigma = max(\sigma, 1/10)$. The noise is computed like this: during the coarse-to-fine optimization framework, we use the Gaussian filter to pre-filter I before downsampling it at each scale, to construct a pyramid of images [1]. Hence, at each pyramid level, we consider noise as the difference of the denoised and the noisy color image I.

This scheme is helpful to modify the denoising performance due to two advantages: (1) in contrast to the fixed manner [5], it adjusts the smoothing parameter σ_{PC} accord with the noise degree of the input image I. Since the noise degree between different images is completely different, a fixed smoothing parameter is not suitable for all kinds of images; (2) comparing to the non-local filters [15,16] which select the smoothing parameter based on $\sigma_{PC} = 10\sigma$, our scheme computes the smoothing parameter more precise. For heavy noisy image the smoothing parameter will be enlarged, while for low noisy image the smoothing parameter will be decreased. This principle satisfies the basic denoising feature. Table 2 demonstrates the effectiveness of this scheme.

Due to the ICPSM, our modified weighted non-local term — we refer to it as PatchWMF, is much more robust to the noisy pixels. The boundary blurring is reduced and the accuracy of the estimated flow field is modified.

4 Implementation

We follow the optimization framework of [5] to compute the flow field, more importantly, some useful practices are used for further modification.

Edge-Preserving Smoothness. To preserve edges, we redefine the smoothness term as [9]:

$$E(\mathbf{u}, \mathbf{v}) = \sum_{i,j} \omega(i, j)(\rho_S(\| \nabla \mathbf{u} \|) + \rho_S(\| \nabla \mathbf{v} \|)) \quad (15)$$

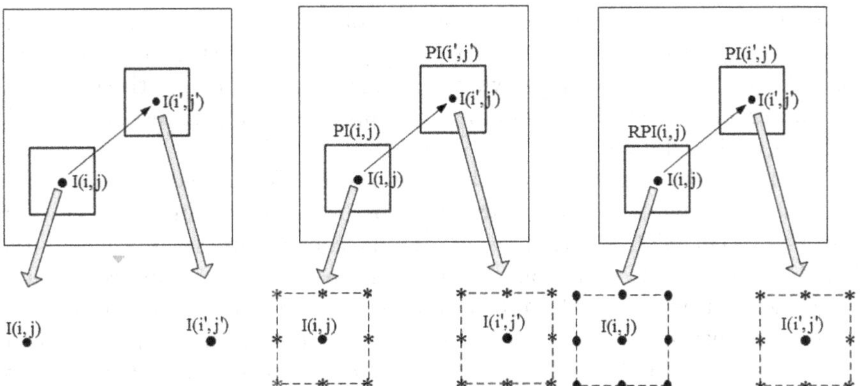

Fig. 1. Three color weight measures. **From Left to Right**: (a) Pixel measure. (b) Patch measure. (c) Replicated patch measure (Color figure online).

the edge-preserving term $\omega(i, j)$ is a structure adaptive map which contains motion discontinuity [9,10]:

$$\omega(i, j) = \exp(-\|\nabla \mathrm{I}_1\|^k) \tag{16}$$

where we set $k = 0.8$.

Large Displacements Handling. The traditional coarse-to-fine framework is good at estimating large displacements of relatively large objects, however, it performs poorly on fine scale structures with motions larger than their size. That because fine scale structures may disappear in coarse scales, leading to no valid matching information in the coarse level can be propagated to finer scale, hence, these structures cannot be well recovered. To handle large displacements while preserve motion details, similar as [10], we first use approximate nearest neighbor fields (NNF) to compute an initial dense correspondence field. Furthermore, we employ the SIFT feature detection and selection method of [9] to obtain some reliable sparse matches. Then, we incorporate the dense NNF and the sparse SIFT matches through the Quadratic Pseudo-Boolean Optimization (QPBO) fusion method [20] to get an improved NNF. After that, during the coarse-to-fine optimization, before the first warping step on each pyramid level, we fuse the improved NNF and the coarser lever computed continuous flow field ($\mathbf{u}$, $\mathbf{v}$) as flow initialization.

Occlusion Detection and Post-processing. Occlusion detection is a notoriously difficult problem, since displacement vectors for occluded pixels generally cannot be determined due to the lack of correspondences. Current optical flow models are not yet powerful enough to handle this problem, thus it is beneficial to tackle occlusions in the post-processing. We employ the mapping uniqueness criterion of [21] to detect occlusions, and the occlusion state is expressed as:

$$Occ(i, j) = \min(\frac{\max(N(i + u_{i,j}, j + v_{i,j}) - 1, 0)}{2}, 1) \tag{17}$$

where $N(i+u_{i,j}, j+v_{i,j})$ denotes the number of pixels in the reference image I_1 that corresponds to a pixel located at $(i+u_{i,j}, j+v_{i,j})$ in the target image I_2. We regard the pixel as occluded pixel when $Occ(i, j) \geq 0.5$. To remove these artifacts while preserving the object boundaries, we apply the joint bilateral filter to fill the detect occluded pixels.

For numerical calculation, we adopt the 3-stage Graduated Non-Convexity (GNC) scheme and perform 5 warping steps on each pyramid level at GNC stage 2. At other GNC stages, due to large motions require more warping iterations [5], we perform 10 warping steps if the sequence is dominated by large displacements, if not we perform 5 warping steps. Other implementation methods and optimization steps are same as [5]. All experiments are performed on a Laptop with an Intel Core i5-2410M 2.30 GHz processor and 4 GB memory. Regarding the running time, in our current CPU implementation, the whole program takes 520 s to compute a high quality flow field for an image pair with resolution 640480 in, for instance, the Urban sequence.

5 Experiments

In this section, we test our method, referred to as PatchWMF-OF, on three public challenging optical flow benchmarks the Middlebury benchmark [3], the MIT benchmark [24], and the MPI Sintel benchmark [23]. Both quantitative comparison in terms of two standard error measures the average angular error (AAE) and the average endpoint error (EPE), and visual analysis compares with other related techniques are performed.

5.1 Evaluation of PatchWMF Technique

We evaluate the proposed PatchWMF technique by testing whether the three presented schemes that aim to improve the color similarity measure are effective, and by quantitatively comparing it with the baseline methods – WMF [5]. In particular, the PatchWMF technique is a combination of the RPColWMF approach and the smoothing parameter selection (Eq. (14)) strategy. Table 1 shows the AAE and EPE results on 8 synthetic sequences from the Middlebury training set. The error statistics display that the three schemes are useful, leading to the PatchWMF outperforms the WMF.

5.2 Evaluation of Noisy Pixels Handling

To further evaluate the noisy pixels handling ability of our PatchWMF technique, we synthesize the 8 training sequences from the Middlebury benchmark by adding Gaussian noise with variance $\sigma_n = [10, 20, 30]$ respectively. From Table 2, we can see that the proposed PatchWMF performs much better than the WMF. Comparing Table 2 with Table 1, it is clear that for a same sequence but with different noise level, the motion estimation accuracy improvement (i.e. AAE and EPE modification) obtained from our PatchWMF on the noisy

Table 1. AAE/EPE of the eight training sequences from the Middlebury benchmark with different color measures for the WMF

Method	WMF($\sigma_C = 7$)	PColWMF($\sigma_{PC} = 7$)	RPColWMF($\sigma_{PC} = 7$)	PatchWMF
RubW.	2.351/0.073	**2.253/0.071**	2.429/0.074	2.400/0.072
Venus	3.327/0.237	3.421/0.243	3.363/0.238	**3.227/0.232**
Dime.	2.570/0.131	2.595/0.132	2.586/0.132	**2.380/0.121**
Hydra.	1.829/0.151	**1.785/0.145**	1.866/0.155	1.837/0.153
Urban2	2.082/0.221	2.095/0.227	2.073/**0.218**	**2.054**/0.221
Urban3	2.600/0.394	2.754/0.391	**2.583**/0.388	2.660/**0.387**
Grove2	1.498/0.104	1.601/0.112	1.509/0.104	**1.433/0.099**
Grove3	4.955/0.463	5.079/0.478	4.957/0.462	**4.829/0.460**
Avg.	2.652/0.222	2.700/0.225	2.670/0.221	**2.600/0.218**

Table 2. Comparison of the AAE and EPE of the Middlebury training sequences with different added Gaussian noise level for the WMF/PatchWMF techniques

Method	$\sigma_n = 10$		$\sigma_n = 20$		$\sigma_n = 30$	
	AAE	EPE	AAE	EPE	AAE	EPE
RubW.	5.122/**4.975**	0.154/**0.148**	8.703/**7.899**	0.262/**0.237**	11.97/**10.89**	0.351/**0.323**
Venus	4.245/**3.953**	0.302/**0.282**	5.423/**5.238**	0.421/**0.406**	**7.197**/7.294	0.546/**0.535**
Dime.	2.819/**2.615**	0.140/**0.131**	4.574/**4.251**	0.229/**0.214**	7.183/**7.122**	0.347/**0.340**
Hydra.	2.379/**2.299**	0.214/**0.208**	3.482/**3.202**	0.328/**0.303**	4.299/**3.984**	0.423/**0.390**
Urban2	2.945/**2.845**	**0.276**/0.279	**4.387**/4.447	**0.386**/0.393	6.286/**6.142**	0.514/**0.508**
Urban3	**3.778**/3.817	**0.475**/0.480	**5.325**/5.387	0.637/**0.630**	7.971/**7.965**	0.872/**0.870**
Grove2	1.751/**1.697**	0.126/**0.120**	2.275/**2.185**	0.163/**0.155**	3.211/**3.101**	0.231/**0.223**
Grove3	5.521/**5.520**	0.525/**0.521**	**6.243**/6.249	**0.608**/0.610	7.333/**7.295**	**0.688**/0.698
Overall improve	2.95 %	1.95 %	3.85 %	2.83 %	3.00 %	2.25 %

Table 3. AAE/EPE of two noisy training sequences from the MIT benchmark [24]

Method	Cameramotion		Fish	
	AAE	EPE	AAE	EPE
WMF	6.408	0.566	26.109	0.731
PatchWMF	6.285	0.550	25.064	0.692
Improve	2.0 %	2.8 %	4.0 %	5.4 %

part is much higher than on the clean part. For example, for the original RubberWhale sequence (without adding noise), the AAE/EPE of the PatchWMF is approximate to the AAE/EPE of the WMF; in contrast, for the noise added RubberWhale sequences, the AAE/EPE of the PatchWMF is significantly decreased compare to the corresponding AAE/EPE of the WMF. The AAE improvement of $\sigma_n = 20$ and $\sigma_n = 30$ is about 3 %. The results well demonstrate the effectiveness of our ICPSM, and making our PatchWMF is much more robust to against noise than the WMF. Additionally, Figs. 2 and 3 show two visual comparison.

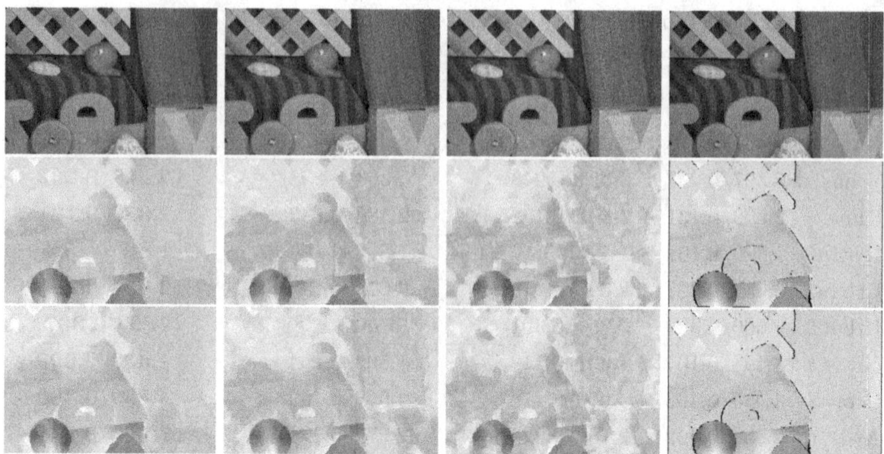

Fig. 2. Visual comparison on the Gaussian noise added RubberWhale sequence [5]. **From Top to Bottom:** RubberWhale sequences, flow results of WMF, flow results of PatchWMF. **From Left to Right:** flow with added Gaussian noise $\sigma_n = 10$, $\sigma_n = 20$, $\sigma_n = 30$, and the ground truth flows.

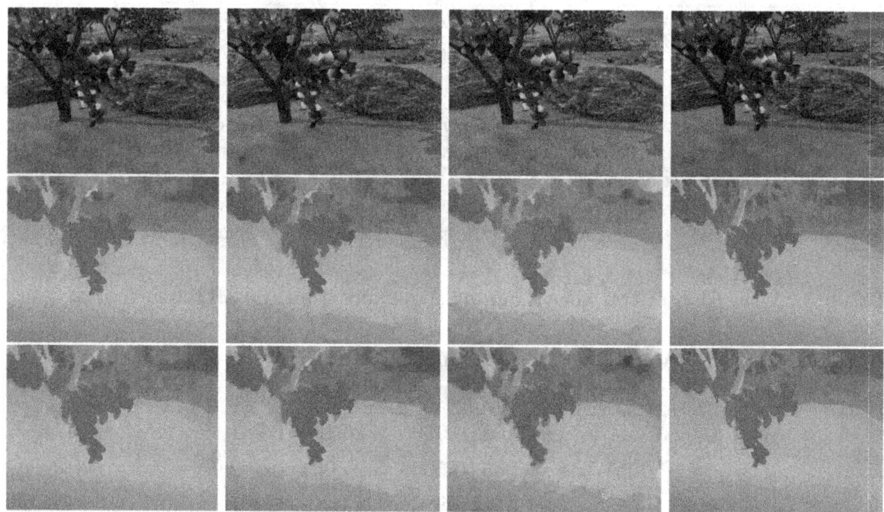

Fig. 3. Visual comparison on the Gaussian noise added Grove2 sequence [5]. **From Top to Bottom:** Grove2 sequences, flow results of WMF, flow results of PatchWMF. **From Left to Right:** flow with added Gaussian noise $\sigma_n = 10$, $\sigma_n = 20$, $\sigma_n = 30$, and the ground truth flows.

The motion boundaries of our flow fields are more accurately preserved. In contrast, due to the disturbance of the noisy pixels, the WMF fails to recover edges, resulting in a lot of errors that are produced by motion blurring distribute at edge regions.

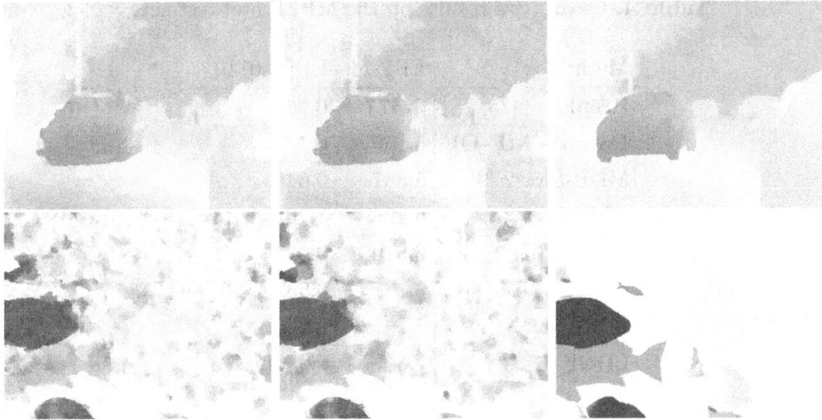

Fig. 4. Visual comparison on two heavy noisy real-world sequences from the MIT benchmark [24]. **From Top to Bottom:** estimated flow fields of cameramotion, estimated flow fields of fish. **From Left to Right:** estimated flow fields with WMF, estimated flow fields with PatchWMF, and the ground truth flows.

Quantitative comparison (Table 3) and visual comparison (Fig. 4) of the denoising results of the WMF and our PatchWMF according to two heavy noisy sequences – cameramotion and fish are conducted. Table 3 reveals that our PatchWMF is superior to WMF to obtain more accurate motion field. In Fig. 4, since the two sequences are fully filled with noisy pixels, the WMF is badly violated and it performs poor on object boundaries. Contrastively, the presented ICPSM helps the WMF robustly reject outliers, thus the motion blurring is reduced in our estimated flow fields.

5.3 Results on MPI Sintel Benchmark

To evaluate the overall performance of our PatchWMF-OF method, we test it on the challenging MPI Sintel benchmark [23]. This benchmark contains long photo-realistic video sequences with extremely difficult cases, e.g., large motions, specular reflections, motion blur, defocus blur, and atmospheric effects. The evaluation is conducted on two kinds of frames, namely clean pass and final pass. EPE all measures the EPE over all pixels, and s0–10 measures pixels with a speed between 10 and 40 pixels (similarly for s10–40 and s40+). Tables 4 and 5 compare our method to state-of-the-art algorithms on the test set of the MPI Sintel benchmark. At the time of submission, for EPE all, it is ranked 7th on the clean pass and 11th on final pass; while for s0–10, it is ranked 1th on the clean pass and 7th on final pass. More importantly, it outperforms current published methods (the huge memory consumption of the DeepFlow [25] prevents itself from practical applications, thus it should be rule out). The results illustrate that our method performs topmost for both large and small displacement optical flow estimation in a unified framework, especially for small motion (i.e. s0–10).

Table 4. Clean pass results on the MPI Sintel test set

Method	EPE all	EPE s0–10
DeepFlow [25]	**5.377**	0.960
PatchWMF-OF	5.550	**0.581**
MDP-Flow2 [9]	5.837	0.640
EPPM	6.494	1.402
S2D-Matching	6.510	0.622
Classic+NLP [5]	6.731	0.638
MLDP-OF	7.297	0.600
LDOF	7.563	0.936

Table 5. Final pass results on the MPI Sintel test set

Method	EPE all	EPE s0–10
DeepFlow [25]	**7.212**	1.284
S2D-Matching	7.872	**1.172**
PatchWMF-OF	7.971	1.279
MLDP-OF	8.287	1.312
Classic+NLP [5]	8.291	1.208
EPPM	8.377	1.834
MDP-Flow2 [9]	8.445	1.420
LDOF	9.116	1.485

In contrast to the baseline method [5], our algorithm performs much better on estimating large motions, which demonstrates our large displacements handling scheme is effective and necessary. On the other side, our method also performs better on small motion estimation. For the clean pass, the EPE of s0–10 is reduced from 0.638 to 0.581, the improvement is about 10 %; for the final pass, the EPE of s0–10 is changed from 1.208 to 1.279, nearly the same. Why our method performs worse on the final pass than on the clean pass? Since the final pass is rendered with motion blur, defocus blur and atmospheric effects while the clean pass are not, and the motion blur and defocus blur do not affect the accuracy of the results too much [26], thus the reason for degradation is due to the synthetic atmospheric effects, not because of noisy pixels. This fact indicates that our ICPSM based WMF is superior to the WMF [5] for rejecting noisy pixels, and outliers can be removed more accurately. Figure 5 shows representative results of the final pass sequences. It is easy to find that our method preserves edges and motion boundaries better than other two related algorithms [5,9], and it also well captures both large and small motions. In particular, comparing to [5], boundary blurring due to noisy pixel perturbation is reduced.

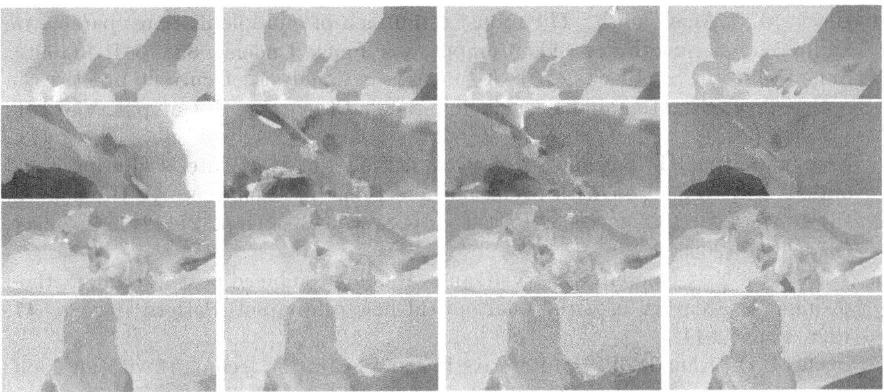

Fig. 5. Visual comparison on the final pass of the MPI Sintel test set. **From Top to Bottom:** shaman1, ambush3, cave3, wall. **From Left to Right:** MDP-Flow2 [9], Classic+NLP [5], PatchWMF-OF(Ours), ground truth flows.

6 Conclusion

This paper addresses the problem of flow field outliers removing depends on the median filter. We present an improved color patch similarity measure to modify the robustness of the WMF to noise. By using the patch difference to replace the pixel difference, the violation due to the noisy pixels is reduced. Additionally, to further improve the noise rejection performance of the patch scheme, a replicated patch method is proposed. Moreover, we introduce an adaptive smoothing parameter selection method to calculate the appropriate smoothing parameter according to the noise degree of the input image. Experiments in this paper have demonstrated that the improved color patch similarity measure is effective to reduce the noise affection – the color difference between a noisy pixel and its neighboring pixel may similar, but the color difference between a replicated patch of a noisy pixel and a patch of its neighboring pixel cannot be similar, leading to the improved WMF denoises intermediate flow fields more accurately.

Acknowledgements. This publication was supported by the Dutch national program COMMIT.

References

1. Horn, B., Schunck, B.: Determining optical flow. Artif. Intell. **17**, 185–203 (1981)
2. Brox, T., Bruhn, A., Papenberg, N., Weickert, J.: High accuracy optical flow estimation based on a theory for warping. In: Pajdla, T., Matas, J.G. (eds.) ECCV 2004. LNCS, vol. 3024, pp. 25–36. Springer, Heidelberg (2004)
3. Baker, S., Scharstein, D., Lewis, J.P., Roth, S., Black, M.J., Szeliski, R.: A database and evaluation methodology for optical flow. Int. J. Comput. Vis. **92**, 1–31 (2011)

4. Black, M.J., Anandan, P.: The robust estimation of multiple motions: parametric and piecewise smooth flow elds. Comput. Vis. Image Underst. **63**, 75–104 (1996)
5. Sun, D., Roth, S., Black, M.J.: A quantitative analysis of current practices in optical flow estimation and the principles behind them. Int. J. Comput. Vis. **106**, 115–137 (2014)
6. Xiao, J., Cheng, H., Sawhney, H.S., Rao, C., Isnardi, M.: Bilateral filtering-based optical flow estimation with occlusion detection. In: Leonardis, A., Bischof, H., Pinz, A. (eds.) ECCV 2006, Part I. LNCS, vol. 3951, pp. 211–224. Springer, Heidelberg (2006)
7. Tu, Z., Aa, N., Gemeren, C.V., Veltkamp, R.C.: A combined post-filtering method to improve accuracy of variational optical flow estimation. Pattern Recogn. **47**, 1926–1940 (2014)
8. Lucas, B.D., Kanade, T.: An iterative image registration technique with an application to stereo vision. In: Proceedings of the International Joint Conference on Artificial Intelligence, pp. 674–679 (1981)
9. Xu, L., Jia, J., Matsushita, Y.: Motion detail preserving optical flow estimation. IEEE Trans. Pattern Anal. Mach. Intel. **16**, 1744–1757 (2012)
10. Chen, Z., Jin, H., Lin, Z., Cohen, S., Wu, Y.: Large displacement optical flow from nearest neighbor fields. In: Proceedings of the IEEE Computer Society Conference on Computer Vision and Pattern Recognition, pp. 2443–2450 (2013)
11. Wedel, A., Pock, T., Zach, C., Bischof, H., Cremers, D.: An improved algorithm for TV-L^1 optical flow. In: Cremers, D., Rosenhahn, B., Yuille, A.L., Schmidt, F.R. (eds.) Statistical and Geometrical Approaches to Visual Motion Analysis. LNCS, vol. 5604, pp. 23–45. Springer, Heidelberg (2009)
12. Wedel, A., Pock, T., Cremers, D.: Structure- and motion adaptive regularization for high accuracy optic flow. In: Proceedings of the IEEE International Conference on Computer Vision, pp. 1663–1668 (2009)
13. Rashwan, H.A., Garca, M.A., Puig, D.: Variational optical flow estimation based on stick tensor voting. IEEE Trans. Image Process. **22**, 2589–2599 (2013)
14. Buades, A., Coll, B., Morel, J.: A review of image denoising algorithms, with a new one. SIAM Multiscale Model. Simul. **4**, 490–530 (2005)
15. Chaudhury, K.N., Singer, A.: Non-local Euclidean medians. IEEE Sig. Process. Lett. **19**, 745–748 (2012)
16. Sun, Z., Chen, S.: Analysis of non-local Euclidean medians and its improvement. IEEE Sig. Process. Lett. **20**, 303–306 (2013)
17. Aharon, M., Elad, M., Bruckstein, A.M.: The K-SVD: an algorithm for designing of over complete dictionaries for sparse representation. IEEE Sig. Process. Lett. **54**, 4311–4322 (2006)
18. Chatterjee, P., Milanfar, P.: Patch-based near-optimal image denoising. IEEE Trans. Image Process. **21**, 1635–1649 (2012)
19. Greenberg, S., Kogan, D.: Improved structure-adaptive anisotropic filter. Pattern Recognit. Lett. **27**, 59–65 (2006)
20. Rother, C., Kolmogorov, V., Lempitsky, V.S., Szummer, M.: Optimizing binary MRFS via extended roof duality. In: Proceedings of the IEEE Computer Society Conference on Computer Vision and Pattern Recognition, pp. 1–8 (2007)
21. Kim, T.H., Lee, H.S., Lee, K.M.: Optical flow via locally adaptive fusion of complementary data costs. In: Proceedings of the IEEE International Conference on Computer Vision, pp. 3344–3351 (2013)
22. Zhang, Q., Xu, L., Jia, J.: 100+ times faster weighted median filter (WMF). In: Proceedings of the IEEE Computer Society Conference on Computer Vision and Pattern Recognition (2014)

23. Butler, D.J., Wulff, J., Stanley, G.B., Black, M.J.: A naturalistic open source movie for optical flow evaluation. In: Fitzgibbon, A., Lazebnik, S., Perona, P., Sato, Y., Schmid, C. (eds.) ECCV 2012, Part VI. LNCS, vol. 7577, pp. 611–625. Springer, Heidelberg (2012)
24. Liu, C., Freeman, W.T., Adelson, E.H., Weiss, Y.: Human-assisted motion annotation. In: Proceedings of the IEEE Computer Society Conference on Computer Vision and Pattern Recognition, pp. 1–8 (2008)
25. Weinzaepfel, P., Revaud, J., Harchaoui, Z., Schmid, C.: DeepFlow: large displacement optical flow with deep matching. In: Proceedings of the IEEE International Conference on Computer Vision, pp. 1385–1392 (2013)
26. Bao, L., Yang, Q., Jin, H.: Fast edge-preserving patchmatch for large displacement optical flow. In: Proceedings of the IEEE Computer Society Conference on Computer Vision and Pattern Recognition (2014)

Efficient Pose-Based Action Recognition

Abdalrahman Eweiwi[1(✉)], Muhammed S. Cheema[1], Christian Bauckhage[1,3], and Juergen Gall[2]

[1] Bonn-Aachen International Center for IT, University of Bonn, Bonn, Germany
eweiwi@bit.uni-bonn.de

[2] Computer Vision Group, University of Bonn, Bonn, Germany

[3] Multimedia Pattern Recognition Group, Fraunhofer IAIS, Sankt Augustin, Germany

Abstract. Action recognition from 3d pose data has gained increasing attention since the data is readily available for depth or RGB-D videos. The most successful approaches so far perform an expensive feature selection or mining approach for training. In this work, we introduce an algorithm that is very efficient for training and testing. The main idea is that rich structured data like 3d pose does not require sophisticated feature modeling or learning. Instead, we reduce pose data over time to histograms of relative location, velocity, and their correlations and use partial least squares to learn a compact and discriminative representation from it. Despite of its efficiency, our approach achieves state-of-the-art accuracy on four different benchmarks. We further investigate differences of 2d and 3d pose data for action recognition.

1 Introduction

Human action recognition has recently drawn an increasing interest in computer vision owing to its applications in many fields including human computer interaction, surveillance and multimedia indexing. This interest has derived a rapid development in terms of the problem scale, the efficiency of the proposed algorithms, and even the data representations of human actions. Early approaches for action recognition used the human pose as a high level representation of actions and used joint trajectories for action and gait recognition [1,2]. However, in these days, obtaining accurate measurements of body poses and joint locations required special setups that were often tedious and very expensive.

Consequently, efforts deviated toward alternative low and mid level representations of pose, motion, visual appearance, or particular combinations of them for better action models. For instance, [3,4] rely majorly on motion cues to identify similar action sequences under static or moving camera setups. Others utilized the human appearance as the basic building blocks in discriminating actions [5–7]. The introduction of interest points in video sequences [8,9] led towards a successful adaption of the bag-of-words model for human action recognition [10–12]. Despite encouraging results of low and mid level features for action recognition on several datasets, they suffer from variations of view point,

D. Cremers et al. (Eds.): ACCV 2014, Part V, LNCS 9007, pp. 428–443, 2015.
DOI: 10.1007/978-3-319-16814-2_28

subject, scale, and appearance. Moreover, they lack of a semantic meaning making the interpretation of the results sometimes difficult. In contrast, high level representations (e.g. 3d pose-based) abstract away most variation factors and can provide a semantic interpretation of the results.

The recent advances in both depth sensors and human pose estimation have recently rekindled interest in high level human representations for action and behavior analysis [13]. Although current algorithms for pose estimation from monocular images [14], depth sensors [15], or multi-view setups [16] still have some limitations in terms of accuracy, several recent studies [16–20] point to the utility of pose estimation for improving the accuracy of action recognition systems. Reference [17] utilize polar coordinates of joints in a sparse reconstruction framework to classify human actions in realistic video datasets. Their evaluation clarifies the implication of accurate pose estimation on action recognition and identifies the potential of current pose estimation approaches for improving action recognition. Similar observations are reported in [16,18] on larger and more complex datasets. In particular, [18] showed that in some scenarios high-level features extracted by a current pose estimation algorithm [14] already outperform a state-of-the-art low level representation based on dense trajectories [11].

Some of the most successful approaches for action recognition from 3d pose data perform feature mining for training. For instance, [20] propose to learn a set of the most distinctive joints. While [21] weight poses of actions based on a mutual information criteria, [19] mine for most occurring temporal and spatial structures of body joints for classification. Mining meaningful poses [21], joints [20], or temporal and spatial joints structures [19], however, is usually time consuming.

In this work, we propose an algorithm for pose-based action recognition that is faster and more efficient for training and testing than existing works. Yet, it achieves on popular datasets for action recognition from 3d pose or RGB-D videos like [22,23], state-of-the-art performance and outperforms other related pose-based approaches. The efficiency is achieved by simplicity in design. Each joint is modeled by a single feature vector that encodes only the most essential information to characterize an action: the relative location of the joint, the velocity of the joint, and the correlation between location and velocity. Inspired by [17], the information over a short video clip is encoded by histograms. Based on these features, a compact and discriminative representation is learned using partial least squares (PLS) [24–28]. The representation can then be used with any classifier like SVM or Kernel-PLS (KPLS) [29].

In our experimental evaluation, we show that for a high-level representation based on 3d pose an expensive training approach as in [19–21] is not necessary to achieve very accurate recognition results. We further investigate the performance of our approach for action recognition from 2d pose data. Since 2d pose data is ambiguous and not view-invariant, the performance drops in comparison to 3d pose data. However, given some training pairs of 2d pose and corresponding 3d pose, a mapping from 2d to 3d can be learned using a standard regression

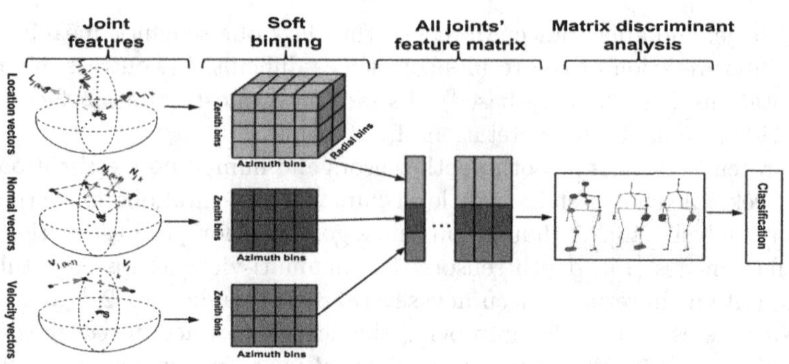

Fig. 1. Overview of the framework.

approach like Kernel partial least squares regression [29]. Although the regression does not provide very accurate 3d poses, our experiments show that features computed on the regressed 3d poses outperform the features computed from the 2d poses directly. This indicates that 3d pose estimation instead of 2d pose estimation from monocular videos has the potential to improve action recognition.

2 High Level Pose Representation

For representing actions by a high level pose-based representation, a sequence of extracted 2d or 3d pose per frame is given. In order to be flexible and learn the importance of a single joint, our representation consists of a feature for each joint as depicted in Fig. 1. Each joint feature, which are discussed in Sect. 2.1 in more detail, models the distributions of the locations, velocities, and geometric orientation of the movements within a video clip or fixed number of frames as histograms. The histograms for each joint are then concatenated to build the feature matrix and matrix discriminant analysis is performed to obtain a set of of discriminant eigenvectors, which are used as high-level representation of the video clip. The representation can then be used with any classifier for classification.

2.1 Joint Features

To increase the robustness of the features to variations caused by different body shapes or even foreshortening in case of 2d pose, the relative joint positions and other vectors are converted into a spherical coordinate system. 2d vectors from 2d poses are represented by the length r and the orientation angle $\theta \in [0, 360]$. For a 3d skeleton representation, the horizontal orientation or azimuth $\alpha \in [0, 360]$ and the vertical orientation or zenith $\phi \in [0, 180]$ are used. A vector $v = (x, y, z) \in \mathcal{R}^3$ is then converted into spherical coordinates (r, α, ϕ) by:

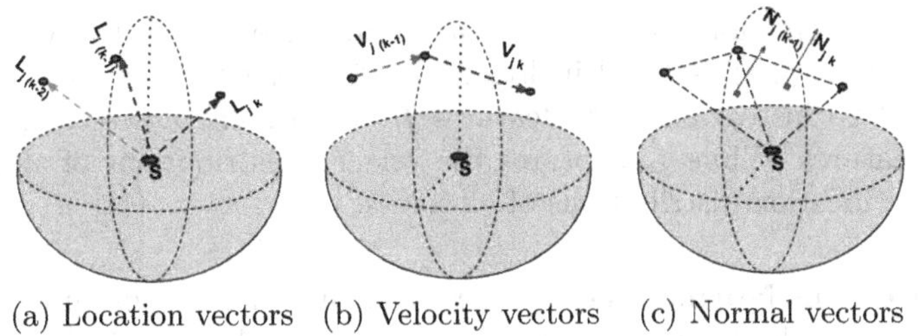

(a) Location vectors (b) Velocity vectors (c) Normal vectors

Fig. 2. Illustration of the locations feature f_l, velocities feature f_v, and the normals feature f_n for a single joint j. For each frame k or frame pair $(k, k+1)$, the vectors l_{jk}, v_{jk}, and n_{jk} are converted into spherical coordinates and added to a histogram as shown in Fig. 1.

$$r = \sqrt{x^2 + y^2 + z^2} \tag{1}$$

$$\phi = \frac{180}{\pi} \times \left(\arccos\left(\frac{z}{r}\right)\right) \tag{2}$$

$$\alpha = \frac{180}{\pi} \times (\text{atan2}(y, x) + \pi) \tag{3}$$

Using spherical coordinates, we use three features that represent distributions over a fixed set of K frames as 3d or 2d histograms. For each feature, we indicate if it applies to 2d and 3d poses or both:

Joint Locations Feature f_l (2d and 3d): The f_l features resemble their 2d counterparts presented in [17]. But with 3d skeletons, our representation includes the azimuth α and zenith ϕ angles along with the joint displacement r from a reference point. For each sequence, we establish a local coordinate system whose origin is located at the *spine* s, which naturally corresponds to the center of the body. For a given location x_{jk} of a joint j at frame k, we quantize the polar coordinates (r, α, ϕ) of the joint location vector $l_{jk} = x_{jk} - s$ into a 3d histogram $(R \times O_{lv} \times O_{lh})$, where R, O_{lv}, O_{lh} are the number of bins for radius, vertical, and horizontal angle. The location vectors of all frames but of a single joint are accumulated in a single 3d histogram. The joint location vectors for three frames and one joint are illustrated in Fig. 2(a). Thus, the locations feature f_l consists of J 3d histograms, where J is the number of joints. In case of 2d pose, the histograms are 2d corresponding to the 2d coordinates (r, θ) for each 2d vector.

Joint Velocities Feature f_v (2d and 3d): The joint locations features do not encode any temporal information, which is important for classifying actions. Given the locations of a joint j at successive frames l_{jk} and $l_{j(k+1)}$, we convert the velocity vector $v_{jk} = l_{j(k+1)} - l_{jk}$ into spherical coordinates without radius (α, ϕ). The radius is not taken into account to be invariant to different execution speeds of an action among subjects. The velocity vectors for all $K-1$ frame pairs are then added to the 2d histogram $O_{vv} \times O_{vh}$, where O_{vv} and O_{vh} are the numbers of bins for vertical and horizontal angle. The velocity vectors for two frame pairs are illustrated in Fig. 2(b). The velocities feature f_l therefore consists of J 2d histograms. The features f_l are in many cases complimentary to the f_v features. While f_v captures the velocity distributions of all joints, f_l captures the location distributions of all joints.

Joint Movement Normals Feature f_n (3d only): The joint movement normals feature models the correlation of location and velocity, which corresponds to the cross product between the location vector l_{jk} and the velocity vector v_{jk} or the cross product of the locations of two consecutive frames as $n_{jk} = l_{jk} \times l_{j(k+1)}$. Up to a scaling factor, n_{jk} corresponds to the normal of the plane spanned by the three points s and the joint positions at the two frames k and $k+1$. Since the length of the normal vector is anyway one, we convert n_{jk} into spherical coordinates (α, ϕ) without r. The normals of the $K-1$ frames are quantized as the velocities feature into a 2d histogram and we obtain J 2d histograms for f_n. The movement normals for two frame pairs are illustrated in Fig. 2(c). All three features model only the most essential information to characterize an action: the relative locations of the joints, the velocities of the joints, and the correlations between locations and velocities. However, combined with a discriminative approach to learn a basis for the features, which is detailed in Sect. 2.2, we achieve state-of-the-art performance and outperform features that are much more expensive to compute.

Normalization and Soft-Binning. To reduce any binning artifacts and to be more robust against style variations, we perform soft-binning. This is achieved by adding a quantized vector to all neighboring bins. The weights for the bins are given by a Gaussian kernel with $\sigma = 1$. To handle sequences of different length, the histograms are normalized by the L2-norm.

Temporal Pyramid. In addition, a temporal pyramid can be used. Instead of having a single histogram per video clip, it can be subdivided into smaller temporal segments. Since the videos in the datasets are short, we use a pyramid with only two layers. The second layer divides the video in three equally sized parts. The three histograms of the second layer and the histogram of the first layer are then concatenated.

2.2 Learning Discriminative Action Features

Not all joints have the same importance for action recognition as illustrated in Fig. 3. It is therefore important to learn a compact and discriminative representation for action recognition. Since we have defined the features per joint, we can define a pose feature $\mathbf{f_p} \in \mathbb{R}^D$ as a weighted sum of all joint features $\{f_j \in \mathbb{R}^D\}_{j=1}^J$:

$$\mathbf{f_p} = \sum_{j=1}^{J} w_j f_j, \tag{4}$$

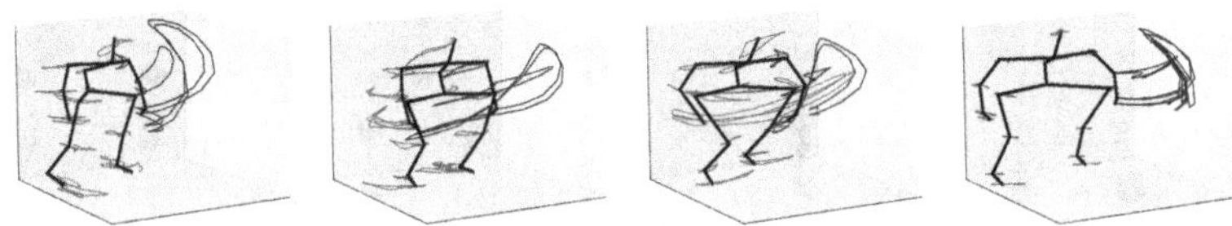

Fig. 3. Examples of joint trajectories for the *hammering* action from *MSR-Action3D* dataset [22]. The action can be well described by the trajectories of the left arm (blue), while the other joints (red) are less relevant. The trajectories also show the variations among subjects in the dataset (Color figure online).

which can be expressed in matrix form as:

$$\mathbf{f_p} = \mathbf{F}\mathbf{w}, \tag{5}$$

where columns of $\mathbf{F} \in \mathbb{R}^{(D \times J)}$ corresponds to the joint features as illustrated in Fig. 1 and $\mathbf{w} \in \mathcal{R}^J$ defines their corresponding weights. The weights $\mathbf{w}$ can be learned by partial least squares (PLS) [24], which has been recently adopted in computer vision for different applications including pose estimation and regression [25], image classification [26], pedestrian detection [27], and multi-view learning [28].

Given M training samples $(\mathbf{x}_i, \mathbf{y}_i)_{i=1}^M$ where $\mathbf{x}_i \in X$ and $\mathbf{y}_i \in Y$, PLS learns two linear projections $s_i = \mathbf{w}^T(\mathbf{x}_i - \overline{\mathbf{x}})$ and $t_i = \mathbf{v}^T(\mathbf{y}_i - \overline{\mathbf{y}})$ that maximize the sampling covariance between $\mathcal{X} = \{x_i\}_i$ and $\mathcal{Y} = \{y_i\}_i$ [26]:

$$\max \left\{ \frac{\left(\frac{1}{M}\sum_i s_i t_i\right)^2}{(\mathbf{w}^T\mathbf{w})(\mathbf{v}^T\mathbf{v})} \right\}, \tag{6}$$

where $\overline{\mathbf{x}}$ and $\overline{\mathbf{y}}$ are the corresponding means. When $\mathcal{Y}$ contains only class labels as in our case, $\mathbf{v}$ is not relevant and only $\mathbf{w}$ is estimated, which is equivalent to solving an eigenvalue problem [24,26]:

$$\mathbf{\Sigma_b}\mathbf{w}^* = \lambda\mathbf{w}^*. \tag{7}$$

In our case, $\mathbf{\Sigma_b}$ is given by

$$\mathbf{\Sigma_b} = \frac{1}{M}\sum_{k=1}^{K} M_k \left[(\overline{\mathbf{F_k}} - \overline{\mathbf{F}})\right]^T \left[(\overline{\mathbf{F_k}} - \overline{\mathbf{F}})\right], \tag{8}$$

where M_k denotes the videos for class k, $\overline{\mathbf{F}}$ the mean feature matrix, and $\overline{\mathbf{F_k}}$ the mean feature matrix for class k. For the P largest eigenvalues λ, we use the corresponding eigenvectors $\mathbf{w}$ as representation. Hence, the final feature $\mathbf{f_p}$ of a video sample i is given by projecting its feature matrix $\mathbf{F_i}$ to the learned P largest projections as $\mathbf{f_p} = [(\mathbf{F_i}\mathbf{w}_1)^T(\mathbf{F_i}\mathbf{w}_2)^T \cdots, (\mathbf{F_i}\mathbf{w}_P)^T]^T$ where $\mathbf{f_p} \in \mathbb{R}^{D*P}$.

Figure 4 depicts the first seven eigenvectors learned using PLS on the *MSR-Action3D*. Notice that most of the eigenvectors focus on joints that are relevant and can discriminate between the performed actions. So in this dataset, only

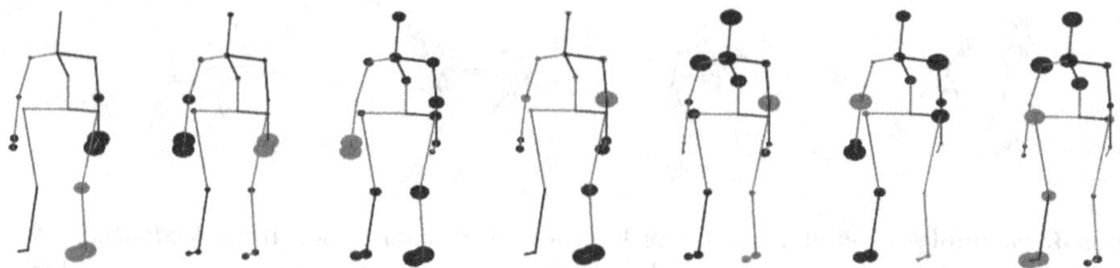

Fig. 4. The first 7 discriminative projections of joint features extracted using PLS from *MSR-Action3d*. Blue indicates positive weights and red negative weights for $\mathbf{w}_1, \ldots, \mathbf{w}_7$. Notice that only few part combinations in this dataset are relevant while some joints like the hips are irrelevant for human actions, which is indicated by the small size of of the joints (Color figure online).

a few body part combinations are relevant where some joints like the hips are irrelevant for the human actions, which is indicated by the small size of the joints.

2.3 Classification

The obtained action features $\mathbf{f_p}$ can be classified using any off-the-shelf classifier like SVM. In our experiments, we use a non-linear classifier based on PLS, namely Kernel-PLS (KPLS) [27,29]. As training data, we have for each video clip the label and the feature vector $\mathbf{f_p}$ which are transformed so that all its entries are positive. While the features define the set $\mathcal{X}$, the class labels are encoded by the set $\mathcal{Y}$. As kernel, we use the intersection kernel defined as $K_{i,j} = \sum_l \min\left(\mathbf{f_{p_i}}(l), \mathbf{f_{p_j}}(l)\right)$.

3 Datasets and Experiments

We choose four challenging datasets to evaluate our approach for human action recognition. The datasets are *MSR-Action3D* [22], *3D Action Pairs* [23], *MSR-DailyActivity3D*[1], and *TUM Kitchen* dataset [30]. For all the experiments in the following sections, we used the same parameters (number of bins) to construct our pose features. Empirically, we evaluated the impact of feature quantization and measured the average classification accuracy over three different splits only for the *MSR-Action3D* dataset for various quantizations of length r, azimuth α, and zenith ϕ of the joint locations, joint velocities, and joint movement normals. The results are shown in Fig. 5. While several configurations give a good performance, we chose 5, 18, and 9 as the number of bins for length, azimuth, and zenith, respectively. Our experiments use these configurations for feature extraction on all pose datasets. For all experiments, we learn the classifier parameters using 5-fold cross validation. This also includes the number of eigenvectors.

[1] http://research.microsoft.com/en-us/um/people/zliu/ActionRecoRsrc/.

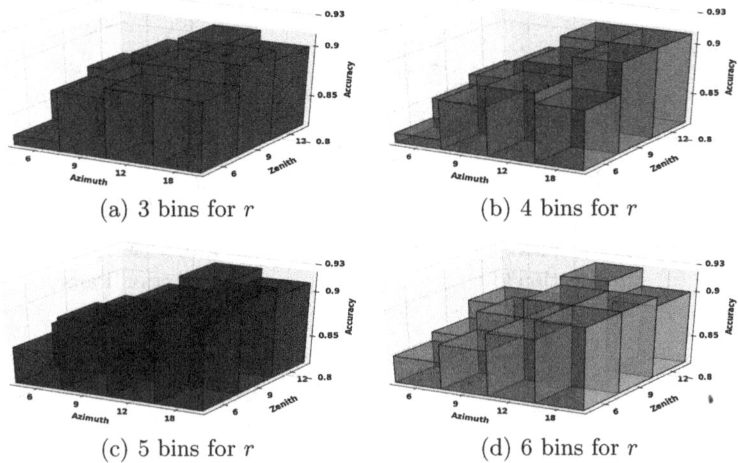

(a) 3 bins for r (b) 4 bins for r

(c) 5 bins for r (d) 6 bins for r

Fig. 5. Recognition accuracy for different feature quantizations for length r, azimuth α, and zenith ϕ. The plots show the accuracy when the number of bins changes. There are several configurations that give a good performance. Among them we use 5, 18, and 9 as the number of bins for length, azimuth, and zenith, respectively.

3.1 MSR-Action3D

The MSR-Action3d dataset is an action dataset captured with a RGB-D camera and designated for gaming-like interactions. It consists of 567 temporally segmented action sequences and contains 20 actions, each performed 2 – 3 times by 10 different subjects. The actions are: *high-arm-wave, horizontal-arm-wave, hammer, hand-catch, forward-punch, high-throw, draw-x, draw-tick, draw-circle, hand-clap, two-hand-wave, side-boxing, bend, forward-kick, side-kick, jogging, tennis-swing, tennis-serve, golf-swing, pick-up and throw*. We exclude 10 sequences as in [20] and operate on the X,Y screen coordinates along with their corresponding depth.

For evaluation, we follow the work in [20, 23] and consider two evaluation tasks: (i) The cross-subject setup where we train our model using the actions of subjects 1,3,5,7,9 and report the results on the rest [20]. (ii) The second task reports the system performance on the average accuracy on all **252 (5-5)** cross-subject splits [23]. Using the first task, Fig. 6(a) shows the individual contribution of each joint feature with respect to the number of projection vectors obtained by PLS. The combinations of the three features f_l, f_v, and f_n, which capture joint location, velocity, and their correlation, clearly boost the performance in comparison to each single feature or feature pair. Using all three features and 10 PLS-projections, an accuracy of **92.3%** is achieved.

We further evaluated the impact of soft-binning in Fig. 7(a). Without soft-binning the descriptor is more sensitive to style variations and binning artifacts. Soft-binning therefore improves the results by a margin.

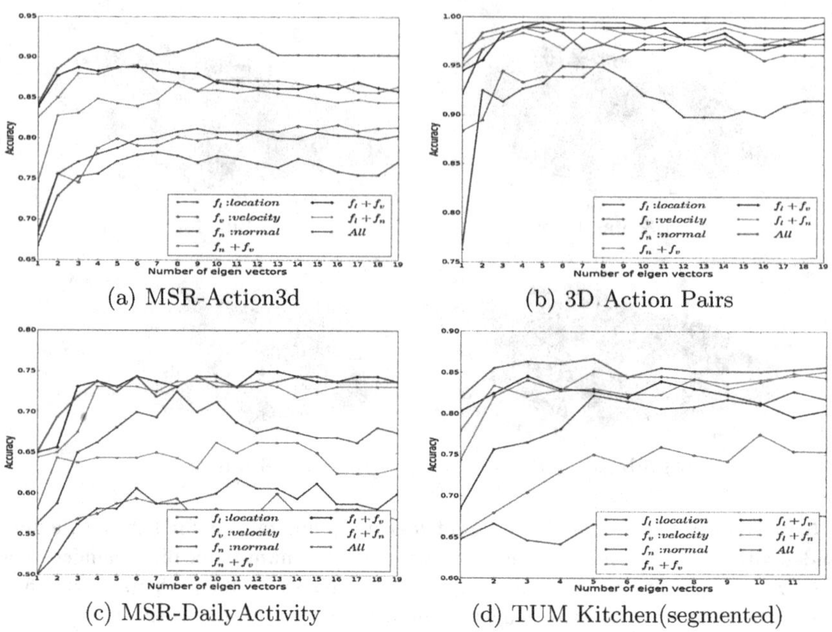

Fig. 6. Recognition accuracies for different numbers of eigenvectors and various feature combinations.

Figure 7(b) compares PLS with linear discriminant analysis (LDA) [31,32]. While PLS relies only on the between-class covariance matrix [26], which results in (8), LDA also takes the intra-class covariances for each class into account. In practice, however, the matrix based on intra-class covariances can be often singular, specially in cases where the number of training samples is less than the feature dimension. This can be observed in Fig. 7(b) where the performance drops when the number of eigenvectors increases. In contrast, PLS does not suffer from singularities. However, both approaches perform better than a baseline that concatenates the joint features described in Sect. 2.1 without learning a compact representation as described in Sect. 2.2 and that uses a SVM for classification. For the SVM and KPLS, we use an intersection kernel. Figure 7(c) also compares KPLS and SVM using our representation described in Sect. 2.2 for a varying number of eigenvectors.

Table 1 compares our approach with the state-of-the-art on this dataset. In this case, the number of eigenvectors is estimated on the training data by 5-fold cross validation. Our approach achieves an accuracy of **91.5** %. It performs comparable to the state-of-the-art [33] and performs better than most other skeleton-based approaches. The temporal pyramid does not improve the results since the dataset contains short, well-defined actions where temporal invariance is beneficial. We verify further the robustness of our features against different subjects by evaluating our features on all **252 (5-5)** possible splits. In this task we achieved a mean accuracy of **88.38** % and standard deviation of **0.027**

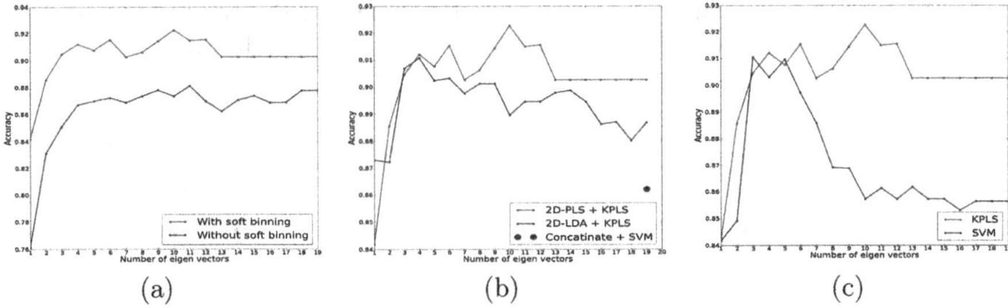

(a) (b) (c)

Fig. 7. Performance evaluation on *MSR-Action3D* dataset. (a) Impact of soft binning (b) Comparison of LDA and PLS (c) Comparison of KPLS and SVM classifiers

Table 1. Recognition accuracy for *MSR-Action3D* dataset. The methods use different data modalities where **S** denotes skeleton data and **D** depth. **TP** denotes the use of a temporal pyramid.

Method	[33]	[20]	[34]	[23]	[12]	[21]	[19]	[35]	Ours	Ours(TP)
Modality	**D+S**	**D+S**	**D**	**D**	**D**	**S**	**S**	**S**	**S**	**S**
Accuracy(%)	92.67	88.2	86.5	88.36	89.3	91.7	90.22	89.48	**91.5**	**90.1**

compared to **82.15 %** $\pm$ **4.18** in [23] establishing our method's robustness against cross-subject variations for human action recognition.

The training and testing time on the *MSR-Action3D* standard split is 27 and 14 seconds, respectively. More precisely, the classification time required for a video clip comprising 55 frames is 161ms where the feature extraction step takes 148 ms. The approach [21] provides comparable results in terms of classification time, however, the training time is much more expensive since each frame is classified by a kNN classifier. We also compared with the recent approach [35], which uses dynamic time warping and requires many mappings between Lie group and tangential space. Using the provided source code [35], classification of a single video clip of 58 frames requires around 20 seconds. All the experiments were conducted on an Intel Core i7 CPU with 3.40 GHz and 8 Gbyte RAM. This shows that our approach is both very efficient for training and testing.

3.2 3D Action Pairs Dataset

This dataset emphasizes on particular scenarios where motion and shape cues are highly correlated. It comprise of six pairs of actions, such that within each pair the motion and the shape cues are similar, but their temporal correlations vary. The action pairs are: *Pick up a box/Put down a chair, Lift a box/Place a box, Push a chair/Pull a chair, Wear a hat/Take off hat, Put on a backpack/Take off a backpack, and Stick a poster/Remove a poster.* We evaluate our framework using the same cross-subject evaluation protocol as in *MSR-Action3D*.

Figure 6(b) shows the individual performance of each feature for different projections. For the datasets, the correlation features f_n outperform the location

Table 2. Recognition accuracy for 3D Action Pairs. The methods use different data modalities where **S** denotes skeleton data and **D** depth. **TP** denotes the use of a temporal pyramid.

Method	MMTW [33]	Actionlets [20]	HON4D [23]	Ours	Ours(TP)
Modality	**D+S**	**D+S**	**D**	**S**	**S**
Accuracy(%)	97.22	82.22	96.67	**92.0**	**99.4**

and velocities features since they capture temporal-spatial correlations of the action classes better. The best performance is, however, achieved when all features are used.

We compare our approach with the state-of-the-art on this dataset in Table 2. As for the other dataset, the number of eigenvectors is estimated on the training data by 5-fold cross validation. Our algorithm achieves **92.0** %. When a temporal pyramid is used, it achieves **99.4** % and outperforms the other methods. The performance boost of the pyramid can be explained by the classes. These are activities that consist of smaller sub-actions in a specific order, which can be well captured by the temporal pyramid.

3.3 MSRDailyActivity

This dataset has been captured with an RGB-D camera to mimic daily human activities in a living room. There are 16 different actions, each performed by 10 subjects twice, once standing and the other while sitting. The actions are: *drink, eat, read book, call cellphone, write on a paper, use laptop, use vacuum cleaner, cheer up, sit still, toss paper, play game, lie down on sofa, walk, play guitar, stand up, sit down.* The standard task for this dataset aims at cross subject evaluation as in *MSR-Action3D*, where we train on the odd numbered subjects and test on the rest. Figure 6(c) shows the individual accuracies of the different features. Unlike *MSR-Action3D* and *3D Action Pairs* datasets, the joints location feature (f_l) in this dataset outperforms both velocity and normal features. This is because many actions in this dataset are of static or merely static nature (e.g. *call cellphone, play game, use laptop*). However, our combined features outperform the individual features and achieve an overall accuracy of **70.0** %. With a temporal pyramid, the accuracy is further improved to **73.1** % accuracy. Compared to previous work [20], our method outperforms their results of **68.0** % by **5.1** %.

3.4 TUM Kitchen Dataset

The *TUM kitchen* dataset focuses on a home-monitoring scenario using a multi-view camera setup (4 cameras). The dataset provides 3d human pose data estimated by a markerless full-body tracker. Our evaluation criteria considers two tasks: (i) *segmented* test data and (ii) *unsegmented* test data as in [16]. On both

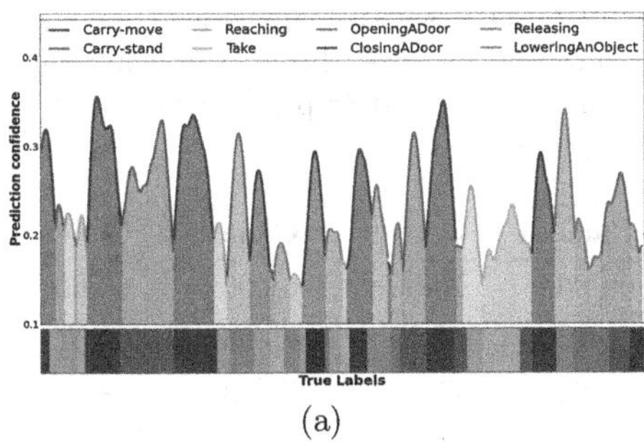

(a)

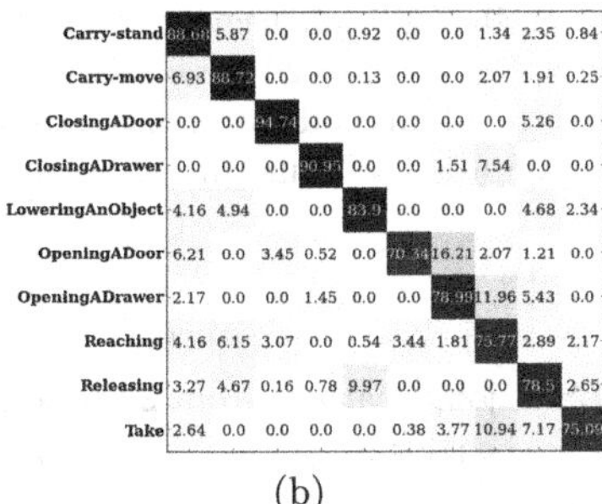

(b)

Fig. 8. Evaluation results on the *TUM Kitchen* dataset (a) Sample frame-level prediction where the x-axis shows the time span of the video sequence with ground-truth annotations and the y-axis shows the predicted class label with confidences. (b) Confusion matrix of the unsegmented video sequence of the *TUM Kitchen* dataset (Best viewed in colors) (Color figure online).

tasks, we used the episodes 0-2,0-8,0-4,0-6,0-10,0-11,1-6 for testing and the remaining 13 for training. However, in the first task we assume that the videos are already segmented while in the second task we perform continuous classification. The evaluation criteria for the unsegmented case follows the protocol described in [16], where the average class accuracies is measured on a frame-level. We use the skeleton with 13 joints for evaluation and do not count the errors at the transition frames between annotations with a margin of 4 frames on both sides as in [16]. For the first task, Fig. 6(d) presents a detailed overview of the average recognition accuracies over all classes for each feature along with their combination. Our algorithm achieves for this task an average accuracy of **86.65** % over all classes.

On the second task, we evaluated the performance of our approach using a fixed sliding window of 30 frames that was determined empirically. This task is more challenging as the dataset stands for actions of arbitrary time stamps ranging from 10 to 150 frames. The evaluation considers the average accuracy on frame level over all classes. Our algorithm achieves an average accuracy of **82.5** % as compared to **80.03** % in [16]. Figure 8(a) depicts the prediction of our model for an unsegmented action sequence from the *TUM* dataset. While Fig. 8(b) shows the confusion matrix for all classes.

3.5 2D vs. 3D Pose

Recent advances in pose estimation introduce new opportunities towards action recognition in challenging environments. For example, several applications in [16–18] show that pose estimation is vital towards generalizable, robust, and efficient action recognition. However, most estimation methods reconstruct 2d poses from monocular views, failing to provide view-invariant descriptors for action recognition.

Table 3. Recognition accuracy (%) for the *TUM* dataset. We compare a 2d appearance based approach [16], 2d versions of our features, 3d features obtained by mapping the 2d pose to 3d, and 3d features computed from the provided 3d poses, which have been estimated using all four camera views.

Camera	Camera 1	Camera 2	Camera 3	Camera 4
HF + 2d appearance features [16]	68.00	70.00	68.00	65.00
KPLS + joint features from 2d pose	65.66	65.19	63.95	62.51
KPLS + joint features from 3d pose estimated from 2d pose of one camera view	77.61	77.78	78.23	78.47
KPLS + joint features from 3d pose estimated from all camera views	82.5			

We therefore compare action recognition using 3d pose features and 2d pose features. To this end, we project the 3d pose of each frame to the 4 camera views and perform action recognition with our 2d pose features as described in Sect. 2.1. The evaluation protocol is the same as for the unsegmented sequences of *TUM*.

Table 3 shows the classification accuracies obtained for each of the four camera views. As opposed to the previously reported result for 3d pose features, action recognition accuracies in 2d show a significant drop of almost **20** % in recognition rates on all 4 cameras. The performance is also lower than the one reported for the 2d appearance approach [16], which does not use high-level features but low-level features based on optical flow and gradients.

In order to investigate if the performance loss comes from the inherent depth ambiguity of 2d poses or the view sensitiveness of the representation based on 2d poses, we learn a mapping from 2d to 3d pose by non-linear regression. Given a set of 2d training poses of J joints $\mathbf{x} \in \mathbb{R}^{2*J}$ and their corresponding 3d poses $\mathbf{y} \in \mathbb{R}^{3*J}$, we linearly scale the individual body parts so that the distance between the central shoulder and the central hip joint is constant. Then we learn a mapping function $\Phi : \mathcal{R}^{2*J} \rightarrow \mathcal{R}^{3*J}$ that maps the observed 2d poses of one camera view to their 3d representation. The non-linear regression is implemented by KPLS [29] with a radial basis kernel, where $\mathcal{X} = \mathbb{R}^{2*J}$ and $\mathcal{Y} = \mathbb{R}^{3*J}$. The bandwidth of the kernel is $\sigma = 0.01$.

Instead of encoding 2d poses by a discriminative representation learned from 2d pose features, we can also predict for a single camera and each frame the 3d pose from the observed 2d pose. The predicted 3d poses are then used for learning the discriminative representation from 3d pose features as described in Sect. 2.2. Table 3 compares the obtained accuracies. Since the predicted 3d poses from a single camera are not as accurate as the 3d poses provided by the dataset, which have been estimated by a multi-view human pose estimation algorithm, also the recognition accuracy with the features computed from the predicted poses is lower. However, the representation based on the predicted 3d poses shows a significant performance boost over the corresponding representation based on 2d poses. It is also interesting to note that the performance is around 78 % for all views while the 2d features show more performance variation among views. Furthermore, the 2d appearance-based approach of [16] is outperformed. This result underlines the benefit of view-invariant pose features and indicates that 3d pose estimation instead of 2d pose estimation from monocular videos has the potential to improve action recognition.

4 Conclusion

We have presented a framework for action recognition from 2d and 3d poses. The approach is very efficient for training and testing and achieves state-of-the-art performances on several datasets. This has been achieved by focusing on the the most essential information that characterizes an action, namely the relative locations of the joints, the velocities of the joints, and the correlations between locations and velocities denoted as movement normals. Together with a discriminative approach to learn a basis for the features, we obtain an action representation that outperforms other representations that are much more expensive to compute. We finally compared 2d and 3d pose features and conclude that learning a mapping from 2d pose to 3d pose to obtain view-invariant features can boost the performance significantly.

Acknowledgment. This work was carried out in the project automatic activity recognition in large image databases which is funded by the German Research Foundation (DFG). The authors would also like to acknowledge the financial support provided by the DFG Emmy Noether program (GA 1927/1-1).

References

1. Campbell, L., Bobick, A.: Recognition of human body motion using phase space constraints. In: ICCV (1995)
2. Bissacco, A., Chiuso, A., Ma, Y., Soatto, S.: Recognition of human gaits. In: CVPR (2001)
3. Wu, S., Oreifej, O., Shah, M.: Action recognition in videos acquired by a moving camera using motion decomposition of Lagrangian particle trajectories. In: ICCV (2011)
4. Efros, A., Berg., A., Mori, G., Malik, J.: Recognizing action at a distance. In: CVPR (2003)
5. Thurau, C., Hlavac, V.: Pose primitive based human action recognition in videos or still images. In: CVPR (2008)
6. Ikizler-Cinbis, N., Cinbis, R., Sclaroff, S.: Learning actions from the web. In: ICCV (2009)
7. Eweiwi, A., Cheema, M.S., Bauckhage, C.: Discriminative joint non-negative matrix factorization for human action classification. In: Weickert, J., Hein, M., Schiele, B. (eds.) GCPR 2013. LNCS, vol. 8142, pp. 61–70. Springer, Heidelberg (2013)

8. Laptev, I.: On space-time interest points. IJCV **64**, 107–123 (2005)
9. Willems, G., Tuytelaars, T., Van Gool, L.: An efficient dense and scale-invariant spatio-temporal interest point detector. In: Forsyth, D., Torr, P., Zisserman, A. (eds.) ECCV 2008, Part II. LNCS, vol. 5303, pp. 650–663. Springer, Heidelberg (2008)
10. Laptev, I., Marszalek, M., Schmid, C., Rozenfeld, B.: Learning realistic human actions from movies. In: CVPR (2008)
11. Wang, H., Kläser, A., Schmid, C., Liu, C.L.: Dense trajectories and motion boundary descriptors for action recognition. Int. J. Comput. Vis. **103**, 60–79 (2013)
12. Xia, L., Aggarwal, J.: Spatio-temporal depth cuboid similarity feature for activity recognition using depth camera. In: CVPR (2013)
13. Ye, M., Zhang, Q., Wang, L., Zhu, J., Yang, R., Gall, J.: A survey on human motion analysis from depth data. In: Grzegorzek, M., Theobalt, C., Koch, R., Kolb, A. (eds.) Time-of-Flight and Depth Imaging. LNCS, vol. 8200, pp. 149–187. Springer, Heidelberg (2013)
14. Yang, Y., Ramanan, D.: Articulated human detection with flexible mixtures of parts. IEEE Trans. Pattern Anal. Mach. Intell. **35**, 2878–2890 (2013)
15. Shotton, J., Girshick, R.B., Fitzgibbon, A.W., Sharp, T., Cook, M., Finocchio, M., Moore, R., Kohli, P., Criminisi, A., Kipman, A., Blake, A.: Efficient human pose estimation from single depth images. IEEE Trans. Pattern Anal. Mach. Intell. **35**, 2821–2840 (2013)
16. Yao, A., Gall, J., van Gool, L.: Coupled action recognition and pose estimation from multiple views. Int. J. Comput. Vis. **100**, 16–37 (2012)
17. Tran, K.N., Kakadiaris, I.A., Shah, S.K.: Modeling motion of body parts for action recognition. In: BMVC (2011)
18. Jhuang, H., Gall, J., Zuffi, S., Schmid, C., Black, M.: Towards understanding action recognition. In: ICCV (2013)
19. Wang, C., Wang, Y., Yuille, A.: An approach to pose-based action recognition. In: CVPR (2013)
20. Wang, J., Liu, Z., Liu, Y., Yuan, J.: Mining actionlet ensemble for action recognition with depth cameras. In: CVPR (2012)
21. Zanfir, M., Leordeanu, M., Sminchisescu, C.: The moving pose: an efficient 3D kinematics descriptor for low-latency action recognition and detection. In: ICCV (2013)
22. Wanqing, L., Zhengyou, Z., Zicheng, L.: Action recognition based on a bag of 3D points. In: CVPRW (2010)
23. Oreifej, O., Liu, Z.: Hon4d: Histogram of oriented 4D normals for activity recognition from depth sequences. In: CVPR (2013)
24. Barker, M., Rayens, W.: Partial least squares for discrimination. J. Chemometr. **17**, 166–173 (2003)
25. Hajd, M.A., Gonzlez, J., Davis, L.: On partial least squares in head pose estimation: how to simultaneously deal with misalignment. In: CVPR (2012)
26. Harada, T., Ushiku, Y., Yamashita, Y., Kuniyoshi, Y.: Discriminative spatial pyramid. In: CVPR (2011)
27. Schwartz, W.R., Kembhavi, A., Harwood, D., Davis, L.S.: Human detection using partial least squares analysis. In: ICCV (2009)
28. Sharma, A., Jacobs, D.: Bypassing synthesis: PLS for face recognition with pose, low-resolution and sketch. In: CVPR (2011)
29. Rosipal, R., Be, P.P., Trejo, L.J., Cristianini, N., Shawe-Taylor, J., Williamson, B.: Kernel partial least squares regression in reproducing Kernel Hilbert space. JMLR **2**, 97–123 (2001)

30. Tenorth, M., Bandouch, J., Beetz, M.: The TUM Kitchen data set of everyday manipulation activities for motion tracking and action recognition. In: ICCV Workshops (2009)
31. Li, M., Yuan, B.: 2D-LDA: a statistical linear discriminant analysis for image matrix. Pattern Recogn. Lett. **26**, 527–532 (2005)
32. Bauckhage, C., Käster, T.: Benefits of separable, multilinear discriminant classification. In: ICPR (2006)
33. Wang, J., Wu, Y.: Learning maximum margin temporal warping for action recognition. In: ICCV (2013)
34. Wang, J., Liu, Z., Chorowski, J., Chen, Z., Wu, Y.: Robust 3D action recognition with random occupancy patterns. In: Fitzgibbon, A., Lazebnik, S., Perona, P., Sato, Y., Schmid, C. (eds.) ECCV 2012, Part II. LNCS, vol. 7573, pp. 872–885. Springer, Heidelberg (2012)
35. Vemulapalli, R., Arrate, F., Chellappa, R.: Human action recognition by representing 3D skeletons as points in a lie group. In: CVPR (2014)

Tracking Multiple People Online and in Real Time

Ergys Ristani(✉) and Carlo Tomasi

Duke University, Durham, USA
ristani@cs.duke.edu

Abstract. We cast the problem of tracking several people as a graph partitioning problem that takes the form of an NP-hard binary integer program. We propose a tractable, approximate, online solution through the combination of a multi-stage cascade and a sliding temporal window. Our experiments demonstrate significant accuracy improvement over the state of the art and real-time post-detection performance.

1 Introduction

In many surveillance or monitoring applications, one or more cameras view several people that move in an environment. Multi-person tracking amounts to using the videos from these cameras to determine who is where at all times.

Abstractly, a multi-person tracker takes as its input a set of *observations*. At the lowest level, these are *detections* computed on each video frame by a person detection algorithm, and consist of a bounding polygon that encloses the person, together with an image position, a time stamp, an estimate of the person's velocity, and an appearance descriptor. For the sake of efficiency, intermediate stages within the tracker may form higher-level observations by grouping detections. The tracker then partitions the input observations into sets, with the intent that each set corresponds to one person and *vice versa*. The literature calls these sets *identities* or—when the linear time ordering of detections in a set needs emphasis—*trajectories*.

Two major pairs of conflicting challenges make multi-person tracking hard. Observations are *ambiguous* in that different people that look alike may be confused with each other. Conversely, changing lighting, viewpoint, and other circumstances may cause *variance of appearance* for a given person, which may not be recognized to be the same in different observations. In the other pair of challenges, person *occlusions*—whether caused by limited field of view, visual obstacles between camera and person, or algorithm failure—generate gaps in the input observations that make tracking harder. Conversely, overactive person detectors may generate *spurious observations* that confuse the tracker. All of these challenges already show up in the convenient nutshell of the single-camera case, on which this paper is focused.

D. Cremers et al. (Eds.): ACCV 2014, Part V, LNCS 9007, pp. 444–459, 2015.
DOI: 10.1007/978-3-319-16814-2_29

1.1 Overview of the Proposed Approach

Our tracker reasons about evidence for or against any two observations being *co-identified*, that is, being assigned to the same identity. If the appearance descriptors of two observations are similar and their times and locations are consistent with typical walking speeds, evidence for their co-identity is positive. If two observations look different or occur at nearby time instants at faraway locations, evidence is negative. In the limit, "hard" evidence may be available: Simultaneous observations at faraway locations cannot possibly correspond to the same person, and yield "infinitely negative" evidence. "Infinitely positive" evidence, on the other hand, denotes an irreversible commitment to a co-identification. Infinite evidence, positive or negative, is equivalent to hard constraints on the solution.

We associate evidence to the edges of an *evidence graph* that has one node per observation and one edge for each pair of observations for which co-identity evidence is available. Multi-person tracking then becomes a *graph partitioning* problem.[1] Specifically, the set of nodes is partitioned into subsets—one subset per person identity—such that edges within sets accumulate high positive evidence, and edges between sets accumulate high negative evidence. Casting multi-person tracking as a graph partitioning problem is one of the main contributions of our paper. As described later, the resulting problem is a Binary Integer Program (BIP) when the input is finite.

Solving a BIP is NP hard. To address complexity, we introduce a cascade with two phases that operate respectively on a short (one second) and a longer (several seconds) time horizon. Each phase is in turn composed of two stages. The first stage forms groups of weakly related observations safely, reasoning about space and time in the first phase, and about appearance in the second. Once these opportunistic and conservative groups are inexpensively formed, the second stage in each phase partitions each group of observations into identities by solving the corresponding BIP, enforcing *both* space-time and appearance criteria optimally and simultaneously.

The input video in most surveillance or monitoring applications has no bounded duration. Because of this, we embed the cascade above into an online algorithm that slides a temporal window over the video stream and works in real-time.

We compare our approach with closely related literature in Sect. 2. Section 3 describes our approach, Sect. 4 discusses experimental results, and Sect. 5 closes with concluding remarks and a discussion of future work.

2 Relationship to Prior Work

Multi-person tracking in video has a long history. In this Section, we compare our method with other approaches based on evidence graphs.

[1] Graph partitioning is often called *graph clustering* in the literature. We avoid this term to prevent confusion with other types of clustering we do in this paper.

Problem Formulation. Several methods limit evidence to pairs of observations that are consecutive in time and can achieve polynomial complexity. These formulations involve maximum-weight vertex-disjoint path cover [1,2], a maximum weight independent set problem [3], bipartite matching [4–8] or some variant of network flow [9–13]. Methods that use stronger and more comprehensive evidence have demonstrated superior performance. These methods consider evidence from all observation pairs [14], observation triplets [15] or higher order relationships [16–19]. The better performance however comes at a cost of increased computational complexity due to the problem's combinatorial nature.

Problem Decomposition. Despite these difficulties, several strategies have been proposed in the literature to address computational complexity, such as (i) approximating the problem formulation, (ii) approximating the solution of the problem [1,3,14,20,21], (iii) limiting the number of edges in the observation graph [10,11], (iv) relaxing constraints in the BIP [22–24] or (v) solving the problem in stages for efficiency [3,12,14,20,21].

We stick to the original problem formulation and propose a tractable, approximate solution for real-time multi-person tracking from a single video stream of indefinite duration. Our approximation decomposes the full problem into smaller subproblems and in two separate phases that examine short- and long-term time horizons respectively. These smaller problems can be solved exactly with a BIP solver, and the resulting solutions are pieced together *post facto*. This decomposition results into a theoretically suboptimal solution. The key challenge is then to define the decomposition so as to make partition errors unlikely. As we show in Sect. 3.3, many opportunities arise to perform a preliminary partitioning of observations based on position and velocity in the short-term phase, and on visual appearance in the long-term phase. If these opportunities are taken conservatively, partition errors are infrequent, as we demonstrate empirically in Sect. 4.

Online Algorithm. Several real-time multi-person tracking methods have been proposed [3,10,11,21], but they buy speed at a noticeable cost in terms of tracking accuracy. Similarly to previous work [1,2,21], we use a sliding temporal window to work online. However, our extended cascade lets us process much longer windows, and thereby achieve significantly higher accuracy and resilience to occlusion. We can process video in real time at 25 frames per second on a single PC while simultaneously improving over the state of the art on existing data benchmarks. We share several technical aspects of our solution with existing approaches. Nonetheless, the multi-stage formulation and how the specific algorithms are used in each stage make our cascade novel.

The work most similar to ours is that of Zamir *et al.* [14], who formulate multi-person tracking as a sequential Generalized Minimum Clique Problem (GMCP) decomposition of a complete graph of observations. As it is common in the literature, they also decompose computation into two stages for computational efficiency, and can incorporate hard constraints on co-identity. We both allow for evidence edges between *any* two observations, and both formulations are NP-hard. However, we differ in two aspects. First, we formulate multi-person tracking jointly for all identities, while Zamir *et al.* handle identities sequentially and greedily. Second, the formulation of Zamir *et al.* mandates that one person must have exactly one observation per time frame in order to form a clique. GMCP adds one hypothetical node for every time frame where the person is missing. In scenarios of lengthy video and short person presence in the scene, most observations in a person's clique are hypothetical nodes outside the field of view, unnecessarily increasing the problem complexity. In contrast, our formulation is more general and considers only available evidence, and as a result complexity depends solely on the number of observations, not sequence length.

In summary, the contributions of this paper consist of (i) a new, general graph partitioning problem formulation which considers all the evidence between any pair of observations at once; (ii) a generic approximation method for real-time, online processing; and (iii) thorough experiments with an analysis of the trade-offs in multi-person tracking and improvements in the state of the art.

3 Multi-person Tracking

Section 3.1 introduces a batch formulation of the multi-person tracking problem in terms of a Binary Integer Program (BIP) that partitions the nodes of a graph we call the *evidence graph*. Section 3.2 discusses how to compute the weights on the edges of this graph. These weights measure evidence for or against two observations being of the same identity ("co-identity"), and the intent is that each of the sets in the computed partition corresponds to one identity. The BIP in Sect. 3.1 is too large to solve for realistic input, and Sect. 3.3 describes a four-stage cascade that computes the partition through successive refinements from a single input set. The input set contains all the person detections from an off-the-shelf detector. Section 3.4 then introduces a sliding-window method for transforming the batch solution into an online algorithm that can process video for an unbounded amount of time.

3.1 Tracking as a Graph Partitioning Problem

Consider a set V of n observations that could be individual outputs from a person detector, or the results of aggregating co-identical detections with some other method. For a pair of observations u, v in V, let w_{uv} be a measure of the evidence for or against the hypothesis that u and v are co-identical. Section 3.2 shows how this evidence can be computed from data. For now, it suffices to say that evidence is quantified by a *correlation*, that is, a number in the set $\{-\infty, [-1, 1], +\infty\}$. Positive values indicate evidence for co-identity, negative values indicate evidence against, zero denotes indifference, and infinite values correspond to definitive evidence (hard constraints).

Let the *evidence graph* $G = (V, E, W)$ be a weighted graph[2] on V. If a correlation is available for a pair of observations in V, an edge is added to set E

[2] The graph can be directed from past to future in time, if simultaneous observations cannot be co-identical, or undirected otherwise.

for that pair, and its correlation is added to set W. In the following, we think of G as being a complete graph, but nothing in our formulation depends on this.

A multi-person tracker partitions V into sets believed to refer to distinct identities. Specifically, the partition maximizes the sum of the rewards w_{uv} assigned to edges that connect co-identical observations and the penalties $-w_{uv}$ assigned to edges that straddle identities. This graph partition problem can be rephrased as the following BIP:

$$\arg\max_{X} \sum_{(u,v)\in E} w_{uv} x_{uv} \tag{1}$$

subject to

$$x_{uv} \in \{0,1\} \qquad \forall (u,v) \in E \tag{2}$$

$$x_{uv} + x_{vt} \leq 1 + x_{ut} \qquad \forall (u,v),(v,t),(u,t) \in E. \tag{3}$$

The set X is the set of all possible combinations of assignments to the binary variables x_{uv}, with the interpretation that x_{uv} is 1 iff the observations u and v are co-identical. The constraints in Eq. (3) enforce co-identity to be transitive: If u and v are co-identical and so are v and t, then u and t must be co-identical as well.

Considering all pairwise correlations has the advantage that even when some edges carry negative correlation, the nodes they connect can still be co-identical if the overall reward of the set is positive, and *vice versa*.

Finding an optimal solution to this BIP is NP-hard [25] and the problem is also hard to approximate [26]. The best known approximation algorithm achieves an approximation ratio of 0.7664 [27], but its semi-definite program formulation makes it slow for practical consideration. Other algorithms exist and we describe one of them in Sect. 4.4, but they come with no quality guarantees. These results suggest that one needs to look at the special properties of the multi-person tracking problem to find an efficient solution, as we do in Sect. 3.3. In Sect. 3.2, we first consider how to compute the correlations w_{uv}.

3.2 Features and Measures of Evidence

To manage computational complexity, the BIP defined in Sect. 3.1 is solved first over individual person detections within small time horizons, and then within longer time horizons and over short trajectories called "tracklets," as explained in Sect. 3.3 below. In this section, we show how observations of both types are described, and how correlations are computed for pairs of them.

Each person detection $D = (\phi, \mathbf{p}, t, \mathbf{v})$ is described by its appearance feature ϕ, position $\mathbf{p}$, time stamp t, and estimated velocity[3] $\mathbf{v}$. We use an HSV color histogram to describe a person's appearance, but different descriptors can be used with no other modification of the proposed methods.

Co-identity evidence from space and time information comes mainly from the assumption that people are limited in their speed, and reasoning about person

[3] Velocity is a vector, and its norm is called the *speed*.

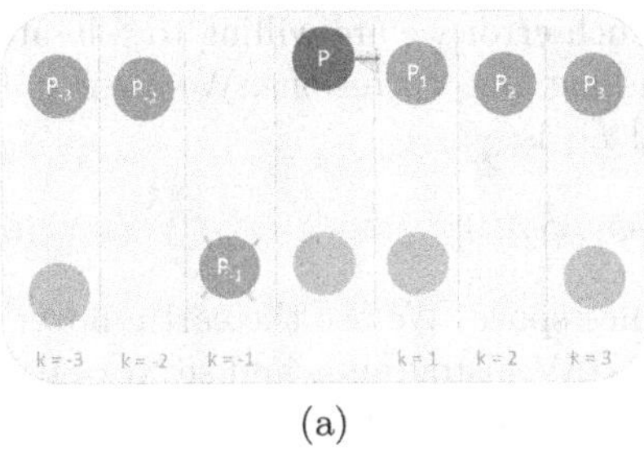

(a)

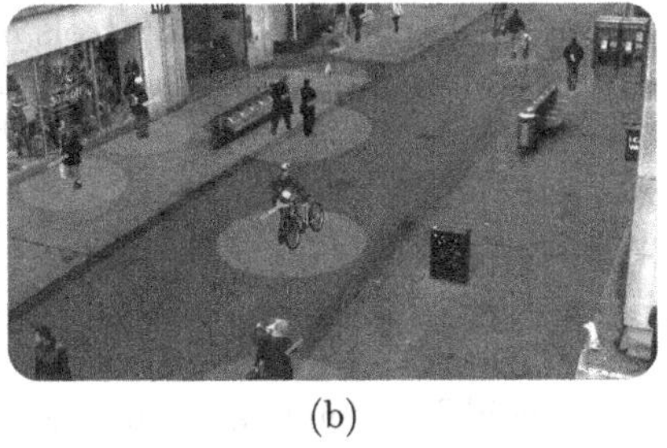

(b)

Fig. 1. (a) Velocity estimation of the blue detection for $m = 3$. Circles are detections, the horizontal dimension is time, and the vertical one stands for 2D space. Green detections are the nearest detections in space to the blue detection for each k. Detections in grey are not considered for velocity estimation. Detection $\mathbf{p}_{-1}$ is discarded because the speed required to reach the blue detection from it exceeds a predefined limit. The green vectors are the velocities computed for each blue-green detection pair and the blue vector is the estimated velocity. (b) Circles enclose disjoint space-time groups, found from assumed bounds on walking speed (Color figure online).

speed requires converting image coordinates to world coordinates. To this end, we assume that people move on a planar region and that a homography is available between the world and the image.

The velocity of a detection at position $\mathbf{p}$ in video frame i is estimated as follows. For each frame k in $[i-m, i+m]$ (where m is a small integer) and $k \neq i$, determine the detection $\mathbf{p}_k$ that is nearest (in space) to $\mathbf{p}$. Compute the velocities from each pair $(\mathbf{p}, \mathbf{p}_k)$, and discard those that violate a predefined speed limit. The velocity estimate for the detection at $\mathbf{p}$ is then the component-wise median of the remaining velocities. See Fig. 1(a).

Tracklets (short trajectories of detections) have somewhat more complex descriptors than individual detections, because they extend over time. Specifically, a tracklet descriptor $\tilde{T} = \{\tilde{\boldsymbol{\phi}}, \tilde{\mathbf{p}}^s, \tilde{\mathbf{p}}^e, \tilde{t}^s, \tilde{t}^e, \tilde{\mathbf{v}}\}$ contains an appearance feature $\tilde{\boldsymbol{\phi}}$ that is equal to the median appearance of its detections. The descriptor also contains the start point $\tilde{\mathbf{p}}^s$ and end point $\tilde{\mathbf{p}}^e$ of the tracklet, its start time $\tilde{t}^s$ and end time $\tilde{t}^e$, and its velocity $\tilde{\mathbf{v}}$. Since tracklets are short, we assume that their detections are on a straight line and we approximate the velocity of the tracklets as follows:

$$\tilde{\mathbf{v}} = \frac{\tilde{\mathbf{p}}^e - \tilde{\mathbf{p}}^s}{\tilde{t}^e - \tilde{t}^s} . \tag{4}$$

Given two detections $D_1 = (\boldsymbol{\phi}_1, \mathbf{p}_1, t_1, \mathbf{v}_1)$ and $D_2 = (\boldsymbol{\phi}_2, \mathbf{p}_2, t_2, \mathbf{v}_2)$, we first define two simple space-time and appearance affinity measures for them in $[0, 1]$, and then combine the affinities into a single correlation measure.

Specifically, the space-time affinity of D_1 and D_2 is:

$$s_{st} = \max[1 - \beta\,(e(D_1, D_2) + e(D_2, D_1)), 0] \tag{5}$$

where $e(D_1, D_2) = \|\mathbf{q}_1 - \mathbf{p}_2\|_2$ measures the error between the position $\mathbf{p}_2$ of detection D_2 and the estimated position $\mathbf{q}_1 = \mathbf{p}_1 + \mathbf{v}_1(t_2 - t_1)$ of detection D_1

at time t_2. The parameter β controls how much error we are willing to tolerate. Setting a lower value for β is helpful for handling long occlusions. We use $\beta = 1$.

The appearance affinity between D_1 and D_2 is:

$$s_a = \max[1 - \alpha\, d(\phi_1, \phi_2), 0] \tag{6}$$

where $d(\cdot)$ is a distance function in appearance space. We use the earth mover's distance [28] in our experiments to compare HSV histograms, and set $\alpha = 1$.

A sigmoid function maps affinities to correlations smoothly, except in extreme cases:

$$w = \begin{cases} -\infty & \text{if } s_a s_{st} = 0 \\ +\infty & \text{if } s_a s_{st} = 1 \\ -1 + \frac{2}{1+\exp(-\lambda(s_a s_{st} - \mu))} & \text{otherwise} \end{cases}. \tag{7}$$

The parameter λ determines the width of the transition band between negative and positive correlation, and μ is the value that separates them. We use $\mu = 0.25$, assuming that $s_a = s_t = 0.5$ indicates indifference.

The definition of appearance affinity remains the same for tracklets, once appearance descriptors are modified as explained earlier. For space-time affinities, the position error $e(\cdot, \cdot)$ is redefined to measure the discrepancy between a tracklet's start point and the estimated start point as determined from the end point of the other tracklet: $e(\tilde{T}_1, \tilde{T}_2) = \|\tilde{\mathbf{q}}_1^s - \tilde{\mathbf{p}}_2^s\|_2$ where $\tilde{\mathbf{q}}_1^s = \tilde{\mathbf{p}}_1^e + \tilde{\mathbf{v}}_1(\tilde{t}_2^s - \tilde{t}_1^e)$.

3.3 The Cascade

In preparation for the online method of Sect. 3.4, we describe a cascade that allows solving the graph partitioning problem defined in Sect. 3.1 approximately and efficiently over a *temporal window* several seconds long. The longer the window, the longer the occlusions through which identities can be retained. Although we lose theoretical guarantees of optimality, we exploit the special structure of multi-person tracking to decompose the large BIP problem from Sect. 3.1 into manageable chunks that are unlikely to take us far from the optimal solution.

Our cascade has two simpler phases divided into two stages each. The first phase partitions detections over short time horizons and results into *tracklets*, short sequences of detections that can be safely connected to each other based on both appearance and space-time affinities. The second phase reasons over the

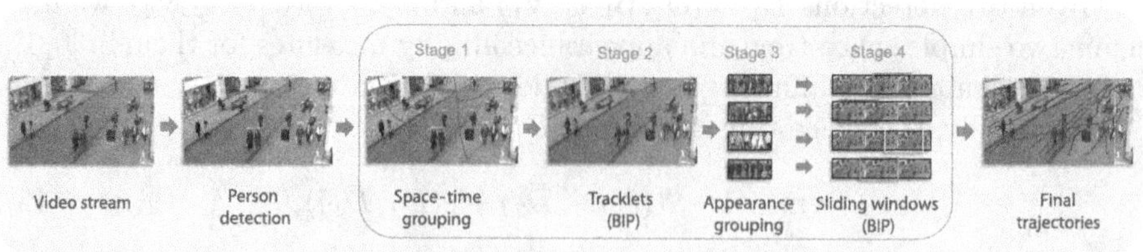

Fig. 2. The proposed processing pipeline.

entire temporal window, and partitions tracklets into identities (a.k.a. trajectories). Each phase has in turn a first stage that does a preliminary partitioning done safely by simple means in order to reduce the size of the BIP in that phase, and a second stage that solves a BIP exactly to utilize all evidence optimally. The four stages are now described in turn.

Space-Time Groups. The first stage divides the entire video sequence into 1-second intervals and uses hierarchical agglomeration [29] to group detections within each interval into *space-time groups* (Fig. 1(b)). Initially, each detection is in a separate group. The algorithm then repeatedly merges the pair of groups that are closest to each other in space until k_i space-time groups are formed for time interval i. We set k_i to one half of the expected number of visible people in the given time interval, estimated as the ratio between the total number of detections and the number of frames in the interval. Because of the conservative choice of k_i, it is unlikely that observations that belong together end up in different groups. Even if they do, one person will end up split into different identities, and the trajectory stage, described later, has an opportunity to undo the split.

Tracklets. The second stage solves a BIP exactly for the observations of each space-time group, using the correlations (7) for evidence. The resulting partitions are called *tracklets*, and are at most one second long by construction. Solving exact BIPs on space-time groups ensures that both appearance and space-time evidence are used optimally within this short time horizon. Missing detections are recovered using interpolation or extrapolation and tracklets shorter than 0.2 s are discarded as false positives.

Appearance Groups. The third stage reasons in appearance space and groups tracklets from the entire temporal window into appearance groups that will be processed independently of each other in the fourth stage. Non-parametric methods for discovering appearance groups [30] are a good fit for this stage. However, we use k-means and set the number k of clusters manually for simplicity.

The wholesale splitting of identities across different appearance groups is an irrecoverable error. However, appearance grouping is again conservative, in that two observations are grouped whenever they are even just loosely similar. The main assumptions in this stage are that a person's appearance can have only short-lived variations (*e.g.*, partial occlusions or shadows) and that person appearance does not change suddenly and dramatically (*e.g.*, a person putting on a rain coat while hidden behind an obstacle). The conservative nature of this stage typically prevents identity-split errors, and a few incorrectly assigned observations can be handled similarly to false positives and false negatives.

Trajectories. The last stage in the cascade solves a separate BIP (exactly) for all the tracklets in each appearance group and within the entire temporal window, again using both space-time consistency and appearance similarity as evidence. Missing tracklets for each trajectory are inferred using interpolation, and very short trajectories (shorter than 2 s) are discarded as false positives. The reduction in the size of the BIPs in the second and fourth stage of our cascade allows processing long temporal windows of data in real time, as Sect. 4 illustrates experimentally.

3.4 Unlimited Time Horizon

Typical surveillance video streams are unbounded in length and require real-time, online processing. To turn the method described so far into an online algorithm we employ a sliding temporal window. The temporal extent of the window is set ahead of time—and depending on application—so that the observations in it can be processed in real time. Video frames stream in continuously, and an off-the-shelf person detector provides the needed detections. One-second-long tracklets are continuously formed by stages 1 and 2 of the cascade, and added to the input data. Once a window is processed completely as explained next, it is advanced by half its temporal extent.

All the tracklets that are at least partially contained in the first window are fed to the second phase of the cascade. Stages 3 and 4 form partial trajectories, and missing and spurious observations are handled as explained in Sect. 3.3. Partial trajectories are never undone, but they can be extended from data in subsequent windows. In windows after the first, the elementary input observations for stage 3 are all the tracklets and all the partial trajectories whose temporal extents overlap the current window. Except for this difference, the computations are the same as in the first window. This process repeats forever. Figure 2 illustrates the complete processing pipeline.

The experiments in Sect. 4 illustrate that the cascade allows processing rather long windows. As a consequence, we can often successfully connect people identities across much longer occlusions than in previous literature, because corresponding tracklets before and after an occlusion are more likely to occur together in some window. For instance, our experiments show that for a medium crowded scene the sliding window can be as long as 32 s if tracklets are split into ten appearance groups, while still achieving real-time performance.

4 Experiments

4.1 Datasets and Performance Measures

We evaluate our algorithm on three standard single-camera datasets for multi-person tracking: PETS2009 [31], Town Center [21] and Parking Lot [14]. We used the PETS2009-S2L1 View 1 sequence, which has a resolution of 768×576 pixels and consists of 798 frames at 7 fps (117 s). The scene is not heavily crowded, but the low predictability in people's motion and a few long occlusions behind a lamp post makes the sequence challenging. The Town Center sequence is more challenging because it is longer, more crowded, and has longer occlusions. Occlusions in this sequence are mainly caused by people walking very close to each other. The sequence has a resolution of 1920×1080 pixels and consists of 4500 frames at 25 fps (180 s). The Parking Lot sequence consists of 998 frames at 30 fps (33.26 s) and has a resolution of 1920×1080 pixels. This sequence is challenging because it is filmed from an oblique angle and several people have similar appearance. Also, people walk close to each other in parallel causing long occlusions, both partial and full.

Table 1. Multi Object Tracking Accuracy (MOTA) and ID switches on three standard datasets. MOTA variance for the Town Center sequence is a result of the randomness of the k-means clustering algorithm, which in different runs yields differences in appearance groups.

	PETS2009	
	MOTA	IDsw
Berclaz [11]	80.00	28
Shitrit [10]	81.46	19
Andriyenko [20]	81.84	15
Henriques [6]	87.95	10
Izadinia [12]	90.70	-
Zamir [14]	91.50	8
Ours	**93.34**	1

	Town Center	
	MOTA	IDsw
Benfold [21]	64.9	259
Zhang [13]	65.7	114
Leal-Taixe [33]	67.3	86
Izadinia [12]	75.70	-
Zamir [14]	75.59	-
McLaughlin [7]	76.46	-
Ours	**78.43±0.29**	**68**

	Parking Lot	
	MOTA	IDsw
Izadinia [12]	88.90	-
Zamir [14]	92.27	1
Ours	**94.20**	**1**

We use the standard Multiple Object Tracking Accuracy (MOTA) score [32] to evaluate the performance of our algorithm. This score combines the number of false positives $f_p(t)$, false negatives $f_n(t)$, and identity switches $id(t)$ over all frame indices t as follows:

$$MOTA = 1 - \frac{\sum_t (f_p(t) + f_n(t) + id(t))}{\sum_t g(t)} \quad (8)$$

where $g(t)$ is the ground-truth number of people in frame t. MOTA is widely accepted in the field as one of the principal indicators of a tracker's performance.

In Table 1 we present results for all sequences. We outperform state of the art methods in MOTA and identity switches. For a fair comparison, we use the detections used in previous work [14], courtesy of the authors. All evaluations are done using the CLEAR MOT evaluation script [34] and we use the standard 1 m acceptance threshold.

In the PETS2009 sequence we use a long temporal window of 20 s and one appearance group since the scene is not crowded. We allow tracklets to be at most 10 frames in this sequence due to its low frame rate. The total running time of our method, not accounting for person detection, is 38 s. In the Town Center sequence we use a temporal window of 12 s and 5 appearance groups because the sequence is more crowded. Tracklets have lengths of at most 20 frames. The total running time on this sequence is 176 s, 120 of which were spent finding all tracklets. In the Parking Lot sequence we use a temporal window of 6 s and tracklets are at most 20 frames long. We used one appearance group in this sequence since it is short. The total running time on this sequence is 34 s.

4.2 Window Length, Accuracy, and Runtime

Figures 3(a) and (b) show the dependency of tracking accuracy and running time on the length of the sliding window for the Town Center Sequence with 10 appearance groups. We ran several experiments on this sequence by progressively elongating the temporal window.

Figure 3(a) shows that after the temporal window length is increased beyond 3 s, which corresponds to the typical occlusion length in the scene, there is no

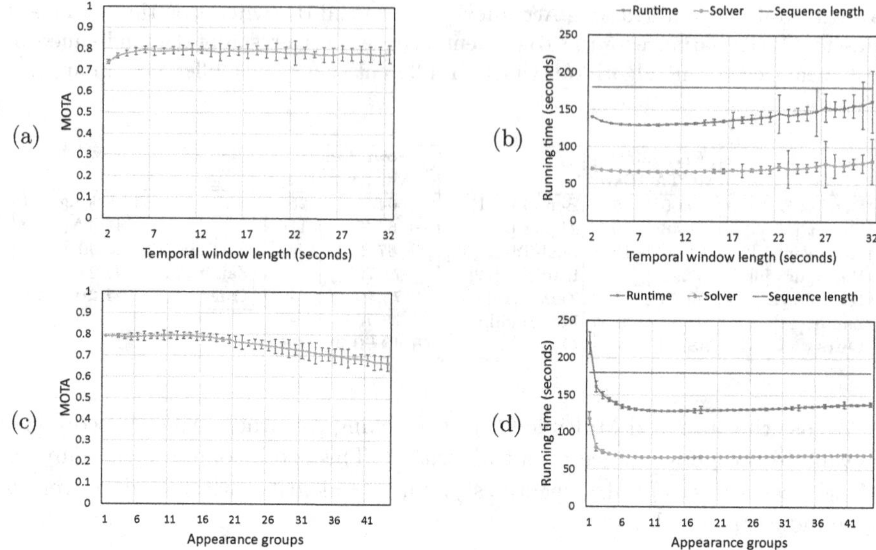

Fig. 3. MOTA scores (a, c) and running times (b, d) as functions of the length of the sliding window (a, b) and the number of appearance groups (c, d) for the Town Center sequence. Solver time indicates how much time was spent for assembling and solving all the Binary Integer Programs. The total running time also includes the time for computing correlations, but does not account for person detection. Figures (a) and (b) are for ten appearance groups, and Figures (c) and (d) are for 8-second sliding windows. Best viewed on screen.

significant improvement in the quality of the solution. The variations in the graph are caused by differences in the appearance groups that the k-means algorithm finds in each window. The slight decrease in the scores for windows longer than 19 s is because the parameter β in Eq. (5) also influences how large partitions can grow in time.

Figure 3(b) shows how the sliding window length affects the running time. Appearance grouping allows us to achieve an unprecedented temporal window length for real-time computation.

4.3 Appearance Groups, Accuracy, and Runtime

Figures 3(c) and (d) show the dependency of tracking accuracy and running time on the number of appearance groups for the Town Center sequence with a temporal window of 8 s.

Figure 3(c) shows that even a moderately high number of appearance groups, around 20, has negligible harmful effects on the accuracy of the tracker. When the number of appearance groups is increased further, the accuracy measure starts to decay because identities are split into separate groups. The fluctuations in the graph are again caused by the k-means algorithm, which over-clusters in windows that contain few tracklets.

Figure 3(d) shows that the overall running time is greatly reduced when we go from 1 to about 5 appearance groups, while the MOTA score only drops from 79 % to 78.4 % (Fig. 3(c)). Increasing the number of appearance groups further yields marginal reductions in running time. The slight increase in total runtime for more than 20 appearance groups is caused by the k-means algorithm, whose complexity increases with k.

4.4 Approximate and Exact Graph Partitioning Solvers

We explore the trade-off between accuracy and runtime for different combinations of solvers for graph partitioning. We demonstrate that approximating the solution of multi-person tracking by piecing together exact solutions of small subproblems is qualitatively better than algorithms with no optimality guarantees, while still achieving real-time performance.

Three algorithms for graph partitioning have been recently proposed in the literature [35], namely: Expand-and-Explore, Swap-and-Explore, and Adaptive Label Iterative Conditional Modes (AL-ICM). We use the latter in our experiment because of its speed and ability to scale to large problems. Given a labeling vector $L = \{1, 2, \ldots\}^n$ the algorithm assigns a label l_u to observation u so as to minimize the following energy function:

$$E(L) = \sum_{uv} w_{uv} \mathbf{1}_{[l_u \neq l_v]} \tag{9}$$

where $\mathbf{1}_{[P]}$ is 1 when P is true and 0 otherwise. Minimizing this energy function is equivalent to maximizing rewards and minimizing penalties in Eq. (1). This energy is lowered when observations supported by negative correlation are labeled differently and when observations supported by positive correlation are labeled identically. This discrete energy minimization formulation has the advantage that the labeling vector L consists of n variables whereas the co-identity matrix X in our formulation consists of n^2 variables. This allows AL-ICM to scale to $n \geq 100,000$ observations.

AL-ICM is a greedy search algorithm. In each iteration, every variable is assigned the label that minimizes the energy, conditioned on the current label of the other variables. While ICM requires a fixed number of labels [36], AL-ICM handles a varying number of labels as follows: conditioned on the current labeling, each observation is assigned to the most rewarding partition, or to a new partition if penalized by all current partitions. The algorithm terminates either when the energy cannot be minimized further or when a predefined number of iterations is reached.

We construct two methods based on this algorithm. Method AL-ICM uses the greedy algorithm in stages 2 and 4 of the cascade, and space-time and appearance grouping in stages 1 and 3. Method AL-ICM-NoGroup uses the greedy algorithm but no grouping, thus only stages 2 and 4 of the full cascade.

We refer to our full algorithm as BIP, and we compare it also to a method we call BIP-NoGroup, that is, stages 2 and 4 of the cascade without space-time and

Table 2. Different combinations of solvers evaluated on three standard datasets. The length of each sequence is 117, 180 and 33.26 s respectively. Solver time indicates how many seconds were spent for solving graph partitioning problems in each sequence. The total running time also includes the time for computing correlations, but does not account for person detection.

	Method	PETS2009			Town Center			Parking Lot		
		MOTA	Runtime	Solver	MOTA	Runtime	Solver	MOTA	Runtime	Solver
	Izadinia [12]	90.70	-	-	75.70	-	-	88.90	-	-
	Zamir [14]	91.50	-	-	75.59	-	-	92.27	-	-
Ours	AL-ICM	91.34	**9.33**	**0.31**	77.78 ± .35	**107.54**	**3.52**	93.33	**15.69**	**0.39**
Ours	AL-ICM-NoGroup	92.20	10.68	0.45	78.46	284.73	18.86	93.92	28.00	1.11
Ours	BIP	**93.18**	17.06	8.06	78.43 ± .29	177.17	73.10	**94.20**	33.59	20.40
Ours	BIP-NoGroup	**93.18**	27.43	16.87	**78.87**	25725.82	23444.58	**94.20**	334.45	307.39

appearance grouping. Performance metrics for all methods on three sequences are presented in Table 2.

Accuracy. All our methods consistently outperform the state of the art. Even method AL-ICM is on par, if not better than the state of the art, although it can be penalized by mistakes due to grouping heuristics and the suboptimal greedy algorithm. The differences in accuracy between our methods that use grouping and their corresponding version without grouping is minimal. This confirms that stages 1 and 3 of our cascade can be used in practice, safely and with negligible harmful effects. It is also worth noting that piecing together optimal solutions of small problems is superior to combining approximate solutions of small problems, which is common in the literature: Both BIP and BIP-NoGroup perform better than AL-ICM and AL-ICM-NoGroup, respectively.

Runtime. It is not surprising that the AL-ICM algorithm is much faster than the BIP solver. AL-ICM is a greedy algorithm and does not require assembling and solving a BIP with a quadratic number of variables and a combinatorial number of constraints. We note that the use of grouping heuristics is crucial for improving runtime performance; methods that do not use heuristics need to compute large and full correlation matrices. While the best time performance is that of AL-ICM, our BIP method is also fast enough to work in real-time at 25 fps.

Trade-offs. Considering the trade-offs between accuracy and runtime, the BIP approach is appropriate when accuracy is important and the scene has medium crowd density. The AL-ICM variant is more appropriate for time-critical applications or more crowded scenes, but comes with a cost in terms of accuracy. In the absence of heuristics, which are not useful when the scene is crowded or all appearances look the same, AL-ICM-NoGroup is the only method from the above set that can be used to meet weaker time constraints.

4.5 Implementation

We implemented our algorithm in MATLAB and we used the Gurobi Optimizer to solve the Binary Integer Programs. All experiments were done on a PC with Intel i7-3610 2.3 GHz processor and 6 GB of memory. The results for the BIP-NoGroup method in Table 2 were produced on a Linux machine with Intel Xeon

E5540 2.53 GHz processor and 96 GB memory in order to solve very large Binary Integer Programs. The code and data to reproduce the above results are available on the authors' website.

5 Concluding Remarks and Future Work

We developed a general, efficient, online method for multiple person tracking that outperforms the state of the art and can be used with any person detector, appearance feature, space-time heuristic, or similarity metric. Our graph partitioning formulation accounts properly for evidence both for and against co-identity, and can both force and forbid co-identity through hard constraints. A cascade of stages that reason over short- and long-term time horizons exploits safe groupings by space-time and appearance opportunistically to reduce computational complexity. We improve over the state of the art and achieve real-time, online performance thanks to a sliding window approach. The windows can be made long enough to handle very significant occlusions successfully.

Future improvements include replacing the k-means algorithm for appearance grouping with clustering-forest techniques, which are more appropriate for online data association; replacing appearance and space-time affinities with more sophisticated metrics that depend on context; and making the temporal window length adapt to data complexity in real time. We are also looking at how additional constraints related to people entering and exiting the scene affect our algorithm. In the long term, we plan to extend our methods to tracking from multiple cameras.

Acknowledgements. This work was supported by the Army Research Office under Grant No. W911NF-10-1-0387 and by the National Science Foundation under Grants IIS-10-17017 and IIS-14-20894.

References

1. Shafique, K., Shah, M.: A noniterative greedy algorithm for multiframe point correspondence. In: PAMI (2005)
2. Javed, O., Shafique, K., Rasheed, Z., Shah, M.: Modeling inter-camera space-time and appearance relationships for tracking across non-overlapping views. In: CVIU (2008)
3. Brendel, W., Amer, M., Todorovic, S.: Multiobject tracking as maximum weight independent set. In: CVPR (2011)
4. Breitenstein, M.D., Reichlin, F., Leibe, B., Koller-Meier, E., Van Gool, L.: Robust tracking-by-detection using a detector confidence particle filter. In: ICCV (2009)
5. Shu, G., Dehghan, A., Oreifej, O., Hand, E., Shah, M.: Part-based multiple-person tracking with partial occlusion handling. In: CVPR (2012)
6. Henriques, J.F., Caseiro, R., Batista, J.: Globally optimal solution to multi-object tracking with merged measurements. In: ICCV (2011)
7. McLaughlin, N., del Rincon, J.M., Miller, P.: Online multiperson tracking with occlusion reasoning and unsupervised track motion model. In: AVSS (2013)

8. Bae, S.H., Yoon, K.J.: Robust online multi-object tracking based on tracklet confidence and online discriminative appearance learning. In: CVPR (2014)
9. Pirsiavash, H., Ramanan, D., Fowlkes, C.C.: Globally-optimal greedy algorithms for tracking a variable number of objects. In: CVPR (2011)
10. Ben Shitrit, H., Berclaz, J., Fleuret, F., Fua, P.: Tracking multiple people under global appearance constraints. In: ICCV (2011)
11. Berclaz, J., Fleuret, F., Turetken, E., Fua, P.: Multiple object tracking using k-shortest paths optimization. In: PAMI (2011)
12. Izadinia, H., Saleemi, I., Li, W., Shah, M.: $(MP)^2T$: multiple people multiple parts tracker. In: Fitzgibbon, A., Lazebnik, S., Perona, P., Sato, Y., Schmid, C. (eds.) ECCV 2012, Part VI. LNCS, vol. 7577, pp. 100–114. Springer, Heidelberg (2012)
13. Zhang, L., Li, Y., Nevatia, R.: Global data association for multi-object tracking using network flows. In: CVPR (2008)
14. Roshan Zamir, A., Dehghan, A., Shah, M.: GMCP-Tracker: global multi-object tracking using generalized minimum clique graphs. In: Fitzgibbon, A., Lazebnik, S., Perona, P., Sato, Y., Schmid, C. (eds.) ECCV 2012, Part II. LNCS, vol. 7573, pp. 343–356. Springer, Heidelberg (2012)
15. Butt, A.A., Collins, R.T.: Multiple target tracking using frame triplets. In: Lee, K.M., Matsushita, Y., Rehg, J.M., Hu, Z. (eds.) ACCV 2012, Part III. LNCS, vol. 7726, pp. 163–176. Springer, Heidelberg (2013)
16. Andriyenko, A., Schindler, K., Roth, S.: Discrete-continuous optimization for multi-target tracking. In: CVPR (2012)
17. Arora, C., Globerson, A.: Higher order matching for consistent multiple target tracking. In: ICCV (2013)
18. Yang, B., Nevatia, R.: An online learned crf model for multi-target tracking. In: CVPR (2012)
19. Wen, L., Li, W., Yan, J., Lei, Z., Yi, D., Li, S.Z.: Multiple target tracking based on undirected hierarchical relation hypergraph. In: CVPR (2014)
20. Andriyenko, A., Schindler, K.: Multi-target tracking by continuous energy minimization. In: CVPR (2011)
21. Benfold, B., Reid, I.: Stable multi-target tracking in real-time surveillance video. In: CVPR (2011)
22. Jiang, H., Fels, S., Little, J.J.: A linear programming approach for multiple object tracking. In: CVPR (2007)
23. Leibe, B., Schindler, K., Van Gool, L.: Coupled detection and trajectory estimation for multi-object tracking. In: ICCV (2007)
24. Butt, A.A., Collins, R.T.: Multi-target tracking by lagrangian relaxation to min-cost network flow. In: CVPR (2013)
25. Bansal, N., Blum, A., Chawla, S.: Correlation clustering. In: Foundations of Computer Science (2002)
26. Tan, J.: A Note on the Inapproximability of Correlation Clustering. Elsevier, Amsterdam (2008)
27. Swamy, C.: Correlation clustering: maximizing agreements via semidefinite programming. In: ACM-SIAM Symposium on Discrete algorithms (2004)
28. Rubner, Y., Tomasi, C., Guibas, L.J.: A metric for distributions with applications to image databases. In: ICCV (1998)
29. Anderberg, M.R.: Cluster Analysis for Applications. Technical report, DTIC Document (1973)
30. Liu, C., Gong, S., Loy, C.C., Lin, X.: Person re-identification: what features are important? In: Fusiello, A., Murino, V., Cucchiara, R. (eds.) ECCV 2012 Ws/Demos, Part I. LNCS, vol. 7583, pp. 391–401. Springer, Heidelberg (2012)

31. Ferryman, J.: Proceedings (pets 2009). In: Eleventh IEEE International Workshop on Performance Evaluation of Tracking and Surveillance (2009)
32. Keni, B., Rainer, S.: Evaluating multiple object tracking performance: the CLEAR MOT metrics. J. Image Video Process, **2008**, Article 1, 10 p. (2008). doi:10.1155/2008/246309
33. Leal-Taixé, L., Pons-Moll, G., Rosenhahn, B.: Everybody needs somebody: modeling social and grouping behavior on a linear programming multiple people tracker. In: ICCV Workshops (2011)
34. Bagdanov, A.D., Del Bimbo, A., Dini, F., Lisanti, G., Masi, I.: Posterity logging of imagery for video surveillance (2012)
35. Bagon, S., Galun, M.: Large scale correlation clustering optimization. arXiv preprint arXiv:1112.2903 (2011)
36. Besag, J.: On the statistical analysis of dirty pictures. J. R. Stat. Soc. Ser. B (Methodological) **48**, 259–302 (1986)

Optimizing Storage Intensive Vision Applications to Device Capacity

Rohit Girdhar(✉), Jayaguru Panda, and C. V. Jawahar

IIIT-Hyderabad, Hyderabad, India
rohit.girdhar@students.iiit.ac.in

Abstract. Computer vision applications today run on a wide range of mobile devices. Even though these devices are becoming more ubiquitous and general purpose, we continue to see a whole spectrum of processing and storage capabilities within this class. Moreover, even as the processing and storage capacity of devices are increasing, the complexity of vision solutions and the variety of use cases create greater demands on these resources. This requires appropriate adaptation of the mobile vision applications with minimal changes in the algorithm or implementation. In this work, we focus on optimizing the memory usage for storage intensive vision applications.

In this paper, we propose a framework to configure memory requirements of vision applications. We start from a gold standard desktop application, and reduce the size for a given the memory constraint. We formulate the storage optimization problem as mixed integer programming (MIP) based optimization to select the most relevant subset of data to be retained. For large data sets, we use a greedy approximate solution which is empirically comparable to the optimal MIP solution.

We demonstrate the method in two different use cases: (a) Instance retrieval task where an image of a query object is looked up for instant recognition/annotation, and (b) Augmented reality where computational requirement is minimized by rendering and storing precomputed views. In both the cases, we show that our method allows a reduction in storage by almost 5× with no significant performance loss.

1 Introduction

With the advancement in computing power, data driven methods have gained popularity in solving many challenging computer vision problems. Just as years of visual experience enables humans to make sense out of sparse, noisy and ambiguous local scene measurements, data-driven methods use multiple examples to train the machine (or just remember them) and help in solving the challenging vision problems. Many computer vision techniques use data (eg. images or features from images) for training the vision solution [1,2]. Often, the data is also required at the testing/inferring stage in these applications (eg. support vectors in kernel SVMs, image patches and dictionaries for inpainting). The situation is more challenging if one uses a template based solution, such as an

D. Cremers et al. (Eds.): ACCV 2014, Part V, LNCS 9007, pp. 460–475, 2015.
DOI: 10.1007/978-3-319-16814-2_30

exemplar SVM [3] or a nearest neighbour scheme [4]. There have been many previous attempts in pruning the templates [5] or support vectors [6] in the pattern recognition literature. Most recently, Misra *et al.* [7] proposed a technique to compact the set of exemplars used in Exemplar SVM. However, such attempts do not get enough attention as the storage capabilities of desktop machines have increased rapidly in the last few years. This also led to an increased interest in the methods that use large number of images or feature representations at the run time to obtain better quality of results. This resulted in dictionaries or databases of image [8], patches [9], or even feature vectors [10] becoming popular in a wide spectrum of vision applications. In this work, we focus on pruning the storage requirements of such vision applications to suite the mobile device capabilities. *Our focus is not to design a novel mobile vision algorithm.* Rather we start with a vision solution that runs on desktops (considering it as a standard reference), and demonstrate how the memory/storage requirements can be reduced to practically design compact but equally powerful mobile vision applications.

There are many applications that require large visual data at the test stage. For example, Video Google [10] is a object retrieval system designed to find identical instances (images or parts) in large collection of images and videos. This technique has now emerged as the backbone of many product search solutions [11]. Popular and commercial implementations still continue to use a client server implementation where the mobile client is used only for capturing the image and displaying of the product information. A more challenging implementation can compute features and compact representations on the mobile and minimize the communication overheads [12,13]. In instance retrieval, typically one needs to retain multiple exemplars of the same instance for acceptable performance. The major challenge in such systems is to decide the number of images or feature representations that needs to be maintained in the database. Panda *et al.* [14] demonstrate the instance retrieval on reasonably large dataset (50 K) on common mobile phones. However, when the dataset (number of images to be indexed) increases beyond 100 K, even this method fails. Focus of [14] was limited to pruning the vocabulary size (or representation) without modifying the dataset of images to be indexed. The problem of automatic selection of relevant exemplar images or their representations still remains as an open problem. A solution to this can result in easy adaptation of the software without changes in the algorithm or even implementation.

Vision on mobile and wearable computers has garnered a lot of interest in the last half a decade. Recent research in this direction is focussing on data-driven and on-device computing approaches. Paucher *et al.* [15] perform indoor localization and pose estimation for AR on mobile devices using a database of images of the environment taken from different locations. As we also show in the experimental section, reducing storage helps in reducing the computational requirement on devices, which have multiple purposes (unlike a dedicated computer). There has been work in optimizing memory and computation of visual search and recognition to work on-device [11,14,16]. Computational photography applications on mobile are also focussing on memory optimized design for tasks such as panorama stitching [17]. Pollefeys *et al.* propose novel approaches overcome the underlying hardware limitations of mobile to accomplish extremely heavy tasks such as live 3D reconstruction [18,19]. Some systems, however, still choose to offload heavier recognition and detection tasks to servers, while running tracking on the device [20–22].

In this work, we address the problem of developing computer vision applications that can be customized to work on different devices having varying hardware capabilities. We specifically target standalone apps which do all the computations on the device itself, and require large amounts of data to be stored on device. We attempt to reduce the size of such datasets to suit the device capability, without any significant loss in quality of the solution. Consider a standalone, product search application that needs to support more than 100 K products, with 10 M exemplars require an index typically of size 40 GB in size [23]. Current cloud or server based infrastructure can support this much memory and would be able to answer queries within less than a second. Modern desktops usually support less than 4 GB of RAM, but can flatten the dataset to disk, leading to response times of the order 15–35 s. High end mobile devices (such as iPhone) support much less disk space (8–16 GB), hence can not use the index from disk, and must use an index over a subset. Though 10 M examples are collected for 100 K products for excellent retrieval performance, we notice that a subset of these images can actually be pruned without any significant loss in performance.

Our main contribution is a fast and simple optimization framework that works for various computer vision problems to select a near-optimal subset of data required for the task to be stored on device. Note that our solution runs on a desktop/server and provides the image/dataset selection information that can lead to an application that fits a specific memory limit. We formulate this selection problem as a mixed integer program (MIP) to select the most relevant subset of data. Integer optimization being NP Hard, the MIP quickly becomes intractable and hence, we use a greedy approximation of the same for larger datasets. We validate our approach in two different vision applications: instance retrieval, and mobile augmented reality for low end devices, by storing and rendering precomputed views.

Even though storage is not a major concern on modern desktops or servers, and in fact leads to more accurate performance, it does become a concern on low-end mobile devices. Moreover, the advent of wearable computing devices in the form of glasses and watches further aggravates the problem, as these typically support even weaker hardware. For example, Google Glass currently support only 682 MB of RAM [24]. Therefore, even though the capabilities of mobile devices have been increasing as a consequence of Moore's law, appearance of computers in miniature formats and growing popularity of data intensive applications still leaves plenty of opportunity in optimizing applications for weaker devices. Even as of today, a significant percentage of mobile devices in the world are incapable of storing or processing large amounts of data to perform complex computer vision tasks. Figure 1 illustrates this fact by giving the percentage market share of android based mobile devices with respect to disk space, RAM and processing power.

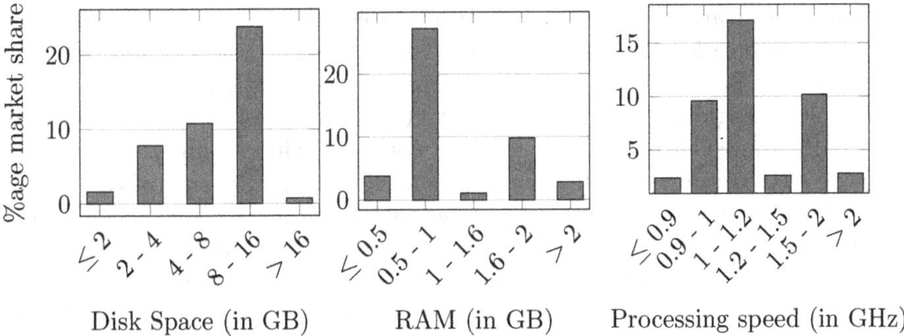

Fig. 1. Market share of android mobile devices by disk space, RAM and processing power in 2014. Even in 2014 we have large number devices with less than 1 GB RAM, and less than 4 GB of disk space. Data from *gsmarena.com* and [25].

We investigate the problem of extracting the most relevant information from a large dataset of visual data. The common theme in most of the work in this direction is to represent the similarity between images in the form of a graph and selecting the nodes that can approximate for the others. One of most relevant works in this direction is by Simon *et al.* on scene summarization [26]. They extract a canonical subset of images as a visual summary of a scene from a large collection of images sourced from the internet. Li *et al.* in [27] further build upon this work to use iconic scene graph with the number of geometrically consistent matches as the edge weights to cluster the images and extract 'iconic' views, which they further use for visualization and search. Crandall *et al.* [28] use a similar approach for organizing large photo collections. A more scalable approach to clustering images at world-scale was described in [29]. Irschara *et al.* [30] use a similar approach to compress 3D scene representation. Chum *et al.* [31] propose similarity measures for detecting near-duplicate images.

In this paper, we propose a simple scalable scheme that can help pruning the dictionaries to suite the mobile devices. We empirically show that pruning can even result in improving the performance in some cases. As an example, we take the instance retrieval and mobile AR problems. In both the cases, we prune dataset of images, with no practical loss in performance. We report a reduction in the number of images to be retained by a factor of 5.

2 Optimizing Memory Usage

2.1 Memory Reduction as Subset Selection

Given a vision solution that uses a database of images $V = \{v_1, v_2, \cdots, v_n\}$ and a given set of possible tasks $T = \{t_1, t_2, \cdots, t_m\}$, we are interested in finding a subset $K \subseteq V$ such that $|K| \leq k$, and can solve the task $t_i, 1 \leq i \leq m$ with minimal impact on accuracy compared to when using the complete set V. For the case of instance recognition, V corresponds to the set of all images available for indexing, and we are interested automatically selecting in the subset K that gives good performance for the task t_i of recognizing specific products. Performance is measured as precision @ 1 (P_1) for the instance recognition.

Instance recognition and retrieval tasks typically use a lot of examples that are usually sourced from the Internet or collected with minimal supervision. They are also incrementally updated in many situations. Because of the nature of this database and its growth, they tend to contain images that have no role in instance recognition. To verify this, we did a small experiment on the Oxford Buildings dataset [23] consisting of images of famous Oxford landmarks sourced from Flickr. We used a Bag of Words (BoW) representation and observed that almost 33 % of the images in this dataset never appear in the top-10 for any of the given queries. In other words, if one uses P_1 as a measure for the recognition accuracy, these images can be pruned from the database with no loss in performance. Figure 2 shows some of them. These images are of two broad types: (i) Images that are redundant, as a better example is sufficient for the recognition. (ii) Images that are really outliers and have not much visual information of interest.

We also observe that the tasks (the possible/popular set of queries) are also not arbitrary. In a typical recognition setting of buildings, users often want recognition of frontal images and not top views. The prior knowledge about the possible tasks t_i can help in computing the loss or cost of a failure due to the pruning of the database. Database can now be designed to support these popular queries and can be compacted further.

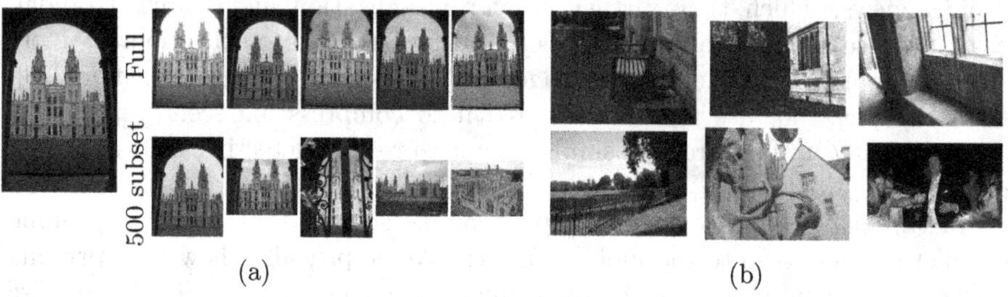

Fig. 2. (a) shows the IR results for the left most query, using the full set and a 500 image subset. Note that the top few results in both cases are relevant and sufficient for recognition. (b) shows some of the outlier images in the set.

Hence, we focus on the problem of selecting a k size subset from the dataset V of all elements required for the task, where k depends on the device capability. When the dataset is a simple collection of images, the selection is easy to appreciate. Even when the dataset is computed from a large population (as in the case of a dictionary computed with K-Means [10]), pruning can be used [14]. In our case, the question of *computing* a reduced size dictionary does not really arise since we start with a database of images, and we can only prune it.

2.2 Selecting Useful Images

We now represent the problem as a mixed-integer optimization (MIP) to select a canonical subset (K) of size k that best approximates the complete set (V). The number k would depend on the disk space and memory available on the device. We define e_i as a measure of error incurred when i^{th} image of V is approximated using K. We limit our attention to problems in which a specific image is approximated using only one other image. If the image v_i is an outlier and does not contribute to the performance of the solution, one can trivially remove v_i directly. However, removal of an image that has some utility is more tricky. In this case, the images selected in the attempt to approximate its role can lead to a possibly poorer performance. This quality reduction is represented in e_i.

As discussed earlier, in many situations the tasks are already known, and can be used to drive the optimization to a solution that is optimal for those specific tasks. Let W_{ij} be the weight of image i with respect to task t_j. For example, if task j is product search, W_{ij} will be high for images i that correspond to the most popular views of the product. Now, as our objective is to minimize the total error incurred in approximating set V using set K, for a given task j, it can be represented as:

$$Objective : \min \sum_{i=1}^{|V|} W_{ij} e_i \tag{1}$$

We weigh the error values with W_{ij} to ensure good approximations for more important views. However, this kind of a prior knowledge is usually hard to determine and needs to be inferred from very large set of case studies and user logs. Hence, for the remainder of this problem, we will consider all images to be equally weighted for the task, and take $W_{ij} = 1, \forall i, j$.

Now, for each image in the set V, we define a binary variable x_i, which equals 1 if it is selected to the subset. Let E_{ij} be the error incurred when i^{th} image is approximated using j^{th} image. Since it can not be actually computed, we define it as based on similarity between v_i and v_j. E_{ij} would be task specific, for instance in IR, it could be the distance between GIST descriptors of the images. In case of 3D object augmentation, we can use an image representation over feature tracks to compute the error. Since each feature track corresponds to a 3D point, a low error would ensure same 3D pose is visible in both the images. For even greater accuracy, we could use the distance between extrinsic camera parameters of the two, if such information is available.

In order to control e_i using E_{ij}s, we need to introduce a binary variable Z_{ij} which equals 1 if image i is approximated using image j. Finally, we need to enforce the following constraints: (i) Total number of selected images is limited by k (see Eq. 2), (ii) An image can approximate for another image if it itself gets selected (see Eq. 4), (iii) An image may be approximated using only one other image (see Eq. 3), and (iv) The error e_i should be determined from E_{ij}, corresponding to the image j that is used to approximate image i (see Eq. 5).

These translate to the following constraints:

$$\sum_{i=1}^{|V|} x_i \leq k \tag{2}$$

$$\sum_{j=1}^{|V|} Z_{ij} = 1 \forall i \tag{3}$$

$$Z_{ij} \leq x_j \qquad \forall i, j \tag{4}$$

$$e_i \geq \sum_{j=1}^{|V|} E_{ij} Z_{ij} \qquad \forall i \tag{5}$$

Equation 5 enforces the constraint (iv) as $Z_{ij} = 1$ for a unique value of $j = j'$ for a given i (as an image is approximated by only one other image), and hence, Eq. 5 reduces down to $e_i \geq E_{ij'}$, which is what is required by the constraint. The variable x at the minimal value of objective will give the optimal subset of given data set to be selected that would give least approximation error summed over all images. The MIP as described above can be easily transformed into a standard format (such as CPLEX) and solved using existing IP solvers.

2.3 Scaling to Large Sets

Even though MIP is easy to formulate and able to select the optimal subset to store on device, solving itself becomes intractable as the size of the original set increases. We observed that using one of the fastest non-commercial solvers, SCIP [32], the time taken and memory usage for the memory optimization grows exponentially as size of original set ($|V|$) increases. Even though this optimization is an offline task and can be performed using powerful servers, optimizing even over sets of a few hundred thousand images could take few weeks for each device, a timeline typically unacceptable to software application developers.

This motivated us to use a greedy algorithm to get an approximate solution to the above problem. The algorithm starts with an empty K set. At every iteration, we choose the image that leads to maximum reduction in the objective (Q), i.e., the unselected image that best approximates the remaining unselected images, and add it to the selected set. We keep going till k images get selected, and output the final K set. Algorithm 1 formally presents our approach.

Figure 3 compares the performance of MIP optimization vs the Greedy approximate solution. We observed for selecting a subset of $\frac{N}{2}$ from a set of size N, the time taken to optimize MIP (using SCIP) and the memory used in this process increases exponentially. On a desktop with 4 GB of RAM, we could not optimize over a set with more than 600 images. The greedy approach, on other hand, was extremely light and fast. The computation time in this case scaled linearly, and we could easily optimize over tens of thousands of images. Moreover, the final objective value at optima in both the cases were comparable for small sets,

Algorithm 1. Greedy algorithm to select representative subset

$K \leftarrow \emptyset$
while $|K| < k$ **do**
  for all $v \in V - K$ **do**
    $Q_v \leftarrow Q(K) - Q(K \cup v)$
    $Q_{v*} \leftarrow \min(Q_{v*}, Q_v)$
  if $Q_{v*} \leq 0$ **then**
    break
  $K \leftarrow K \cup v*$

showing the near-optimality of the greedy approximation. Hence, we use our greedy approach for the further analysis in Sect. 3, and compare with MIP for smaller subsets where ever possible.

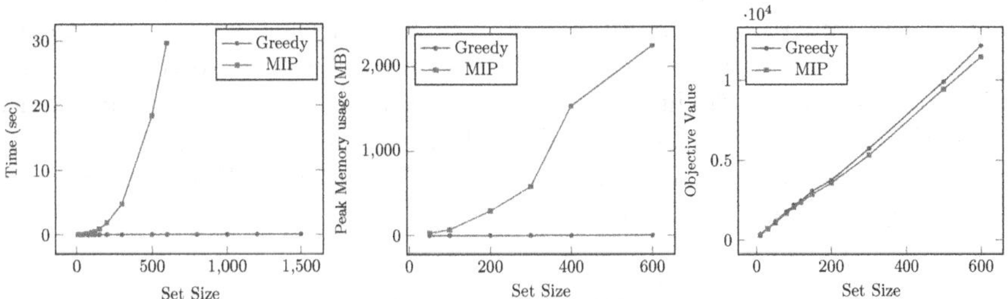

Fig. 3. These plots compare running time, memory usage and objective value for greedy and MIP to select a subset of size $\frac{N}{2}$ from N size sets. Greedy is quite comparable to MIP in performance. MIP, however, takes much more time and memory to compute.

3 Experimental Results

3.1 Example Use Cases

We validate our approach using two popular mobile vision applications, product search using instance retrieval and 3D object augmentation. Instance recognition focusses on recognizing an image related to a specific object given a query from widely varying imaging conditions. Most of the existing IR literature uses variants of bag of words based approaches for the task [10,23,33] by matching local image features that represent image geometry to those in database. Image recognition mobile devices also has several successful examples such as Google Goggles, Amazon Snaptell etc., but most of these applications rely on a remote server for matching within large image databases. Some of these optimize on the network communication by sending compressed feature representations to the server [13,34–36]. Prior work on offline IR on mobile focusses on reducing memory footprint of search index and includes [14,37–39]. Though mean average precision (mAP) is used as the measure to quantify the retrieval quality, precision at k (P_k) with $k = 1$ or even 3 or 5 are better suited for the instance recognition task that we are interested in. Since product search or image annotation applications typically use top 1 or 3 matches for recognition, we believe mean precision (mP) to be a better indicator of the performance of our system.

3D object augmentation, on the other hand, involves augmenting natural 3D scenes with virtual objects. The standard approach in such problems is to register the query image with respect to the 3D structure of the scene. The camera parameters thus obtained are then used to transform, render and merge the object onto the query scene. Camera calibration for the query image is the computationally heaviest step in this pipeline, typically achieved by first computing 2D-3D correspondences between the image and 3D structure, and using these to compute camera parameters using RANSAC. As these computations are usually too heavy for a low-end mobile device, we design an approximate solution that can easily be configured to the device capabilities. We pre-compute the augmentation snapshots for a database set of images of the scene. At the test time, the precomputed views of the virtual objects are merged with the input image. If the camera parameters of the precomputed view is very close to that of real one, visually the result is indistinguishable. However, storing thousands of views of a structure might become a bottleneck on lower end devices. Hence, there is a need to prune this database set of views to select best k views to store (where k depends on the amount of disk space available). We use our subset selection technique for the same.

3.2 Experiments and Results

Comparing MIP and Greedy Over IR. We first compare IR performance over the subsets selected using MIP optimization and the greedy method. We use a bag of words based approach over SIFT vectors quantized into visual words using a 1M vocabulary computed using Approximate K-Means [23]. The scores for ranking are computed using the tf-idf statistic over the visual words, and we further refine the ranklist using spatial consistency constraints, i.e., fitting a fundamental matrix and re-ranking based on number of inliers (we ignore the matches if number of inliers $<$15). We evaluate it over a 480 image subset of Oxford Buildings dataset, consisting of the images of All Souls, Ashmolean and Balliol, and their corresponding 15 queries. Number of SIFT inliers is popularly used as a similarity measure between images, and we use its reciprocal to compute the approximation error matrix (E) in both the subset selection approaches. As we can observe from Fig. 4, the subsets selected by both MIP optimization and greedy give comparable mP at 3,5 and 10 (though MIP does little better than greedy on average), justifying the usage of greedy for larger sets.

Greedy Subset Selection Over Complete Dataset. We evaluate the above IR algorithm over the complete Oxford Buildings dataset, consisting of 5062 images of 11 Oxford landmarks with ground truth for 55 queries. We segregate the images into a test set (containing the 55 query images) and a training set (containing the rest 5007 images), and compute the index over the subsets of

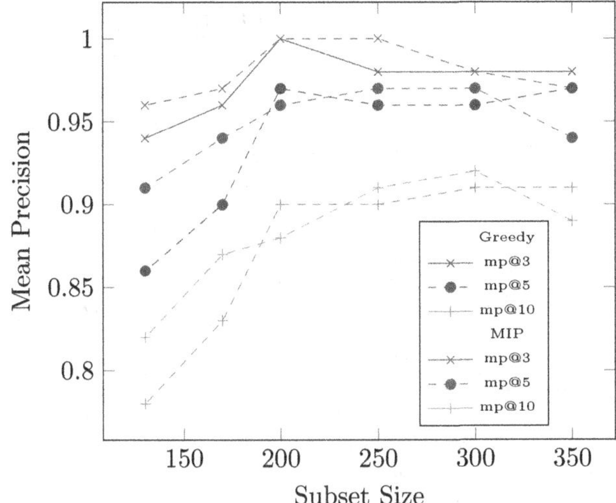

Fig. 4. Graph compares the P_3, P_5, P_{10} values over 480 images subset of Oxford buildings, using both MIP and greedy approaches. Both perform comparably, though MIP is little better on the average.

training set. This helps in evaluating the performance of the system in the real-world product search scenario, where the database does not contain the query images.

We experimented with two different values for E_{ij}. GIST [40] is a popular global descriptor for representing scenes, and quite relevant for our problem of removing the similar and outlier images of products. We used the euclidean distance between 512D GIST descriptors as E_{ij}. Another possible way to define similarity between images is as the number of geometrically consistent inlier matches. We also experimented with using reciprocal of this number as the error metric. As we can observe from Fig. 5, SIFT inliers are able to model similarity better than GIST, and hence give better mean precision results.

In both cases, we observe from Table 1 that the size of index and computation time goes down almost linearly. This makes our approach suitable for configuring IR applications to mobile devices with all kinds of storage capacities.

Comparing MIP vs Greedy for Augmented Reality. In this case, we use a slightly more complex definition of E to ensure images with similar pose incur less error. Hence, we compute SIFT feature tracks across all images, each of which corresponds to a 3D feature point on the structure being augmented (using VisualSfM [41]). Now, we use the images of these feature points to compute the error incurred by using homography to approximate one of these images, by the other. For every 3D point P visible in image i and j, let x and y be the images of P in i and j respectively. Now, E_{ij} is defined as the Euclidean distance between x, and the point obtained by transforming y by the homography between these images, averaged over all such P.

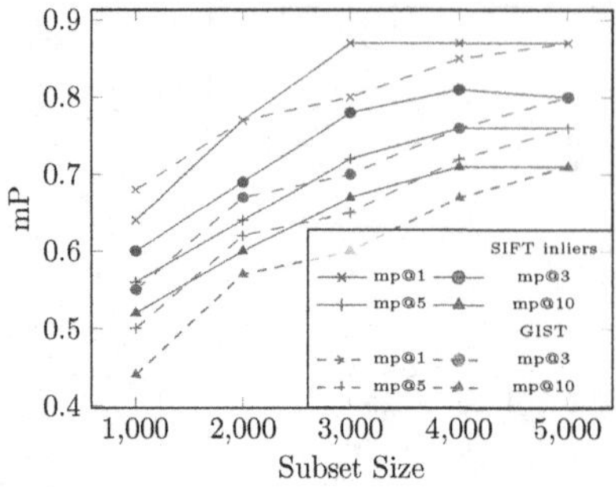

Fig. 5. Greedy subset selection results on Oxford Buildings Dataset. We compare the mean precision (mP) at positions 1,3,5 and 10 for GIST and SIFT inliers as the similarity measures between images. In both the cases, size of index stored on device and time taken for search comes down almost linearly.

Table 1. Size and speed with subset size

Subset size (K)	Index size (MB)	Time (s)
500	7.33	0.47
1000	12.78	0.76
2000	23.065	1.3
3000	31.221	1.75
4000	38.39	2.17
4500	41.65	2.31
5007	44.62	2.56

For experimentation and analysis, we created our own dataset of a toy 3D object in the lab setting. We collected 96 images of the object from different viewpoints, and hand-picked 15 images as the test set. We used a 3D model of a cap to augment the structure, and precomputed the augmentation snapshots of the cap for all the database views. Figure 6 gives a visualization of the same.

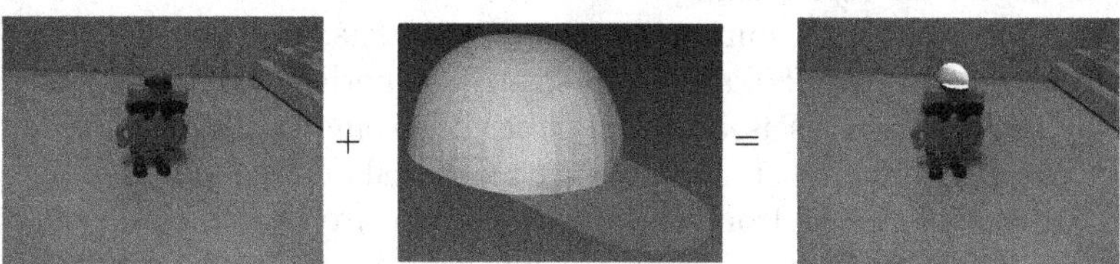

Fig. 6. An image of the toy 3D model from our dataset, and a snapshot of the cap used for augmentation. A snapshot of the cap corresponding to the first image is used to generate the final result

We used the greedy and MIP optimization strategies of Sect. 2 to select subset from the remaining 81 images. We quantitatively evaluate the performance using mean reconstruction error over test images, defined in a similar way as E. Reconstruction error for image i is defined as

$$\min_{j \in K} E_{ij}$$

and is averaged over all test images to get the mean (E_{ij} is defined in Sect. 2.2). We compute the mean reconstruction error for the 15 test images and plot it against the subset sizes in Fig. 7. Interestingly, the greedily selected subset at times gives even lesser error than the MIP optimized subset. This is because MIP tends to overfit the solution to the training data, giving the most optimal subset that can reconstruct the other training images, with no consideration to test images. Greedy, on the other hand, does not have such tight constraints and hence tends to generalize better. We also show qualitative results of augmentation with different subset sizes in Fig. 7.

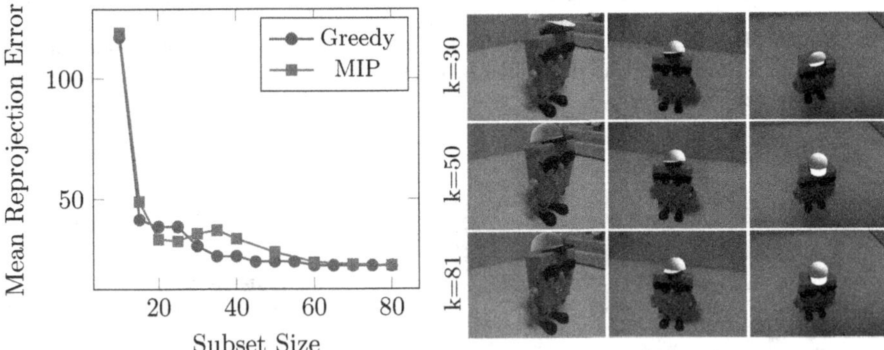

Fig. 7. The graph shows the variation of reprojection error as we use smaller sets of precomputed views. We also show augmentation results for 3 different views of our 3D object at different values of subset size k. Clearly, reducing the size of selected subset has marginal effect on quality of augmentation.

3.3 Applications in Digital Heritage

Recently, there has been a rising interest in building computer vision applications for digitally preserving and promoting cultural heritage, such as the Great Buddha Project [42], HeritageApp [43] etc. The 3D augmentation system too has a natural application in digital heritage, especially in augmenting 3D structures with parts that no longer exist. Stone Chariot at Hampi is a famous historical monument in India (Fig. 8). Its structure went through various changes over the course of history; the most prominent one being the removal of a dome like super-structure from top of the monument. With the objective of preserving this cultural heritage, a 3D model was built that captures the structure in its former glory (Fig. 9) We aim to make this visualization accessible to people on their mobile devices. Our application allows any tourist to see the missing parts augmented over the original structure, using any mobile device. Some of the results of our homography based approach are shown in Fig. 10.

This dataset consists of 1505 images of a heritage monument taken from different viewpoints and the precomputed augmentation snapshots occupy nearly 420 MB on disk. We reduce this requirement using the greedy subset selection to enable it to run on devices with low disk space. Figure 11 shows the marginal

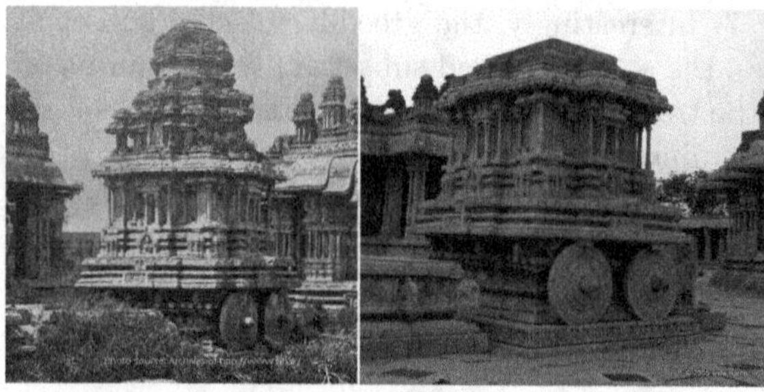

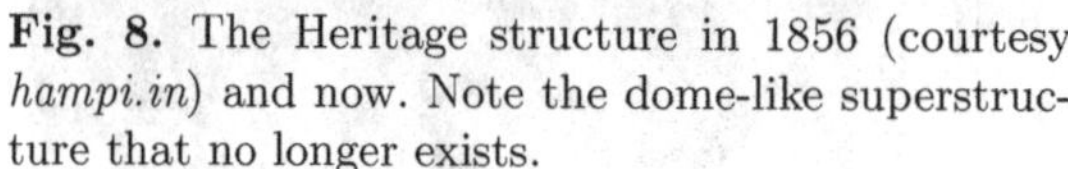

Fig. 8. The Heritage structure in 1856 (courtesy *hampi.in*) and now. Note the dome-like superstructure that no longer exists.

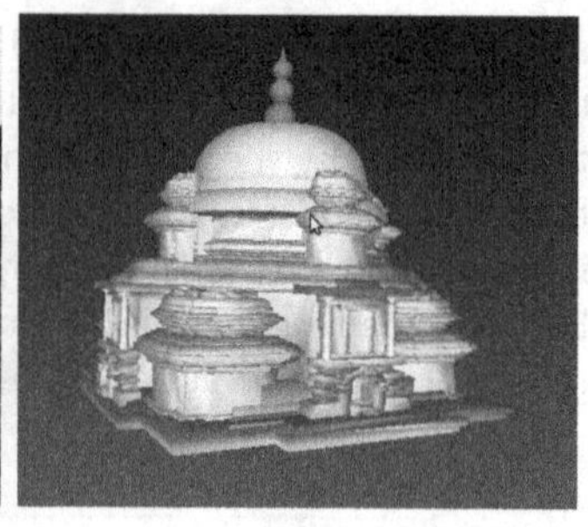

Fig. 9. The 3D model of the missing dome constructed by architects.

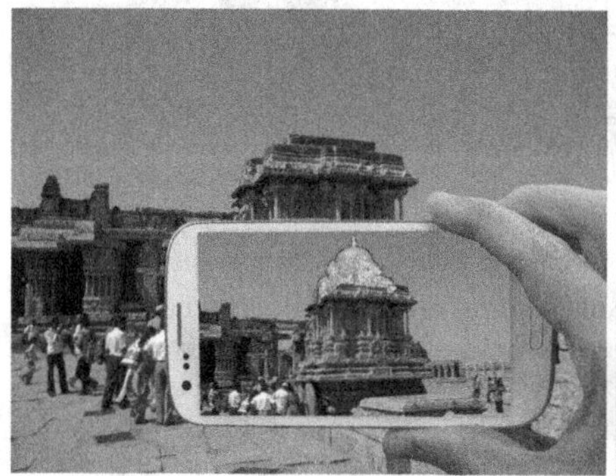

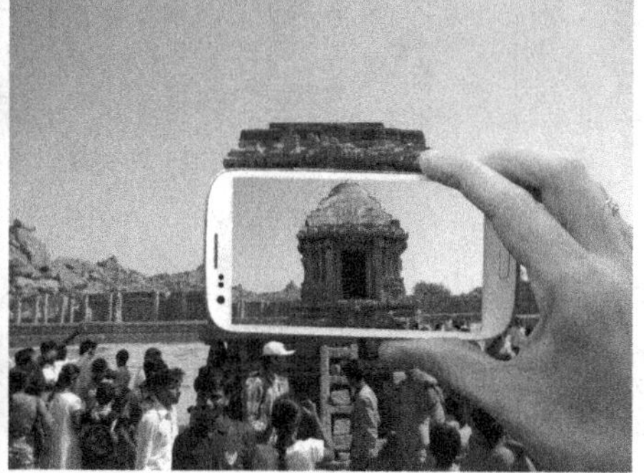

Fig. 10. Example use of our application to augment the missing parts.

increase in reprojection error with reduction in size of subset using the greedy approach. Table 2 lists the various specifications of the app for different subset sizes for a Lenovo s820 mobile device. These include the disk space occupied by precomputed snapshots, size of the search index used for localization, startup time of the app to read data into memory, time in instance retrieval over database views for localization and finally the time to compute matching, homography and warping and merging the precomputed snapshot onto the query. As expected, total computation time and memory load decreases with decrease in the subset size.

3.4 Discussions

Apart from low processing power, less memory capacity, small screen size and limited connectivity, another major challenge faced by mobile devices is limited battery power. Even as the memory and processing power continue to grow

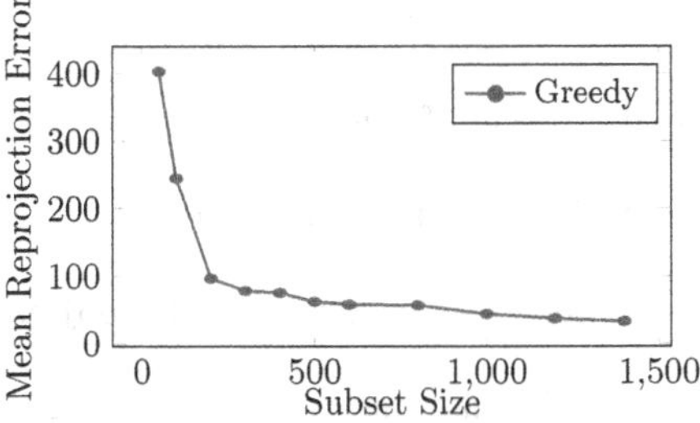

Fig. 11. The graph of mean reprojection error with subset size shows for the 1505 image heritage monument dataset. The table lists our app specifications for different subset sizes.

Table 2. AR Mobile app specs

Subset size	500	1000	1505
Snapshots (MB)	140	278	422
Search Index (MB)	7.3	12.7	18.6
Startup Time (s)	0.7	1.2	1.6
Localization (s)	0.03	0.07	0.1
Augmentation (s)	0.6	0.6	0.6

exponentially according to the Moore's law, growth in battery technology has been much slower. For instance, while Apple claims that the iPhone 5S delivers 56× faster graphics and 40× faster CPU than original iPhone [44], the battery capacity of 5S has grown by only 15 % from the original [45].

Clearly, such a situation warrants the need for more battery conscious applications. Fortunately, our configurable application approach fits this scenario well, too. Since using smaller subset of visual data requires lesser computation and hence lesser battery consumption, a smart application can automatically shift to using a smaller subset as the device goes low on power. The different subsets may either be stored on device or can be retrieved on the fly over the network. Once the device charges up again, the application can again shift to using complete data for more accurate performance.

4 Conclusion

In this work, we successfully formulate a fast and simple approach for pruning datasets required by storage intensive applications, enabling them to work across a spectrum of devices with varying capabilities. Even though finding the most optimal such subset is computationally infeasible, we show that a greedy approach can closely approximate that performance. We validate this approach over popular vision applications, IR and Augmented Reality, showing significant reductions in storage and computation requirements while nearly preserving the accuracy of performance. We also demonstrate its application in digital heritage, by enabling low end mobile devices to visualize the parts of heritage monuments that were lost over time.

Acknowledgement. This work was partly supported by the Indian Digital Heritage Project of the DST.

References

1. Dalal, N., Triggs, B.: Histograms of oriented gradients for human detection. In: CVPR (2005)
2. Judd, T., Ehinger, K., Durand, F., Torralba, A.: Learning to predict where humans look. In: ICCV (2009)
3. Malisiewicz, T., Gupta, A., Efros, A.A.: Ensemble of exemplar-SVMs for object detection and beyond. In: ICCV (2011)
4. Zhang, H., Berg, A., Maire, M., Malik, J.: SVM-KNN: discriminative nearest neighbor classification for visual category recognition. In: CVPR (2006)
5. Fayed, H.A., Atiya, A.F.: A novel template reduction approach for the k-nearest neighbor method. IEEE Trans. Neural Netw. **20**(5), 890–896 (2009)
6. Liang, X.: An effective method of pruning support vector machine classifiers. IEEE Trans. Neural Netw. **21**(1), 26–38 (2010)
7. Misra, I., Shrivastava, A., Hebert, M.: Data-driven exemplar model selection. In: Winter Conference on Applications of Computer Vision (2014)
8. Hays, J., Efros, A.A.: Scene completion using millions of photographs. In: ACM SIGGRAPH (2007)
9. Peyr, G.: Sparse modeling of textures. J. Math. Imag. Vis. **34**(1), 17–31 (2009)
10. Sivic, J., Zisserman, A.: Video google: a text retrieval approach to object matching in videos. In: ICCV (2003)
11. Shen, X., Lin, Z., Brandt, J., Wu, Y.: Mobile product image search by automatic query object extraction. In: Fitzgibbon, A., Lazebnik, S., Perona, P., Sato, Y., Schmid, C. (eds.) ECCV 2012, Part IV. LNCS, vol. 7575, pp. 114–127. Springer, Heidelberg (2012)
12. Rublee, E., Rabaud, V., Konolige, K., Bradski, G.: ORB: an efficient alternative to SIFT or SURF. In: ICCV (2011)
13. Chandrasekhar, V., Takacs, G., Chen, D.M., Tsai, S.S., Reznik, Y., Grzeszczuk, R., Girod, B.: Compressed histogram of gradients: a low-bitrate descriptor. IJCV **96**(3), 384–399 (2012)
14. Panda, J., Brown, M.S., Jawahar, C.: Offline mobile instance retrieval with a small memory footprint. In: ICCV (2013)
15. Paucher, R., Turk, M.: Location-based augmented reality on mobile phones. In: CVPR Workshop (2010)
16. He, J., Feng, J., Liu, X., Cheng, T., Lin, T.H., Chung, H., Chang, S.F.: Mobile product search with bag of hash bits and boundary reranking. In: CVPR (2012)
17. Xiong, Y., Pulli, K.: Fast image stitching and editing for panorama painting on mobile phones. In: CVPR Workshop (2010)
18. Kolev, K., Tanskanen, P., Speciale, P., Pollefeys, M.: Turning mobile phones into 3d scanners. In: CVPR (2014)
19. Tanskanen, P., Kolev, K., Meier, L., Camposeco, F., Saurer, O., Pollefeys, M.: Live metric 3d reconstruction on mobile phones. In: ICCV (2013)
20. Dantone, M., Bossard, L., Quack, T., Van Gool, L.: Augmented faces. In: ICCV Workshops (2011)
21. Gammeter, S., Gassmann, A., Bossard, L., Quack, T., Van Gool, L.: Server-side object recognition and client-side object tracking for mobile augmented reality. In: CVPR Workshop (2010)
22. Kumar, S.S., Sun, M., Savarese, S.: Mobile object detection through client-server based vote transfer. In: CVPR (2012)

23. Philbin, J., Chum, O., Isard, M., Sivic, J., Zisserman, A.: Object retrieval with large vocabularies and fast spatial matching. In: CVPR (2007)
24. Google glass. en.wikipedia.org/wiki/Google_Glass. Accessed 19 June 2014
25. Top android phones. http://www.appbrain.com/stats/top-android-phones. Accessed 03 June 2014
26. Simon, I., Snavely, N., Seitz, S.M.: Scene summarization for online image collections. In: ICCV (2007)
27. Li, X., Wu, C., Zach, C., Lazebnik, S., Frahm, J.-M.: Modeling and recognition of landmark image collections using iconic scene graphs. In: Forsyth, D., Torr, P., Zisserman, A. (eds.) ECCV 2008, Part I. LNCS, vol. 5302, pp. 427–440. Springer, Heidelberg (2008)
28. Crandall, D.J., Backstrom, L., Huttenlocher, D., Kleinberg, J.: Mapping the world's photos. In: WWW (2009)
29. Quack, T., Leibe, B., Van Gool, L.: World-scale mining of objects and events from community photo collections. In: International Conference on Content-based Image and Video Retrieval (2008)
30. Irschara, A., Zach, C., Frahm, J.M., Bischof, H.: From structure-from-motion point clouds to fast location recognition. In: CVPR (2009)
31. Chum, O., Philbin, J., Zisserman, A.: Near duplicate image detection: min-hash and tf-idf weighting. In: BMVC (2008)
32. Achterberg, T.: Scip: Solving constraint integer programs. Math. Program. Comput. **1**(1), 1–41 (2009)
33. Nister, D., Stewenius, H.: Scalable recognition with a vocabulary tree. In: CVPR (2006)
34. Girod, B., Chandrasekhar, V., Chen, D.M., Cheung, N.M., Grzeszczuk, R., Reznik, Y., Takacs, G., Tsai, S.S., Vedantham, R.: Mobile visual search. SPM **8**(3), 86–94 (2011)
35. Chandrasekhar, V., Reznik, Y., Takacs, G., Chen, D., Tsai, S., Grzeszczuk, R., Girod, B.: Quantization schemes for low bitrate compressed histogram of gradients descriptors. In: CVPR (2010)
36. Chen, D.M., Tsai, S.S., Chandrasekhar, V., Takacs, G., Singh, J., Girod, B.: Tree histogram coding for mobile image matching. In: DCC (2009)
37. Jégou, H., Douze, M., Schmid, C.: Packing bag-of-features. In: ICCV (2009)
38. Jégou, H., Perronnin, F., Douze, M., Sánchez, J., Pérez, P., Schmid, C.: Aggregating local image descriptors into compact codes. In: TPAMI (2012)
39. Zhang, X., Li, Z., Zhang, L., Ma, W.Y., Shum, H.Y.: Efficient indexing for large scale visual search. In: ICCV (2009)
40. Oliva, A., Torralba, A.: Modeling the shape of the scene: a holistic representation of the spatial envelope. IJCV **42**(3), 145–175 (2001)
41. Wu, C.: Visualsfm: a visual structure from motion system (2011)
42. Ikeuchi, K., Oishi, T., Takamatsu, J., Sagawa, R., Nakazawa, A., Kurazume, R., Nishino, K., Kamakura, M., Okamoto, Y.: The great buddha project: digitally archiving, restoring, and analyzing cultural heritage objects. Int. J. Comput. Vis. **75**(1), 189–208 (2007)
43. Panda, J., Sharma, S., Jawahar, C.V.: Heritage app: annotating images on mobile phones. In: ICVGIP (2012)
44. Heath, A.: iphone 5s is 56x faster than original iphone with 64-bit a7 chip. http://www.cultofmac.com/244572/iphone-5s-is-56x-faster-than-original-iphone-with-64-bit-a7-chip/. Accessed 5 June 2014
45. Drang, D.: The small improvement in iphone battery capacity. http://www.leancrew.com/all-this/2013/10/the-small-improvement-in-iphone-battery-capacity/. Accessed 5 June 2014

MTS: A Multiple Temporal Scale Tracker Handling Occlusion and Abrupt Motion Variation

Muhammad Haris Khan(✉), Michel F. Valstar, and Tony P. Pridmore

Computer Vision Laboratory, School of Computer Science,
University of Nottingham, Nottingham, UK
{psxmhk,michel.valstar,tony.pridmore}@nottingham.ac.uk

Abstract. We propose visual tracking over multiple temporal scales to handle occlusion and non-constant target motion. This is achieved by learning motion models from the target history at different temporal scales and applying those over multiple temporal scales in the future. These motion models are learned online in a computationally inexpensive manner. Reliable recovery of tracking after occlusions is achieved by extending the bootstrap particle filter to propagate particles at multiple temporal scales, possibly many frames ahead, guided by these motion models. In terms of the Bayesian tracking, the prior distribution at the current time-step is approximated by a mixture of the most probable modes of several previous posteriors propagated using their respective motion models. This improved and rich prior distribution, formed by the models learned and applied over multiple temporal scales, further makes the proposed method robust to complex target motion through covering relatively large search space with reduced sampling effort. Extensive experiments have been carried out on both publicly available benchmarks and new video sequences. Results reveal that the proposed method successfully handles occlusions and a variety of rapid changes in target motion.

1 Introduction

Visual tracking is one of the most important unsolved problems in computer vision. Though it has received much attention, no framework has yet emerged which can robustly track across a broad spectrum of real world settings. Two major challenges for trackers are abrupt variations in target motion and occlusions. In some applications, e.g. video surveillance and sports analysis, a target may undergo abrupt motion changes and be occluded at the same time.

While many solutions to the occlusion problem have been proposed, it remains unsolved. Some methods [1–3] propose an explicit occlusion detection and handling mechanism. Reliable detection of occlusion is difficult in practice, and often produces false alarms. Other methods, e.g. those based on adaptive appearance models [4,5], use statistical reasoning to handle occlusions indirectly, by learning how appearance changes over time. Occlusions can, however, contaminate the appearance models, as such methods use blind update strategies.

D. Cremers et al. (Eds.): ACCV 2014, Part V, LNCS 9007, pp. 476–492, 2015.
DOI: 10.1007/978-3-319-16814-2_31

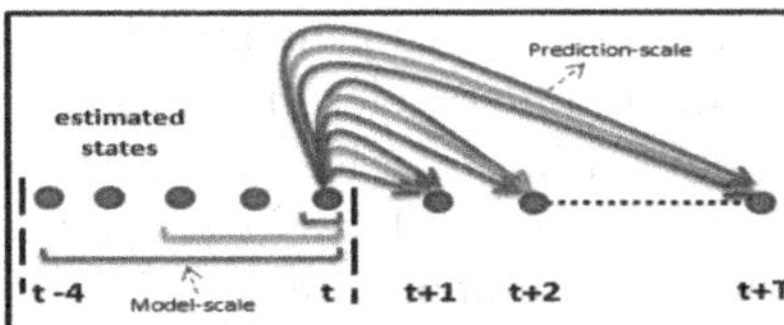

(a) Multiple motion models are learned from the recent history of estimated states at different temporal scales, and each model is applied to multiple temporal scales in the future.

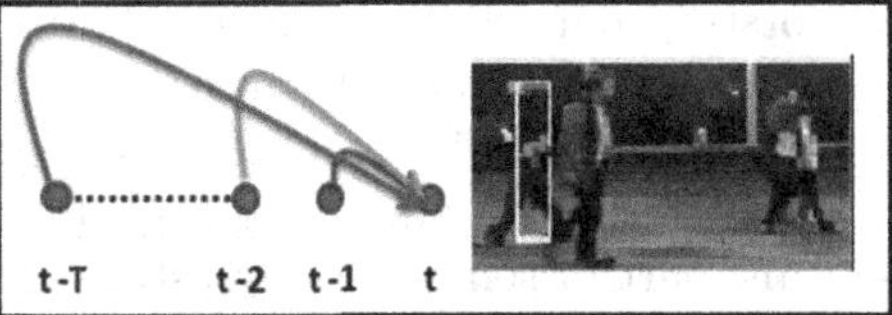

(b) This means that, when determining target state, multiple sets of motion models are available to make predictions. Each set includes models learnt at multiple model-scales. In the proposed framework one model per set is selected to propagate particles.

Fig. 1. Visual tracking over multiple temporal scales.

Abruptly varying motion can be addressed using a single motion model with a large process noise. This approach requires large numbers of particles and is sensitive to background distractors. Alternative approaches include efficient proposals [6], or hybrid techniques with hill climbing methods [7] to allocate particles close to the modes of the posterior. These approaches can, however, be computationally expensive.

We propose a new tracking method that is capable of implicitly coping with partial and full target occlusion and non-constant motion. To recover from occlusion we employ a flexible prediction method, which estimates target state at temporal scales similar to the expected maximum duration of likely occlusions. To achieve this, motion models are learnt at multiple model-scales and used to predict possible target states at multiple prediction-scales ahead in time. The model-scale is the duration of a sequence of recently estimated target states over which a motion model is learnt. The prediction-scale is the temporal distance, measured in frames of the input image sequence, over which a prediction is made. Reliable recovery of tracking after occlusions is achieved by extending the bootstrap particle filter to propagate particles to multiple prediction-scales, using models learnt at multiple model-scales. Figure 1 summarises the approach.

The proposed framework can handle variable motion well due to the following: In predictive tracking, learnt motion models describe the recent history of target state —the most recent section of the target's path across the image plane. Trackers using, for example, a single linear motion model effectively represent target path as a straight line. By building multiple motion models at multiple model scales, the proposed framework maintains a much richer description of target path. The diverse set of models produced captures at least some of the complexity of that path and, when used to make predictions, the model set represents variation in target motion better than any single model.

The contributions of this work are three-fold. **(1)** We propose and evaluate the idea of tracking over multiple temporal scales to implicitly handle occlusions of variable lengths and achieve robustness to non-constant target motion. This is accomplished by learning motion models at multiple model-scales and applying them over multiple prediction-scales. Consequently, the proposed framework does not require an explicit occlusion detection, which could be difficult to achieve reliably in practice. **(2)** We propose a simple but generic extension of the bootstrap particle filter to search around the predictions generated by the motion models. **(3)** Current trackers typically adopt a first-order Markov Chain assumption, and predict a target's state at time t using only its state at time $t-1$. That is, they all work on a single temporal scale i.e. $[t-1,t]$. We propagate important part of some recently estimated posteriors to approximate prior distribution at the current time-step through combining the above two proposals in a principled way. The resulting formulation is a tracker operating at multiple temporal scales that has not been proposed before to the best of our knowledge.

2 Related Work

Occlusion handling may be explicit or implicit. Implicit approaches can be divided into two categories. The first is based on adaptive appearance models which use statistical analysis [4,5,8] to reason about occlusion. The appearance models can, however, become corrupt during longer occlusions due to the lack of an intelligent update mechanism. Approaches in the second category divide the target into patches and either use a voting scheme [9] or robust fusion mechanism [10] to produce a tracking result. These can, however, fail when the number of occluded patches increases. The proposed approach also handles occlusion implicitly, but using a fixed and very simple appearance model.

Explicit occlusion handling requires robust occlusion detection. Collins et al. [1] presented a combination of local and global mode seeking techniques. Occlusion detection was achieved with a naive threshold based on the value of the objective function used in local mode seeking. Lerdsudwichai et al. [2] detected occlusions by using an occlusion grid with a drop in similarity value. This approach can produce false alarms because the required drop in similarity could occur due to natural appearance variation. To explicitly tackle occlusions, Kwak et al. [3] trained a classifier on the patterns of observation likelihoods in a completely offline manner. In [11,12], an occlusion map is generated by examining trivial coefficients, this is then used to determine the occlusion state of a target candidate. Both these methods are prone to false positives where it is hard to separate the intensity of the occluding object from small random noise. The proposed approach here does not detect occlusions explicitly, as it is difficult to achieve reliably.

Some approaches address domain-specific occlusion of known target types. Lim et al. [13] propose a human tracking system based on learning dynamic appearance and motion models. A three-dimensional geometric hand model was proposed by Sudderth et al. [14] to reason about occlusion in a non-parametric belief propagation tracking framework. Others [15,16] attempt to overcome occlusion using multiple cameras. As most videos are shot with a single camera, and multiple cameras bring additional costs; this is not a generally applicable solution. Furthermore, a domain-agnostic approach is more widely applicable.

Recently, some methods exploited context along with target description [17–19], and a few exploited detectors [20,21] to overcome occlusions. Context-based methods can tackle occlusions, but rely on the tracking of auxiliary objects.

Approaches based on detector could report false positives in the presence of distractors, causing the tracker to fail. Our approach does not search the whole image space, instead multiple motion models define relatively limited search spaces of variable size where there is high target probability. This results in reduced sampling effort and lower vulnerability to distractors.

When target motion is difficult to model, a common solution is to use a single motion model with a large process noise. Examples of such models are random-walk (RW) [7,22] and nearly constant velocity (NCV) [23,24]. Increased process noise demands larger numbers of particles to maintain accurate tracking, which increases computational expense.

One approach to the increased variance in estimation caused by high process noise is to make an efficient and informed proposal distribution. Okuma et al. [6] designed a proposal distribution that mixed hypotheses generated by an AdaBoost detector and a standard autoregressive motion model to guide a particle filter based tracker. Reference [25] formulated a two-stage dynamic model to improve the accuracy and efficiency of the bootstrap PF, but their method fails during frequent spells of non-constant motion. Kwon and Lee [8] sampled motion models generated from the recent sampling history to enhance the accuracy and efficiency of MCMC based sampling process. We also learn multiple motion models, but at different model-scales instead of a single scale and use recently estimated states history in comparison to sampling history.

Several attempts have been made to learn motion models offline. Isard and Blake [26] use a hardcoded finite state machine (FSM) to manage transitions between a small set of learned models. Madrigal et al. [27] guide a particle filter based target tracker with a motion model learned offline. Pavlovic et al. [28] switch between motion models learned from motion capture data. Their approach is application specific, in that it learns only human motion. Reference [29] classifies videos into categories of camera motion and predicts the right specialist motion model for each video to improve tracking accuracy, while we learn motion models over multiple temporal scales in an online manner to generate better predictions. An obvious limitation of offline learning is that models can only be used to track the specific class of targets for which they are trained.

To capture abrupt target motion, which is difficult for any motion model, [30] combined an efficient sampling method with an annealing procedure, [31] selects easy-to-track frames first and propagates density from all the tracked frames to a new frame through a patch matching technique, and [32] introduced a new sampling method into the Bayesian tracking. Our proposed method tries to capture reasonable variation in the target's path.

Two approaches that at first glance appear similar to ours are [33,34]. Mikami et al. [33] use the entire history of estimated states to generate a prior distribution over the target state at immediate and some future time-steps, though the accuracy of these prior distributions relies on strict assumptions. In [34], offline training is required prior to tracking and thus it cannot be readily applied to track any object. Our approach learns multiple simple motion models at relatively short temporal scales in a completely online setting, and each model predicts the target state at multiple temporal scales in the future.

In contrast to previous work, we learn motion models over multiple model-scales, whose predictions are pooled over multiple prediction-scales to define the search space of a single particle filter. Hence, this is an online learning approach not restricted to any specific target class, and a novel selection criterion selects suitable motion models without the need for a hardcoded FSM.

3 Bayesian Tracking Formulation

Our aim is to find the best state of the target at time t given observations up to t. State at time t is given by $\mathbf{X}_t = \{X_t^x, X_t^y, X_t^s\}$,where X_t^x, X_t^y, and X_t^s represent the x, y location and scale of the target, respectively. In a Bayesian formulation, our solution to tracking problem comprises two steps: update(1), and prediction (2).

$$p(\mathbf{X}_t|\mathbf{Y}_{1:t}) \propto p(\mathbf{Y}_t|\mathbf{X}_t)p(\mathbf{X}_t|\mathbf{Y}_{1:t-1}). \tag{1}$$

where $p(\mathbf{X}_t|\mathbf{Y}_{1:t})$ is the posterior probability given the state $\mathbf{X}_t$ at time t, and observations $\mathbf{Y}_{1:t}$ up to t. $p(\mathbf{Y}_t|\mathbf{X}_t)$ denotes the observation model.

$$p(\mathbf{X}_t|\mathbf{Y}_{1:t-1}) = \int_{\mathbf{X}_{t-1}} p(\mathbf{X}_t|\mathbf{X}_{t-1})p(\mathbf{X}_{t-1}|\mathbf{Y}_{1:t-1})d\mathbf{X}_{t-1}. \tag{2}$$

where $p(\mathbf{X}_t|\mathbf{Y}_{1:t-1})$ is the prior distribution at time t, and $p(\mathbf{X}_t|\mathbf{X}_{t-1})$ is a motion model.

In this work, we improve the accuracy of the posterior distribution at a given time t by improving the prior distribution. Here, the prior distribution is approximated by a mixture of the most probable modes of T previous posteriors propagated by the T selected motion models, which are generated using information from up to T frames ago. The Eq. 2 in the standard Bayesian formulation can now be written as:

$$p(\mathbf{X}_t|\mathbf{Y}_{1:t-1}) = \int_{k=1}^{k=T} \int_{\mathbf{X}_{t-k}} p(\mathbf{X}_t|\mathbf{X}_{t-k})p(\tilde{\mathbf{X}}_{t-k})d\mathbf{X}_{t-k}dk. \tag{3}$$

where $p(\mathbf{X}_t|\mathbf{X}_{t-k})$ is the motion model selected at time t from a set of motion models learned at time $t-k$, and $p(\tilde{\mathbf{X}}_{t-k}) \subset p(\mathbf{X}_{t-k}|\mathbf{Y}_{1:t-k})$ is the most probable mode (approximated via particles) of the posterior at time $t-k$. A relatively rich and improved prior distribution in Eq. 3 allows handling occlusions and abrupt motion variation in a simple manner without resorting to complex appearance models and exhaustive search methods.

The best state of the target $\hat{\mathbf{X}}_t$ is obtained using Maximum a Posteriori (MAP) estimate over the N_t weighted particles which approximate $p(\mathbf{X}_t|\mathbf{Y}_{1:t})$,

$$\hat{\mathbf{X}}_t = \arg\max_{\mathbf{X}_t^{(i)}} p(\mathbf{X}_t^{(i)}|\mathbf{Y}_{1:t})\, for\, i = 1, ..., N_t, \tag{4}$$

where $\mathbf{X}_t^{(i)}$ is the i_{th} particle.

4 Proposed Method

4.1 A Multiple Temporal Scale Framework

To reliably recover the target after occlusion and achieve robustness to non-constant motion, we introduce the concept of learning motion models at a range of model-scales, and applying those over multiple prediction-scales. Furthermore, we contribute a simple but powerful extension of the bootstrap particle filter to search around the predictions generated by the motion models.

The core idea is to construct an improved and rich prior distribution at each time-point by combining sufficient particle sets that at least one set will be valid and allow recovery from occlusion and robustness to non-constant motion. A valid particle set is the most probable mode of an accurate estimation of the posterior probability from some previous time-point, propagated by a motion model generated over an appropriate model-scale and unaffected by occlusion.

Learning and Predicting Motion Over Multiple Temporal Scales. Simple motion models are learned over multiple model-scales and are used to make state predictions over multiple prediction-scales. A simple motion model is characterized by a polynomial function of order d, and represented by $\mathbf{M}$. $\mathbf{M}$ is learned at a given model-scale separately for the x-location, y-location, and scale s of the target's state.[1] This learning also considers how well each state is estimated in a given sequence and how far it is from the most recently estimated state [25]. For instance, an $\mathbf{M}$ of order 1, learned at model-scale m, predicts a target's x-location at time t as:

$$\tilde{x}_t = \beta_o^m + \beta_1^m t, \tag{5}$$

where β_1 is the slope, and β_o the intercept. Model parameters can be learned inexpensively via weighted least squares.

A set of learned motion models at time t is represented by $\mathbf{M}_t^{j=1,\ldots,|\mathbf{M}_t|}$, where $|.|$ is the cardinality of the set. Each model predicts target state $l(\tilde{x}, \tilde{y}, \tilde{s})$ at T prediction-scales. See Figs. 2a and b for an illustration of learning and prediction.

Model Set Reduction. The aim of model set reduction is to establish search regions for the particle filter in which there is a high probability of target being present. This in turn will reduce the sampling effort as search regions corresponding to all the predictions no longer need to be searched.

Suppose there are T sets of motion models available at time t, one from each of T previous time-steps. Each set of models at time t is represented by its corresponding set of predictions. The most suitable motion model from each set is selected as follows.

Let us denote $G = |\mathbf{M}_t|$, and let $\mathbf{l}_t^k = \{l_t^{j,k} | j = 1, ..., G\}$ represent a set of states predicted by G motion models learned at time $t - k$, where $l_t^{j,k}$ denotes

[1] To demonstrate the basic idea of the proposed approach and for the sake of simplicity, x, y, and s part of the target state are considered uncorrelated. They may be correlated, and taking this into account while learning might produce improved models. We would pursue this avenue in future work.

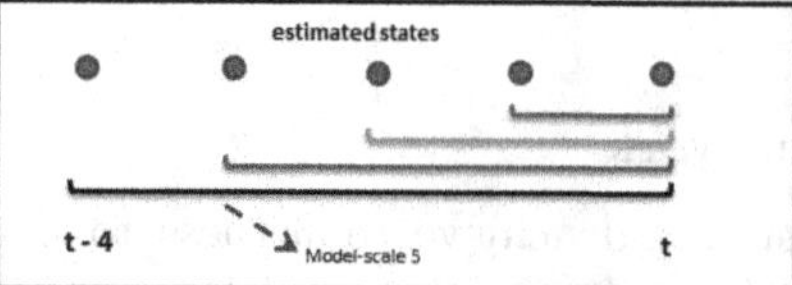

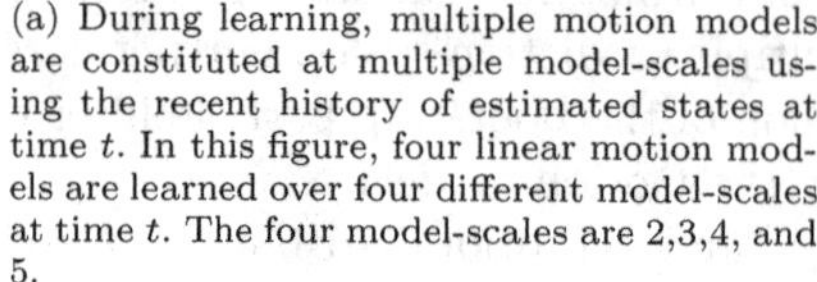

(a) During learning, multiple motion models are constituted at multiple model-scales using the recent history of estimated states at time t. In this figure, four linear motion models are learned over four different model-scales at time t. The four model-scales are 2,3,4, and 5.

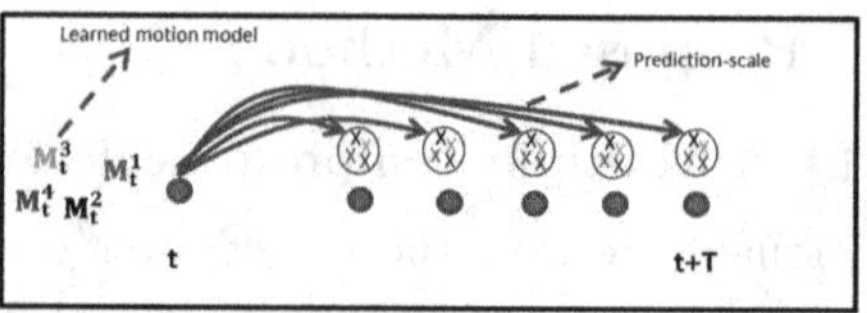

(b) During prediction, a set of learned motion models are used to predict possible target states at T prediction-scales. In this figure, a set comprising four learned motion models is shown at time t. Each motion model predicts possible target state at T prediction-scales.

Fig. 2. Graphical illustration of what happens during learning and prediction.

the predicted state by j_{th} motion model learned at k_{th} previous time-step. As $k = 1, ..., T$, there are T sets of predicted states at time t (Fig. 3(a)). Now the most suitable motion model $\mathbf{R}_t^k$ is selected from each set using the following criterion:

$$\hat{l}_t^k = \arg\max_{l_t^{j,k}} p(\mathbf{Y}_t | l_t^{j,k}) \tag{6}$$

where $\hat{l}_t^k$ is the most suitable state prediction from the set $\mathbf{l}_t^k$, and $p(\mathbf{Y}_t|l_t^{j,k})$ measures the visual likelihood at the predicted state $l_t^{j,k}$. In other words, $\hat{l}_t^k$ is the most suitable state prediction of the most suitable motion model $\mathbf{R}_t^k$. For example, Fig. 3(b) shows the predicted state $\hat{l}_t^1$ of the most suitable motion model $\mathbf{R}_t^1$ chosen from 4 motion models learned at time $t-1$. After this selection process, the T sets of motion models are reduced to T individual models.

Propagation of Particles. In the bootstrap particle filter [35], the posterior probability at time $t-1$ is estimated by a set of particles $\mathbf{X}_{t-1}^{(i)}$ and their weights $\omega_{t-1}^{(i)}, \{\mathbf{X}_{t-1}^{(i)}, \omega_{t-1}^{(i)}\}_{i=1}^N$, such that all the weights in the particle set sum to one. The particles are resampled to form an unweighted representation of the posterior $\{\mathbf{X}_{t-1}^{(i)}, 1/N\}_{i=1}^N$. At time t, they are propagated using the motion model $p(\mathbf{X}_t|\mathbf{X}_{t-1})$ to approximate a prior distribution $p(\mathbf{X}_t|\mathbf{Y}_{t-1})$. Finally, they are weighted according to the observation model $p(\mathbf{Y}_t|\mathbf{X}_t)$, approximating the posterior probability at time t.

Here, particle sets not just from one previous time-step $(t-1)$, but from T previous time-steps are propagated to time t using the T selected motion models. When using first-order polynomial (linear) motion models the most suitable motion model $\mathbf{R}_t^k$ selected from those learnt at the k_{th} previous time-step will propagate a particle set from the k_{th} previous time-step as follows

$$X_{t,k}^x = X_{t-k}^x + g(\mathbf{R}_t^k)k + \mathcal{N}(0, \sigma_x^2 k), \tag{7}$$

where X^x is the horizontal part of the target state, $g()$ indicates the slope of the model, and $\mathcal{N}(0, \sigma_x)$ is a Gaussian distribution with zero-mean and σ_x^2 variance. For instance, in Fig. 3(c), the most suitable motion model $\mathbf{R}_t^1$, is used to propagate a particle set from time $t-1$ to time t.

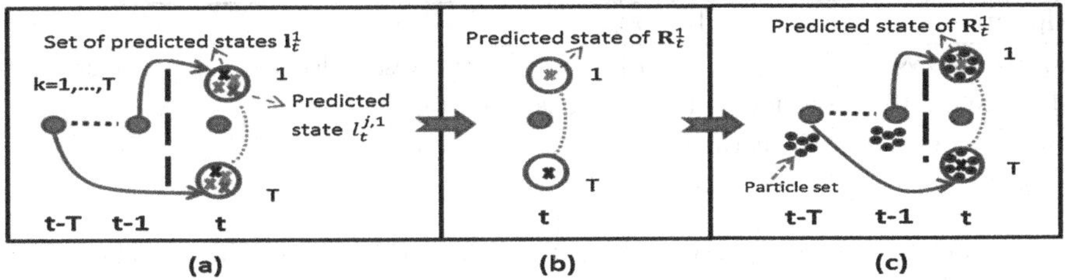

Fig. 3. (a) Before model set reduction, there exist T different sets of predicted states at time t, where each set $\mathbf{l}_t^k$ comprises G states predicted by G motion models learned at k_{th} previous time-step. In Fig. 3(a), $\mathbf{l}_t^1$ is a set composed of 4 states predicted by 4 motion models learned at time $t-1$. (b) **Model Set Reduction.** T sets of motion models available at time t, represented by the corresponding T sets of predicted states, are reduced to T individual models. Figure 3(b) shows the predicted state $\hat{l}_t^1$ of the most suitable motion model $\mathbf{R}_t^1$ selected from 4 motion models learned at time $t-1$. (c) **Propagation of Particles.** T selected motion models, one from each of the T preceding time-steps, are used to propagate particle sets from T preceding time-steps to time t. In Fig. 3(c), the most suitable motion model $\mathbf{R}_t^1$, is used to propagate particle set from time $t-1$ to time t.

Propagation from the last T time-steps, generates T particle sets at time t. All particles are weighted using the observation model $p(\mathbf{Y}_t|\mathbf{X}_t)$ to approximate the posterior probability $p(\mathbf{X}_t|\mathbf{Y}_{1:t})$. If the target was occluded for less than or equal to $T-1$ frames, it may be recovered by a set of particles unaffected by the occlusion. To focus on particles with large weights, and reduce computational cost, we retain the first N particles after the resampling step. The proposed framework is summarised in Algorithm 1.

5 Experimental Results

In the proposed method, the appearance model used in all experiments was the colour histogram used in [36].[2] The Bhattacharyya coefficient was used as the distance measure. As simple motion model the first-order polynomial (linear) model with model-scales of 2, 3, 4, and 5 frames was used (four models in total).

MTS-L denotes the proposed method applied over a first-order polynomial (linear) motion model (Algorithm 1). We also apply our proposed framework to the two-stage model of [25], which is denoted by MTS-TS, to show its generality[3].

[2] We investigate the power of using multiple temporal scales of motion model generation and application to deal with visual tracking problems related to occlusion and abrupt motion variation. To evaluate this hypothesis independently of the appearance model, a simple appearance model is used on purpose.

[3] MTS-TS is identical to MTS-L except that the propagation of particles takes place through a different model instead of the model proposed in Eq. 7 and the variance of the best state (estimated through particles) is reduced by combining it with the highest likelihood motion prediction. See the supplementary material for the details of this application.

Algorithm 1. A Multiple Temporal Scale Tracker

Input: Let $\mathbf{W} = \{W_{t-1}, ..., W_{t-T}\}$ represent the resampled sets of particles after estimation of the posterior from T previous time-steps, where $W_{t-1} = \{\mathbf{X}_{t-1}^{(i)}, \frac{1}{N}\}_{i=1}^{N}$.
Output: Best state $\hat{\mathbf{X}}_t$ at time t.

for $k = 1$ *to* T
  for $j = 1$ *to* G
    - Measure visual likelihood $p(\mathbf{Y}_t | l_t^{j,k})$, where $l_t^{j,k}$ denotes the predicted state at time t by j_{th} motion model from k_{th} previous time-step.
  end
  - Select the most suitable motion model $\mathbf{R}_t^k$ at time t using Eq. 6.
  - Propagate the particle set from k_{th} previous time-step $W_{t-k} = \{\mathbf{X}_{t-k}^{(i)}, \frac{1}{N}\}_{i=1}^{N}$ using Eq. 7 by taking the slope of selected motion model $\mathbf{R}_t^k$ to time t.
end
- Assign weights to all the particles to approximate the posterior $\{\mathbf{X}_t^{(i)}, \omega_t^{(i)}\}_{i=1}^{N \times T}$.
- Calculate the best state $\hat{\mathbf{X}}_t$ using Eq. 4.
- Retain first N particles after the resampling step.
- Learn simple motion models using the recent history of estimated states.

In MTS-TS, the β parameter of the two-stage model was fixed at 10, giving high weight to the rigid velocity $\hat{v}$, estimated by the simple motion model, and very low weight to the internal velocity v. As a result, it becomes strongly biased towards the predicted location, but still allows some deviation.

We compared the proposed method to three baseline and seven state-of-the-art trackers. The first two baseline trackers, T_{RW} and T_{NCV}, were colour based particle filters from [36], but use different motion models. T_{RW} used a random-walk model while T_{NCV} used a nearly constant velocity model. The third baseline tracker T_{TS} was the two-stage dynamic model proposed by [25]. The parameters, K and β, in [25] were set to 5 and 10, respectively. The state-of-the-art trackers are SCM [37], ASLA [38], L1-APG [12], VTD [5], FragT [9], SemiBoost [21], and WLMCMC [30]. The minimum and maximum number of samples used for WLMCMC, VTD, SCM, ASLA, and L1-APG was 600 and 640, respectively. Our proposed tracker is implemented in MATLAB and runs at about 3 frames/sec with 640 particles. The source code and datasets (along with ground truth annotations) will be made available on the authors' webpages.

We chose state-of-the-art trackers keeping in view two important properties: their performance according to the CVPR'13 benchmark [39], and their ability to handle occlusions (partial and full) and abrupt motion variations. SCM and ASLA both have top ranked performance on the CVPR'13 benchmark. SCM combines a sparsity based classifier with a sparsity based generative model and has a occlusion handling mechanism, while ASLA is based on a local sparse appearance model and is robust to partial occlusions. In L1-APG, the coupling of L1 norm minimization and an explicit occlusion detection mechanism makes it robust to partial as well as full occlusions. The integration of two motion models having different variances with a mixture of template-based object models lets VTD explore a relatively large search space, while remaining robust to a wide

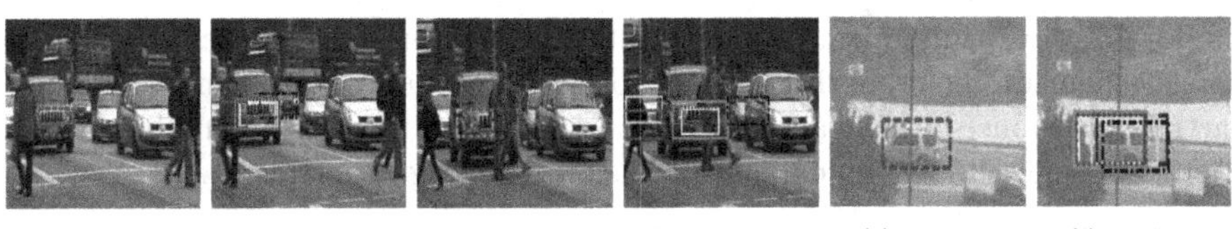

(a) TU-Cr♯46 (b) TU-Cr♯46 (c) TU-Cr♯124 (d) TU-Cr♯124 (e) car♯169 (f) car♯169

Fig. 4. Tracking through multiple partial occlusions. MTS-TS(magenta), MTS-L (cyan), SCM(green) FragT(white), Semi(yellow), L1-APG(blue), VTD(red), WLMCMC (black), and ASLA(purple) (Color figure online).

range of appearance variations. FragT was chosen because its rich, patch-based representation makes it robust to partial occlusion. SemiBoost was picked as it searches the whole image space once its tracker loses target, and thus, it can re-locate the target after full occlusions. WLMCMC searches the whole image space by combining an efficient sampling strategy with an annealing procedure that allows it to capture abrupt motion variations quite accurately and re-locate the target after full occlusions.

Eleven video sequences were used. Seven are publicly available (*PETS 2001 Dataset 1*[4], *TUD-Campus* [40], *TUD-Crossing* [40], *Person* [41], *car*[5] [39], *jogging* [39], and *PETS 2009 Dataset S2*[6]) and four are our own (*squash*, *ball1*,*ball2*, and *toy1*). All involve frequent short and long term occlusions (partial and full) and/or variations in target motion. We used three metrics for evaluation: centre location error, Pascal score [42], and precision at a fixed threshold of 20 pixels [43].

5.1 Comparison with Competing Methods

Quantitative Evaluation: Table 1 summarises tracking accuracy obtained from sequences in which the target is occluded. MTS-L outperformed competing methods in most sequences, because it efficiently allocated particles to overcome occlusions. VTD performed badly because inappropriate appearance model updates during longer occlusions causes drift from which it cannot recover. Although SemiBoost uses explicit re-detection once the target is lost, its accuracy was low due to false positive detections. With the ability to search the whole image space using an efficient sampling scheme, WLMCMC produced the lowest error in the *TUD-Campus* and *jogging* sequences. In sequences containing partial occlusions (Fig. 4), SCM produced the lowest error in the *car* sequence, while both SCM and L1-APG had the best performance in the *TUD-Crossing* sequence. SCM uses a sparse based generative model that considers spatial relationship among local patches with an occlusion handling scheme, and L1-APG

[4] *PETS 2001 Dataset 1* is available from http://ftp.pets.rdg.ac.uk/.
[5] We downsampled original *car* sequence by a factor of 3 to have partially low frame rate.
[6] *PETS 2009 Dataset S2* is available from http://www.cvg.rdg.ac.uk/PETS2009/.

employs a robust minimization model influenced by an explicit occlusion detection mechanism. Thus, both these approaches are quite effective in overcoming partial occlusions. In contrast, MTS-L and MTS-TS use a very simple, generic appearance model, and no explicit occlusion handling mechanism[7].

Table 1. Tracking accuracy in the presence of occlusion

(a) Mean centre location error in pixels is given, averaged over all frames of all videos showing occlusions. Each tracker was run five times and the results were averaged. The best results are marked in bold. T denotes the prediction-scales, and N is the number of particles propagated from $t-k$ to t in our proposed method. N is fixed at 20, and N_t is the total number of particles accumulated at time t in our proposed method. The number of particles used in baseline trackers was equal to N_t.

Sequence	SCM	ASLA	L1	VTD	Semi	FragT	WL	T_{NCV}	T_{RW}	T_{TS}	MTS-L	MTS-TS	T	N_t=N×T
ball2	76	71	71	66	78	106	37	91	71	125	17	**16**	32	640
TUD-Camp	186	180	100	186	61	112	**22**	141	119	31	24	**22**	9	180
TUD-Cross	**2**	6	**2**	63	62	5	50	43	75	106	25	21	25	500
PETS 2001	61	63	60	83	114	67	90	43	131	112	25	**21**	32	640
Person	91	80	103	85	177	84	25	90	33	95	10	**8**	20	400
PETS 2009	35	13	81	94	29	10	91	75	37	56	7	**6**	14	280
car	**8**	31	31	47	38	15	28	37	43	87	25	25	20	400
toy1	88	85	111	98	99	107	30	74	134	76	**21**	22	30	600
jogging	110	104	45	70	30	94	**19**	27	24	100	25	24	20	400

(b) A(B): A - the percentage of correctly tracked frames based on Pascal Score [42]; B - Precision at a fixed threshold of 20 pixels. Pascal score is computed by assessing to what extent the tracking template overlaps the ground truth template as a ratio. If the Pascal score is greater than 0.5 in a certain frame, that frame is counted as a correctly tracked frame. Precision is computed by dividing the number of frames, where estimated target location was not beyond the fixed threshold distance of 20 pixels of the ground truth, by the total number of frames in a video sequence. The best results are marked in bold.

Sequence	SCM	ASLA	L1	VTD	Semi	FragT	WL	MTS-L	MTS-TS
ball2	12(0.21)	9(0.17)	7(0.21)	9(0.11)	7(0.13)	9(0.09)	28(0.53)	31(0.8)	**36(0.8)**
TUD-Camp	14(0.17)	10(0.14)	19(0.21)	25(0.25)	38(0.34)	27(0.27)	46(**0.61**)	55(0.57)	**57**(0.46)
TUD-Cross	**100(1)**	99(0.9)	**100(1)**	24(0.23)	41(0.42)	87(1)	25(0.23)	61(0.59)	69(0.65)
PETS 2001	23(0.33)	23(0.27)	22(0.25)	20(0.25)	17(0.2)	16(0.31)	19(0.52)	58(0.65)	**66(0.7)**
Person	45(0.46)	44(0.45)	10(0.12)	43(0.45)	20(0.2)	38(0.41)	49(0.86)	79(0.93)	**80(0.94)**
PETS 2009	26(0.36)	36(0.7)	21(0.26)	21(0.21)	27(0.45)	65(0.73)	7(0.23)	70(0.97)	**71(0.96)**
car	**92(0.93)**	62(0.64)	66(0.65)	66(0.65)	55(0.46)	80(0.76)	62(0.52)	71(0.72)	73(0.72)
toy1	18(0.19)	19(0.2)	15(0.15)	16(0.18)	16(0.18)	3(0.09)	**49(0.8)**	43(0.8)	38(0.78)
jogging	21(0.22)	22(0.22)	21(0.21)	22(0.22)	**60(0.61)**	21(0.21)	42(**0.61**)	20(0.44)	21(0.45)

Tracking accuracy was also measured when the target was occluded and underwent motion variation at the same time (Tables 2a and b). MTS-L produced higher accuracy than the other methods. The allocation of particle sets with different spreads from multiple prediction scales in regions having probable local maxima lets MTS-L capture increased search space with relatively smaller sampling effort. VTD performed well in *squash* sequence because it combines two motion models of different variances to form multiple basic trackers which search a large state space efficiently. WLMCMC produced the second best accuracy on *ball1* as it searches the whole image space using an efficient sampling mechanism to capture abrupt target motion.

[7] We admit that a more complex system complete with more advanced appearance models would obtain a higher overall tracking accuracy, but we believe that for the sake of scientific evidence finding employing such a system would obfuscate attribution of our experimental results to the original hypothesis.

Table 2. Accuracy through simultaneous motion variation and occlusion

(a) Mean centre location error (pixels).

Sequence	SCM	ASLA	L1	VTD	Semi	FragT	WL	T_{NCV}	T_{RW}	T_{TS}	MTS-L	MTS-TS	T	N_t=N×T
squash	40	34	60	20	68	35	22	27	52	41	12	**10**	5	100
ball1	91	96	124	69	66	188	23	74	87	98	15	**14**	14	280

(b) A(B): A - the percentage of correctly tracked frames based on Pascal Score; B - Precision at a fixed threshold of 20 pixels.

Sequence	SCM	ASLA	L1	VTD	Semi	FragT	WL	MTS-L	MTS-TS
squash	60(0.62)	38(0.56)	9(0.11)	68(0.78)	44(0.7)	37(0.5)	50(0.75)	71(0.92)	**75(0.96)**
ball1	6(0.06)	3(0.04)	2(0.05)	19(0.22)	19(0.33)	2(0.02)	35(0.79)	40(0.83)	**41(0.89)**

Qualitative Evaluation: Tracking is particularly difficult when the time between consecutive occlusions is small. In *TUD-Campus*, the tracked person suffers two occlusions only 17 frames apart (Fig. 5a). MTS-L and WLMCMC recover the target after each occlusion, while other methods fail due to incorrect appearance model updates, or being distracted by the surrounding clutter. Video surveillance data often requires tracking through partial and/or full occlusions. In the *PETS 2001 Dataset 1* sequence (Fig. 5b) the target (car) first stays partially occluded for a considerable time, and is then completely occluded by a tree. MTS-L successfully re-acquires the target. Occlusions of varying lengths are common in real-world tracking scenarios. In the *person* sequence, a person moves behind several trees and is shot with a moving camera. As shown in Fig. 6, competing methods lose the target after first occlusion(Frame # 238) or second occlusion(Frame # 329), while MTS-L shows robustness in coping with varying lengths of occlusions.

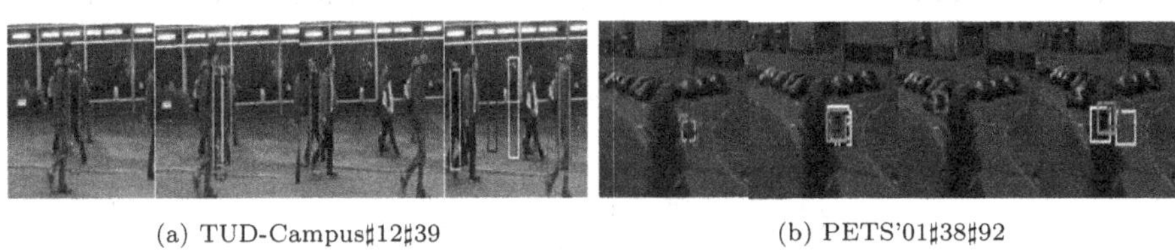

(a) TUD-Campus♯12♯39 (b) PETS'01♯38♯92

Fig. 5. Tracking results in a crowded (a) and a surveillance environment (b).

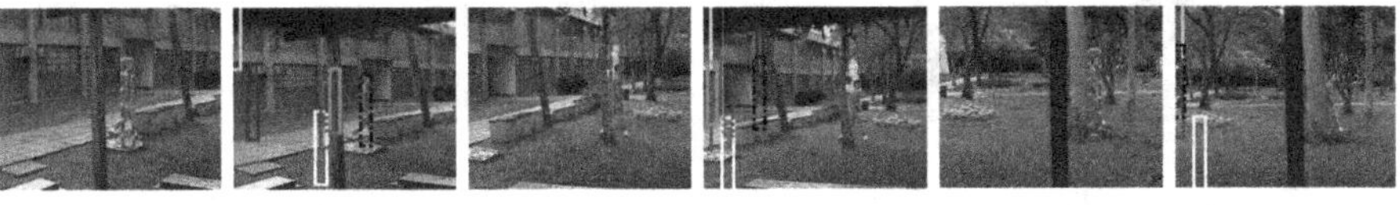

(a) Person♯238 (b) Person♯238 (c) Person♯329 (d) Person♯329 (e) Person♯457 (f) Person♯457

Fig. 6. Tracking results with occlusions of different lengths.

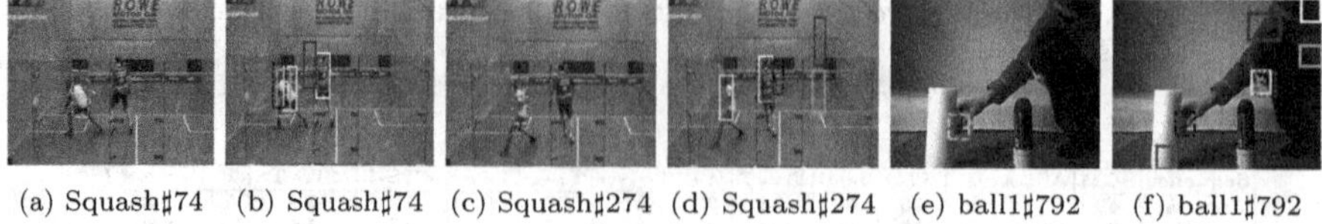

(a) Squash♯74 (b) Squash♯74 (c) Squash♯274 (d) Squash♯274 (e) ball1♯792 (f) ball1♯792

Fig. 7. Tracking results in case of motion variations and frequent occlusions.

The ability of MTS-L to cope with simultaneous occlusion and non-constant target motion was tested by making two challenging sequences: *squash* and *ball1*. In these sequences, the target accelerates, decelerates, changes direction suddenly, and is completely occluded multiple times. Figure 7 illustrates tracking results. MTS-L provided more accurate tracking than the other methods on both sequences. This is because the efficient allocation of particles at multiple prediction-scales allows a wider range of target motion to be handled. WLM-CMC shows good accuracy in the *ball1* sequence as it is aimed at handling abrupt target motion.

5.2 Analysis of the Proposed Framework

Without Multiple Prediction-Scales. The proposed framework was tested without employing multiple prediction-scales. We designed MTSWPS-L in which the target state is predicted only 1 frame ahead i.e. $T = 1$. For evaluation, at first, the number of particles in MTSWPS-L was kept equal to N_t and the process noise σ_{xy} was same as used for MTS-L between two consecutive time-steps. To analyze further, later, both the number of particles N_t and the process noise σ_{xy} were doubled and tripled. Figure 8(left) reveals the performance of the proposed framework with and without multiple prediction-scales in five video sequences

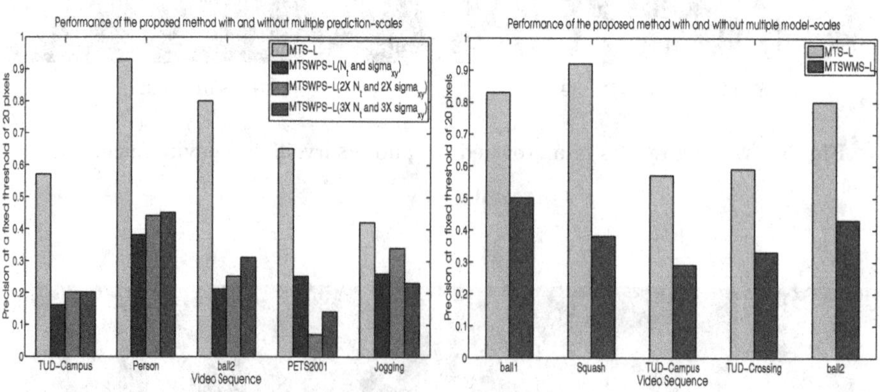

Fig. 8. (left)Performance of the proposed framework with and without multiple prediction-scales. (right)Performance of the proposed framework with and without multiple model-scales.

involving occlusions. As can be seen, MTSWPS-L has poor performance compared to MTS-L in all 5 sequences even after increasing the sampling effort and the process noise by three times of the original. Therefore, we can say that operation over multiple prediction-scales allows the proposed method to reliably handle occlusions in a principled way.

Without Multiple Model-Scales. The proposed framework was also analyzed without learning over multiple model-scales. MTSWMS-L denotes the proposed framework in which a linear motion model is learned over model-scale 2 only. As a result, there is no need to select models from each of the previous time-steps at the current time-step since only 1 model is learned over a single model-scale. As can be seen in Fig. 8(right), MTS-L has superior performance over MTSWMS-L in all 5 sequences. This shows that by constructing motion models over multiple model-scales MTS-L maintains a richer description of the target's path, which is not possible with a single scale model. Furthermore, this diverse set of models produces temporal priors that ultimately develops into a rich prior distribution required for reliably recovery of tracking after occlusions.

Experimental results show the robust performance of the proposed framework during occlusions, but it can fail when faced with very long duration occlusions. In addition, it can be distracted by visually similar objects after occlusion, if the state estimations during the period of occlusion are poor.

6 Conclusion

We propose a tracking framework that combines motion models learned over multiple model-scales and applied over multiple prediction-scales to handle occlusion and variation in target motion. The core idea is to combine sufficient particle sets at each time-point that at least one set will be valid, and allow recovery from occlusion and/or motion variation. These particle sets are not, however, simply spread widely across the image: each represents an estimation of the posterior probability from some previous time-point, predicted by a motion model generated over an appropriate model-scale.

The proposed method has shown superior performance over competing trackers in challenging tracking environments. That there is little difference between results obtained using linear and two-stage motion models suggests that this high level of performance is due to the framework, rather than its components.

References

1. Yin, Z., Collins, R.T.: Object tracking and detection after occlusion via numerical hybrid local and global mode-seeking. In: IEEE Conference on Computer Vision and Pattern Recognition, CVPR 2008, pp. 1–8. IEEE (2008)
2. Lerdsudwichai, C., Abdel-Mottaleb, M., Ansari, A.: Tracking multiple people with recovery from partial and total occlusion. Pattern Recogn. **38**, 1059–1070 (2005)
3. Kwak, S., Nam, W., Han, B., Han, J.H.: Learning occlusion with likelihoods for visual tracking. In: 2011 IEEE International Conference on Computer Vision (ICCV), pp. 1551–1558. IEEE (2011)

4. Ross, D.A., Lim, J., Lin, R.S., Yang, M.H.: Incremental learning for robust visual tracking. Int. J. Comput. Vis. **77**, 125–141 (2008)
5. Kwon, J., Lee, K.M.: Visual tracking decomposition. In: 2010 IEEE Conference on Computer Vision and Pattern Recognition (CVPR), pp. 1269–1276. IEEE (2010)
6. Okuma, K., Taleghani, A., de Freitas, N., Little, J.J., Lowe, D.G.: A boosted particle filter: multitarget detection and tracking. In: Pajdla, T., Matas, J.G. (eds.) ECCV 2004. LNCS, vol. 3021, pp. 28–39. Springer, Heidelberg (2004)
7. Naeem, A., Pridmore, T.P., Mills, S.: Managing particle spread via hybrid particle filter/kernel mean shift tracking. In: BMVC, pp. 1–10 (2007)
8. Kwon, J., Lee, K.M.: Tracking by sampling trackers. In: 2011 IEEE International Conference on Computer Vision (ICCV), pp. 1195–1202. IEEE (2011)
9. Adam, A., Rivlin, E., Shimshoni, I.: Robust fragments-based tracking using the integral histogram. In: 2006 IEEE Computer Society Conference on Computer Vision and Pattern Recognition, vol. 1, pp. 798–805. IEEE (2006)
10. Han, B., Davis, L.S.: Probabilistic fusion-based parameter estimation for visual tracking. Comput. Vis. Image Underst. **113**, 435–445 (2009)
11. Mei, X., Ling, H., Wu, Y., Blasch, E., Bai, L.: Minimum error bounded efficient l1 tracker with occlusion detection. In: 2011 IEEE Conference on Computer Vision and Pattern Recognition (CVPR), pp. 1257–1264. IEEE (2011)
12. Bao, C., Wu, Y., Ling, H., Ji, H.: Real time robust l1 tracker using accelerated proximal gradient approach. In: 2012 IEEE Conference on Computer Vision and Pattern Recognition (CVPR), pp. 1830–1837. IEEE (2012)
13. Lim, H., Camps, O.I., Sznaier, M., Morariu, V.I.: Dynamic appearance modeling for human tracking. In: 2006 IEEE Computer Society Conference on Computer Vision and Pattern Recognition, vol. 1, pp. 751–757. IEEE (2006)
14. Sudderth, E.B., Mandel, M.I., Freeman, W.T., Willsky, A.S.: Distributed occlusion reasoning for tracking with nonparametric belief propagation. In: Advances in Neural Information Processing Systems, pp. 1369–1376 (2004)
15. Dockstader, S.L., Tekalp, A.M.: Multiple camera tracking of interacting and occluded human motion. Proc. IEEE **89**, 1441–1455 (2001)
16. Fleuret, F., Berclaz, J., Lengagne, R., Fua, P.: Multicamera people tracking with a probabilistic occupancy map. IEEE Trans. Pattern Anal. Mach. Intell. **30**, 267–282 (2008)
17. Grabner, H., Matas, J., Van Gool, L., Cattin, P.: Tracking the invisible: Learning where the object might be. In: 2010 IEEE Conference on Computer Vision and Pattern Recognition (CVPR), pp. 1285–1292. IEEE (2010)
18. Yang, M., Wu, Y., Hua, G.: Context-aware visual tracking. IEEE Trans. Pattern Anal. Mach. Intell. **31**, 1195–1209 (2009)
19. Dinh, T.B., Vo, N., Medioni, G.: Context tracker: Exploring supporters and distracters in unconstrained environments. In: 2011 IEEE Conference on Computer Vision and Pattern Recognition (CVPR), pp. 1177–1184. IEEE (2011)
20. Kalal, Z., Mikolajczyk, K., Matas, J.: Tracking-learning-detection. IEEE Trans. Pattern Anal. Mach. Intell. **34**, 1409–1422 (2012)
21. Grabner, H., Leistner, C., Bischof, H.: Semi-supervised on-line boosting for robust tracking. In: Forsyth, D., Torr, P., Zisserman, A. (eds.) ECCV 2008, Part I. LNCS, vol. 5302, pp. 234–247. Springer, Heidelberg (2008)
22. Perez, P., Vermaak, J., Blake, A.: Data fusion for visual tracking with particles. Proc. IEEE **92**, 495–513 (2004)
23. Shan, C., Tan, T., Wei, Y.: Real-time hand tracking using a mean shift embedded particle filter. Pattern Recogn. **40**, 1958–1970 (2007)

24. Pernkopf, F.: Tracking of multiple targets using online learning for reference model adaptation. IEEE Trans. Syst. Man Cybern., B **38**, 1465–1475 (2008)
25. Kristan, M., Kovačič, S., Leonardis, A., Perš, J.: A two-stage dynamic model for visual tracking. IEEE Trans. Syst. Man Cybern. B **40**, 1505–1520 (2010)
26. Isard, M., Blake, A.: A mixed-state condensation tracker with automatic model-switching. In: Sixth International Conference on Computer Vision, pp. 107–112. IEEE (1998)
27. Madrigal, F., Rivera, M., Hayet, J.-B.: Learning and regularizing motion models for enhancing particle filter-based target tracking. In: Ho, Y.-S. (ed.) PSIVT 2011, Part II. LNCS, vol. 7088, pp. 287–298. Springer, Heidelberg (2011)
28. Pavlovic, V., Rehg, J.M., MacCormick, J.: Learning switching linear models of human motion. In: NIPS, Citeseer, pp. 981–987 (2000)
29. Cifuentes, C.G., Sturzel, M., Jurie, F., Brostow, G.J., et al.: Motion models that only work sometimes. In: British Machive Vision Conference (2012)
30. Kwon, J., Lee, K.M.: Tracking of abrupt motion using wang-landau monte carlo estimation. In: Forsyth, D., Torr, P., Zisserman, A. (eds.) ECCV 2008, Part I. LNCS, vol. 5302, pp. 387–400. Springer, Heidelberg (2008)
31. Hong, S., Kwak, S., Han, B.: Orderless tracking through model-averaged posterior estimation. In: 2013 IEEE International Conference on Computer Vision (ICCV), pp. 2296–2303. IEEE (2013)
32. Zhou, X., Lu, Y., Lu, J., Zhou, J.: Abrupt motion tracking via intensively adaptive markov-chain monte carlo sampling. IEEE Trans. Image Process. **21**, 789–801 (2012)
33. Mikami, D., Otsuka, K., Yamato, J.: Memory-based particle filter for face pose tracking robust under complex dynamics. In: IEEE Conference on Computer Vision and Pattern Recognition, CVPR 2009, pp. 999–1006. IEEE (2009)
34. Li, Y., Ai, H., Lao, S., et al.: Tracking in low frame rate video: A cascade particle filter with discriminative observers of different lifespans. In: 2007 IEEE Conference on Computer Vision and Pattern Recognition, pp. 1–8 (2007)
35. Arulampalam, M., Maskell, S., Gordon, N., Clapp, T.: A tutorial on particle filters for online nonlinear/non-gaussian bayesian tracking. IEEE Trans. Signal. Proc. **50**, 174–188 (2002)
36. Pérez, P., Hue, C., Vermaak, J., Gangnet, M.: Color-based probabilistic tracking. In: Heyden, A., Sparr, G., Nielsen, M., Johansen, P. (eds.) ECCV 2002, Part I. LNCS, vol. 2350, pp. 661–675. Springer, Heidelberg (2002)
37. Zhong, W., Lu, H., Yang, M.H.: Robust object tracking via sparsity-based collaborative model. In: 2012 IEEE Conference on Computer Vision and Pattern Recognition (CVPR), pp. 1838–1845. IEEE (2012)
38. Jia, X., Lu, H., Yang, M.H.: Visual tracking via adaptive structural local sparse appearance model. In: 2012 IEEE Conference on Computer Vision and Pattern Recognition (CVPR), pp. 1822–1829. IEEE (2012)
39. Wu, Y., Lim, J., Yang, M.H.: Online object tracking: A benchmark. In: 2013 IEEE Conference on Computer Vision and Pattern Recognition (CVPR), pp. 2411–2418. IEEE (2013)
40. Andriluka, M., Roth, S., Schiele, B.: People-tracking-by-detection and people-detection-by-tracking. In: IEEE Conference on Computer Vision and Pattern Recognition, CVPR 2008, pp. 1–8. IEEE (2008)
41. Dihl, L., Jung, C.R., Bins, J.: Robust adaptive patch-based object tracking using weighted vector median filters. In: 2011 24th SIBGRAPI Conference on Graphics, Patterns and Images (Sibgrapi), pp. 149–156. IEEE (2011)

42. Santner, J., Leistner, C., Saffari, A., Pock, T., Bischof, H.: Prost: Parallel robust online simple tracking. In: 2010 IEEE Conference on Computer Vision and Pattern Recognition (CVPR), pp. 723–730. IEEE (2010)
43. Babenko, B., Yang, M.H., Belongie, S.: Visual tracking with online multiple instance learning. In: IEEE Conference on Computer Vision and Pattern Recognition, CVPR 2009, pp. 983–990. IEEE (2009)

Video Annotation by Incremental Learning from Grouped Heterogeneous Sources

Han Wang(✉), Hao Song, Xinxiao Wu, and Yunde Jia

Beijing Lab of Intelligent Information Technology and the School of Computer Science, Beijing Institute of Technology, Beijing 100081, China
wanghan@bjfu.edu.cn, {songhao,wuxinxiao,jiayunde}@bit.edu.cn

Abstract. Transfer learning has shown promising results in leveraging loosely labeled Web images (source domain) to learn a robust classifier for the unlabeled consumer videos (target domain). Existing transfer learning methods typically apply source domain data to learn a fixed model for predicting target domain data once and for all, ignoring rapidly updating Web data and continuously changes of users requirements. We propose an incremental transfer learning framework, in which heterogeneous knowledge are integrated and incrementally added to update the target classifier during learning process. Under the framework, images (image source domain) queried from Web image search engine and videos (video source domain) from existing action datasets are adopted to provide static information and motion information of the target video, respectively. For the image source domain, images are partitioned into several groups according to their semantic information. And for the video source domain, videos are divided in the same way. Unlike traditional methods which measure relevance between the source group and the whole target domain videos, the group weights in this paper are treated as latent variables for each target domain video and learned automatically according to the probability distribution difference between the individual source group and target domain videos. Experimental results on the two challenging video datasets (*i.e.*, CCV and Kodak) demonstrate the effectiveness of our proposed method.

1 Introduction

The rise of personal hand-held cameras and video sharing websites such as YouTube has resulted in massive amounts of consumer videos online. The ability to rapidly analyze and annotate the event from these unconstrained videos is a challenging computer vision task due to three main issues. First, these videos are generally captured by mobile devices at random and thus containing considerable camera motion, occlusion, cluttered background, and large intraclass variation, making the videos within the same type of event appear different and less discriminant. Second, the labels of these videos are usually meaningless due to users' random noting and subjective understanding, posing a great challenge to traditional learning methods which requires sufficient labeled videos to learn robust event classifiers. Third, the data on the internet updated every second,

D. Cremers et al. (Eds.): ACCV 2014, Part V, LNCS 9007, pp. 493–507, 2015.
DOI: 10.1007/978-3-319-16814-2_32

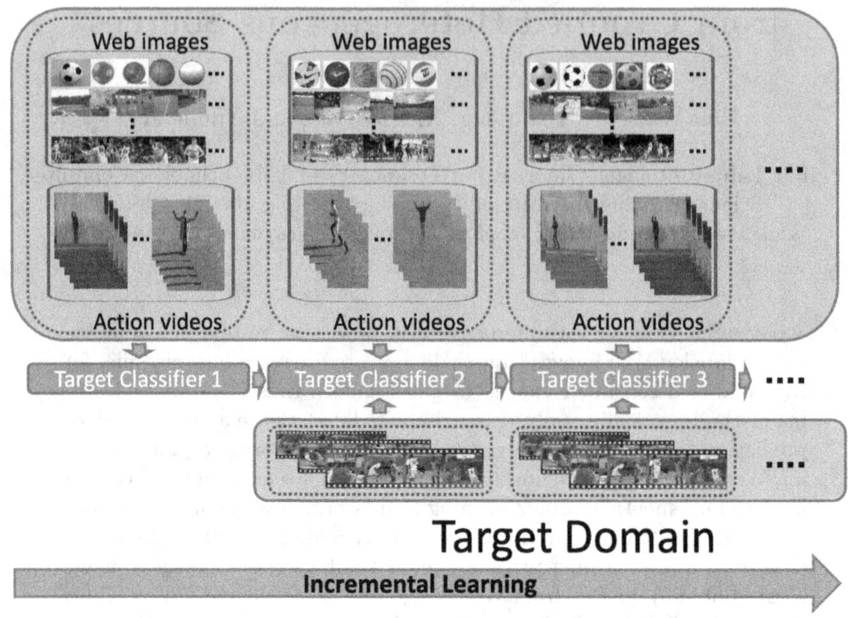

Fig. 1. Illustration of our framework.

and fixed model trained on the pre-defined data may not work well for predicting new coming data. How to acquire sufficient knowledge while freeing the labor from burdensome annotation process is an important problem for event annotation in consumer videos.

Many researchers have tried to seek other sources of labeled data and transfer the related knowledge from these data to videos [1–4]. Most of previous work focuses on learning a fix model from a set of predefined images or videos (source domain) to predict the events in the complex videos (target domain). It is natural to ask if such fixed models would work well in the scenario that the Web data changes with each passing day. To deal with the fast updating of the source data, we propose a novel incremental learning framework for consumer video annotation. Under the framework, the classifiers learned on the source domains can be incrementally updated to capture the changes of both source and target domains and thereby facilitate the annotation task of real-world videos.

In this paper, we propose to acquire the source knowledge from the increasingly mature Web image search engines as well as existing labeled action datasets (e.g. KTH [5] and Weizmann [6]), which is based on the following observations: (1) the duration of videos on the Web are relatively long, so it will take more time and labor to analyze a video than an image. Obviously, it is more efficient to query images from the Web than directly search videos from the Web; (2) Besides the static information provided by Web images, temporal information provided by action videos is also beneficial for recognizing some key actions in consumer videos; (3) The action videos in the two datasets are relatively simple (the time spend on these videos is relatively less) but can provide basic human action information (e.g., running, waving) for complex social event; (4) All the action video datasets are well labeled by researchers and do not need additional labeling efforts.

Though it is beneficial to learn from Web images and action datasets, noise knowledge of little relevance with consumer videos still exists due to random noting and subjective understanding. To handle this negative transfer, we propose to organize the source samples in groups, and each group stands for one event-related semantic concept. Given the groups for each event class, we can leverage these groups by assigning different weights to different groups according to their relevance to target domain data. Besides irrelevant source domain data, the intra-class variation of the target domain videos also must not be overlooked. In other words, one piece of knowledge which is irrelevant to one video may be useful to identify another video, even through both videos belonging to the same event class. To deal with above problem, the relevance between the source and the target should be measured not only according to the event class variation but also to the video itself. In this paper, we measure the relevance between a set of the source groups and an individual target domain sample, the relevance are described by using group weights. Instead of fix the group weight for every target domain sample, we treat the weights as latent variables and try to optimize the group weights and the group templates simultaneously in a latent structural learning framework.

As mentioned before, the knowledge on the Web is updating rapidly, one cannot learn a fixed model for consumer video annotation once and for all. The emerging images and videos make the fixed model hard to be well generalized. Besides changes of the Web data, continuously changes of users' needs also require updating the classifiers for annotating videos. An incremental transfer learning work is introduced by acquiring new knowledge of new added data from both the source and target domain while retaining the knowledge learned before. Our incremental transfer learning work is based on a latent structural model which minimizes the difference in a marginal probability measure between the new added source and target domain data. To make the learned model more stable on target domain data, we biasing the new target classifier close to the hyperplanes of old ones during incremental process. At the same time, smooth assumptions on two regularizers and different groups are imposed to enhance the target classifier more adaptable to the target domain data.

Figure 1 illustrates the framework of our method. The contributions of this paper are three folds. (1) We develop a principle framework for annotating consumer videos by incrementally updating the model using heterogenous sources. (2) We propose a latent structural model by treating the groups weights as latent variables to capture the relevance between the source domain groups and the target domain samples. (3) We introduce two constraints in our incremental learning process by biasing the hyperplane on the target domain close to those learn earlier.

1.1 Related Work

Recently, applying domain adaptation to multimedia content analysis has attracted more attentions [1–4]. Yang *et al.* [7] proposed an Adaptive SVM method to learn a new SVM classifier for the target domain, which is adapted from a pre-trained classifier from a source domain. Duan *et al.* [8] proposed to simultaneously learn the optimal linear combination of base kernels and the target classifier by minimizing a regularized structural risk function. And then, they proposed A-MKL [9] to add the pre-learned classifiers as the prior. Their methods mainly focus on the single source domain setting. To utilize numerous labeled source domain data, multiple source domain adaptation methods [4,10–12] are proposed to leverage different pre-computed classifiers learned from multiple source domains. In these methods, different weights are assigned to different source domains without taking account of intrinsic semantic relations between source domains. In this paper, we propose leveraging different groups of source domain training data according to their semantic meanings. We insure that the data in each group are of the same concept, and different groups within the same event are correlated to each other.

Several recent methods have been proposed to investigate the knowledge transform from Heterogeneous domain adaptation methods. In [13], Web images are incrementally collected to learn classifiers for action video recognition. Tang *et al.* [14] introduced a novel self-paced domain adaptation algorithm to iteratively adapt the detector from source images to target videos. Duan *et al.* [4] developed a domain selection method to select the most relevant source domains. In these existing works, the pre-learned classifiers are primarily using training data from different source domains and then the target classifiers are learned from pre-learned classifiers in a late-fuse fashion. In contrast, our work can simultaneously learn the optimal classifiers and weights of different source-domain groups to construct the target classifier in an incremental way. [15] is closely related to our work, which deals with heterogeneous feature spaces and aims at transferring knowledge from labeled source domain images and videos to unlabeled target domain videos. However, in our method group weights are treated as latent variables which can explicitly describe the contribution of different groups for different target domain samples.

2 Problem Setting and Definitions

To obtain the Web images of the image source domain, we first manually define a semantic concept collection as $\mathcal{C} = \{C_1, C_2, ..., C_G\}$, where C_i represents one event-related concept. In this paper, we use 73 semantic concept keywords, including event names (e.g. "play basketball"), action related concepts (e.g. "waving"), object related concepts (e.g. "ball"), and scene related concepts (e.g. "basketball court"). For each concept, a group of images are collected by querying a keyword to the Web image search engine. And for action videos in the video source domain, videos are clustered into groups according to their action labels in the corresponding datasets (e.g. "waving", "running", etc.). The image source domain and video source domain form the source domain. Following this grouping strategy, and G groups of heterogeneous data including web images and action videos consist the source domain, and each group is represented by one type of features (i.e. image feature for the image source domain or motion feature for the video source domain). As for the target domain, each consumer video is represented by two types of feature: motion features (i.e. STIP features) extracted from the whole video, as well as image features (i.e. SIFT features) extracted from the keyframes.

Formally, for each event class, we are given a set of groups $\{(x^s_{g_i}, y^s_{g_i})|_{i=1}^{N_g}\}, g \in \{1, ..., G\}$ including both images and videos from the source domain $\mathcal{D}^s$, where N_g is the total number of samples in the g-th group and $x^s_{g_i}$ is the i-th sample in the group with its label $y^s_{g_i} \in \{-1, 1\}$. A set of pre-learned source classifiers $f^s_g(x^s_g) = \widetilde{w'_g}\varphi_g(x^s_g)$ are learned by using the training data from each individual group. φ_g is the feature mapping function for the g-th group. Also, we are provided with a set of unlabeled consumer videos $\{x^t_i|_{i=1}^{N_t}\}$ from the target domain $\mathcal{D}^t$.

In our setting of incremental learning, there are two types of information in the source domain. First, we have a set of group classifiers f^s_g that are obtained from initial G groups of images in the source domain. Since in incremental learning there is no access to the samples used to train the initial source classifiers, we encoded these source models as a set of G hyperplanes represented in a matrix form as $\widetilde{W} = [\widetilde{w_1}, \widetilde{w_2}, ..., \widetilde{w_G}]$. Second, for every incremental stage, we are given a set of new Web images or action videos from the source domain and a small set of consumer videos in the target domain. Our goal is to use the newly given source domain data to boost the annotation performance on the newly given target domain videos. It should be noted that the newly given source domain data may belong original groups or new groups, which means new concept can be learned during the incremental transfer learning process.

3 Incremental Learning from Heterogeneous Sources

Unlike traditional multi-source adaptation methods, our method treats the combination coefficients (group weights) of different groups as latent variable rather than fixes them for each incoming target video. To this end, we learn the following target classifier f^t for any consumer video sample x^t_i, which fuses the decisions from multiple sources according to the latent weights:

$$f^t(x^t_i) = \sum_{g=1}^{G} w'_g \phi(\theta_{i_g}, \varphi_g(x^t_i)), \tag{1}$$

where w_g is the template for the g-th group data; $\theta_{i_g}, i \in \{1, ..., N_t\}$ and $g \in \{1, ..., G\}$ is the g-th latent group weight for consumer video x^t_i, and φ_g is the feature mapping function for the target video x^t_i on the g-th group.

Once there are new target domain videos available, we update the target classifier to make it more adaptable for these newly coming videos. In other words, the aim of our incremental approach is to find a new combination (i.e. $\Theta_i = [\theta_{i_1}, \theta_{i_2}, ..., \theta_{i_G}]$) of a new set of hyperplanes (i.e. $W = [w_1, w_2, ..., w_G]$), such that (1) performance on newly coming target data improves by transferring knowledge from both the original source models and new source domain data, (2) efficiency of learning additional information improves without any access to the original data used to train the existing classifiers, and (3) the model is able to accommodate new event class introduced with new data. Thanks to the development of the Internet, we can easily obtain new labeled source domain data to incrementally update knowledge.

3.1 Learning

Although the explosion of Web data can bring new knowledge, the random noting and subjective understanding of images make the noise images unavoidable. To prevent negative transfer brought by the newly coming data, we enforce the new learned hyperplanes W to remain close to the original hyperplanes $\widetilde{W}$ using the term $\| W - \beta\widetilde{W} \|^2$. This term enforces the target model W to be relatively close to the original model $\widetilde{W}$, using coefficient vector $\beta = [\beta_1, ..., \beta_G]^T$. Besides the constraints on the hyperplane, we also enforce a smooth assumption on the single group decision value, i.e., different group classifiers belonging to the same event should have similar decision values on the target domain data. In our work, this constraint is implemented using the regularizer $\sum_{g=1}^{G} \theta_{i_g} \sum_{k \neq g}^{G} \|w_g f_g^s(x_i^t) - w_k f_k^s(x_i^t)\|^2$. For example, if the g-th group and the k-th group represent different concepts of the same event, we ensure that $f_s^k(x)$ should be close to $f_s^g(x)$. Actually, we introduce this term to penalize those groups far from major event-related groups. For domain adaptation, we similarly assume that the pre-learned classifiers in the source domain should have similar decision values on the unlabeled samples in the target domain.

Since the group weights are treated as latent variables, our goal is to learn a prediction rule of the following form:

$$\begin{aligned} f^t(x) &= \arg\max_{\Theta, y} F(x, y, \Theta) \\ &= \arg\max_{\Theta, y} W \cdot \Phi(x, y, \Theta), \end{aligned} \tag{2}$$

where $\Phi(x, y, \Theta)$ is a joint feature vector that describes the relationship among the input consumer video x, output event class label y, and latent group weights Θ.

In order to learn the group weights Θ_i for each newly coming target video x_i^t and simultaneously update the group templates W, we introduce above constraints into a latent structural objective function as follows:

$$\min_{W} \frac{1}{2} \| W - \beta\widetilde{W} \|^2 + \lambda_1 \sum_{i=1}^{N_t} \xi_i + \lambda_2 \sum_{j=1}^{N_t} \zeta_j, \tag{3}$$

$$\text{s.t. } \xi_i = l(\max_{\Theta_i} F(x_i^t, y_i^t, \Theta_i) - \max_{\widetilde{\Theta}_i, \widetilde{y}_i} \widetilde{F}(x_i^t, y_i^t, \Theta_i)), \tag{4}$$

$$\zeta_j = \sum_{g=1}^{G} \theta_{j_g} \sum_{k \neq g}^{G} \| f_g^s(x_j^t) - f_k^s(x_j^t) \|^2, \tag{5}$$

$$\sum_{g=1}^{G} \theta_{i_g} = 1, \tag{6}$$

where λ_1, λ_2 are tradeoff parameters. Here $l(t)$ is the hinge loss function defined by $l(t) = max(0, 1-t)$. We use this loss function to enforce the decision value of the newly learned target classifier not far away from that of the original classifier. We argue that such supervision is very important for our incremental adaptation problem. The reason is two-fold: (a) There is a certain amount of overlap between the updated target classifier and the original target classifier, so it is very possible that decisions on these two types of classifier would not be too far from each other; (b) We do not have any labeled data in the target domain, so the performance of updated classifier will become much worse without having the constraints in Eq. 4. Our experiments demonstrate the strength of this constraint.

The optimization problem in Eq. 3 can be solved in many different ways. In our implementation, we adopt a non- convex cutting plane method proposed in [16]. First, it is easy to show that Eq. 3 is equivalent to $\min_W L(w) = \frac{1}{2} \| W - \beta\widetilde{W} \|^2 + \sum_{i=1}^{N_t} R(W)$ where $R(W)$ is a loss function defined as

$$\begin{aligned} R(W) =& \lambda_1 l(\max_{\Theta_i} F(x_i^t, y_i^t, \Theta_i) - \max_{\widetilde{\Theta}_i, \widetilde{y}_i} \widetilde{F}(x_i^t, y_i^t, \Theta_i)) \\ &+ \lambda_2 \sum_{g=1}^{G} \theta_{g_i} \sum_{k \neq g}^{G} \| f_g^s(x_i^t) - f_k^s(x_i^t) \|^2. \end{aligned} \tag{7}$$

The non-convex cutting plane method [16] aims to iteratively build an increasingly accurate piecewise quadratic approximation of $L(W)$ based on its sub-gradient $\partial_W L(W)$. The key issue here is how to compute the sub-gradient $\partial_W L(W)$. We define

$$\begin{aligned} \Theta_i^* &= \arg\max_{\Theta} \widetilde{F}(x_i^t, y_i^t, \Theta_i), \forall y \in \mathcal{Y}, \\ y^{t*} &= \arg\max_{y} \widetilde{F}(x_i^t, y_i^t, \Theta_i^*). \end{aligned} \tag{8}$$

The inference problem in Eq. 8 will be described in Sec. 4.2. It is easy to show that $\partial L(W)$ can be calculated as follows:

$$\begin{aligned} \partial_W L(W) = W - \beta\widetilde{W} + \sum_{i=1}^{N_t} \Theta_i \Phi(x_i^t, y_i^t, \Theta_i) \\ - \sum_{i=1}^{N_t} \Theta_i^* \Phi(x_i^t, y_i^{t*}, \Theta_i^*) + \sum_{i=1}^{N_t} \Theta_i \Omega_i. \end{aligned} \tag{9}$$

Here

$$\Omega_i = \{\Omega_i^1, ..., \Omega_i^g, ..., \Omega_i^G\} \tag{10}$$

and

$$\Omega_i^g = \sum_{k=1,k\neq g}^{G} \phi(x_i^t)(f_g^s(x_i^t) - f_k^s(x_i^t)) \tag{11}$$

Given the sub-gradient $\partial_W L(W)$ according to Eq. 9, we can minimize $L(W)$ using the method in [16].

3.2 Inference

Given the group templates W, we need to solve the following inference problem for each target domain sample x_i^t:

$$\Theta_i = \arg\max_{\theta_{i_g}} \sum_{g=1}^{G} w'_g \phi(\theta_{i_g}, \varphi_g(x_i^t)) \qquad \forall y \in \mathcal{Y}. \tag{12}$$

As we know, the key issue of transfer learning approach is to measure the relevance between the source domain data and the target domain data. Motivated by MMD [17–19], we infer the group weights $\Theta_g = [\Theta_i, ...\Theta_{N_t}]$ for the target domain samples by measuring the marginal probability distribution difference between two sets of samples:

$$\Theta_g = \|\frac{1}{N_g}\sum_{j=1}^{N_g} \phi(x_{g_j}^s) - \frac{1}{N_t}\sum_{i=1}^{N_t} \theta_{g_i}\phi(x_i^t)\|_{\mathcal{H}}^2. \tag{13}$$

We stress that the criterion above is defined according to source domain groups which are a subset of the source domain, as the sample mean is computed only

---

Algorithm 1. Incremental Heterogeneous Domain Adaptation.

Require:

$\{X^g\}_{g=1}^G$: the set of source domain groups;
X^t : unlabeled target videos;
$\widetilde{W}$: original source domain hyperplane set;

Ensure:

W: Updated target classifiers;

repeat
  Calculate $F(\cdot)$ and $\widetilde{F(\cdot)}$ for x_i^t
  Compute group smooth constraint Ω_i
  Infer the latent group weight Θ_i for x_i according to Eq. (13)
until All target domain samples are involved
Use cutting plane method to minimize Eq. (3) to update W
return W

---

on the semantic related instances. This is much different from the other MMD approaches that have used similar nonparametric techniques for comparing distributions. There they make stronger assumptions that all data points in the source domain need to be collectively distributed similarly to the target domain. Furthermore, in our inference problem, different weights are assigned to different target domain samples. Our results below will show that these differences are crucial to the success of our approach. Our incremental learning method is summarized in Algorithm 1.

3.3 Datasets

We evaluate our method on two consumer video datasets: CCV [20] and Kodak [21].

CCV dataset contains a training set of 4, 659 videos and a testing set of 4, 658 videos which are annotated to 20 semantic categories. Since our work focuses on event annotation, we do not consider the non-event categories (*i.e.*, "playground", "bird", "beach", "cat" and "dog"). In order to facilitate the keyword based image collection using the Web search engine, the events of "wedding ceremony", "wedding reception"and "wedding dance" are merged into one event as "wedding". The events of "non-music performance" and "music performance"are merged into "performance". Finally, twelve event categories: "basketball", "baseball", "soccer", "iceskating", "biking", "swimming", "skinning", "graduation", "birthday", "wedding", "show", and "parade" are conducted in our experiment.

Kodak dataset is collected by Kodak from about 100 real users over one year, consisting of 195 consumer videos with their ground truth labels of six event classes (*i.e.*, "wedding", "birthday", "picnic", "parade", "show"and "sports").

To construct clearly labeled source domain videos, we apply two widely used action video datasets (i.e. KTH [5] and Weizman [6]).

KTH action video dataset contains six types of human actions: walking, jogging, running, boxing, hand waving and hand clapping. These actions are performed several times by twenty-five subjects in four different scenarios.

Weizmann action video dataset consists of about 90 low-resolution video sequences showing nine different subjects, each performing 10 actions including bending, jumping, running, skipping, galloping, walking and waving.

Web image dataset covers thirteen events: "basketball", "baseball", "soccer", "iceskating", "biking", "swimming", "graduation", "birthday", "wedding", "skinning", "show", "parade" and "picnic". In our experiment, we use the Google image search engine to collect images, and for each input keyword, the top ranked 300 images are downloaded and the corrupted images with invalid URLs are discarded. Finally, total 76 event-related semantic keywords are used to query images from Web image search engine and 16, 708 images are collected.

3.4 Experimental Setup

For videos in both domains, we extract 162-dimensional 3D Space-Time Interest Point (STIP) in which 72-dimensional Histograms of Oriented Gradient (HOG) and 90-dimensional Histograms of Optical Flow (HOF) are extracted by using the online tool from [22]. For consumer videos in the target domain, we additionally extract image features by randomly sampling five frames from each video as its keyframe and extracting 128-dimensional SIFT features from salient regions on each frame detected by the Difference of Gaussians (DoG) detectors [23]. The bag-of-words representation is used for both image and video features. Specifically, we cluster the SIFT descriptors extracted from all the training Web images and keyframes, into 2,000 words by using k-means clustering method. Each image (video keyframe) is then represented as a 2,000-dimensional token frequency (TF) feature by quantizing its SIFT descriptors with respect to the visual codebook. Similarly, we cluster the STIP features extracted from consumer videos and action videos into 2000 words using k-means, and the motion feature of each video is then represented by a 2000-dimensional token frequency feature. Finally, two types of feature is used for videos in the target domain, and one type of feature is sued for images and videos in the source domain, respectively.

To pre-learn a classifier for each group of each event, the positive samples are constructed by the samples belonging to the corresponding group in the corresponding event class and the negative samples consist of randomly selected 300 samples in the same type of any other groups. At the training stage, for the CCV dataset the training set defined by [20] is used as the unlabeled target domain. For the Kodak dataset, all the 195 target domain videos are used as unlabeled training data. Consequently, the training data includes the heterogeneous groups from the source domain and unlabeled videos from the target domain.

We compare our transfer learning method with several state-of-the-art methods, including the standard SVM (S_SVM), the single domain adaptation methods of Domain Adaptive SVM (DASVM) [24], the multi-domain adaptation methods of Domain Adaptation Machine (DAM) [25], Conditional Probability based Multi-source Domain Adaptation (CPMDA) [26], Domain Selection Machine (DSM) [4] and Multi-domain Adaptation with Heterogeneous Sources (MDA-HS) [15]. Since the S_SVM can only handle data from a single group, we merge the training samples represented by same type of features into one source to train SVM classifier. Consequently, two types of SVM classifiers based on SIFT and STIP features are obtained for Web images and action videos, respectively. The final S_SVM classifier is obtained by equally fusing these two types of source classifiers. For DASVM, which is semi-supervised learning method and also cannot handle the multi-group setting, the target classifiers are trained using the labeled source domain samples and the keyframes of unlabeled videos from the target domain. Similar to S_SVM, we employ the same fusing strategy to obtain the target classifier for DASVM. The traditional multi-source adaptation methods CPMDA, DAM and DSM can not directly handle the heterogeneous sources problem, so we perform these multi-source leveraging strategies on single feature type and then average the decision values to obtain the final decision.

In our incremental learning setting, the source domain data is partitioned into two parts: an initial set used for learning the initial source group classifiers and the remaining sets added successively for updating. More specifically, about 3000 source domain samples are used for updating the target model at each incremental stage. And for the testing data, we evaluate the annotation performance on all the input target domain videos (including the new videos in the current step and the videos used before). For all the methods, Average Precision (AP) is used for performance evaluation and mean Average Precision (mAP) is defined as the mean of APs over all event classes.

3.5 Results

We first compare our method with existing approaches and report the per-event APs of all the methods on the CCV and Kodak datasets in Figs. 2 and 3, respectively. We also show the mAPs of all methods on these datasets in Table 1.

Table 1. Comparison of mAPs (%) between our method and other methods on the CCV and Kodak datasets.

Method	S_SVM	DASVM [24]	CPMDA [26]	DAM [25]	DSM [4]	MDA [15]	**Ours**
CCV	7.43	8.08	8.46	11.59	11.10	10.47	**17.05**
Kodak	12.95	17.78	21.58	30.25	23.38	25.18	**35.63**

From the results, we notice that:

- Our method achieves the best results on both datasets, which shows that our incremental weighting strategy is beneficial to positive transform. Multi-source adaptation methods (i.e. CPMDA, DAM, DSM, MDA and our method) generally outperform the single source methods (i.e. S_SVM and DASVM), which clearly reveals that it is helpful to weight different sources for knowledge transfer. The contribution of different sources may be different, by this means, the weighting strategy becomes particularly important.
- Our method is better than MDA, which illustrates the benefit of using latent video-specific weights for domain adaptation. A possible explanation is that the events in real-world vary dramatically, so fixed group weights can not capture the relevance information between different groups in various situations in every situation.
- It is also interesting to notice that our method performs better than DSM, which indicates that the data from all groups querying by associational keywords can benefit understanding video events to some extend.
- In terms of per-event average precisions, there is no consistent winner among these methods. This indicates the existence of the irrelevant data which hinds these transfer learning methods to acquire good target classifiers. Our method achieves more stable performance, which demonstrates that latent weighting strategy can effectively cope with noisy data in the source domain.

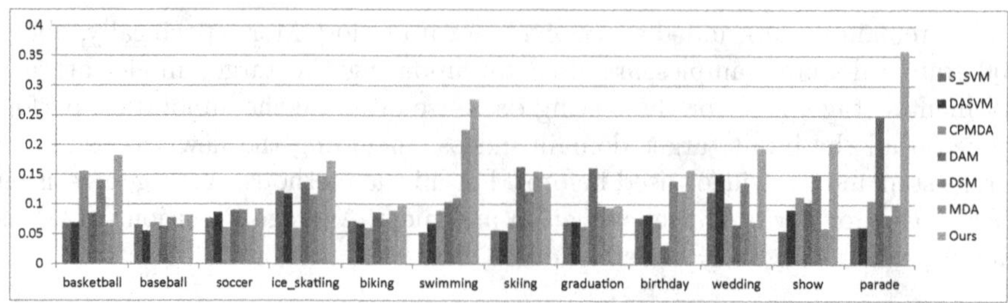

Fig. 2. Per-event Average Precisions (APs) (%) of all methods on the CCV dataset.

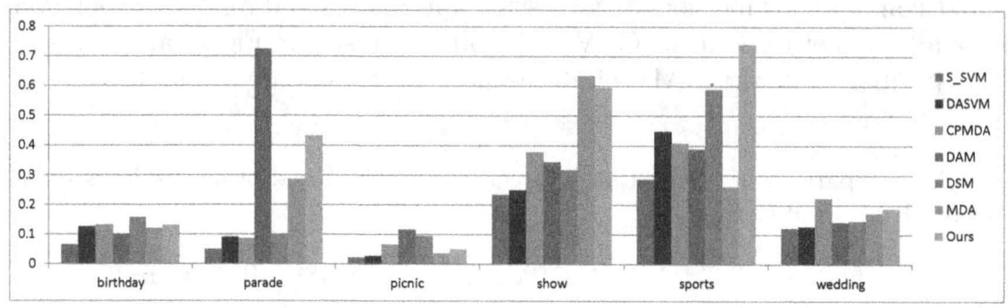

Fig. 3. Per-event Average Precisions (APs) (%) of all methods on the Kodak dataset.

We also investigate the effects of each constraint in our optimization function in Eq. (3) for learning knowledge from the source. The column of $\theta_{i_g} = \theta_{j_g}$ reports the performance of annotating when group weights for all the target video are equal. The objective function is given by

$$\min_{W} \frac{1}{2} \parallel W - \beta\widetilde{W} \parallel^2 + \frac{1}{2} \parallel \Theta \parallel^2 + \sum_{l=1}^{N_s} \parallel \sum_{g=1}^{G} f_g^s(x_l^s)) - y_l^s \parallel^2$$
$$+ \sum_{j=1}^{N_t} \sum_{g=1}^{G} \theta_g \sum_{k \neq g}^{G} \|f_g^s(x_j^t) - f_k^s(x_j^t)\|^2,$$
$$s.t. \sum_{g=1}^{G} \theta_g = 1, \tag{14}$$

where θ_g stands for the group weights of the g-th group. In the objective function, group weights are treated as explicit variable and simultaneously optimized with the group templates W. As shown is the results, the annotation performance degrades dramatically when group weights are not treated as latent variables for each target domain video. A possible explanation is that large intra-class variations within the same type of events exist in the target domain videos, making their visual cues highly variable. The relevance between the different groups and the individual target video cannot be accurately represented by a unified group weight. The performance is degraded when all groups are

Table 2. Evaluation on different components of the optimal function using mAPs (%).

Method	$\theta_{i_g} = \theta_{j_g}$	$\theta_g = 1/G$	$\lambda_1 = 0$	$\lambda_2 = 0$	*Ours*
CCV	9.94	15.21	15.20	7.87	17.05
Kodak	32.81	15.09	29.3	28.72	35.63

Table 3. The efficiency of our incremental method on the Kodak and CCV dataset.

	Kodak		CCV	
	mAP (%)	Time (min)	mAP (%)	Time (min)
Non-incremental	31.90	14.19	7.25	54.32
Incremental	35.63	11.34	17.05	38.21

treated equally($\theta_g = 1/G$), which demonstrates that the contributions of different groups are different to the target classifier. This further indicate the relevance between the source and target is crucial for processing positive knowledge transfer (Table. 2).

Finally, we evaluate the efficiency of our incremental domain adaptation method. Figures 4 and 5 give the per-event comparison of non-incremental results and incremental results on both datasets. Table 3 shows mAP and computational time in minutes of our incremental method. As shown in the table, the non-incremental method degrades a lot, especially on the CCV dataset. A possible

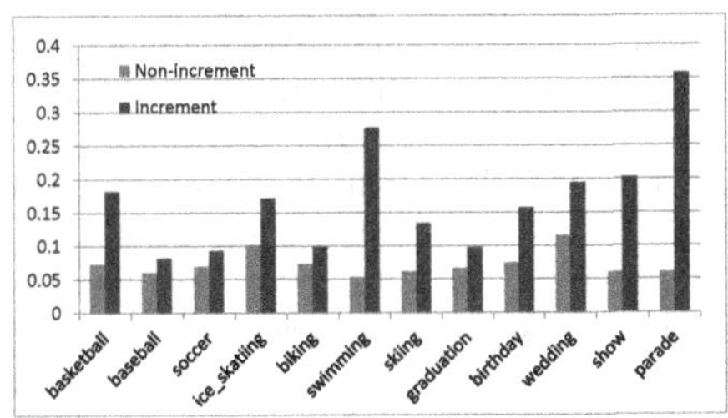

Fig. 4. Evaluation on the incremental efficiency on CCV dataset.

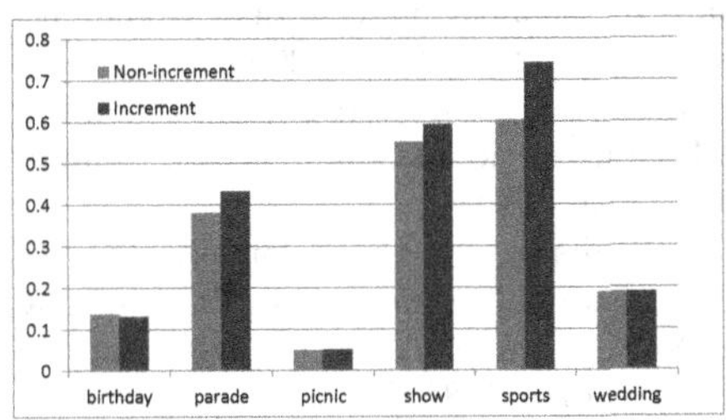

Fig. 5. Evaluation on the incremental efficiency on Kodak dataset.

explanation is that the videos in the CCV dataset are much more than those in the Kodak, which is more close to the real-world situation. This also confirms our claim that the incremental method is more suitable for modeling consumer videos.

4 Conclusion

In this paper, we have presented a new framework for consumer video event annotation by leveraging a large number of freely available labeled sources (i.e. images from Google and action videos from lab). By introducing a new incremental learning method and a new latent weighting scheme, our method, called Incremental Learning with Latent Groups Weights, can simultaneously seek and update the optimal group weights and group templates by using data from both domains. Comprehensive experiments on two benchmark datasets demonstrate the effectiveness of our method for video event annotation without requiring any labeled consumer videos.

Acknowledgements. The research was supported in part by the Natural Science Foundation of China (NSFC) under Grant No. 61203274, the Specialized Research Fund for the Doctoral Program of Higher Education of China (20121101120029), the Specialized Fund for Joint Building Program of Beijing Municipal Education Commission, and the Excellent young scholars Research Fund of BIT.

References

1. Bergamo, A., Torresani, L.: Exploiting weakly-labeled web images to improve object classification: a domain adaptation approach. In: Advances in Neural Information Processing Systems (NIPS) (2010)
2. Gopalan, R., Li, R., Chellappa, R.: Domain adaptation for object recognition: an unsupervised approach. In: ICCV, pp. 999–1006 (2011)
3. Kulis, B., Saenko, K., Darrell, T.: What you saw is not what you get: domain adaptation using asymmetric kernel transforms. In: CVPR, pp. 1785–1792 (2011)
4. Duan, L., Xu, D., Tsang, Chang, S.F.: Exploiting web images for event recognition in consumer videos: a multiple source domain adaptation approach. In: CVPR, pp. 1959–1966 (2012)
5. Schuldt, C., Laptev, I., Caputo, B.: Recognizing human actions: a local svm approach. In: Proceedings of the 17th International Conference on Pattern Recognition. ICPR 2004, vol. 3, pp. 32–36. IEEE (2004)
6. Blank, M., Gorelick, L., Shechtman, E., Irani, M., Basri, R.: Actions as space-time shapes. In: Tenth IEEE International Conference on Computer Vision. ICCV 2005, vol. 2, pp. 1395–1402. IEEE (2005)
7. Yang, J., Yan, R., Hauptmann, A.: Cross-domain video concept detection using adaptive svms. In: International Conference on Multimedia, pp. 188–197 (2007)
8. Duan, L., Tsang, I., Xu, D., Maybank, S.: Domain transfer svm for video concept detection. In: CVPR, pp. 1375–1381 (2009)
9. Duan, L., Xu, D., Tsang, I., Luo, J.: Visual event recognition in videos by learning from web data. In: CVPR, pp. 1959–1966 (2010)

10. Wang, H., Wu, X., Jia, Y.: Video annotation via image groups from the web. IEEE Trans. Multimedia **16**, 1282–1291 (2014)
11. Doretto, G., Yao, Y.: Boosting for transfer learning with multipple auxiliary domains. In: CVPR (2010)
12. Schweikert, G., Widmer, C., Schölkopf, B., Rätsch, G.: An empirical analysis of domain adaptation algorithms for genomic sequence analysis. In: NIPS (2009)
13. Ikizler-Cinbis, N., Cinbis, R., Sclaroff, S.: Learning actions from the web. In: CVPR, pp. 995–1002 (2009)
14. Tang, K., Ramanathan, V., Fei-Fei, L., Koller, D.: Shifting weights: adapting object detectors from image to video. In: Advances in Neural Information Processing Systems, pp. 647–655 (2012)
15. Chen, L., Duan, L., Xu, D.: Event recognition in videos by learning from heterogeneous web sources. In: 2013 IEEE Conference on Computer Vision and Pattern Recognition (CVPR), pp. 2666–2673. IEEE (2013)
16. Do, T.M.T., Artières, T.: Large margin training for hidden markov models with partially observed states. In: Proceedings of the 26th Annual International Conference on Machine Learning, pp. 265–272. ACM (2009)
17. Borgwardt, K.M., Gretton, A., Rasch, M.J., Kriegel, H.P., Schölkopf, B., Smola, A.J.: Integrating structured biological data by kernel maximum mean discrepancy. Bioinformatics **22**, e49–e57 (2006)
18. Gretton, A., Borgwardt, K., Rasch, M.J., Scholkopf, B., Smola, A.J.: A kernel method for the two-sample problem. In: NIPS (2008)
19. Sriperumbudur, B.K., Gretton, A., Fukumizu, K., Schölkopf, B., Lanckriet, G.R.: Hilbert space embeddings and metrics on probability measures. J. Mach. Learn. Res. **99**, 1517–1561 (2010)
20. Jiang, Y., Ye, G., Chang, S., Ellis, D., Loui, A.: Consumer video understanding: a benchmark database and an evaluation of human and machine performance. In: ICMR, p. 29 (2011)
21. Loui, A., Luo, J., Chang, S., Ellis, D., Jiang, W., Kennedy, L., Lee, K., Yanagawa, A.: Kodak's consumer video benchmark data set: concept definition and annotation. In: Workshop on Multimedia Information Retrieval, pp. 245–254 (2007)
22. Laptev, I., Marszalek, M., Schmid, C., Rozenfeld, B.: Learning realistic human actions from movies. In: CVPR, pp. 1–8 (2008)
23. Lowe, D.: Distinctive image features from scale-invariant keypoints. IJCV **60**, 91–110 (2004)
24. Bruzzone, L., Marconcini, M.: Domain adaptation problems: a dasvm classification technique and a circular validation strategy. PAMI **32**, 770–787 (2010)
25. Duan, L., Xu, D., Tsang, W.H.: Domain adaptation from multiple sources: a domain-dependent regularization approach. IEEE Trans. Neural Networks Learn. Syst. **23**, 504–518 (2012)
26. Chattopadhyay, R., Sun, Q., Fan, W., Davidson, I., Panchanathan, S., Ye, J.: Multisource domain adaptation and its application to early detection of fatigue. ACM Trans. Knowl. Discov. Data (TKDD) **6**, 18 (2012)

A Novel Group-Sparsity-Optimization-Based Feature Selection Model for Complex Interaction Recognition

Luyu Yang[1], Chenqiang Gao[1](✉), Deyu Meng[2], and Lu Jiang[3]

[1] Chongqing Key Laboratory of Signal and Information Processing, Chongqing University of Posts and Telecommunications, Chongqing, China
gaochenqiang@gmail.com

[2] School of Mathematics and Statistics, Xi'an Jiaotong University, Xi'an, China

[3] School of Computer Science, Carnegie Mellon University, Pittsburgh, USA

Abstract. Interaction recognition is an important part of action recognition and has various applications such as surveillance systems, human computer interface, and machine intelligence. In this paper, we propose a novel group-sparsity-optimization-based feature selection model for complex interaction recognition. Firstly multiple local and global features are concatenated into a feature pool, and then based on the group sparsity optimization, different feature types are automatically selected to fit specific interaction categorization. We test our method on the benchmark dataset: the UT-interaction dataset. Experimental results substantiate the effectiveness of the proposed method on complex interaction recognition tasks as compared with current state-of-the-art methods.

1 Introduction

Action recognition aims to recognize the ongoing action from an unknown video. This technique has a variety of potential applications, such as intelligent surveillance systems, human computer interface, machine intelligence et al. In the past decades, the research focus was mainly on the task of single-person action recognition [1,2] and good performance was achieved. In some typical datasets [3,4], the recognition accuracy has reached over 90 % [5,6]. Good progress for single-person action recognition makes many researchers devote efforts to the interaction recognition which is a more complex recognition task. Besides the challenges of background clutter, partial occlusion and the perspective effect, compared with single-person action recognition, the interactive action recognition task additionally suffers from: (1) variations within an interaction among different performers; (2) similar patterns among different interactions or with background interference.

D. Cremers et al. (Eds.): ACCV 2014, Part V, LNCS 9007, pp. 508–521, 2015.
DOI: 10.1007/978-3-319-16814-2_33

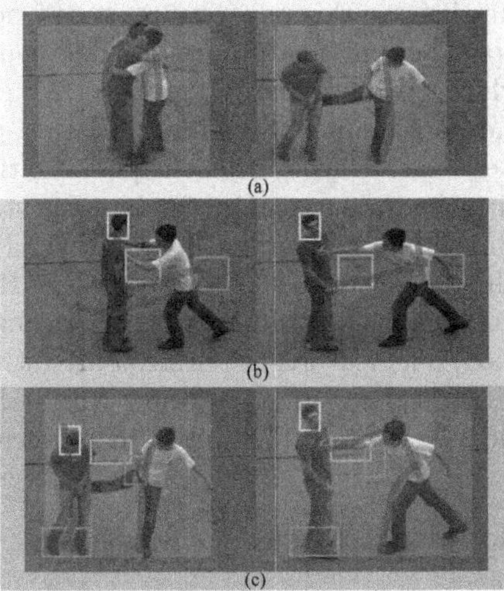

Fig. 1. Three image pairs demonstrate one-vs-one interaction classification of (a) "hug" and "kick"; (b) "punch" and "push"; (c) "kick" and "push". The bigger shadowed-areas and smaller bounding boxes respectively indicate global and local regions containing discriminative information for classification. Each pair of bounding boxes of comparison is colored differently. The strokes around human torsos indicate the interaction pose of two performers.

Various methods [7–9] have been proposed to address this challenge in recent years. Among them, methods under the framework of machine learning have received more attention. Most of such methods try to recognize various interactions using only one feature or one concatenation of features. Although good performance can be achieved among classes with more prominent discrimination, classes with obscure discrimination were always recognized poorly. It is a challenging task to improve accuracy on interactions with obscure discrimination while still keep high accuracy on interactions with prominent discrimination. In [10], the recognition accuracy of interactions "hug" and "kick" were above 95 %, but only around 70 % for "punch" and "push". One reason is that the former two interactions are different from other interactions in a more prominent way, while the latter two interactions have more obscure discriminative information. As shown in Fig. 1, between "hug" and "kick", the region which provides discriminative information is prominent and large, so a global feature such as the popular dense trajectory would be sufficient. However, between "punch" and "push", discriminative information is obscure and exists only in small local areas. In this case, local features around those areas have to be rationally utilized to provide effective description. Differently, in "kick" and "push", both global and local areas can provide some discriminative information, but not typical enough when being considered separately. Therefore, it is more reasonable to combinationally consider multiple feature types here. Faced with various classes of interactions, the questions are, **which** types of features should be chosen and **how** can this choice be made automatically.

To answer these questions, in this paper we propose a novel feature selection model for interaction recognition. The proposed model automatically learns to select feature types which optimize the recognition. We choose multiple local and global features and concatenate them into a feature pool, and our model selectively learns the best feature types from the pool. To the best of our knowledge, it is new to utilize the group sparsity for human interaction recognition. We test our method on the interaction benchmark, the UT-interaction dataset, and experimental results demonstrate the effectiveness of the proposed method.

The rest of paper is organized as follows: Sect. 2 reviewed related methods of interaction recognition. The features we utilized are introduced in Sect. 3. In Sect. 4, how our model selects feature types and why it has feature selection capability are explained. Finally, Sect. 5 exhibits experimental results.

2 Related Work

As compared with the action recognition problem, which has been investigated for more than a decade, the interaction recognition has not attracted much attention until the first attempt by Oliver et al. [11]. This method handled the interaction recognition problem by employing motion trajectories obtained from blob-tracking of human. Another remarkable milestone is the successful use of a new spatio-temporal feature detector [12] in action recognition which received much attention in the field [13–16]. Its invariability under illumination change and noisy background has largely benefited the action recognition task under real-world scenes. Recognition based on key frames [17,18] is also a widely-used method in interaction recognition. These methods analyzed descriptors extracted from key frames of a video, trying to model the relations between interactions and poses of key frames, while somewhat underused the contextual information of motion trajectory. To utilize contextual information within an interaction, a respectable amount of works have been presented to model the context of interactions [19,20]. By presenting interactions by action context descriptors, in [20], action context was encoded by interactive phrases which were composed of atomic actions of elementary movements, namely attributes. Their method obtained improvement compared with previous methods. However, in this method, the attributes need to be manually labeled and specified to certain data sets, which makes the method less automatic in recognition and less scalability onto other data sets. In many works, fusion of multiple features was used to balance the contribution of each feature type. In [21], training scores of each feature type were employed as an input to learn the fusion weight vector. However, these methods tend to lose the discriminative description of combined features at the early-fusion stage. Our method capitalizes on selecting feature types using the group sparsity technique and feature types are selected before training. To realize group sparsity, a weight vector indicating the importance of all sample features is involved. The $L_{2,1}$-norm is imposed on these weights to enforce its group sparsity on simultaneously selecting certain scales of features. Results show that our feature selection model makes feature-fusion more effective. Although there exist some feature selection models [22,23], it is new to use group sparsity to achieve the feature selection goal in interaction recognition.

3 Interaction Representation

We utilize five scales of features as a feature pool, including three features for local context and two for global context. The local features are extracted based on images. We use the pedestrian detector [24] to detect each interacting person and his body parts in one image and thus 1 full-body bounding box and a group of 8 body-part bounding boxes for one person can be obtained. The first and second local features are the HOG of full-body bounding box and body-part bounding boxes, respectively. The third local feature is the configuration of body-part bounding boxes. The global features are extracted along the complete video based on dense trajectory. It should be noted that our method represents a general implementation scheme, and any other local or global features can be readily integrated to further extend its capability.

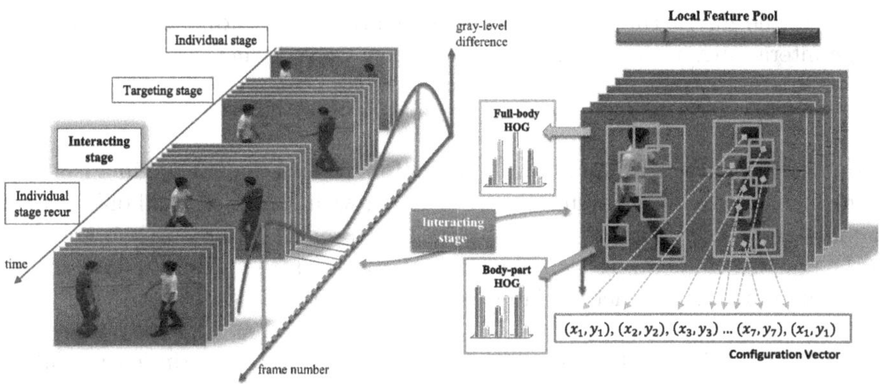

Fig. 2. The left demonstrates Interacting Stage Detection process: Frame-sequences of the four stages are represented and the right-side curve corresponds to the changes of gray-level differences during the stages. The right shows how local features: full-body HOG, body-part HOG and body-part configuration vector are extracted from the interacting stage. On top of the right is the concatenated local features.

3.1 Local Feature Representation

Local feature representations are important in interaction recognition, since in some interactions the discriminative information is obscure and exists only in small local regions with few frames. In order to properly recognize these interactions, we need to make full use of discriminative information of local regions. In our work, we utilized three types of features as the representation of local regions.

Instead of using the whole video for local feature extraction, the core part of video is used in this paper. According to our observation, most interactions can be regarded as a four-stage sequential transition including: individual stage, targeting stage, interacting stage, and individual stage recurrence. Only the interacting stage, which provides more prominent in this state is to our interest. This is mainly due to two reasons. Firstly, when a video is regarded as frames, the other three stages, including individual stage, targeting stage and individual stage recurrence, might appear very similar among different interactions, which inclines to reduce the distinguishability among interaction classes. Secondly, the other three stages are of much randomness, and may not be contributory to the classification since how performers would like to act before or after they interact is much up to their willingness.

Interacting Stage Detection. Figure 2 demonstrates the process of the interacting stage detection. In order to automatically detect the third interacting stage, for each video we compute the gray-value difference between each two consecutive frames and the difference value of each pixel is added up, thus obtaining a gray-value difference curve. According to our experience, the curve is saddle-shaped with two peaks which respectively indicates the starting and ending frames of the interacting stage. To get the starting and ending frame numbers of the interacting stage, we employ an n-degree curve fitting

$$y = ax^n + bx^{(n-1)} + cx^{(n-2)} + ... + dx + e \tag{1}$$

to smooth the curve with an initial $n = 10$. If more than 2 local maxima is found in the fitted curve, we continue the curve fitting with increased n till only 2 local maxima are left. The frame numbers which correspond to the maxima are used as the starting and ending frames of the interacting stage. Frames between the two frames are those which we later extract local feature from.

Local HOG. We try to detect the local regions where discriminative information is more likely to exist. So features are extracted only in regions where full-body and body-part bounding boxes are detected.

Histogram of gradients (HOG) [25] is a powerful description of texture in action recognition [24,26,27], so we use it as a feature of the detected local regions. We resize each bounding box to 64×128 using nearest neighbor interpolation, and then an 8×8 grid is superimposed upon each full-body bounding box and body-part bounding box corresponding to each interacting person. Finally, a full-body local descriptor with a size of $S_f = 8 \times 16 \times 31$ and a body-part local descriptor with a size of $S_p = 64 \times 16 \times 31$ are obtained for each interacting person.

Body-Part Configuration. Besides texture description using HOG, spatial information of tracked body-part is another type of description for local regions. Figure 2 demonstrates the extraction process of this local feature. According to our observations, the configuration of body-part bounding boxes is discriminative among different interactions. In some obscurely discriminative interactions, such spatial information of body parts can be important clues when texture of local regions appears similar. We employ the relative location of detected body-part as a representation of configuration. Concatenation of coordinate centers (x_b, y_b) of 8 body-part bounding boxes, where $b = (1, 2, ..., 8)$ is used in our work and thus a configuration vector of length 2×8 is obtained.

In order to cover the discriminative regions as much as possible, three types of local features are used, including full-body HOG, body-part HOG and body-part configuration covered both texture and spatial description. Moreover, the texture description is of both larger and smaller local regions which is more comprehensive compared with [18,21], in which texture descriptions were only refined to the full-body scale.

3.2 Global Feature Representation

In videos, motion is a most informative cue for action recognition, and the motion trajectory is one of ways to describe motion. The dense trajectory extraction method described in [28] is popular in action recognition in recent years. We employ this method in interaction recognition to obtain a good representation of interaction trajectory. In our work, interactive motion is tracked, which forms a trajectory of interest points, and descriptors are extracted along the trajectory. The more detailed process includes three steps. Firstly, densely sampled points at multiple scales are tracked using the optical flow method used in [29]. Secondly, we track the sampled points to form trajectories. Finally, descriptors are computed by space-time volume around the trajectory. We utilize state-of-art descriptors including HOGHOF which shows prominent performance on various datasets [15,30], and the motion boundary histogram (MBH) [31] which can capture the relative motion between pixels both vertically and horizontally. The two descriptors are computed in the same parameter setup as in [28]. As a result, two types of global features based on trajectory are obtained with the size of 204 for HOGHOF and 192 for MBH.

All together we used 5 types of features of both local and global representation. Each type of feature has different representation capability, and by utilizing them, we try to capture discriminative information which might exist in texture, brightness and spatial locations. Before we concatenate them into a feature pool, a powerful fisher vector tool [32] is employed to encode each type of feature. Therefore, the final feature pool consists of 5 types of encoded features.

4 Intrinsic Feature Selection Model

With multiple types of features obtained, the easiest way is to concatenate all of them into one feature and directly use it as an input of a machine learning model. However, as we analyze earlier in Sect. 2, the recognition complexity is not always on the same level among different interactions. For interactions with prominent discriminative information such as “hug” and “kick”, features at global scale would be sufficient, but such features are not sufficient for those with obscure discriminative information such as "punch" and "push" which share similar patterns that can even be confused by human eyes. So in order to achieve good performance among interactions with obscurely discriminative information, we have to utilize local features to make up for or even replace the insufficient description of global features. However in practice, interactions are not just divided into two poles of complexity. There exist different mixtures of discriminative information which correspond to the concatenation of different feature types, and it is difficult to decide which feature types should be selected. To address this problem, we formulate the feature selection into a learning process, in which feature types are selected according to how well they perform. Aiming at effective feature selection, our method uses the group sparsity technique [33] and feature types are selected to optimize the recognition performance. The samples as well as features can also be simultaneously selected during training based on the intrinsic mechanism of SVM. More details are presented as follows.

4.1 Formulation of Our Model

Given an input video, we extract K types of features from it and formulate a concatenation of K types of features with total dimension $d = d_1 + d_2 + ... + d_k$. In order to enable the model with feature selection capability, we define a weight vector $\boldsymbol{\alpha} = (\alpha_1, \alpha_2, ..., \alpha_d)^T$, where the elements of $\boldsymbol{\alpha}$ can be grouped into $(\boldsymbol{\alpha_1}, \boldsymbol{\alpha_2}, ..., \boldsymbol{\alpha_k})$ according to the lengths of K feature types. Hence the weighted feature group is presented as $\boldsymbol{\alpha} \odot \boldsymbol{x}$. Given the ith sample $\boldsymbol{x_i}$ with label y_i, the interaction recognition problem can be formulated as an optimization problem:

$$min_{\boldsymbol{\omega},b,\boldsymbol{\alpha}} \frac{1}{2}\|\boldsymbol{\omega}\|^2 + C\sum_i (1 - y_i(b + \boldsymbol{\omega}^T(\boldsymbol{\alpha} \odot \boldsymbol{x_i})))_+^2 \qquad s.t. \qquad \|\boldsymbol{\alpha}\|_{2,1} \leq s, \quad (2)$$

where $\boldsymbol{\omega}$ is the model parameter, b is the offset value, C is the cost coefficient and s is the constraint of $\|\boldsymbol{\alpha}\|_{2,1}$. In Eq. 2, $L_{2,1}$-norm of $\boldsymbol{\alpha}$ can be written as

$$\|\boldsymbol{\alpha}\|_{2,1} = \sum_{k=1}^{K} \|\boldsymbol{\alpha}_k\|_2.$$

By optimizing Eq. 2, we can simultaneously make the calculated $\boldsymbol{\omega}$ and $\boldsymbol{\alpha}$ sparse. $\boldsymbol{\alpha}$ is sparse among K feature groups while dense within each type of features, which indicates that this model can have both sample selection and feature selection capability.

4.2 Learning and Inference

Inference: Given the model parameters $\boldsymbol{\omega}$, $\boldsymbol{\alpha}$ and b, the inference problem is to find the right interaction class label y for a test video $\boldsymbol{x}$. We define the following function to score $\boldsymbol{x}$.

$$y = b + \boldsymbol{\omega}^T(\boldsymbol{\alpha} \odot \boldsymbol{x}). \quad (3)$$

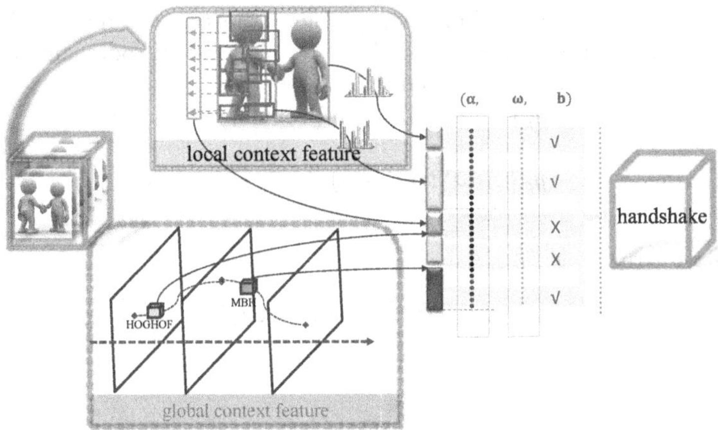

Fig. 3. The testing procedure: two global features (shown at the bottom) and three local features (shown on the top) are extracted from the test sample, and a concatenation of five features is shown as the rectangular patches in five colors in the middle. A set of trained $\boldsymbol{\alpha}$ which corresponds to feature selection, $\boldsymbol{\omega}$ and b, correspond to a test score calculated with the score function. The class which has the highest score is the test result of this video. The recognition result is "handshake"as shown, which rightly matches the interaction class.

The complete inference procedure is demonstrated in Fig. 3. Five features are extracted from the test video to form a feature pool. We employ the one-vs-one classification method in the learning phase, so between each two interaction classes there is a set of trained $\boldsymbol{\omega}$, $\boldsymbol{\alpha}$ and b, corresponding to a test score calculated with Eq. 3. The class which has the highest score is the test result of this video.

Learning: Given N training samples $(x_n, y_n)(n = 1, 2, ..., N)$, the training task is to learn the model parameters $\boldsymbol{\omega}$, $\boldsymbol{\alpha}$ and b. Our optimization algorithm includes mainly two steps to iteratively learn these three parameters.

(1) Holding $\boldsymbol{\alpha}$ fixed, the optimization problem is:

$$min_{\omega,b}\frac{1}{2}\|\boldsymbol{\omega}\|^2 + C\sum_i(1 - y_i(b + \boldsymbol{\omega}^T(\boldsymbol{\alpha} \odot \boldsymbol{x_i})))_+^2, \tag{4}$$

which can be written as

$$min_{\omega,b}\frac{1}{2}\|\boldsymbol{\omega}\|^2 + C\sum_i(1 - y_i(b + \boldsymbol{\omega}^T Q^T \boldsymbol{x_i}))_+^2,$$

where Q =

$$\begin{pmatrix} \alpha_1 & 0 & 0 \\ 0 & \ddots & 0 \\ 0 & 0 & \alpha_d \end{pmatrix}$$

is a diagonal matrix. The optimization problem above is a standard SVM [34] model and can be directly solved by virtue of off-the-shelf tools, among which LIBSVM described in [35] is adopted.

(2) Holding $\boldsymbol{\omega}$, b fixed, the optimization problem is,

$$min_{\boldsymbol{\alpha}} \sum_i (1 - y_i(b + \boldsymbol{\omega}^T(\boldsymbol{\alpha} \odot \boldsymbol{x_i})))_+^2 \qquad s.t. \qquad \|\boldsymbol{\alpha}\|_{2,1} \leq s, \tag{5}$$

which can be written as:

$$min_{\boldsymbol{\alpha}} \sum_i (1 - y_i(b + \boldsymbol{\alpha}^T P^T \boldsymbol{x_i}))_+^2 \qquad s.t. \qquad \|\boldsymbol{\alpha}\|_{2,1} \leq s, \tag{6}$$

where P =

$$\begin{pmatrix} \omega_1 & 0 & 0 \\ 0 & \ddots & 0 \\ 0 & 0 & \omega_d \end{pmatrix}$$

is a diagonal matrix and s is constraint parameter that controls sparsity level.

For being better solvable, the constrained optimization problem of the Eq. 6 is transformed into a unconstrained optimization problem with Lagrangian expression as follows:

$$L(\boldsymbol{x_i}, y_i, \boldsymbol{\alpha}, \boldsymbol{\lambda}) = \sum_i (1 - y_i(b + \boldsymbol{\omega}^T(\boldsymbol{\alpha}^T P^T \boldsymbol{x_i})))_+^2 + \boldsymbol{\lambda}\|\boldsymbol{\alpha}\|_{2,1}, \tag{7}$$

Under certain $\boldsymbol{\lambda}$, this is a convex optimization model with respect to $\boldsymbol{\alpha}$, and can be readily solved by gradient descent method [36]. We can then derive $\boldsymbol{\alpha}$ based on the obtained result. The appropriate $\boldsymbol{\lambda}$ can be properly specified by cross-validation.

5 Experiments

We test our method on the UT-Interaction dataset. This dataset consists of 20 videos in total, containing 6 classes of human-human interactions: "handshake", "hug", "kick", "point", "punch" and "push". On average, there are 8 instances of interactions per video and each video contains at least one instance. According to the filming condition, the dataset is divided into two sets. Set 1 is recorded at a parking plot with a stationary background, and Set 2 is recorded on a lawn with slight background movement and camera jitter. In accordance with experimental settings of the recognition task described in High-level Human Interaction Recognition Challenge [37], bounding boxes are used and the performance of our method is evaluated using leave-one-out cross validation on each set. The information of main actors (standing on the left or right side) is provided in the dataset as ground-truth. However, we did not use this information since it is hard to be obtained in realistic situations.

5.1 Implementation Details

By using the interacting stage detection method mentioned in Sect. 3, we obtain frames of the interacting stage upon which we detect a full human body and 8 body parts of each interacting person using the deformable part-based model [24]. To ensure at least two interacting person detection results, we set the detection score threshold at a lower $threshold = -1.5$ compared with the default $threshold = -0.5$. And the Top two detection results of the rank list are chosen as the interacting person detection results.

We compute HOG of each full-body bounding box and body-part bounding boxes as described in [24]. Next we compute HOGHOF descriptor and MBH descriptor as described in [28]. Fisher vector is utilized to generate a codebook for each feature type.

When generating codebooks, the number of Gaussians G in Gaussian mixture model is an important parameter, so we evaluate a variety of G on UT-interaction dataset with HOGHOF, MBH and their combinations. We process parameter search, and it turned out the best performance is obtained when $G = 65$. Model parameter C and $\boldsymbol{\lambda}$ are optimized using cross validation.

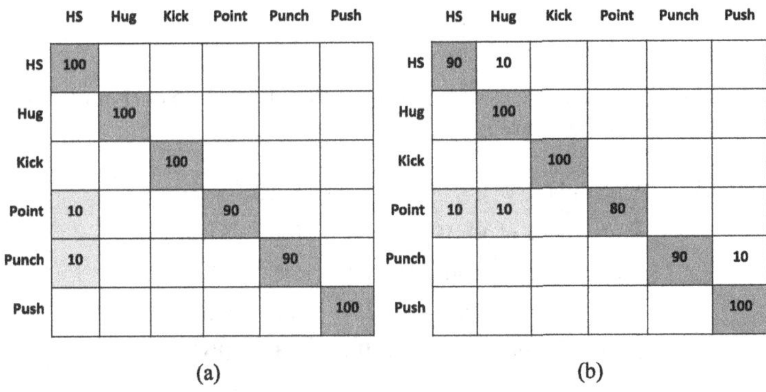

Fig. 4. (a) Confusion matrix of our method on Set 1 of UT-interaction dataset. (b) Confusion matrix of our method on Set 2. Note that "HS" stands for "Handshake".

5.2 Results

Figure 4 shows the confusion matrix of the Set 1 and Set 2 in the UT-interaction dataset. It can be seen from Fig. 4 that the interactions "hug", "kick" and "push" are recognized better than other interactions, and achieve 100 % recognition precision. In addition, the interactions "handshake" and "punch" which are usually regarded as interactions with obscure discriminative information with lower average precision [10,37], also achieve precision above 90 % for our method. Relatively, "point" is the difficulty-recognized class, with a precision of 85 %, since it is a special class in the dataset, with only one performer performing the action. Performance on Set 2 is not as good as on Set 1 in "handshake" and "point",

Table 1. Per-class precision (%) on UT-interaction dataset. 7 previous methods are compared with ours according to their average degree of precision. Average precision is listed in the last column.

Methods	Handshake	Hug	Kick	Point	Punch	Push	Average
Ryoo et al. [37]	75	87.5	75	62.5	50	75	70.8
Waltisberg et al. [10]	60	95	**100**	**100**	75	60	81.5
Yu et al. [14]	**100**	65	75	**100**	85	75	83.3
Ryoo et al. [26]	80	90	90	80	**90**	80	85
Patron-Perez et al. [21]	95	95	85	-	65	85	85
Kong et al. [20]	**100**	90	**100**	80	**90**	90	91.67
Vahda et al. [18]	85	**100**	95	95	80	95	92
Our Method	95	**100**	**100**	85	**90**	**100**	**95**

since Set 2 is filmed with camera jitter and partial occlusions of the background. Among the interactions with obscure discriminative information, "handshake" is slightly confused with "hug" in Set 2, and "punch" is misclassified as "push" in Set 2, which indicates that clutter increases the difficulty of recognizing interactions.

Table 2. Average precision (%) on UT Interaction Dataset Set 1 and Set 2. Three state-of-art methods are compared.

Methods	Set1	Set2	Average
Waltisberg et al. [10]	83	80	81.5
Patron-perez et al. [21]	84	86	85
Vahdat et al. [18]	93	90	92
Our Method	**96.7**	**93.3**	**95**

We also compare our classification accuracy in each interaction class with the methods proposed in [10,14,18,20,21,26,37] and the results are listed in Table 1. From Table 1 we can see that our method keeps high accuracy among interactions with prominent discrimination such as "hug" and "kick", meanwhile improves accuracy among interactions with obscure discrimination such as "punch" and "push". Best average precision is achieved using our method compared to the other 7 competing methods as well as best accuracy among four interactions out of six. Among interactions with obscure discriminative information, our method prominently outperforms state-of-art methods, especially in "punch" and "push" which demonstrates bad performance in most previous methods. However, "point" does not show strong performance in our method. This is since "point" is an exceptional class in the UT-interaction dataset, containing only one person performing the activity with no interaction information.

Since our model is specifically designed for capturing interaction information between humans, it might not be so appropriate for this specific class. Yet our method still gets a reasonable result on this class (85 %), comparable to most current methods along this line.

The average precision of all competing methods on each set are listed in Table 2. Our method achieves 96.7 % and 93.3 % precision on Set 1 and Set 2, respectively, which shows that our method outperforms the state-of-art methods on both sets.

5.3 Conclusion

In this paper, we have proposed a novel group-sparsity-optimization-based feature selection model for complex interaction recognition. We have used various combines of feature types with different representation capacity to recognize interactions with different prominent/obscure discrimination. Aiming at this goal, we have proposed a model which automatically selects feature types for specific interactions. We test our method on interaction benchmark UT-interaction dataset and extensive experimental results show the effectiveness of the proposed method for complex interaction recognition tasks compared to the state-of-the-art methods. Specifically, our method improves accuracy on interactions with obscure discrimination, while still keeps high accuracy on interactions with prominent discrimination.

Acknowledgement. This work is supported by the National Natural Science Foundation of China (No. 61102131, 61373114, 61275099), the Natural Science Foundation of Chongqing Science and Technology Commission (No. cstc2014jcyjA40048), the Project of Key Laboratory of Signal and Information Processing of Chongqing (No. CSTC2009CA2003).

References

1. Gallese, V., Fadiga, L., Fogassi, L., Rizzolatti, G.: Action recognition in the premotor cortex. Brain **119**, 593–609 (1996)
2. Weinland, D., Ronfard, R., Boyer, E.: Free viewpoint action recognition using motion history volumes. Comput. Vis. Image Underst. **104**, 249–257 (2006)
3. Schuldt, C., Laptev, I., Caputo, B.: Recognizing human actions: a local svm approach. In: 2004 IEEE International Conference on Pattern Recognition, vol. 3, pp. 32–36. IEEE (2004)
4. Blank, M., Gorelick, L., Shechtman, E., Irani, M., Basri, R.: Actions as space-time shapes. In: 2005 IEEE International Conference on Computer Vision, vol. 2, pp. 1395–1402. IEEE (2005)
5. Bregonzio, M., Gong, S., Xiang, T.: Recognising action as clouds of space-time interest points. In: 2009 IEEE Conference on Computer Vision and Pattern Recognition, pp. 1948–1955. IEEE (2009)
6. Hoai, M., Lan, Z.Z., De la Torre, F.: Joint segmentation and classification of human actions in video. In: 2011 IEEE Conference on Computer Vision and Pattern Recognition, pp. 3265–3272. IEEE (2011)

7. Joo, S.W., Chellappa, R.: Attribute grammar-based event recognition and anomaly detection. In: 2006 Conference on Computer Vision and Pattern Recognition Workshop, pp. 107–107. IEEE (2006)
8. Khan, S.M., Shah, M.: Detecting group activities using rigidity of formation. In: Proceedings of the 13th ACM international conference on Multimedia, pp. 403–406. ACM (2005)
9. Kitani, K.M., Sato, Y., Sugimoto, A.: Deleted interpolation using a hierarchical bayesian grammar network for recognizing human activity. In: 2005 Joint IEEE International Workshop on Visual Surveillance and Performance Evaluation of Tracking and Surveillance, pp. 239–246. IEEE (2005)
10. Waltisberg, D., Yao, A., Gall, J., Van Gool, L.: Variations of a hough-voting action recognition system. In: Ünay, D., Çataltepe, Z., Aksoy, S. (eds.) Recognizing Patterns in Signals, Speech, Images, and Videos. LNCS, vol. 6388, pp. 306–312. Springer, Heidelberg (2010)
11. Oliver, N., Rosario, B., Pentland, A.: Graphical models for recognizing human interactions. In: Proceedings of International Conference on Neural Information and Processing Systems, pp. 924–930. Citeseer (1998)
12. Dollar, P., Rabaud, V., Cottrell, G., Belongie, S.: Behavior recognition via sparse spatio-temporal features. In: 2nd Joint IEEE International Workshop on Visual Surveillance and Performance Evaluation of Tracking and Surveillance, pp. 65–72 (2005)
13. Wu, X., Ngo, C.W., Li, J., Zhang, Y.: Localizing volumetric motion for action recognition in realistic videos. In: Proceedings of the 17th ACM International Conference on Multimedia, pp. 505–508 (2009)
14. Yu, T.H., Kim, T.K., Cipolla, R.: Real-time action recognition by spatiotemporal semantic and structural forest. In: Proceedings of the British Machine Vision Conference, pp. 52.1–52.12. BMVA Press (2010)
15. Laptev, I., Marszalek, M., Schmid, C., Rozenfeld, B.: Learning realistic human actions from movies. In: 2008 IEEE Conference on Computer Vision and Pattern Recognition, pp. 1–8. IEEE (2008)
16. Choi, W., Savarese, S.: A unified framework for multi-target tracking and collective activity recognition. In: Fitzgibbon, A., Lazebnik, S., Perona, P., Sato, Y., Schmid, C. (eds.) Computer Vision - ECCV 2012. LNCS. Springer, Heidelberg (2012)
17. Laptev, I., Pérez, P.: Retrieving actions in movies. In: IEEE 11th International Conference on Computer Vision, pp. 1–8. IEEE (2007)
18. Vahdat, A., Gao, B., Ranjbar, M., Mori, G.: A discriminative key pose sequence model for recognizing human interactions. In: 2011 IEEE International Conference on Computer Vision Workshops, pp. 1729–1736. IEEE (2011)
19. Lan, T., Wang, Y., Yang, W., Robinovitch, S.N., Mori, G.: Discriminative latent models for recognizing contextual group activities. IEEE Trans. Pattern Anal. Mach. Intell. **34**, 1549–1562 (2012)
20. Kong, Y., Jia, Y., Fu, Y.: Interactive phrases: semantic descriptions for human interaction recognition. IEEE Trans. Pattern Anal. Mach. Intell. **36**, 1775–1788 (2014)
21. Patron-Perez, A., Marszalek, M., Reid, I., Zisserman, A.: Structured learning of human interactions in tv shows. IEEE Trans. Pattern Anal. Mach. Intell. **34**, 2441–2453 (2012)
22. Tan, M., Wang, L., Tsang, I.W.: Learning sparse svm for feature selection on very high dimensional datasets. In: Proceedings of the 27th International Conference on Machine Learning, pp. 1047–1054 (2010)

23. Qian, Y., Zhou, J., Ye, M., Wang, Q.: Structured sparse model based feature selection and classification for hyperspectral imagery. In: 2011 IEEE International Conference on Geoscience and Remote Sensing Symposium, pp. 1771–1774. IEEE (2011)
24. Felzenszwalb, P., McAllester, D., Ramanan, D.: A discriminatively trained, multiscale, deformable part model. In: 2008 IEEE Conference on Computer Vision and Pattern Recognition, pp. 1–8. IEEE (2008)
25. Dalal, N., Triggs, B.: Histograms of oriented gradients for human detection. In: 2005 IEEE Conference on Computer Vision and Pattern Recognition, vol. 1, pp. 886–893. IEEE (2005)
26. Ryoo, M.S.: Human activity prediction: early recognition of ongoing activities from streaming videos. In: 2011 IEEE International Conference on Computer Vision, pp. 1036–1043. IEEE (2011)
27. Dong, Z., Kong, Y., Liu, C., Li, H., Jia, Y.: Recognizing human interaction by multiple features. In: 2011 First Asian Conference on Pattern Recognition, pp. 77–81. IEEE (2011)
28. Wang, H., Klaser, A., Schmid, C., Liu, C.L.: Action recognition by dense trajectories. In: 2011 IEEE Conference on Computer Vision and Pattern Recognition, pp. 3169–3176. IEEE (2011)
29. Farnebäck, G.: Two-frame motion estimation based on polynomial expansion. In: Bigun, J., Gustavsson, T. (eds.) SCIA 2003. LNCS, vol. 2749, pp. 363–370. Springer, Heidelberg (2003)
30. Wang, H., Ullah, M.M., Klaser, A., Laptev, I., Schmid, C., et al.: Evaluation of local spatio-temporal features for action recognition. In: 2009 British Machine Vision Conference, p. 127 (2009)
31. Dalal, N., Triggs, B., Schmid, C.: Human detection using oriented histograms of flow and appearance. In: Leonardis, A., Bischof, H., Pinz, A. (eds.) ECCV 2006. LNCS, vol. 3952, pp. 428–441. Springer, Heidelberg (2006)
32. Oneata, D., Verbeek, J., Schmid, C.: Action and event recognition with fisher vectors on a compact feature set. In: 2013 IEEE International Conference on Computer Vision, pp. 1817–1824. IEEE (2013)
33. Nie, F., Huang, H., Cai, X., Ding, C.H.: Efficient and robust feature selection via joint 2, 1-norms minimization. In: Advances in Neural Information Processing Systems, pp. 1813–1821 (2010)
34. Xu, Z., Dai, M., Meng, D.: Fast and efficient strategies for model selection of gaussian support vector machine. IEEE Trans. Syst. Man Cybern. Part B: Cybern. **39**, 1292–1307 (2009)
35. Chang, C.C., Lin, C.J.: Libsvm: a library for support vector machines. ACM Trans. Intell. Syst. Technol. **2**, 27 (2011)
36. Baird, L., Moore, A.W.: Gradient descent for general reinforcement learning. In: Advances in Neural Information Processing Systems, pp. 968–974 (1999)
37. Ryoo, M.S., Aggarwal, J.K.: Spatio-temporal relationship match: video structure comparison for recognition of complex human activities. In: 2009 IEEE 12th International Conference on Computer Vision, pp. 1593–1600. IEEE (2009)

Boosting-Based Visual Tracking Using Structural Local Sparse Descriptors

Yangbiao Liu, Bo Ma(✉), Hongwei Hu, and Yin Han

Beijing Laboratory of Intelligent Information Technology, School of Computer Science and Technology, Beijing Institute of Technology, Beijing 100081, China
bma000@bit.edu.cn

Abstract. This paper develops an online algorithm based on sparse representation and boosting for robust object tracking. Local descriptors of a target object are represented by pooling some sparse codes of its local patches, and an Adaboost classifier is learned using the local descriptors to discriminate target from background. Meanwhile, the proposed algorithm assigns a weight value, calculated with the generative model, to each candidate object to adjust the classification result. In addition, a template update strategy, based on incremental principal component analysis and occlusion handing scheme, is presented to capture the appearance change of the target and to alleviate the visual drift problem. Comparison with the state-of-the-art trackers on the comprehensive benchmark shows effectiveness of the proposed method.

1 Introduction

Visual tracking is an important problem in computer vision and has a wide range of applications in surveillance, robotics, human computer interaction, and medical image analysis. Although steady progress has been made to the speed, accuracy and robustness of object tracking in recent years, it is still a difficult task due to appearance changes of a target object caused by some factors such as illumination variation, occlusion, background clutter, pose variation and shape deformation.

A lot of tracking methods have been proposed to deal with the challenges mentioned above, and readers can refer to the survey papers [1,2] and a recent benchmark [3]. Most recent tracking algorithms can be roughly categorized as either generative or discriminative approaches. Based on the appearance model of target object, generative tracking methods search the most similar region with the best matching score by some metric. These methods update target appearance model dynamically to make the model fit for the target appearance changes and reduce the drifting problem. Ross *et al.* [4] learned the dynamic appearance of the target via incremental low-dimensional subspace representation to adapt online to changes of target appearance. Recently, numerous tracking algorithms based on sparse representation [5–8] have been proposed due to its robustness to occlusion and noise. In [6], a tracking algorithm was developed with structural local sparse appearance model, using both partial information and spatial information of the target with

D. Cremers et al. (Eds.): ACCV 2014, Part V, LNCS 9007, pp. 522–533, 2015.
DOI: 10.1007/978-3-319-16814-2_34

alignment-pooling method. Wang *et al.* [9] proposed a least soft-thresold squares tracking algorithm by modeling the error term with the Gaussian-Laplacian distribution. However, background information that is critical for effective tracking isn't considered in these generative models.

Discriminative tracking methods [10–14] usually treat tracking as a binary classification task which separates the object from its surrounding background. These methods first train a classifier in an online manner, then the classifier is applied to candidate targets sampled from next frame. Babenko *et al.* [10] used multiple instance learning (MIL) which put the positive and negative samples into some positive and negative bags respectively to learn a discriminative model to solve ambiguity problem. Kalal *et al.* [12] developed a semi-supervised learning approach in which tracking results were regarded as unlabeled and positive and negative samples were selected with structural constraints. Zhang *et al.* [13] utilized a random sparse compressive matrix to reduce dimensionality of Haar-like features, and then trained a naive Bayes classifier with the low-dimensional compressive features. Discriminative trackers are usually more robust against appearance variations than generative trackers under complicated environments, because discriminative trackers take background information into account. Some hybrid methods that combine generative approach and discriminative approach to get a more robust result were proposed, such as [15–17].

Recently, sparse representation has attracted considerable interest in object tracking due to its robustness to occlusion and image noise etc. Moreover, a large number of experiments suggest that sparse representations are effective models to account for appearance change. In this paper, we present an online visual object tracking algorithm using local sparse appearance representation and an Adaboost classifier. The proposed method samples overlapped local image patches inside the object region and then represents each image patch with its sparse code. Different from [18] which represents a target by concatenating the sparse codes of all image patches, our method represents a target using some local descriptors. Each local descriptor is represented by pooling several sparse codes selected from all sparse codes of the target. And then, an Adaboost classifier can be trained using the local descriptors of positive and negative samples collected in the first several frames. A candidate target has a classification score via the Adaboost classifier, but the classification score is not accurate if the candidate target experiences great appearance variations, so the classification score should be adjusted. The proposed algorithm assigns a weight value to each candidate target to adjust its classification score, and the weight value is calculated by structural reconstruction error of the candidate target. In addition, a template update strategy is applied to capture the appearance change of the target.

2 Proposed Tracking Algorithm

In this section, the proposed tracking algorithm is described in detail. We first show how the local descriptors of target are represented with local sparse codes. Next, we give a description of training classifier and calculating weight of candidate target. The update strategy of template and classifier is then introduced.

2.1 Local Descriptors Representation by Local Sparse Codes

Given an object image I, we can extract a set of overlapped local image patches $X = \{x_i | i = 1, 2, \cdots, N\} \in R^{d \times N}$ inside the target region with a sliding window, where x_i is the i-th column vectorized local image patch extracted from image I, d is the dimension of the image vectors and N is the number of local patches. If we have an image set of templates $T = [T_1, T_2, \cdots, T_n]$, we extract local image patches from T in the same way mentioned above, and then a dictionary $D = [d_1, d_2, \cdots, d_{N \times n}] \in R^{d \times (N \times n)}$ used to encode local patches of candidate targets can be obtained, where n is the number of templates. Each item of the dictionary is a d-dimensional vector corresponding to a local patch extracted from T. The process of constructing dictionary is similar to [6] that demonstrates the advantage of constructing dictionary in this way.

The first n ($n = 8$) frames are tracked using other tracking algorithm and the tracking result (normalized to 32×32) of each frame is treated as a template, then we obtain the set of templates T.

Each local image patch x_i in X can be encoded with the dictionary D by solving

$$\min_{\alpha_i} \|x_i - D\alpha_i\|_2^2 + \lambda \|\alpha_i\|_1, \tag{1}$$

where $\alpha_i \in R^{(N \times n) \times 1}$ is the sparse code, corresponding to local patch x_i. λ is a regularization parameter that controls sparsity and reconstruction error. Then the sparse coefficient matrix A of the candidate X can be obtained, i.e. $A = [\alpha_1, \alpha_2, \cdots, \alpha_N] \in R^{(N \times n) \times N}$.

In order to fully describe the candidate X, we generate some local descriptors for X with the sparse coefficients. Detailed process is as follows: Given a candidate object region X, we can extract a set of overlapped local image patches (denoted as $x_1, x_2, \cdots, x_N$), and calculate a sparse code for each local patch according to Eq. 1. We select M local patches from all N local patches of the object region randomly (denoted as $x_{i_1}, x_{i_2}, \cdots, x_{i_M}$) and pool the sparse codes of the selected local patches using average-pooling method (see Eq. 2). Then, we get a local descriptor of the object region, $f_i \in R^{(N \times n) \times 1}$. If different local patches are selected, we can obtain different local descriptors. Therefore, the object region can generate m ($m = C_N^M$) local descriptors in total.

$$f_i = \frac{1}{M} \sum_{j=1}^{M} \alpha_{i_j} \tag{2}$$

where α_{i_j} is the sparse code of the local patch x_{i_j}.

In [19], in order to represent target with local sparse codes, authors use average pooling method for all sparse codes of the target to generate a vector. However, the strategy ignores the spatial layout of local patches. In our paper, each local descriptor which is generated by several sparse codes with average pooling method can keep spatial information to some extent.

2.2 Classifier Learning with Local Descriptors

Adaboost classifier is selected as our classifier for making the best of local descriptors. To initialize the classifier, we need to get training sample set S which is composed of N_p positive samples and N_q negative samples from the first n frames. We draw p ($p = 9$) positive samples around the tracking result of each frame via perturbation of a pixel around the target position, then N_p ($N_p = n \times p$) positive samples are obtained. We select N_q negative samples from the n-th frame further away from the target location with a Gaussian perturbation. Using the same way as Sect. 2.1, each training sample can generate m local descriptors. After that, our Adaboost classifier is learned with the local descriptors of training sample set.

Some training examples are randomly selected from entire training set S according to their weight. Each selected example has m local descriptors, so we can train m weak classifiers based on these local descriptors of selected examples. Next, the best weak classifier of m weak classifiers is selected (having the lowest classification error) according to the classification error of the weak classifier that is estimated to entire training set S. We denote the best weak classifier as $h_1(x)$. Then, all training samples of S are re-weighted so that samples that are misclassified can get more weight. Carrying out the process repeatedly, we can receive some weak classifiers $h_2(x), \cdots, h_k(x)$. The final strong classifier $H(x)$ is as follow,

$$H(x) = \sum_{i=1}^{k} \rho_i h_i(x), \tag{3}$$

where ρ_i is the weight of $h_i(x)$.

In this paper, we use linear classifier as weak classifier that is calculated by solving the following optimization problem [18],

$$w^* = \arg\min_{w} \frac{1}{L} \sum_{i=1}^{L} \log\left(1 + e^{-y_i w^T z_i'}\right) + \frac{\eta}{2} \|w\|_2^2, \tag{4}$$

where w is the classifier parameter, L is the number of selected training examples, $z_i' = [z_i^T, 1]^T$ and $z_i \in R^{(N \times n) \times 1}$ is a local descriptor, y_i represents the property of the local descriptor z_i, i.e., $+1$ for positive training example and -1 for negative training example, η is a regularization term.

2.3 Weight Calculation Based on Reconstruction Error

We draw some samples around the target location in the previous frame as the candidate targets of current frame and each candidate target has a classification score with the strong classifier $H(x)$. A simple approach is that the candidate target with the largest score is treated as tracking result of current frame. However, the classification result is not accurate when the target experiences great appearance variations, because the samples used to train classifier are sampled from the previous frames. In order to improve the accuracy of result, we assign a weight to each candidate target to adjust its classification score. The weight value of a candidate target is calculated based on reconstruction error under the dictionary and reflects the similarity between the candidate target and templates.

From the Sect. 2.1, we know that the dictionary can be denoted as

$$D = \left[d_1, \cdots, d_N, d_{N+1}, \cdots, d_{2N}, \cdots, d_{(n-1)N+1}, \cdots, d_{nN}\right] \in R^{d\times(n\times N)}. \quad (5)$$

If the candidate X is perfect, the local image patch x_i in X should be represented well by sub-dictionary $D_i = \left[d_i, d_{N+i}, \cdots, d_{(n-1)N+i}\right] \in R^{d\times n}, 1 \leq i \leq N$ and the sparse code under D_i is denoted as $\beta^i = \left[\alpha_i^i, \alpha_i^{N+i}, \cdots, \alpha_i^{(n-1)N+i}\right]^T \in R^{n\times 1}$ where α_i^j is the j-th item of α_i. The reconstruction error ε_i of the local image patch x_i under D_i can be calculated by

$$\varepsilon_i = \left\|x_i - D_i\beta^i\right\|_2^2. \quad (6)$$

For purpose of calculating the reconstruction error more conveniently, Eq. 6 can be rewritten as follow,

$$\varepsilon_i = \|x_i - D\left(\omega_i \otimes \alpha_i\right)\|_2^2, \quad (7)$$

where $\alpha_i \in R^{(N\times n)\times 1}$ is the sparse code of x_i under dictionary D, $\otimes$ is the element-wise multiplication,

$$\omega_i = \left[\omega_i^1, \omega_i^2, \cdots, \omega_i^{(N\times n)}\right]^T \in R^{(N\times n)\times 1}, \quad (8)$$

and

$$\omega_i^j = \begin{cases} 1, & j = i, i+N, \cdots, i+(n-1)N \\ 0, & others \end{cases}. \quad (9)$$

Our method of calculating reconstruction error is motivated by the paper [6]. The main advantage of the method is that it takes spatial layout between local patches into account. In order to make full use of the sparse code α_i, we add a penalty term $\|D \cdot ((1-\omega_i) \otimes \alpha_i)\|_1$ to Eq. 7, so Eq. 7 can be rewritten as follow,

$$\varepsilon_i = \|x_i - D\left(\omega_i \otimes \alpha_i\right)\|_2^2 + \gamma\|D \cdot ((1-\omega_i) \otimes \alpha_i)\|_1, \quad (10)$$

where γ controls the strength of the penalty term. If x_i can be represented well by sub-dictionary D_i, the penalty term will be very small, otherwise very large.

After reconstruction errors of all patches in candidate X are obtained, the weight W of X can be calculated by

$$W = \sum_{i=1}^{N} \exp\left(-\beta\varepsilon_i\right), \quad (11)$$

where β is a constant and N is the number of local patches in X.

When partial occlusion happens to target, the occluded patches may have large reconstruction errors, but the other patches still have small reconstruction errors, so the weight of the target still keep a relative big value. If a candidate is bad, its weight is smaller than target because each patch of the bad candidate has large reconstruction error.

2.4 Template and Classifier Update

Templates should be updated dynamically to adapt to appearance changes. In our work, each template T_i has a weight a_i and its initial value is 1. After getting the target of each frame, we update the weight of each template via $a_i = a_i \cdot e^{-\theta}$, where θ is the angle between T_i and target. Template update is carried out every t ($t = 5$) frames and we choose the template with the least weight to be replaced by a new template. The process mentioned above is similar to [5] to some extent.

In [6], authors use sparse representation and incremental subspace learning to reconstruct a new template and then exploit it to replace an old template. It is efficient but it still has a problem. Before a new template is reconstructed, the tracking results are employed to incrementally update the eigenbasis vectors. If noise or occlusion exists in tracking results, the updated eigenbasis vectors will degenerate gradually. Therefore, the occlusion in tracking results should be handled firstly. In this paper, we use the same way as [9] to handle the occlusion in tracking results.

After getting the target of each frame, we reconstruct the target by

$$[\hat{z}, \hat{s}] = \arg\min_{z,s} \frac{1}{2} \|\bar{y} - Uz - s\|_2^2 + \lambda_1 \|s\|_1, \tag{12}$$

where $\bar{y} = y - \mu$, y represents the observation vector, U is composed of PCA basis vectors, μ is the mean vector, z denotes the coefficients of $\bar{y}$ under U and s is the noise term. Then y is reconstructed by

$$y_r^i = \begin{cases} y^i \,, s^i = 0 \\ \mu^i \,, s^i \neq 0 \end{cases}, \tag{13}$$

where y_r^i denotes the i-th item of y_r which is the reconstructed observation vector. The reconstructed observation vector is collected and then we incrementally update U and μ.

When template needs to be updated (every t frames), we firstly compute the coefficient $\hat{z}$ of current observation vector by Eq. 12, then reconstruct a new template by

$$T^* = U\hat{z} + \mu, \tag{14}$$

where T^* is the new template used for updating the template with the least weight.

We draw p ($p = 9$) positive samples around the tracking result of each frame via perturbation of a pixel, then replace some old positive samples, and update the negative samples every t frames via drawing some samples further away from the target location. The Adaboost classifier is then retrained by the updated training sample set.

2.5 Object Tracking by Particle Filter

Our tracking algorithm is implemented based on particle filter framework. Let x_t represents the target state variable and $z_{1:t} = \{z_1, z_2, \cdots, z_t\}$ denotes the observations up to time t. x_t can be estimated by $\hat{x}_t = \arg\max_{x_t} p(x_t|z_{1:t})$, where $p(x_t|z_{1:t})$ is the posterior probability and can be computed by Bayesian theorem,

$$p(x_t|z_{1:t}) \propto p(z_t|x_t) \int p(x_t|x_{t-1})\, p(x_{t-1}|z_{1:t-1}) dx_{t-1}, \tag{15}$$

where $p(x_t|x_{t-1})$ is a dynamic model and $p(z_t|x_t)$ is an observation model. In our algorithm, the target motion is modeled by the affine transformation with six parameters. We apply a Gaussian distribution $p(x_t|x_{t-1}) = \mathrm{N}(x_t; x_{t-1}, \Sigma)$ to represent the dynamic model, where Σ is a diagonal covariance matrix. The observation model is constructed by

$$p(z_t|x_t) \propto W \cdot H(x), \tag{16}$$

where $H(x)$ is the classification score of a candidate and W is the weight.

3 Experimental Results

Our tracking algorithm is tested on 51 challenging videos provided with the recent benchmark [3], and compared with 12 state-of-the-art trackers which show the best performance on the benchmark. The trackers used for comparison are: Struck [11], SCM [15], TLD [12], ASLA [6], CXT [20], VTD [21], VTS [22], CSK [23], LSK [19], DFT [24], LOT [25], OAB [26]. For convenience, we directly use the results of these trackers provided with [3] to conduct comparative experiments with our results.

We use the precision plot and success plot [3] to measure the overall performance. The precision plot indicates the percentage of frames whose center location error (the distance between center location of tracking result and that of ground truth) is less than a given threshold distance. The precision score of each tracker is represented with the score under the threshold = 20 pixels. The success plot demonstrates the radios of successful frames whose bounding box overlap is larger than a given threshold. The AUC (area under curve) of each success plot is used to measure the trackers.

3.1 Experiments Setup

The proposed algorithm is implemented in MATLAB R2012b and runs at 1.1 frames/s on an Intel Core i7 3.4 GHz with 4G memory. The number of templates is 8, training samples and candidate targets are all normalized to 32×32 pixels, and then 9 overlapped 16×16 local patches are extracted within the region with 8 pixels as step length. When representing the local descriptors with local sparse codes, we select 3 local sparse codes from 9 local sparse codes to carry out average pooling, then can get 84 local descriptors. For learning classifier, we collect $N_p = 72$ (9 positive samples per frame and 8 consecutive frames) positive samples and $N_q = 150$ negative samples. We select 2/3 samples randomly from all training samples to get 84 weak classifiers, and then select the best weak

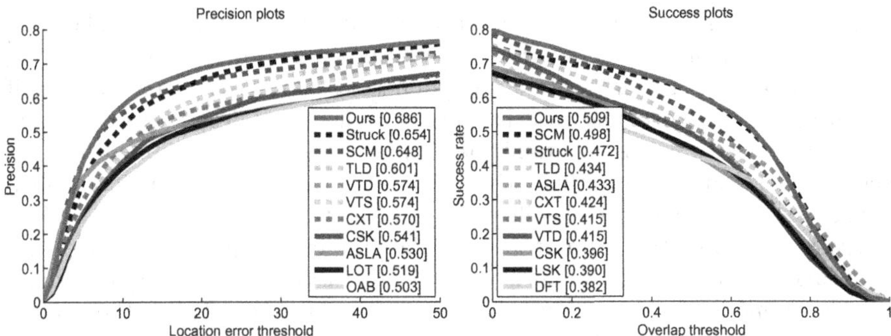

Fig. 1. Precision plots and success plots over all 51 video sequences. The legends in left figure and right figure shows the precision scores and AUC scores for each tracker, respectively.

classifier. After repeat 100 times, we obtain 100 candidate weak classifiers and the number of chosen weak classifier is set to 45. The templates and the Adaboost classifier are updated every 5 frames.

The other parameters are set as follows. The variable λ in Eq. 1, η in Eq. 4, γ in Eq. 10, β in Eq. 11 and λ_1 in Eq. 12 are set to 0.01, 0.1, 0.01, 5 and 0.1 respectively. The affine transformation with six parameters is fixed to [8, 8, 0.005, 0, 0, 0]. The number of particles is set to 600. All the parameters mentioned in this section are fixed for all sequences.

3.2 Overall Performance

Figure 1 shows the precision plots and success plots which illustrate the overall performance of our tracker and the competing trackers on 51 videos. For precision plots, we rank the trackers according to the result at error threshold of 20 pixels. For success plots, the trackers are ranked as the AUC scores. The precision scores and AUC scores for each tracker are shown in the legend of Fig. 1. Only the top 10 of the competing trackers and our tracker are displayed for clarity.

From Fig. 1, we can see that our tracker, Struck and SCM perform well, but our tracker achieves the best performance. In precision plot, our algorithm performs 3.2 % better than Struck, 3.8 % better than SCM. When the error threshold is reduced to 10 pixels, the SCM performs better than Struck but our method still performs best. If the error threshold is set to 5 pixels, our tracker and the SCM perform favorably compared to other trackers. In success plot, our tracker outperforms SCM by 1.1 % and Struck by 3.7 %. When given a specific overlap threshold (e.g. 0.5), our method still achieves the best performance. We can also observe that SCM achieves higher precision when the error threshold is relatively small and higher success rate when the overlap threshold is relatively large. This is because SCM integrates holistic templates and local representations based on sparse code to handle appearance variations. Struck achieves higher precision scores than SCM, but lower AUC scores than SCM. The main reason is that Struck only predicts the location of target and ignores scale variation.

Overall, our tracker performs favorably compared to other trackers. The main reasons are explained as follows. First, the proposed method can generate some structural local descriptors for target which possess good discrimination. Even if the target is partial occluded or contaminated, some local descriptors generated by the parts which are not contaminated still possess good discrimination. Our method can select some discriminative local descriptors to train classifier, which ensures the accuracy of the classifier. Second, the weight value is calculated by structural reconstruction error of the candidate target to adjust the classification score, and a small weight value is assigned to the bad candidate. Therefore, the weight model improves the robustness of our tracker. Third, the update scheme doesn't introduce heavy occlusion and alleviates the drift problem to some extent.

3.3 Attribute Based Performance Analysis

The performance of a tracker is affected by many factors which can be divided into 11 attributes [3]. The 51 videos are annotated with the 11 different attributes and one sequence may be annotated with several attributes, then we can con-

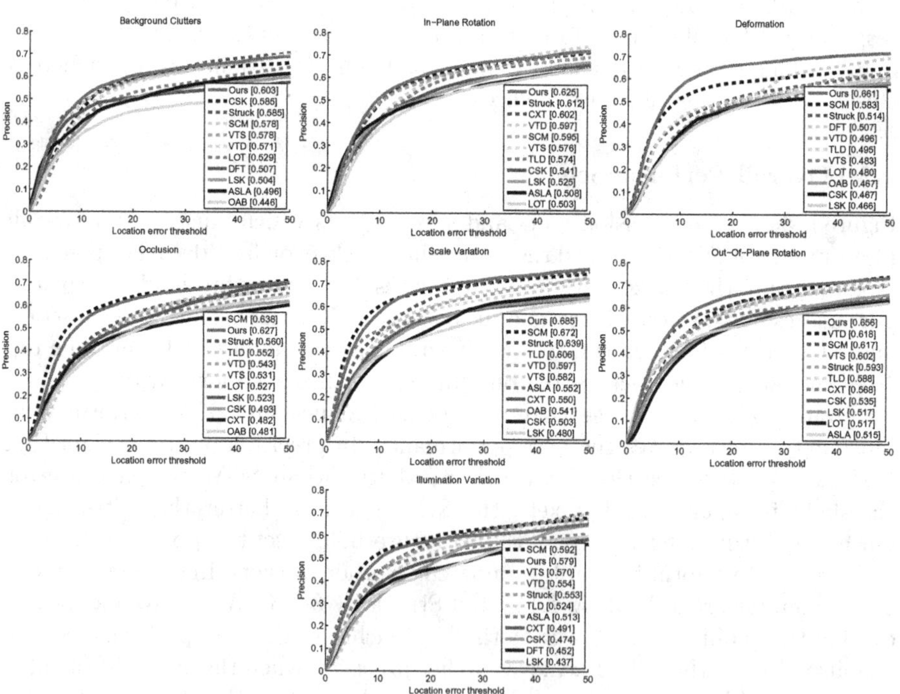

Fig. 2. Attribute based performance analysis using precision plots. These attributes are: background clutters, in-plane rotation, deformation, occlusion, scale variation, out-of-plain rotation, illumination variation.

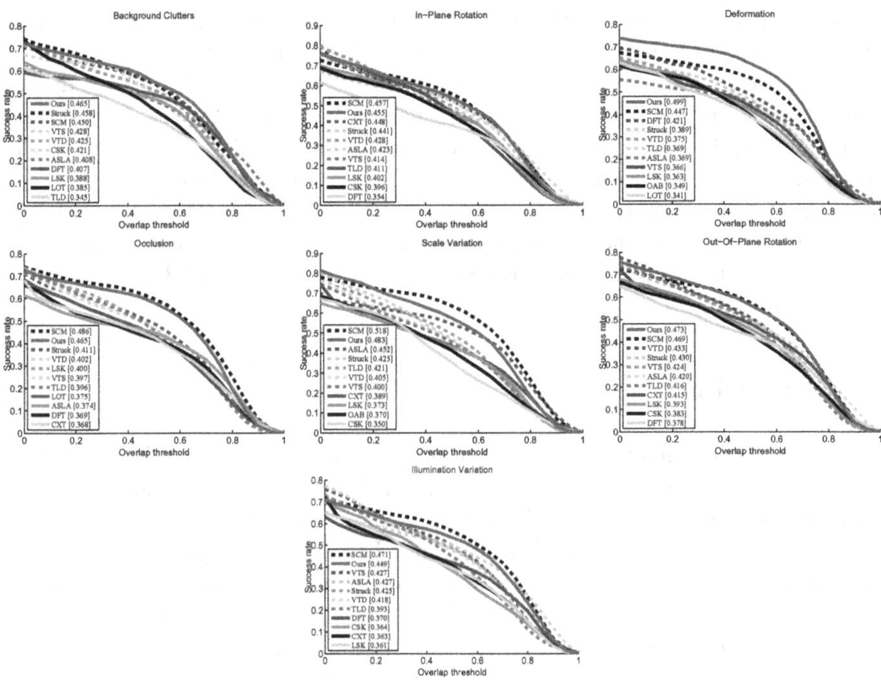

Fig. 3. Attribute based performance analysis using success plots. These attributes are: background clutters, in-plane rotation, deformation, occlusion, scale variation, out-of-plain rotation, illumination variation.

struct 11 subsets based on these attributes. Each subset can be utilized to evaluate the performance of trackers to deal with a specific challenging factor.

We compare our tracker with other methods on the 51 video sequences with respect to the 11 attributes mentioned above. Our tracker performs well in 7 of the 11 video subsets: background clutters, in-plane rotation, deformation, occlusion, scale variation, out-of-plain rotation and illumination variation. Figures 2 and 3 show the precision plots and success plots of our tracker and the competing trackers in these 7 attributes, respectively. These results show that our tracker is robust to appearance changes of a target object caused by some factors. At present, the proposed algorithm can't handle motion blur well.

On the occlusion subset, the SCM and our method perform favorably compared to other trackers. Our some structural local descriptors which are generated by the local patches that are not occluded still possess good discrimination; therefore, our tracker can avoid much influence of occlusion. Meanwhile, the weight model focuses more on the uncontaminated local patches, which makes our tracker more accurate. On the background clutters subset, the SCM, Struck and our method provide much better results. The reason that our method performs well is that our tracker considers the background information and selects some discriminative local descriptors to train classifier, which ensures the accuracy of the classifier. On the illumination variation subset, the SCM and our method perform much better than others. The reason is that the template update strategy, based on incremental PCA and occlusion handing scheme, is able to capture the appearance change due to illumination variation and alleviate the visual drift problem. On the deformation subset, our method provides superior results than others. It may be due to the proposed structural local descriptors that are robust to the deformation of target. However, for the blurry target, the proposed method may fail. The main reason is that the blurry local patches can't be well represented by the dictionary. Therefore, effectiveness of the sparse codes is restricted and the pooled local descriptors may lose discrimination.

4 Conclusion

In this paper, we employ sparse codes of local patches to generate local descriptors of object and then an Adaboost classifier is learned with the local descriptors of training sample set. The classifier is applied to candidate targets to separate the object from its surrounding background. In order to adapt the classifier to appearance change of the target, we assign a weight to each candidate target to adjust its classification score. The weight is computed based on reconstruction error under generative model and it reflects the similarity between the candidate target and templates. In addition, a robust template update scheme is applied. Comparison with the state-of-the-art trackers on the comprehensive benchmark shows effectiveness of the proposed method.

Acknowledgement. This work is supported in part by the National Natural Science Foundation of China (No. 61472036) and the Major State Basic Research Development Program of China (No. 2012CB720003).

References

1. Yilmaz, A., Javed, O., Shah, M.: Object tracking: a survey. ACM Comput. Surv. **38**, 1–45 (2006)
2. Li, X., Hu, W., Shen, C., Zhang, Z., Dick, A., Hengel, A.: A survey of appearance models in visual object tracking. ACM Trans. Intell. Syst. Technol. **4**, 271–288 (2013)
3. Wu, Y., Lim, J., Yang, M.: Online object tracking: a benchmark. In: CVPR, pp. 2411–2418 (2013)
4. Ross, D., Lim, J., Lin, R., Yang, M.: Incremental learning for robust visual tracking. IJCV **77**, 125–141 (2008)
5. Mei, X., Ling, H.: Robust visual tracking using l1 minimization. In: ICCV, pp. 1–8 (2009)
6. Jia, X., Lu, H., Yang, M.: Visual tracking via adaptive structural local sparse appearance model. In: CVPR, pp. 1822–1829 (2012)
7. Zhang, T., Ghanem, B., Liu, S., Ahuja, N.: Robust visual tracking via multi-task sparse learning. In: CVPR, pp. 2042–2049 (2012)

8. Wang, N., Wang, J., Yeung, D.: Online robust non-negative dictionary learning for visual tracking. In: ICCV, pp. 657–664 (2013)
9. Wang, D., Lu, H., Yang, M.:Least soft-threshold squares tracking. In: CVPR, pp. 2371–2378 (2013)
10. Babenko, B., Yang, M., Belongie, S.: Robust object tracking with online multiple instance learning. PAMI **33**, 1619–1632 (2011)
11. Hare, S., Saffari, A., Torr, P.H.: Struck: structured output tracking with kernels. In: ICCV, pp. 263–270 (2011)
12. Kalal, Z., Matas, J., Mikolajczyk, K.: P-n learning: bootstrapping binary classifiers by structural constraints. In: CVPR, pp. 49–56 (2010)
13. Zhang, K., Zhang, L., Yang, M.-H.: Real-time compressive tracking. In: Fitzgibbon, A., Lazebnik, S., Perona, P., Sato, Y., Schmid, C. (eds.) ECCV 2012, Part III. LNCS, vol. 7574, pp. 864–877. Springer, Heidelberg (2012)
14. Yao, R., Shi, Q., Shen, C., Zhang, Y., Hengel, A.: Part-based visual tracking with online latent structural learning. In: CVPR, pp. 2363–2370 (2013)
15. Zhong, W., Lu, H., Yang, M.: Robust object tracking via sparsity-based collaborative model. In: CVPR, pp. 1838–1845 (2012)
16. Dinh, T.B., Medioni, G.G.: Co-training framework of generative and discriminative trackers with partial occlusion handling. In: WACV, pp. 642–649 (2011)
17. Liu, R., Cheng, J., Lu, H.: A robust boosting tracker with minimum error bound in a co-training framework. In: ICCV, pp. 1459–1466 (2009)
18. Wang, Q., Chen, F., Xu, W., Yang, M.: Online discriminative object tracking with local sparse representation. In: WACV, pp. 425–432 (2012)
19. Liu, B., Huang, J., Yang, L., Kulikowsk, C.: Robust tracking using local sparse appearance model and k-selection. In: CVPR, pp. 1313–1320 (2011)
20. Dinh, T.B., Vo, N., Medioni, G.: Context tracker: exploring supporters and distracters in unconstrained environments. In: CVPR, pp. 1177–1184 (2011)
21. Kwon, J., Lee, K.: Visual tracking decomposition. In: CVPR, pp. 1269–1276 (2010)
22. Kwon, J., Lee, K.: Tracking by sampling trackers. In: ICCV, pp. 1195–1202 (2011)
23. Henriques, J.F., Caseiro, R., Martins, P., Batista, J.: Exploiting the circulant structure of tracking-by-detection with kernels. In: Fitzgibbon, A., Lazebnik, S., Perona, P., Sato, Y., Schmid, C. (eds.) ECCV 2012, Part IV. LNCS, vol. 7575, pp. 702–715. Springer, Heidelberg (2012)
24. Sevilla-Lara, L., Learned-Miller, E.G.: Distribution fields for tracking. In: CVPR, pp. 1910–1917 (2012)
25. Oron, S., Bar-Hillel, A., Levi, D., Avidan, S.: Locally orderless tracking. In: CVPR, pp. 1940–1947 (2012)
26. Grabner, H., Grabner, M., Bischof, H.: Real-time tracking via on-line boosting. In: BMVC (2006)

Coupling Multiple Alignments and Re-ranking for Low-Latency Online Multi-target Tracking

Yingkun Xu[1(✉)], Lei Qin[1], and Qingming Huang[1,2]

[1] Key Laboratory of Intelligent Information Processing of Chinese Academy of Sciences (CAS), Institute of Computing Technology, CAS, Beijing, China
{yingkun.xu,lei.qin,qingming.huang}@vipl.ict.ac.cn
[2] University of Chinese Academy of Sciences, Beijing, China

Abstract. Previous works for multi-target tracking employ two strategies: global optimization and online state estimation. In time-critical applications, the former methods have long temporal latency, and the latter can't recover from erroneous association or drifting. In this paper, we combine these two strategies, and propose a new low-latency online tracking approach. Unlike previous multi-hypotheses methods, which are always suffered from combinational explosion, our approach keeps the candidate associations using multiple alignments only in ambiguous cases. The novel features based on previous multi-frame associations are designed for re-ranking of the multiple linkages. The experimental results illustrate the advantage and robustness of these features based on prediction of previously generated tracks, and their discrimination to find optimal ones. Comparison with five state-of-the-art methods proves that our proposed method is competitive to global optimal ones and is superior to other online tracking algorithms.

1 Introduction

Visual multi-target tracking is a very important topic in computer vision. Applications based on visual multi-target tracking can be roughly classified into two categories. One is related with offline analysis after events take place. Mining similar actions and searching specific activities are examples of this category. The other aims to react to the online time-critical scenarios, such as finding abnormal events immediately or predicting dangerous accidents, and so on. Our work aims to promote the performance of multi-target tracking for the second category applications.

Various tracking approaches [1–8] are proposed to handle the tracking problems based on associations of detection responses. Considering the relationships between neighbor detection responses as being linked or not, the detection association can be modeled as network flow problems [1], k-shortest paths optimization [2], or conditional random fields (CRFs) with different constrains [3,4]. There are large feasible solution spaces for these models, and global optimizations are employed to achieve promising performance. In order to employ these global

D. Cremers et al. (Eds.): ACCV 2014, Part V, LNCS 9007, pp. 534–549, 2015.
DOI: 10.1007/978-3-319-16814-2_35

optimization algorithms for online time-critical applications, the temporal sliding windows mechanism is utilized to extend these methods. However, they are suffered from the cost of long latency by the straightforward extension.

In order to implement online multi-target tracking for quick reaction in instantaneous tasks, the frame-by-frame associations using greedy or bipartite matching approaches are employed with well-designed affinity metrics [5,6]. By comparison with global optimization, these approaches are more likely to produce some ambiguous associations at current instants. Because it is more distinguishable considering the linkages of future frames, one possible solution is using the information of next few frames to decide the better association at the present moment. Thus, the current tracking results will be deferred for some frames. If this latency is small enough, for example less than 0.5 s, such as the latency has nearly no effect for online applications, we still can deem the algorithm as online ones. Differing from frame-by-frame online tracking, we call these online methods with small-deferring as low-latency online tracking algorithms. The classic low-latency online tracking algorithms are multi-hypothesis tracking method (MHT) [7] and joint probabilistic data association filter (JPDAF) [8]. However, these two methods are suffered from two problems. The first is combinational explosion when the space of observation increases. The second is the final determination of association is coupled tightly with the local features which cause the ambiguities, thus the erroneous linkages can seldom be corrected. We need global features beyond the local affinities to find a better choice. In our work, we propose a new multi-association based online multi-tracking method. Instead of only using Gaussian kernel similarity of position in MHT, we combine different appearance and motional features in structured output Ranking-SVM framework, and generate multiple hypotheses considering different alignments between tracks and detections. The final association is determined by the multi-frames features considering the previous long temporal multi-frame assignments as illustrated in Fig. 1.

The insight of our approach tries to hybridize the frame-to-frame local affinity and multi-frame associations into one low-latency online tracking framework. We utilize weighted multiple features for frame-to-frame matching as in [6]. Through using multiple alignments, we can explore wider association space, and have more probability to cover correct linkages. We select the best solution using high-order multiple frame features which are more informative and discriminative than frame-to-frame affinity. Those long-term association features are widely used in the CRF model [3,4]. However, it is time-consuming and even intractable to train and to infer the best association status using arbitrarily complex features in CRFs. By comparison, re-ranking the possible associations using these multi-frame association features is more efficient and concise. Thus, the low-latency online solution can be designed using the strategy of local multi-frame associations and global re-ranking. In our method, the weights for combing the multi-frame association features are learned offline, and our approach is based on a hybrid strategy of the online tracking and offline learning.

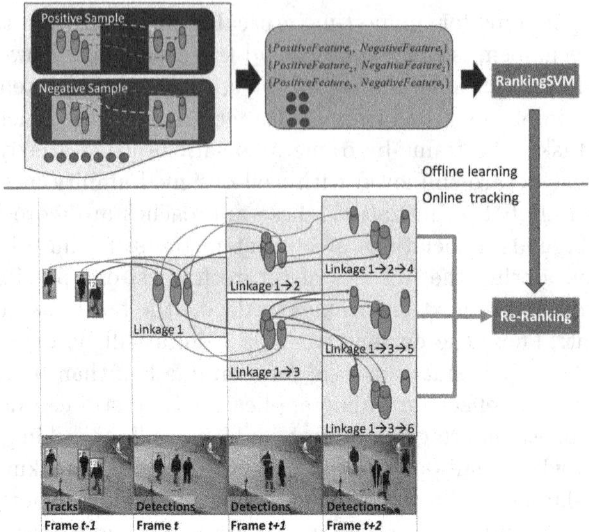

Fig. 1. The framework of our proposed approach. We construct the association pairs from ground truth as training samples to learn Ranking SVM model, and use the model to re-rank the current candidate associations when they can't be decided definitely. The 3 frame associations are composed by 3 step linkages as linked number list (such as linkage $1 \rightarrow 2 \rightarrow 4$) in the figure. The selected association is considered as the best association, and the its first linkage is the t-frame tracking result.

The main contributions of this paper lie in three points. (I) We develop a novel low-latency online multi-target tracking framework using re-ranking strategy. Compared with global optimization, which directly infer the most probable posterior within the CRF or MRF framework, we can use more complex high-order features. (II) We propose a new method to generate online multiple-hypotheses without bringing in the problem of combinational explosion. These multiple hypotheses consider the multiple alignments between tracks and detections, and are only necessary in the case of ambiguous linkage. (III) The discriminative features are proposed for multi-frame association re-ranking. Experimental results prove they are effective for re-ranking of the candidate associations based on previous tracking results.

2 Related Works

The core motivation of our paper is how to integrate the global association into the online tracking framework. Our strategy lies from the spirit of deferring the decision when the online matching is not easy to obtain. We instantiate this strategy in the online multi-target tracking with structured learning and re-ranking algorithm. The related works are outlined in following aspects.

Generating a small set of feasible solutions, and finding the best one after accumulation of evidences is a common strategy in the field of visual computing.

It is multi-stage cascading procedure in essence. The face detection algorithm [9] illustrates its advantages in performance and speed. This strategy is applied for measurement appraisal in the MHT [7] and JPDAF [8]. These approaches depend on the two stages of finding the candidate K-best solutions and choosing the optimal one with largest sum of log-probabilities of leaf-branches after a temporal delay. The cascading algorithms have also been utilized within particle filter framework [10,11]. Different from these algorithms, we combine the re-ranking algorithm to promote the association results of the online structured learning.

Combination of offline global optimization and online updating is utilized in some previous works [12,13]. It has been proved to be effective to improve the tracking performance using the selected features which are trained with large scale dataset. In [12], a most discriminative feature pool is learned beforehand, and they serve as the candidate features for each gallery track segment. In [13], a deep stacked denoising auto-encoder is employed to learn the robust features from an image dataset, and these features are updated in online tracking using additive sigmoid classifiers. By contrast, our proposed approach can be considered as a tradeoff between the global optimization and online multi-target state updating.

There have been some works related with getting M best solutions in probabilistic model [14,15], and deterministic graphic optimization problems [16,17]. In our work, we use different alignments to get at most M best solutions within the framework of structured output learning. Among the candidate M best solutions, we utilize the re-ranking algorithm to score and select the potential best one. Re-ranking algorithms are transferred from natural language processing [18] and information retrieval [19] to the problems of visual tracking [20,21]. In [20], a CRF model is constructed to represent the possible connections between detection responses. RankBoost algorithm is employed to train the model with sampling association pairs. In [21], the weakly supervised ranking algorithm is proposed to learn the weights of appearance features. The graph Laplacian is used to regularize the smoothness of similarities between samples. Different from above methods, we employ the high-order and complex features from multi-frames associations to preferably assess the correctness of the candidate solutions, and appraisal the best one.

3 Online Multi-target Tracking with Multiple Alignments Between Tracks and Detections

Learning multiple features and combining them is an important topic to enhance the robustness of online multi-target tracking. Here, we employ the structured output SVM learning as in [6] to learn the weights for combining multiple features.

Denoting the j-th detection response in frame t as $s_j^t = (b_j^t, o_{j,1}^t, o_{j,2}^t, \dots, o_{j,K}^t)$, where b_j^t is the bounding box and $o_{j,k}^t$ is its k-th feature, the set of detection responses in frame t is $S^t = \{s_j^t\}_{j=1}^n$. Further, we can define the i-th candidate

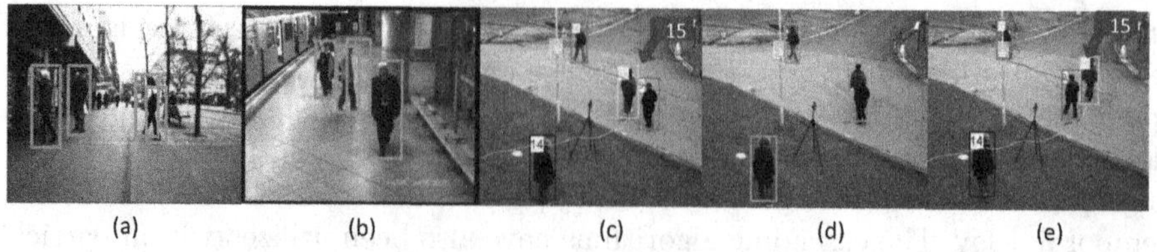

Fig. 2. (a,b) Detection responses are imprecise using two type detectors [23,24]. (c–e) Object 15 has occluded template features. In order to decide the association of object 15 to the detections in (d), the association of next frame in (e) has more distinguishable features.

track till frame $t-1$ as the detection response list $r_i^{t-1} = \{s_i^{t-l}, s_i^{t-l+1}, \ldots, s_i^{t-1}\}$ from the start frame $t-l$ to frame $t-1$. Thus, the set of candidate tracks for frame t is $R^{t-1} = \{r_i^{t-1}\}_{i=1}^m$. Based on the K dimension features defined for each detection response, we can calculate the K-dimensional affinity between r_i^{t-1} and s_j^t denoted as $a_{i,j}^t = \phi(r_i^{t-1}, s_j^t)$, and combine the K-dimensional affinity vector using weight w into one affinity scalar.

In the problem of online multi-target tracking using detection response association, we need to link the candidate tracks R^{t-1} and detection responses S^t for each frame t. Let a binary vector set $\mathcal{Y}_t = \{y_t | y_t = [y_{1,1}^t, \ldots, y_{m,1}^t, y_{1,2}^t, \ldots, y_{m,n}^t]^T\}$ represent the linking result candidates, there should be the constraints $\sum_i y_{i,j} \leq 1$ and $\sum_j y_{i,j} \leq 1$ because one candidate track is matched with one detection response at most. To solve the problem of how to obtain the online association y^t. The optimal bipartite matching method can be employed to obtain y_t by $y_t = \arg\max_{y \in \mathcal{Y}_t} \langle w, y^T \Phi(R^{t-1}, S^t) \rangle$, where the feature matching matrix $\Phi(R^{t-1}, S^t) = [a_{1,1}^t, \ldots, a_{m,1}^t, a_{1,2}^t, \ldots, a_{m,n}^t]^T$. To obtain the optimized weight vector $\tilde{w}$, we utilize the structured output SVM algorithm as in [6]:

$$
\begin{aligned}
\tilde{w} = \arg\min_{w} \quad & \frac{1}{2}\|w\|^2 + \frac{C_1}{N}\sum \xi^t \\
s.t. \ & \max_{y \in \mathcal{Y}_t} \Delta(y, y_t) - \langle w, y_t^T \Phi(R^{t-1}, S^t) - y^T \Phi(R^{t-1}, S^t) \rangle \leq \xi^t \\
& \forall \xi^t \geq 0, t = 1...N
\end{aligned}
\tag{1}
$$

This problem has efficient cutting-plane solution [27] using N collected samples: $\{y_t, \Phi(R^{t-1}, S^t)\}_{t=1}^N$.

The above formulations present an efficient solution for multi-target tracking by offline learning. Same as in [6], we define the loss function $\Delta(y, y_t) \equiv y^T(1-y_t)$ and 42-dimensional features for each detection response. However, there are still some problems needed to be discussed in detail. One of the most important issues is how to define the K-dimensional affinity $a_{i,j}^t = \phi(r_i^{t-1}, s_j^t)$ so that the matching between s_j^t and r_i^t is aligned. In order to design meaningful and effective affinity vector, we should keep the features in tracks and in detections consistent as far as possible. Normally, it is difficult for detectors to obtain complete aligned results. It is also hard to design consistent tracking features using detection pools along tracks, which acts as the templates to match with detections. For example, in Fig. 2, the detectors [23,24] obtain some imprecise results as illustrated in (a) and (b). To match with detection results in the next frame as in (c) and (d), the tracks may utilize their last detected features as their templates because these detections are mostly close to their next matched detections. However, this strategy is not suitable for the case of partial occlusion, in which the features of the last detections may be generated from the occluders rather than from targets themselves as in (d). These misaligned features between tracks and detections make the affinity unreliable for online tracking.

From above discussion, the problems of inconsistent features between tracks and detections can be considered as different cases of misalignments. From the view of tracking, the features of tracks may suffer from unreliability due to pose changing and occlusions, which will cause the feature templates to be ambiguous. These ambiguities can be considered as progressive misalignment. From the view of detections, the bounding boxes of detection response may be skew to one side because of irregular shapes or non-max suppression operations. These skew bounding boxes can be considered as detection misalignment. These two kinds of misalignments are the main problems of how to design the appropriate affinity functions between tracks and detections. Our paper mainly discuss how to obtain the better online association using re-ranking considering these misalignments.

4 Re-ranking of Multi-online Associations with SSVM Learning

4.1 Re-ranking of Multiple Online Associations Using Multi-alignments

To handle the feature misalignment between tracks and detections, a straightforward approach is to infer the best one among the candidate alignments. However, it is nearly intractable to find the optimal alignment because it is hard to predict which trajectories are occluded and whether the detections are irregular. Therefore, we keep the different alignments to cover the optimal one as possible as we could. In our approach, the kept alignments of tracks have two types: the average features and the latest features of their most recent detections. The kept alignments of detections are based on four corners of the bounding box. Therefore, there are at most eight cases for the association in one frame, although in the most frames only one or two of them are different and kept.

To find the best one of the multiple alignments at the frame t, we foresee associations in next Δt frames based on previous ΔT tracking results, and we denote the temporal range from $t - \Delta T$ to $t + \Delta t$ as $[t - \Delta T : t + \Delta t]$. Because the accumulative features are more discriminative than those from single one frame, we accumulate evidences of multiple frame association in these $\Delta T + \Delta t$ frames. Then, we employ the re-ranking algorithm with the accumulative features to select the best candidate multi-frame associations. To simplify

Table 1. Notations for Re-ranking of Multi-frame Associations

Symbols	Description
$[t_a : t_b]$	The discrete set from t_a to t_b. If t_a and t_b is frame number, then the discrete set represent one frame range from t_a to t_b
$R_{[t-\Delta T:t+\Delta t]}$	The trajectory set which are overlapped with the frame range from frame $t - \Delta T$ to frame $t + \Delta t$
$S_{[t-\Delta T:t+\Delta t]}$	The detection set which are detected within the frame range from frame $t - \Delta T$ to frame $t + \Delta t$
$y_{[t:t+\Delta t]}$	The association between trajectory set $R_{[t-\Delta T:t+\Delta t]}$ and detection set $S_{[t:t+\Delta t]}$ within the frame range from t to $t + \Delta t$
$r_k^{[t-\Delta T:t+\Delta t]}$	The k-th trajectory in the trajectory set $R_{[t-\Delta T:t+\Delta t]}$ which has detection set within the frame range from $t - \Delta T$ to $t + \Delta t$
t_s^k, t_e^k	The first frame number and the last frame number of the trajectory $r_k^{[t-\Delta T:t+\Delta t]}$ within the frame range from $t - \Delta T$ to $t + \Delta t$
$s_k^{t_p}$	The detection response at the frame t_p for the trajectory $r_k^{[t-\Delta T:t+\Delta t]}$
$B(r_k^{[t-\Delta T:t]})$	One B-spline curve fitting for the k-trajectory $r_k^{[t-\Delta T:t]}$
$\theta_k^{t_p}$	The motion angle of the k-trajectory $r_k^{[t-\Delta T:t+\Delta t]}$ at frame t_p
$P_k^{t_p}$	The location point of detection bounding box of the k-trajectory $r_k^{[t-\Delta T:t+\Delta t]}$ at frame t_p
$W_k^{t_p}$	The width of detection bounding box of the k-trajectory $r_k^{[t-\Delta T:t+\Delta t]}$ at frame t_p
$v\theta(\Delta t_\tau)_k^{t_p}$	The angle velocity of the k-trajectory $r_k^{[t-\Delta T:t+\Delta t]}$ at frame t_p
$vP(\Delta t_\tau)_k^{t_p}$	The linear velocity of the k-trajectory $r_k^{[t-\Delta T:t+\Delta t]}$ at frame t_p

the detailed explanation of our re-ranking algorithm. We extend the notations in Sect. 3 and list their descriptions in Table 1.

The function to score the multi-frame associations based on above multiple alignments is expressed as:

$$f_{[t-\Delta T:t+\Delta t]}(y_{[t:t+\Delta t]}) = \alpha^T \Psi(R_{[t-\Delta T:t+\Delta t]}, S_{[t-\Delta T:t+\Delta t]}, y_{[t:t+\Delta t]}) \quad (2)$$

where α is the weight of re-ranking features Ψ, $S_{[t-\Delta T:t+\Delta t]}$ is the set of detections in temporal range $[t - \Delta T : t + \Delta t]$, and $R_{[t-\Delta T:t+\Delta t]}$ are trajectories in $[t - \Delta T : t + \Delta t]$ by appending the foresee associations $y_{[t:t+\Delta t]}$. The best association of y_t can be obtained by $y_t = \arg\max_{y \in \tilde{\mathcal{Y}}_t} f_{[t-\Delta T:t+\Delta t]}(y_{[t:t+\Delta t]})$, in which $\tilde{\mathcal{Y}}_t$ is the candidate association set obtained from Sect. 3 considering multi-alignments. Next subsection will discuss how to design the re-ranking features Ψ.

4.2 Re-ranking Features for Multi-frame Associations

The key to find optimal choice of candidate associations is to design appropriate features $\Psi(R_{[t-\Delta T:t+\Delta t]}, S_{[t-\Delta T:t+\Delta t]}, y_{[t:t+\Delta t]})$ for these associations.

Intuitively, the foreseeing short-term associations $y_{[t:t+\Delta t]}$ in frames $[t : t + \Delta t]$ are expected to be consistent with the previous long-term associated trajectories backward to frames. To achieve this point, we design the features in three aspects. First, we expect the observed detection responses in each trajectory between frames $[t : t + \Delta t]$ have consistent appearance and motional trends as its previous part in frames in frames $[t - \Delta T : t]$. Second, the relationship between every two trajectories should have potential consistency with the scenario, while keeping the exclusions between each other. Third, the statistical attributes of the associations should have similar distribution as those in the training dataset. We discuss in detail for these features in following three aspects.

In the first aspect, we consider the features to keep intra-consistency for trajectories from the points of appearance, shape and motion. Given the trajectory set $R_{[t-\Delta T:t+\Delta t]} = \{r_k^{[t-\Delta T:t+\Delta t]}\}_{k=1}^M$, we split the frame length ΔT to N_a parts $[t - \Delta T_i : t - \Delta T_{i+1}]$, $i \in [1..N_a]$, using same log-length frame intervals. We denote the k-th track as the detection list $\{s_k^{t_s^k}, ..., s_k^{t_e^k}\}$. For each interlaced frame $t_j \in [t : 2 : t + \Delta t]$, the appearance intra-consistency feature can be expressed as $\Psi_{i,j}^1$:

$$\Psi_{i,j}^1 = \frac{1}{M} \sum_{k=1}^{M} I(t_s^k < t - \Delta T_i) \max_{t_p \in [t - \Delta T_i : t - \Delta T_{i+1}]} Aff(s_k^{t_p}, s_k^{t_j}) \tag{3}$$

where $I(.)$is indicator function, and $Aff(s_k^{t_p}, s_k^{t_j})$ is the similarity between two detections $s_k^{t_p}$, $s_k^{t_j}$ using Bhattacharyya coefficient. Using three types of appearance information (HSV, LBP, and RGB color), we can obtain 45 dimension features for appearance similarities based on 3 interlaced short-term frames and 64 frames of previously tracking results ($N_a = 5$).

To express the intra-consistency of the shape for trajectories, we expect the smoothness of fitting curves is good as possible as those in ground truth. Thus, fitting the detection points and computing the errors of detection points in the future Δt frames is very important clues. To allow motional changes, we fit the curve for detections within different length frames, with the length as half of the previous length. For example, looking backward 64 frames of previously tracking results, there are 4 groups of curves $B_i(r_k^{[t-\Delta T:t]})$, where the i-th group of curves is obtained from temporal range $[t - 2^i \Delta\tau : t]$, $i \in [1..4]$. Thus, for the i-th group of curves, the smoothness for all tracks can be:

$$\Psi_i^2 = \frac{1}{M} \sum_{k=1}^{M} I(t_s^k < t - 2^{i-1}\Delta\tau) \frac{1}{\Delta t} \sum_{t_j \in [t:t+\Delta t]} \exp(-\lambda_1 \left\| P_k^{t_j} - B_i(r_k^{[t-\Delta T:t]}) \right\|_2) \tag{4}$$

where $\|P - B\|_2$ is the Euclidean distance from the center point P to the curve B.

To illustrate the intra-consistency of motional trend for the trajectories, we consider the motional direction and velocity respectively. Given the directions and locations of the trajectory $r_k^{[t-\Delta T:t+\Delta t]}$ as $\{\theta_k^{t_s^k}, \ldots, \theta_k^{t_e^k}\}$ and $\{P_k^{t_s^k}, \ldots, P_k^{t_e^k}\}$, we can compute their angular velocity and linear velocity at each moment as

$\{v\theta(\Delta t_\tau)_k^{t_i^k} = (\theta_k^{t_i^k} - \theta_k^{t_i^k+\Delta t_\tau})/\Delta t_\tau\}$ and $\{vP(\Delta t_\tau)_k^{t_i^k} = (P_k^{t_i^k} - P_k^{t_i^k+\Delta t_\tau})/\Delta t_\tau\}$ by consideration of different temporal interval Δt_τ. It is helpful to tolerate the misalignments of detections using different Δt_τ because the small perturbations exist in the detection responses. Assuming the angular velocities obey von Mises distribution as in [25] and the linear velocities obey Gaussian distribution, the motion consistencies based on temporal difference Δt_τ are expressed as:

$$\Psi^3_{\Delta t_\tau} = \frac{1}{M}\sum_{k=1}^{M}\frac{1}{\Delta t}\sum_{t_j\in[t:t+\Delta t]}\frac{1}{2\pi I_0(\lambda_2)}\exp(\lambda_2\cos(v\theta(\Delta t_\tau)_k^{t_j})) \tag{5}$$

$$\Psi^4_{\Delta t_\tau} = \frac{1}{M}\sum_{k=1}^{M}\frac{1}{\Delta t}\sum_{t_j\in[t:t+\Delta t]}\exp(-\frac{(vP(\Delta t_\tau)_k^{t_j} - vP(\Delta t_\tau)_k^{t_j-1})^2}{2\sigma_k^2(vP(\Delta t_\tau)_k)}) \tag{6}$$

where I_0 is modified Bessel function of order 0. Using 3 different values for Δt_τ, e.g. (1, 2, 4), we can get 6 dimension features.

In the second aspect, we expect to obtain the features between every two trajectories. These features should reflect the information of mutual exclusion among the trajectories, as well as coincident with context. For example, people always walk along the limited paths since there are not too many roads in one scenario. Thus, some persons will pass along similar paths when there are lots of people walking through. We design the features from the aspects of trajectory shapes. To obtain the features between the trajectory shapes, we compute the chamfer distance between every two trajectories. We keep its 5-bins histogram after normalization by the width of bounding box $\{W_k^{t_s^k},\ldots,W_k^{t_e^k}\}$. The value of i-bin is:

$$\Psi_i^5 = \frac{1}{M(M-1)}\sum_{u\neq v}^{M} I(L(i) < Chd(r_u^{[t-\Delta T:t+\Delta t]}, r_v^{[t-\Delta T:t+\Delta t]}) < H(i)) \tag{7}$$

$$\text{where: } \mathrm{Chd}(\mathrm{r_u},\mathrm{r_v}) = \frac{1}{|\mathrm{r_u}|}\sum_{\mathrm{t_j}\in[\mathrm{t_t^u}:\mathrm{t_e^u}]}\min_{\mathrm{t_l}\in[\mathrm{t_t^v}:\mathrm{t_e^v}]}(\|\mathrm{P_u^{t_j}} - \mathrm{P_v^{t_l}}\|/\mathrm{W_u^{t_j}})$$

where $L(i)$ and $H(i)$ are the low and high boundary for bin i. We set the values as $(0, 0.5, 1, 2, 4)$ and $(0.5, 1, 2, 4, +\infty)$ for 5 bins respectively.

In the third aspect, extra statistic features of the trajectory group in the temporal range $[t - \Delta T : t + \Delta t]$ are calculated according to the ground truth. We expect the features obtained from the test associated trajectories are matched to these statistic values as much as possible. We utilize three statistic features. The first is the average occluded length. Inspired by the work [4], we use Cauchy-Lorentz distribution to model the consecutive occluded frames of each trajectory. The average weighted value is:

$$\Psi^6 = \frac{1}{M}\sum_{k=1}^{M}\prod_{\Delta j\in gaps(r_k^{[t-\Delta T:t]})}\frac{\lambda_3}{\left|r_k^{\Delta j}\right|^2 + \lambda_3^2} \tag{8}$$

where $gaps(r)$ is the occluded segments of track r, and $\left|r_k^{\Delta j}\right|$ is the consecutive frame length for occluded segment Δj.

The second statistic information is the number of started trajectory and the number of terminated trajectory between the temporal range $[t : t + \Delta t]$. We assume they are modeled by exponential distribution. Thus, we obtain the features related with these numbers as:

$$\Psi^7 = \exp(-\lambda_4 \frac{1}{M} \sum_{k=1}^{M} I(t <= t_s^k < t + \Delta t)) \tag{9}$$

$$\Psi^8 = \exp(-\lambda_5 \frac{1}{M} \sum_{k=1}^{M} I(t <= t_e^k < t + \Delta t)) \tag{10}$$

The third statistic information is the length of trajectory. We hope the trajectory extends as long as possible. Thus, too short trajectories are unexpected because they are always obtained by abnormal linkages. We calculate this attribution as following feature:

$$\Psi^9 = \exp(-\lambda_6 \frac{1}{M} \sum_{k=1}^{M} \frac{1}{t_e^k - t_s^k}) \tag{11}$$

Above 9 types of features are appended to appraisal whether the generated trajectories are better or not. The parameters $(\lambda_1, \lambda_2, \ldots, \lambda_6)$ are estimated by the ground truth. Using the length of $\Delta t = 5$ and $\Delta T = 64$, there are 64-dimension features by considering all above three aspects' features. By experiments, they are suitable for discrimination between positive associated tracks and negative ones.

4.3 Ranking SVM Learning of Multi-online Associations

Because our goal is to appraise multi-frame associations obtained using multiple alignments, we need to prioritize them using one score function $f_{[t-\Delta T:t+\Delta t]}(\cdot)$. This is a problem of re-ranking learning for structured output as discussed previously [26]. Given one pair of association results $y^i_{[t:t+\Delta t]}$ and $y^j_{[t:t+\Delta t]}$ such that the former has higher priority than the latter, denoting as $y^i_{[t:t+\Delta t]} \succ y^j_{[t:t+\Delta t]}$, we hope their values using score function have relationship:

$$y^i_{[t:t+\Delta t]} \succ y^j_{[t:t+\Delta t]} \Leftrightarrow f_{[t-\Delta T:t+\Delta t]}(y^i_{[t:t+\Delta t]}) > f_{[t-\Delta T:t+\Delta t]}(y^j_{[t:t+\Delta t]}) \tag{12}$$

Considering the linear weighted formulation defined in Eq.(2) and features defined in above section, we need to obtain the optimal weight vector α. This re-ranking for structured output can be solved efficiently using cutting-plane algorithm [27]. We employ the scaling slack form to learn the weight vector:

$$\alpha = \arg\min_{\alpha} \frac{1}{2} \|\alpha\|^2 + C_2 \sum_{i \in [1:|Q|]} \zeta^i \tag{13}$$

$$s.t.$$

$$\alpha^T (\Psi(R_{[t_i - \Delta T:t_i+\Delta t]}, S_{[t_i - \Delta T:t_i+\Delta t]}, y^{\circ}_{[t:t+\Delta t]}) -$$

$$\Psi(R_{[t_i - \Delta T:t_i+\Delta t]}, S_{[t_i - \Delta T:t_i+\Delta t]}, y_{[t:t+\Delta t]})) \geq 1 - \frac{\zeta^i}{L(y^{\circ}_{[t:t+\Delta t]}, y_{[t:t+\Delta t]})}$$

$$\forall \zeta^i \geq 0, \quad \forall y_{[t:t+\Delta t]} \neq y^{\circ}_{[t:t+\Delta t]} \quad \wedge \quad y_{[t:t+\Delta t]} \in Y_{[t:t+\Delta t]}$$

In our method, we extract the training sample pairs set Q from the ground truth. Each sample in this set is composed by the detections $S_{[t_i - \Delta T:t_i+\Delta t]}$ with at most length $\Delta T + \Delta t$, their association results $y^{\circ}_{[t:t+\Delta t]}$ by changing some linkages in ground truth as introduced in experiments, and the associated tracks $R_{[t_i:t_i+\Delta t]}$. The loss $L(y^{\circ}_{[t:t+\Delta t]}, y_{[t:t+\Delta t]})$ between two associations $y^{\circ}_{[t:t+\Delta t]}$ and $y_{[t:t+\Delta t]}$ are defined as the Hamming loss of the $y_{[t:t+\Delta t]}$ when $y^{\circ}_{[t:t+\Delta t]}$ is same with ground truth, or difference between the Hamming losses of $y_{[t:t+\Delta t]}$ and $y^{\circ}_{[t:t+\Delta t]}$. We use efficient one-slack algorithm [27] to train the weight vector α.

5 Experiments

To evaluate the performance of our proposed method, we utilize three public datasets: PETS09-S2-L1, ETHMS, and TUD. The sequences in these datasets contain different visual conditions, such as static camera and moving camera, partial occlusion and full occlusion, pose variation, and illumination changing, etc. More importantly, the detection results and tracking ground truth of these datasets are opened to public.[1] Thus, we can compare with other methods fairly.

We set the hyper-parameters C_1 and C_2 as 10.0 and 100.0, and estimate other parameters related with specific distributions by training dataset. In experiments, we train the re-ranking of multiple candidate associations using multi-frame features (3)–(11) in offline process. Then, we compare with five state-of-the-art multi-target tracking algorithms with public evaluation metrics.

In the offline training process, we learn the weights α for association features Ψ. We employ the ranking SVM algorithm. First, we need to construct the training dataset Q which is composed by multi-frame association pairs $\{(y^{q1}_{[t:t+\Delta t]}, y^{q2}_{[t:t+\Delta t]})\}_{q=1}^{|Q|}$. In each frame range $[t : t + \Delta t]$, we extract three different associations $y^{GT}_{[t:t+\Delta t]}$, $y^{A}_{[t:t+\Delta t]}$ and $y^{B}_{[t:t+\Delta t]}$, where the first association $y^{GT}_{[t:t+\Delta t]}$ is same as ground truth, and latter two associations $y^{A}_{[t:t+\Delta t]}$ and $y^{B}_{[t:t+\Delta t]}$ are obtained by three different transformation operations to $y^{GT}_{[t:t+\Delta t]}$: switching some detection segments between two tracks, drifting some detections for some tracks, or adding some faked tracks into the association. By using these operations, the constructed associations have such relationship $y^{GT}_{[t:t+\Delta t]} \succ y^{A}_{[t:t+\Delta t]} \succ y^{B}_{[t:t+\Delta t]}$ that we can construct three different pair samples $(y^{GT}_{[t:t+\Delta t]}, y^{A}_{[t:t+\Delta t]})$,

[1] http://iris.usc.edu/people/yangbo/downloads.html.

$(y^{GT}_{[t:t+\Delta t]}, y^{B}_{[t:t+\Delta t]})$ and $(y^{A}_{[t:t+\Delta t]}, y^{B}_{[t:t+\Delta t]})$. The size of training dataset triples the number of frame ranges which we can separate training sequences into. Thus, we construct 1404, 1095 and 114 pair samples from ETHMS, PETS09 and TUD respectively, and verify the tracking results by cross-validation between them.

Our method aims to combine the re-ranking multi-candidate associations into online tracking strategy. As discuss above, we need the cross-validate strategy to evaluate our method using different training set for re-ranking learning. We call our method as re-ranking based low-latency online multi-target tracking (ReRankingLMT). Specifically, the methods based on training datasets, ETHMS, PETS09 and TUD, are named ReRankingLMT-E, ReRankingLMT-P and ReRankingLMT-T respectively. To evaluate the performance of our proposed method using this combining strategy, we need to compare with the methods using online strategy and offline optimization. Using the common ground truth and detection response input, we compare with five state-of-the-art methods. The first two methods are recognition based tracking (PIRMPT) [12] and structured output SVM based method (SSVMMOT) [6]. Similar with our methods, these two algorithms combine the offline learned features to online tracking process. The last three methods are energy based algorithm (EnergyMIN) [22], the method considering exclusion between detections and trajectories (ExcTracking) [4] and the online CRF based method (OnlineCRF) [3]. These three methods construct different CRFs with different constraints, and global optimizations are executed to finding the best association results. It is convincible for our proposed method to compare with these five methods in aspects of both feature learning and long-term association optimization.

To evaluate the quantitative performance, we employ the VACE metrics [3]. These metrics are mainly composed by detection recall (RECALL), detection precision (PREC), the percentage of the mostly tracked objects (MT), the percentage of the partial tracked objects (PT), the percentage of the mostly lost objects (ML), the number of trajectories' interruption by tracking (Frag), and the number of real identities' changes for tracked trajectory (IDS). Because ML is redundant with MT and PT, we omit this item. These metrics can be calculated using public tools [3]. Moreover, we use the harmonic mean (F) of RECALL and PRECISION to reflect the overall metric.

Table 2 gives the results of comparison. By comparison with the similar online algorithms, PIRMPT and SSVMMOT, which utilized offline learned features in the online tracking manner. Our method exceeds them both in recall and integrity of the trajectories. Most true detections are linked to our tracked results and trajectories are generated more completely. By comparison with global optimization methods, EnergyMIN, ExcTracking and OnlineCRF, our approach shows competitive results. In the scenario of the static camera, such as in PETS09, our approach even outperforms these global optimizing algorithms. There are less identity switches and false-alarming tracking fragments. As discussed above, these attribute to the stable distinguishability in ambiguous associations. Besides, different from these global optimizing methods which all

Table 2. Comparison With State-of-the-art Methods

Datasets	METHOD	RECALL	PREC	F	MT	PT	Frag	IDS
PETS-2009-S2-L1	PIRMPT [12]	89.5 %	99.6 %	0.94	78.9 %	21.1 %	23	1
	SSVMMOT [6]	97.2 %	93.7 %	0.95	94.7 %	5.3 %	19	4
	OnlineCRF [3]	93.0 %	95.3 %	0.94	89.5 %	10.5 %	13	0
	ExcTracking [4]	—	—	—	94.7 %	5.3 %	15	22
	EnergyMIN [22]	92.4 %	98.4 %	0.95	91.3 %	4.3 %	6	11
	ReRankingLMT-E	98.9 %	97.5 %	0.98	94.7 %	5.3 %	3	2
	ReRankingLMT-T	98.9 %	97.7 %	0.98	94.7 %	5.3 %	4	2
TUD Stadtmitte	PIRMPT [12]	81.0 %	99.5 %	0.89	60.0 %	30.0 %	0	1
	SSVMMOT [6]	80.0 %	96.7 %	0.88	80.0 %	20.0 %	11	0
	OnlineCRF [3]	87.0 %	96.7 %	0.92	70.0 %	30.0 %	1	0
	ExcTracking [4]	—	—	—	40.0 %	60.0 %	13	15
	EnergyMIN [22]	84.7 %	86.7 %	0.86	77.8 %	22.2 %	3	4
	ReRankingLMT-E	89.0 %	98.6 %	0.94	80.0 %	20.0 %	3	3
	ReRankingLMT-P	89.5 %	98.2 %	0.94	80.0 %	20.0 %	4	3
ETHMS	PIRMPT [12]	76.8 %	86.6 %	0.81	58.4 %	33.6 %	23	11
	SSVMMOT [6]	78.4 %	84.1 %	0.81	62.7 %	29.6 %	72	5
	OnlineCRF [3]	79.0 %	90.4 %	0.84	68.0 %	24.8 %	19	11
	ExcTracking [4]	77.3 %	87.2 %	0.82	66.4 %	25.4 %	69	57
	ReRankingLMT-P	79.7 %	86.4 %	0.83	66.0 %	24.5 %	37	33
	ReRankingLMT-T	78.9 %	86.9 %	0.83	62.8 %	27.7 %	38	27

induce long-time delay when used for online tracking applications, our method only has low latency less than 10 frames.

Figure 3 shows some tracking examples. The first row illustrates some results from the static camera as in PETS09-S2-L1 sequence. There are interactions and short term partial occlusions, such as those of person 11 and person 9 in the 480-th and 510-th frames. Our method appears robust for these partial occlusions, even in the long-time occlusion case for person 3 in the 65-th frame. The second and third rows illustrate the examples when camera is parallel with view field in TUD and ETHMS sequences. There are many inaccurate detection results in TUD sequence, and person 3 and person 8 pass behind others causing full occlusions. Our method obtains correct tracking trajectories for them, although several ID switches are induced such as for track 5 in the 76-th frame. By contrast with TUD, the sequence of ETHMS is taken from moving camera, and there are lots of full occlusions when the persons pass by. Our method can handle them in most cases like in frame 910 to frame 950, where two persons 77 and 78 are full occluded and recovered after person 73 leaves the view of camera.

We implement our method with runtime of about 2.2 FPS using the non-optimized code of Matlab 2013 at the platform of INTEL i7-3632QM and 2.2 GHz CPU. This runtime is slow mostly due to the calculation of multi-frame features for multi-candidate associations. However, it can be promoted in the future since

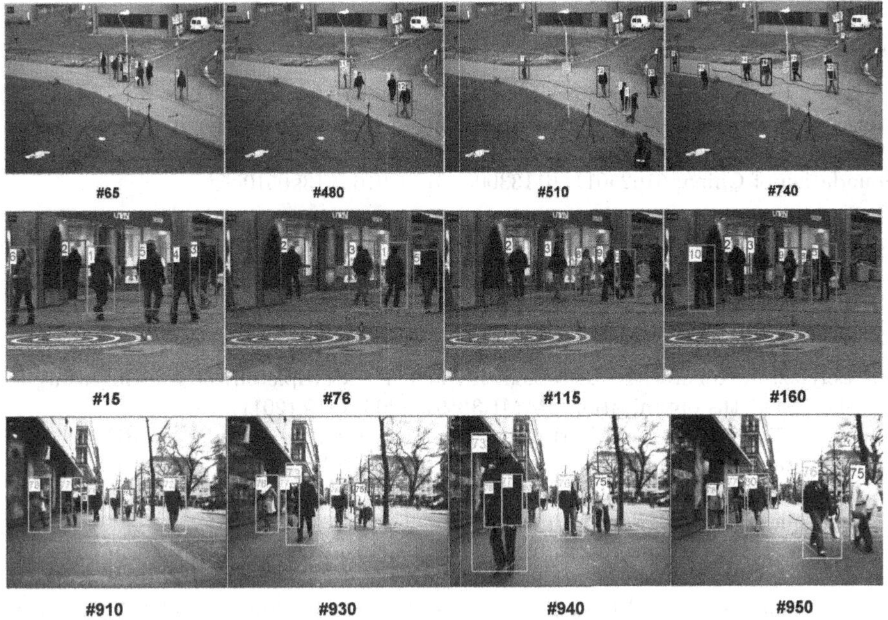

Fig. 3. Tracking examples for (a) PETS09, (b) TUD and (c) ETHMS bahnnof.

most of these calculations are redundant. Another issue is how to handle the problem of occlusion. Because we mainly focus on how to find better candidate association in this paper, we adopt the method in [6] to handle the short-term occlusion problem for each association. Besides, we expect the occlusion gaps are reasonable due to the feature (8). One of the advantages of our method is we can integrate our re-ranking process into the other online tracking frameworks, because our method is not tightly coupled with them, and promote the final performance.

6 Conclusions

In this paper, we propose an online tracking framework combining the global optimization of previous long-term associations. We implement this by re-ranking of multiple short-term associations generated by multiple alignments. The features considering both the trajectory specific self-similarities and mutual relationships between tracks are designed to choose the optimal associations. The experimental results show the discrimination of these weighted features by offline training. By comparison with five state-of-the-art algorithms in three public datasets using common evaluation tools, our method outperforms the other online tracking algorithms and is competitive with global optimal ones. In the future work, we can try to promote the performance by adding more related features, or integrate the possible alignments into an efficient online optimization algorithm by treating them as latent variables, and thus avoiding the re-ranking process.

Acknowledgement. This work was supported in part by National Basic Research Program of China (973 Program): 2012CB316400, in part by National Natural Science Foundation of China: 61025011, 61133003, 61332016, 61390510.

References

1. Zhang, L., Li, Y., Nevatia, R.: Global data association for multi-object tracking using network flows. In: Proceedings of CVPR (2008)
2. Berclaz, J., Fleuret, F., Turetken, E., Fua, P.: Multiple object tracking using k-shortest paths optimization. PAMI **33**(9), 1806–1819 (2011)
3. Yang, B., Nevatia, R.: Multi-target tracking by online learning a CRF model of appearance and motion patterns. IJCV **107**, 203–217 (2013)
4. Milan, A., Schindler, K., Roth, S.: Detection- and trajectory-level exclusion in multiple object tracking. In: Proceedings of CVPR (2013)
5. Yan, X., Wu, X., Kakadiaris, I.A., Shah, S.K.: To track or to detect? an ensemble framework for optimal selection. In: Fitzgibbon, A., Lazebnik, S., Perona, P., Sato, Y., Schmid, C. (eds.) ECCV 2012, Part V. LNCS, vol. 7576, pp. 594–607. Springer, Heidelberg (2012)
6. Kim, S., Kwak, S., Feyereisl, J., Han, B.: Online multi-target tracking by large margin structured learning. In: Lee, K.M., Matsushita, Y., Rehg, J.M., Hu, Z. (eds.) ACCV 2012, Part III. LNCS, vol. 7726, pp. 98–111. Springer, Heidelberg (2013)
7. Reid, D.B.: An algorithm for tracking multiple targets. IEEE Trans. Autom. Control **24**, 843–854 (1979)
8. Bar-Shalom, Y., Formann, T.E.: Tracking and Data Association. Academic Press, San Diego (1988)
9. Viola, P., Jones, M.J.: Robust real-time face detection. IJCV **57**(2), 137–154 (2004)
10. Li, Y., Ai, H., Yamashita, T., Lao, S., Kawade, M.: Tracking in low frame rate video: a cascade particle filter with discriminative observers of different life spans. PAMI **30**, 1728–1740 (2008)
11. Stalder, S., Grabner, H., Van Gool, L.: Cascaded confidence filtering for improved tracking-by-detection. In: Daniilidis, K., Maragos, P., Paragios, N. (eds.) ECCV 2010, Part I. LNCS, vol. 6311, pp. 369–382. Springer, Heidelberg (2010)
12. Kuo, C. H., Nevatia, R.: How does person identity recognition help multi-person tracking? In: Proceedings of CVPR (2011)
13. Wang, N., Yeung, D. Y.: Learning a deep compact image representation for visual tracking. In: NIPS (2013)
14. Fromer, M., Globerson, A.: An LP view of the M-best MAP problem. In: NIPS (2009)
15. Batra, D., Yadollahpour, P., Guzman-Rivera, A., Shakhnarovich, G.: Diverse M-Best solutions in markov random fields. In: Fitzgibbon, A., Lazebnik, S., Perona, P., Sato, Y., Schmid, C. (eds.) ECCV 2012, Part V. LNCS, vol. 7576, pp. 1–16. Springer, Heidelberg (2012)
16. Guerriero, F., Musmanno, R., Lacagnina, V., Pecorella, A.: A class of label-correcting methods for the K shortest paths problem. Oper. Res. **49**, 423–429 (2001)

17. Murty, K.G.: An algorithm for ranking all the assignments in order of increasing cost. Oper. Res. **16**, 682–687 (1968)
18. Collins, M., Koo, T.: Discriminative reranking for natural language parsing. Comput. Linguist. **31**, 25–70 (2005)
19. Liu, T.Y.: Learning to rank for information retrieval. Found. Trends Inf. Retrieval **3**, 225–331 (2009)
20. Yang, B., Huang, C., Nevatia, R.: Learning affinities and dependencies for multi-target tracking using a CRF model. In: Proceedings of CVPR (2011)
21. Bai, Y., Tang, M.: Robust tracking via weakly supervised ranking svm. In: Proceedings of CVPR (2012)
22. Milan, A., Roth, S., Schindler, K.: Continuous energy minimization for multi-target tracking. PAMI **36**, 58–72 (2014)
23. Huang, C., Nevatia, R.: High performance object detection by collaborative learning of joint ranking of granules features. In: Proceedings of CVPR (2010)
24. Felzenszwalb, P.F., Girshick, R.B., McAllester, D., Ramanan, D.: Object detection with discriminatively trained part-based models. PAMI **32**, 1627–1645 (2010)
25. Song, B., Jeng, T.-Y., Staudt, E., Roy-Chowdhury, A.K.: A stochastic graph evolution framework for robust multi-target tracking. In: Daniilidis, K., Maragos, P., Paragios, N. (eds.) ECCV 2010, Part I. LNCS, vol. 6311, pp. 605–619. Springer, Heidelberg (2010)
26. Joachims, T.: Training linear SVMs in linear time. In: KDD (2006)
27. Joachims, T., Finley, T., Yu, C.N.J.: Cutting-plane training of structural SVMs. Mach. Learn. **77**, 27–59 (2009)

Determining Interacting Objects in Human-Centric Activities via Qualitative Spatio-Temporal Reasoning

Hajar Sadeghi Sokeh(✉), Stephen Gould, and Jochen Renz

The Australian National University, Canberra, ACT 0200, Australia
{hajar.sadeghi,stephen.gould,jochen.renz}@anu.edu.au

Abstract. Understanding the activities taking place in a video is a challenging problem in Artificial Intelligence. Complex video sequences contain many activities and involve a multitude of interacting objects. Determining which objects are relevant to a particular activity is the first step in understanding the activity. Indeed many objects in the scene are irrelevant to the main activity taking place. In this work, we consider human-centric activities and look to identify which objects in the scene are involved in the activity. We take an activity-agnostic approach and rank every moving object in the scene with how likely it is to be involved in the activity. We use a comprehensive spatio-temporal representation that captures the joint movement between humans and each object. We then use supervised machine learning techniques to recognize relevant objects based on these features. Our approach is tested on the challenging Mind's Eye dataset.

1 Introduction

Human activity recognition is motivated by the increasing needs of real-world applications. Some of these applications involve recognizing the type of activity or recognizing the object(s) which a person is interacting with. The behaviour of involved objects can be defined as a certain spatial and temporal pattern involving the interactions of a single or multiple actors.

A model can be learnt from a sequence of spatio-temporal features which describes how a person is behaving or interacting with an object for different activities. Accordingly one approach to recognizing activities involves acquiring concepts of what objects mean to them based on the function they perform in activities. In these methods, it is required to initially find the object(s) involved in the activity then consider the spatial changes between objects to recognize the activity. A pre-trained object detector can be used to detect the involved objects [1]. However in many activity recognition tasks, the type of object does not help in identifying the activity. For example, for action *carry*, it is not critical to know that person is carrying a box or a ball.

Spatio-temporal reasoning aims to represent and reason about spatial aspects of the world. It has been argued in AI that a person's form of spatio-temporal

D. Cremers et al. (Eds.): ACCV 2014, Part V, LNCS 9007, pp. 550–563, 2015.
DOI: 10.1007/978-3-319-16814-2_36

reasoning is of a qualitative rather than a quantitative nature [2], and we aim to emulate this in our work. Coarse and vague qualitative representations frequently suffice for us to deal with the problems that we want to solve. For example, to know that the meal is prepared in the kitchen rather than knowing the exact coordinates for this activity.

Most qualitative approaches to spatial and temporal reasoning are based on relations between objects, such as regions or time intervals. Learning activity models can be formulated as the representation of time series data from tracking objects in videos and then, mining these time series for patterns obeying certain constraints. These patterns can be used for analysing videos, activity recognition, anomaly detection and extracting some information about the objects of interest in the video. Sridhar et al. [3,4] proposed the qualitative spatial relations in a graph to naturally represent interactions between objects participating in video activities.

Yao et al. [5], developed a random field model that uses a structure learning method to learn the mutual context of objects and person body parts in human-object interaction activities. Their model discovered the connectivity and spatial relationships between the objects and body parts. Different to our work, Kjellstrom et al. [6] assumed that objects and actions of interests are already categorized. Then the relations are inferred from video data and represented as pairs between action and object classes like "drink-cup". The learned relations can then be used for object and action recognition.

Clearly, recognising objects and identifying activities are related tasks, and solving one informs the other. One motivation of our work is detecting activities without recognising objects. Once the activity is detected, we could add object recognition to identify the type of the involved object. The principal assumption that we make in this work is that it is the collective behaviour and interaction of objects rather than the individual behaviour that make an activity. This is the main reason why we pay more attention in our work to analysing the interactions of the objects using spatio-temporal primitives.

Detecting the relevant objects in human-object activities, regardless of the type of object or the activity, is a very difficult problem in its own right which is the main contribution we are making through this research. Initially, the interacting objects, people and moving objects, are detected. The objects are tracked and their behaviour in relation to each person is analysed. With the classification method used in our work, we are able to differentiate between relevant and irrelevant objects to the activities in each video.

The only input to our system is a video. After detecting the bounding boxes of people and possible relevant objects in each video, we extract statistical information from the computed spatio-temporal features. These features are calculated for each person-object pair. For example, if there are two people and five possible relevant objects in a video, we consider all ten possible relations between them. Then after classification, we calculate a ranked list of objects of interest. We use human-centric videos, which involve at least one person performing an activity. In some of the videos like *running*, *jumping* and *walking*, there is no object involved in the activity, i.e., all other objects in the scene are irrelevant.

2 Spatio-Temporal Features

Our motivation for applying qualitative spatio-temporal features for determining interacting objects in human-object activities is initially analysed before detailing our method.

The changing spatial properties of objects in video and their changing relationships with other objects are often characteristic of particular activities. It is then possible to express some rules in terms of these changes or to learn activities based on similar change patterns [3,7].

As mentioned before, qualitative features contain enough detailed information to permit recognition and reduce the importance of noise existence in real-world applications. There are many calculi defined in the field of *Qualitative Spatial Reasoning* [8] with many applications in high level interpretation of video data [3,4,9]. One of them is CORE-9, proposed by Cohn et al. [10].

CORE-9 is a uniform spatial representation of moving objects that integrates the important aspects of space. This model relies purely on obtaining minimal bounding rectangles of the objects in each video frame.

In CORE-9, the relevant objects and their minimum bounding rectangles are detected and tracked in order to extract qualitative information from the video. For every pair of objects per frame, nine cores are defined as shown in Fig. 1. Then the status of each core is determined and their changes over frames are analysed. All qualitative relations between the pair objects can be inferred using these nine cores.

Topology, size, distance and direction are some of the most important spatial properties of the objects that may change over time. In qualitative reasoning, the relative change of these characteristics is taken into account. In human-object activities, the relative size of interacting objects is important, regardless of their absolute size. For example, when a person is dragging a box, the size of box or person does not make any difference in the activity, since they can be close to the camera and look bigger, or far from the camera and look smaller.

In this work, we use a rectangle representation for objects relevant to the activities, since the applied detection algorithm gives us bounding rectangles for the objects. Extracted features are based on changes of spatio-temporal relations between human and object when the activity is occurring. Some of these features have been chosen from CORE-9. Figure 1 indicates two rectangles A and B and illustrates how their projections define the nine cores in CORE-9. In our work, these two rectangles represent the bounding rectangles around the person and relevant object.

CORE-9 takes into account topology, direction, size, and distance between objects as well as changes of those relations over time. A function called "change function" is defined in [10] which is used for comparing changes in cores and intervals. This function is defined for each variable ν as $ch(\nu) \longmapsto \{<,=,>\}$ where $ch(\nu)$ is '=' if $\nu_t - \nu_{t-1} = 0$, $ch(\nu)$ is '<' if $\nu_t - \nu_{t-1} < 0$ and $ch(\nu)$ is '>' if $\nu_t - \nu_{t-1} > 0$, in which t represents a time spot in a video. The variable ν can be a core or an interval.

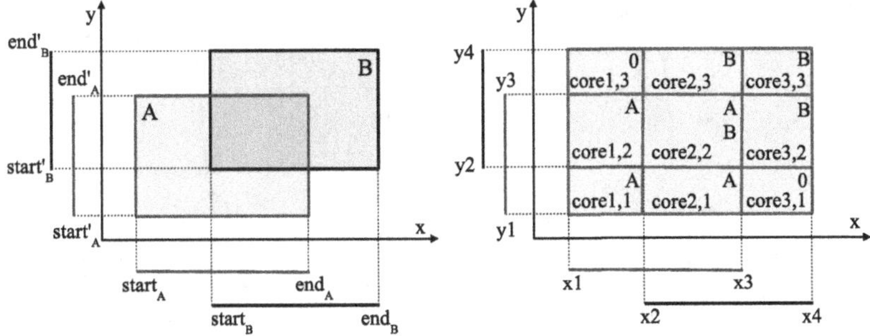

Fig. 1. Pair minimum bounding rectangles of A and B and their projections (left). Defining nine cores and six intervals using the projections in CORE-9 (right).

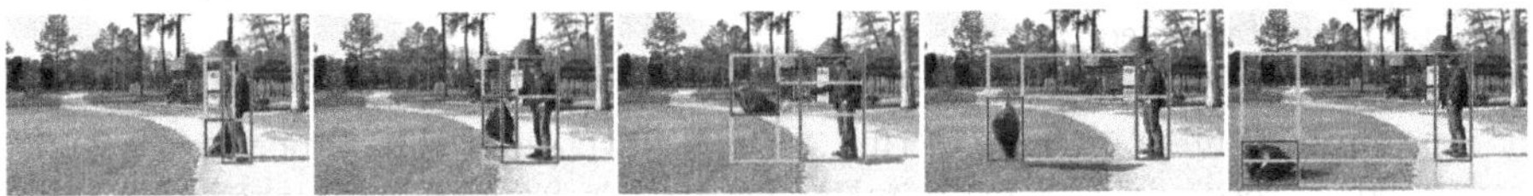

Fig. 2. (Best viewed in colour) Changing of nine cores in CORE-9 when action *throw* happens. (Nine cores of CORE-9, person and the relevant object bounding rectangles are shown by yellow, red and blue, respectively.) (Color figure online)

There are nine changes over time between sets of cores forming rectangles and six for their intervals in CORE-9. These 15 features not only give some information about the size changes for each object, but also provide some knowledge about the direction and distance changes between the bounding rectangles of two interacting objects. Figure 2 shows how these CORE-9 features can describe the changes when a person throws a bag.

We consider distance [11] separately even though it is partially embedded in CORE-9 change features. The idea is that if a person wants to interact with an object, at least in some frames of the video they should be very close to each other and the distance between them shows this closeness.

Two other suitable features for our application are how much the location of each interacting object is changing over time. As many irrelevant moving objects like moving tree leaves, only move slightly around the same location throughout the video. Hence, these features can prune out many irrelevant objects. To remove the effect of object size on these features, we normalized the features by dividing by the object size in the image plane.

Figure 3 shows how the change in distance and location is different for relevant and irrelevant objects. These features are calculated for the same video as Fig. 2. Regarding this figure, the distance between the person and the irrelevant object which is a small part of the tree, is not changing considerably. Instead, the distance between the person and the bag is increasing between frames 42 and 56. There is a noteworthy difference between the location changes for relevant and irrelevant object which is illustrated in Fig. 3(b).

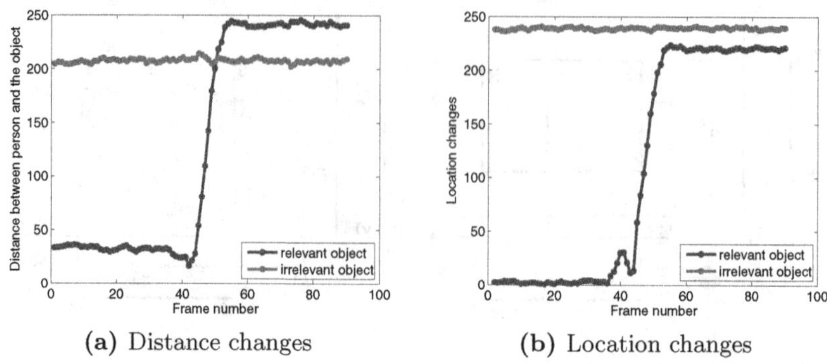

(a) Distance changes

(b) Location changes

Fig. 3. (a) Changing distance between person and the object over frames, (b) Changing the location of the object over frames. (relevant and irrelevant objects are shown by blue and magenta respectively).

The prominent point here is that for the purpose of this paper, we are not interested in recognising what kind of activity is happening in the video. We track behaviour of each moving object in the scene and then label it as relevant or irrelevant. For this aim, we calculate some descriptive statistics to capture important aspects of the distribution of frame-by-frame feature changes.

3 Detecting Human-Object Interactions

Interactions are often the main characteristic of an action. In this section, we discuss the technical steps of our method to detect these interactions.

3.1 People Detection

Detection of people is of prime importance for most activity recognition applications as many interesting activities are done by humans. In order to find the objects involved in the activities, we initially detect humans. The output of most existing people detectors is a bounding rectangle around the person which is suitable for our work.

For collecting the person detections, we use the publicly available implementation of the discriminatively trained deformable part models of Felzenszwalb et al. [12]. This algorithm has been found to outperform many others in numerous competitions. We did not have the ground truth for detections in Mind's Eye dataset, but visually the algorithm worked very well in this dataset and significant number of people were accurately detected.

3.2 Detecting Possible Relevant Objects

Detecting objects involved in human-object activities is a challenging problem in computer vision. In many cases, the relevant object tends to be small or only partially visible. The question here is how we can find the object of interest

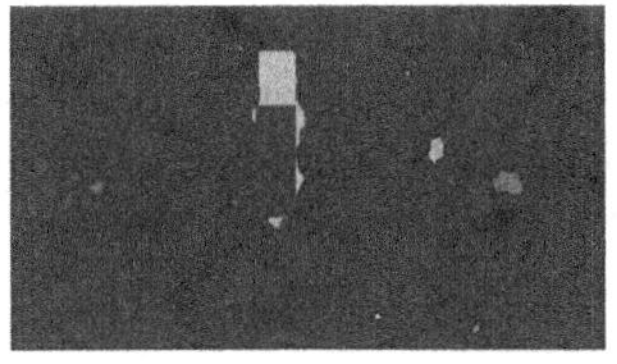

(a) Optical flow

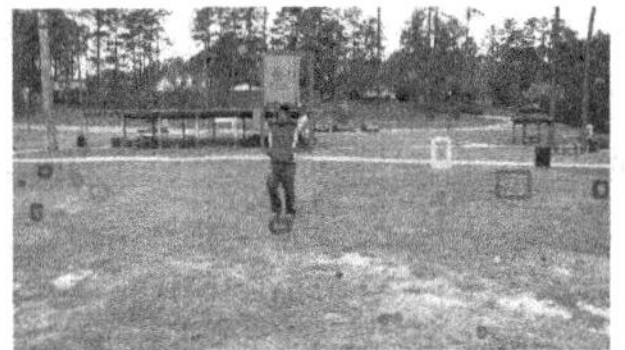

(b) Detected blobs

Fig. 4. (Best viewed in colour) Detected moving blobs out of person bounding rectangle (Color figure online).

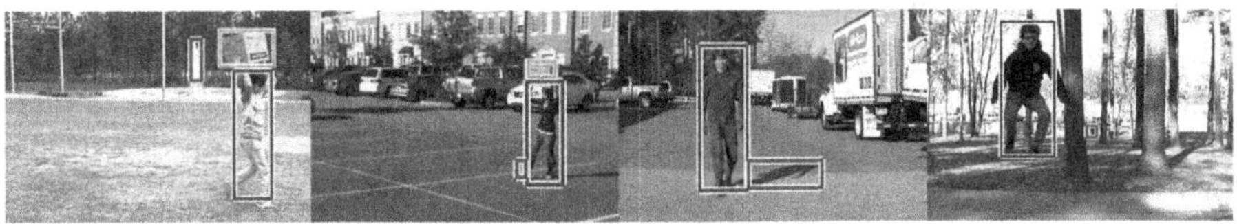

(a) activity *carry* (b) activity *carry* (c) activity *walk* (d) activity *jump*

Fig. 5. (Best viewed in colour) Some examples of relevant and irrelevant objects. (person: blue, relevant object: green, irrelevant object: red) (Color figure online)

in each activity. In many of these interactions, a person changes the interacted object. This change can be in its shape like opening a box or in its location, for example when a person throws an object. Such changes can be detected in videos by investigating the motion of the relevant objects.

Optical flow [13] is used in this work to detect motion on all pixels of each frame except within the boundary rectangle inferred from the person detector. Figure 4 illustrates the detected person and all possible relevant objects in a frame. There are many challenges in using optical flow for detecting the relevant objects. Tree branches moving with the wind, moving parts of human body out of its bounding rectangle, and shadow are among these challenges (see Fig. 5).

We do not consider static objects, as we can not reliably detect them with existing methods. Once static object detection works reliably, we can add these objects to our analysis without having to change our method.

If we have multiple people in the scene, we can determine relevant objects for each person separately, since our features are derived for each human-object pair.

3.3 Tracking and Data Association

After applying optical flow, there are many moving blobs in the video each of which has the possibility of being either relevant or irrelevant to the activity. The relational changes between each blob-person pair is different over time. Therefore, by analysing the spatio-temporal relational changes between each blob and person, we can differentiate between the relevant and irrelevant blobs. For the temporal analysis, each relevant object candidate should be tracked over the frames of the video.

Tracking-Learning-Detection (TLD) [14] is a real-time algorithm for tracking unknown objects in videos. Given a bounding rectangle defining the object of interest in a single frame, the algorithm automatically determines the object's bounding rectangle in other frames or indicates the invisibility of the object. TLD simultaneously tracks the object, learns its appearance and detects it whenever it appears in the video. TLD is capable of handling significant appearance changes and short-term occlusions which is very useful for real world videos such as those used in our experiments.

From the previous optical flow step, we have bounding rectangles for all moving blobs. In this step we give these bounding rectangles to the tracker as the targets to be tracked. In order to capture an object that only starts moving after the first frame, we repeat these steps for all frames of video to calculate tracks for all of possible object candidates.

In each frame we need to check if a moving blob is a new born target or an existing target which is already being tracked. Hence, we need a method to find the relationship between a detected moving blob in a frame and all detections for the previous tracks in the current frame.

A simple approach is to associate the bounding rectangles in a frame to existing targets that have the minimal Euclidean distance. In order to have more robust object association, we have applied two metrics to greatly enhance the results which are detailed as follows.

Assume B_m is a detected bounding rectangle for a moving blob in a frame. This blob can be a new born object which has just started moving in the scene. It can also represent an existing blob, if it is associated with at least one bounding rectangle in an existing track. To be considered as an existing tracked blob, the area of overlap, between B_m and the bounding rectangle of tracked object in the same frame, B_t, must exceed 80 %. Bounding rectangle overlap is defined as the area of intersection divided by the area of union of the bounding rectangles. This criterion is formulated as follows.

$$overlap(B_m, B_t) = \frac{area(B_m \cap B_t)}{area(B_m \cup B_t)} > 0.8 \tag{1}$$

in which $B_m \cap B_t$ denotes the intersection of two bounding rectangles and $B_m \cup B_t$ their union.

We also extract histogram of oriented gradients [15] as a feature descriptor for both bounding rectangles, B_m and B_t. Then using a normalized square distance, we quantified the difference between two bounding rectangles as another criterion with threshold of 0.05 as described in the following:

$$\frac{1}{2}\|HOG(B_m) - HOG(B_t)\|_2^2 < 0.05 \tag{2}$$

Both thresholds of 0.8 and 0.05 were chosen arbitrarily but reasonable. So, for each moving blob in a frame, we look for a bounding rectangle in one of the existing tracks which satisfies the overlap and normalized square distance measures. If there is no such B_t and no association found by the algorithm, the detected blob will be considered as a new-born object in that frame and will be

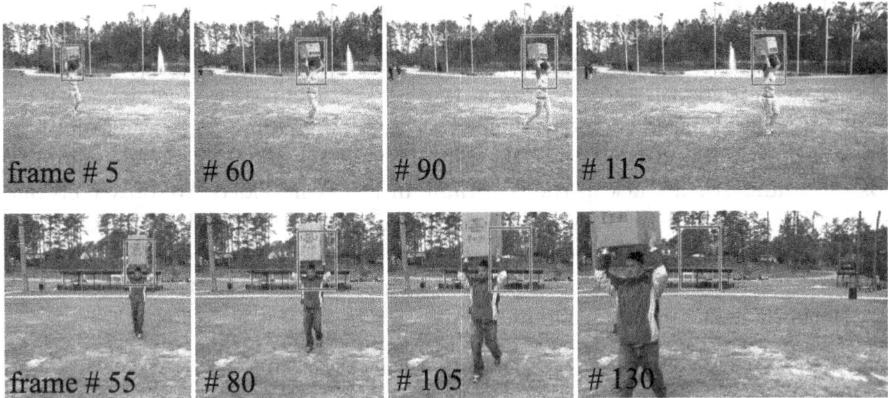

Fig. 6. Good and bad tracking results for two relevant objects in two different videos of activity *Carry*, respectively.

tracked over the subsequent frames. Otherwise, if we find an association, we will disregard the detected moving blob as already being tracked.

The TLD tracker can continue tracking, even when there is no detection by the algorithm for a few frames, which might be due to the occlusion of the object in the scene. In such cases, we generate some linearly interpolated rectangles to represent the missed detections.

The output of this step is a track for each possible relevant object in the video. Figure 6 illustrates some good and bad tracking results for a relevant object in two videos of activity *carry*. The second row of Fig. 6 shows how the tracking algorithm fails in some cases despite the correct initialization of the bounding box. However in the subsequent frames of this video, the object detection algorithm finds the box as a new born object again and continues tracking it.

3.4 Extracting Spatio-Temporal Features

As explained earlier, after detecting all possible relevant objects, we track them. We extract a feature vector of 18 different spatio-temporal features for each human-object pair per frame, and calculate seven statistical descriptors for each spatio-temporal feature vector over frames. These descriptors are the maximum, minimum, mean, median, mode, standard deviation and variance for each feature. As a result, each spatio-temporal feature matrix is converted to a vector of $7 \times 18 = 126$ feature values. The experimental results show that these features can describe the data very well.

Our training data is highly imbalanced, as the class of relevant objects is significantly under-represented compared to the class of irrelevant objects. To overcome this problem, we over-sample positive data using Synthetic Minority Over-sampling Technique (SMOTE) [16]. In this algorithm, the minority class is over-sampled by taking each minority class sample and introducing synthetic examples along the line segments joining all of the k minority class nearest neighbours.

3.5 Evaluation Algorithm

Our evaluation metric is track-based in which the metrics are computed based on each detected track and the ground truth track. We use two metrics, both on simple threshold-based correspondence. For a video, assume B_{ij} is the bounding box in the ith frame from the jth track in that video. BG_i is the bounding box of ground truth track in the ith frame in the same video. We only consider frames where both detected and ground truth objects appear. Both metrics are computed for each frame i, between a detected object track, B_{ij}, and ground truth track, BG_i. The first metric is the same overlap criteria used in data association which can be formulated as:

$$overlap(B_{ij}, BG_i) = \frac{area(B_{ij} \cap BG_i)}{area(B_{ij} \cup BG_i)} > 0.5 \tag{3}$$

In some videos, the relevant object bounding rectangle and the person bounding rectangle in one frame have too much overlap. The only clue we use to detect objects is motion in all parts of the frame except within the bounding box from the person rectangle. Then if there is too much overlap between these two rectangles, i.e. the person and the object bounding rectangle, we can only detect part of the object which is out of person bounding rectangle. In these situations, we define a second metric for the evaluation. If at least 90 % of object bounding rectangle, B_{ij}, is covered by the ground truth bounding rectangle, BG_i, we consider it as a good overlapping bounding rectangle. We formulate this metric as follows:

$$\frac{area(B_{ij} \cap BG_i)}{area(B_{ij})} > 0.9 \tag{4}$$

Based on these metrics, a track is considered covered by a ground truth track if both criteria, described above, are satisfied at least for 50 % of frames in which both detected and ground truth objects appear.

4 Experimental Results and Evaluation

This section outlines the train and test dataset and the obtained results using the metrics discussed in the previous section. Experiments were carried out using the challenging Mind's Eye dataset[1]. A total of 306 video sequences of 11 different activities were evaluated. The actions are: *carry, dig, fall, jump, kick, pickup, putdown, run, throw, turn, walk.* I these videos, different scenes and humans performing the activities and different objects for the same activities are used. We sampled every 5th frame in the videos and resized each frame from 720×1280 to 360×640. We also made a ground truth track corresponding to each of relevant object for each video. The number of detected tracks in all videos was 15694 which were used for training and testing the method.

[1] http://www.visint.org/.

After detecting and tracking the bounding rectangles for the human and all possible interacted objects per video, we extracted the qualitative spatio-temporal features for each frame of object track and the person bounding rectangle in the same frame. Next, we calculate statistical descriptors from the feature matrix, as explained in the last section, which then used for training and testing a classifier.

The key objective of this step is using a learning algorithm to build a predictive model that accurately predicts the probability of being relevant or irrelevant of previously unknown tracks. We use Support Vector Machine (SVM) in LIB-SVM library [17] which is publicly available.

To our best knowledge, there is no other work on the same dataset that addresses the problem of explicit detection of relevant objects. Therefore, we defined our own baseline to compare results against. To develop a strong baseline, we have separately trained the model with each of the 18 features explained before, and distance gave the best results, 63.74 % (see Table 1). This is consistent with our intuition that interacting objects exhibit characteristic patterns in how their relative distance changes over time. The next best feature was *relative speed* with performance of 55.89 %. Quantitative results are shown in Table 1. As the training data is highly imbalanced, the number of *false positives* is much higher than the number of *true positives*. It gives a very low precision. We also report Macro Accuracy as the average of the true positive and true negative rates. Both numbers and percentages are included in the table from which other statistics can be derived.

To indicate the type of learning relevant objects in our work is generic and is not based on some prior knowledge about the types of activities, we performed a leave-one-activity-out cross validation experiment. We trained the classifier on 10 activities and evaluated on the 11th activity for each in turn. We measured the performance of classification for each track using the evaluation procedure detailed before. Quantitative results are presented as a confusion matrix in Table 2. The results are quite reasonable and better than the baseline as the macro accuracy shows almost 12 % improvement and around 5 % improvement in accuracy.

The experimental results show that our model works quite well on unknown activities. Next, we tested our model for the case which some instances of all activities have been seen. We trained SVM with instances from all activity classes to learn how the relevant and irrelevant objects are behaving in relation to the person in each activity. We used a 10-fold cross validation on all tracks of all activities. According to the results in Table 3, almost 81 % of irrelevant objects have been classified correctly as irrelevant. In this work we are interested in the number of *true positives*, i.e. the number of relevant objects which are classified correctly which in our results is more than 93 %. As it is illustrated in the table, the number of irrelevant object tracks is far larger than the number of relevant objects. This imbalance in the data resulted in too many *false positives*, 2877, which is considerably more than the number of *true positives*, 488, which affects our algorithm's precision. As expected, comparing Tables 2 and 3 shows that we get more accuracy by training our model on instances from all activities.

Table 1. The confusion matrix for the baseline algorithm.

Confusion Matrix				Precision	Macro Acc
		Predicted			
		irrelevant	relevant		
Actual	irrelevant	8394(55.33%)	6776(44.67%)	5.58%	63.74%
	relevant	146(27.86%)	378(72.14%)		

Table 2. The confusion matrix for "Leave-one-activity-out".

Confusion Matrix				Precision	Macro Acc
		Predicted			
		irrelevant	relevant		
Actual	irrelevant	11414(75.24%)	3756(24.76%)	10.49%	75.22%
	relevant	130(24.81%)	394(75.19%)		

Table 3. The confusion matrix for "10-fold cross validation".

Confusion Matrix				Precision	Macro Acc
		Predicted			
		irrelevant	relevant		
Actual	irrelevant	12293(81.03%)	2877(18.97%)	16.96%	87.08%
	relevant	36(6.87%)	488(93.13%)		

Table 4. The confusion matrix for "adding activity feature".

Confusion Matrix				Precision	Macro Acc
		Predicted			
		irrelevant	relevant		
Actual	irrelevant	13159(86.74%)	2011(13.26%)	25.46%	92.23%
	relevant	12(2.29%)	512(97.71%)		

Finally, we evaluated our model in scenarios where the activity is known. We presented a new binary indicator feature vector comprised of 11 features; the number of activities. These features were then augmented with the previous feature set. As illustrated in Table 4, using the type of activity improves the accuracy of the system significantly. Only 2.29 % of the relevant data has been mistakenly classified as irrelevant and both precision and accuracy are much higher as expected. This shows that knowing the activity type provides us with more information on the relevancy of the object to the activity.

Figure 7 shows two tracks which are correctly classified by our algorithm. The first row shows a track of an irrelevant object, a fountain in this example, which

PutDown

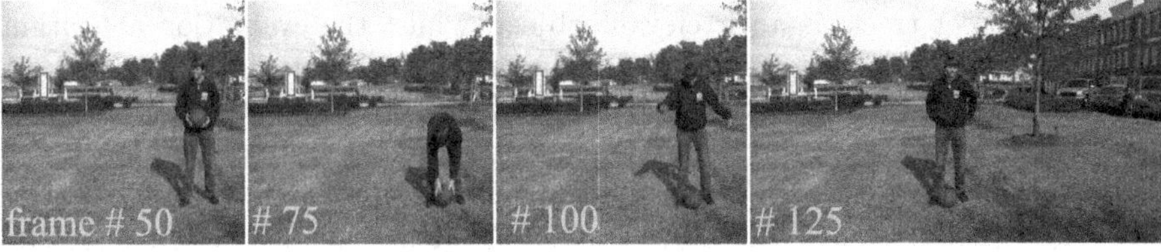

Carry

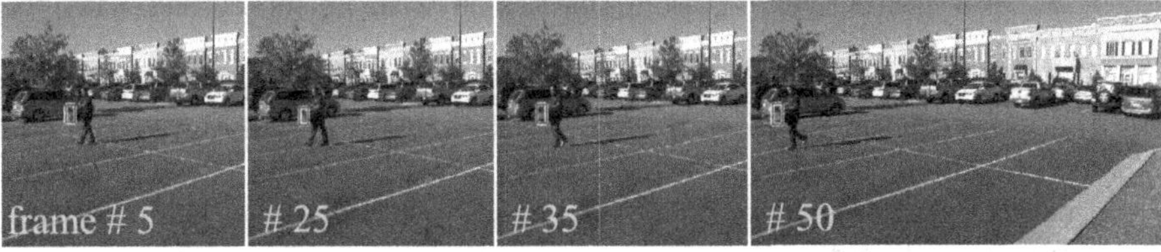

Fig. 7. Some frames of videos which our model correctly classifies. (detected relevant object is shown by red bounding rectangle). The rows are tracks of a true negative and true positive examples in the test data (Color figure online).

PutDown

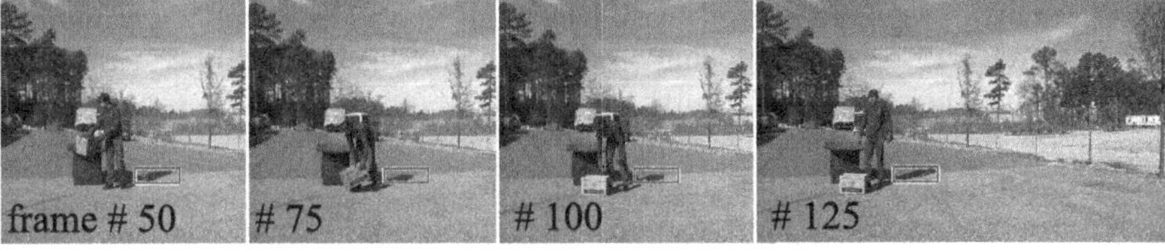

Throw

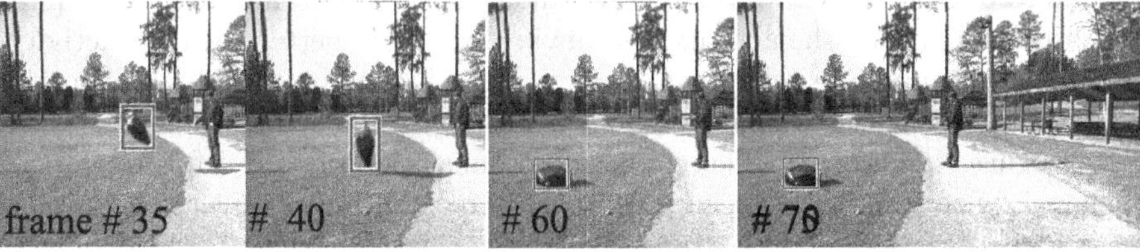

Fig. 8. Some frames of videos which our model wrongly classifies. Rows illustrates a false positive and a false negative example of test tracks, respectively.

has been correctly classified. The second row also demonstrates four sequences of *true positive* tracks which were correctly classified as relevant object track.

Two examples of wrong classification are illustrated in Fig. 8. The first row belongs to a *false positive* track. Based on the extracted spatio-temporal features in this work, this object which is the person's shadow, behaves like a relevant object. For these cases, we can not strongly say if they are irrelevant to the activity since they can be considered as a part of person. This problem can be addressed by applying a semantic reasoning to these tracks to classify them into the negative category.

The second row of Fig. 8 belongs to a *false negative* in which the algorithm finds this object track as an irrelevant object, whilst the evaluation algorithm finds it as a relevant object. After checking all *false negatives*, we found that more than half of them had the same problem. The problem is that the tracking algorithm failed for these objects. Consequently, after detecting the object, the algorithm considers it as a new born target and tracks it. The new track is then classified as an irrelevant object which does not have any interaction with the person. The figure shows that in frame 35, the bag is detected as a new born target which is getting further from the person with no interaction with the person.

Currently our method is implemented in Matlab. There are a number of processing steps in our pipeline. It takes 100 seconds to pre-process each frame to detect the human and extract objects. It then takes less than 1ms per human-object pair to extract the features and almost 3ms per track to be classified either as relevant or irrelevant.

5 Conclusion and Future Work

One approach to identify relevant objects to a particular activity is through qualitative spatio-temporal features. This is the main motivation of our work in this paper. We presented a framework which, given a video involving a human-centric activity, ranks every moving object with how likely it is to be involved in that activity. The extracted features are mostly about how spatial properties of objects are changing over time compared to the people. These changes mainly have a meaningful manner for the relevant objects.

We demonstrated our approach on videos involving different human activities, differentiating relevant and irrelevant objects for unknown activities. Experimental results on the real world videos demonstrate that our method works quite well without knowing the activity, but obviously can do better with the activity.

After discriminating relevant from irrelevant objects, by considering how the spatio-temporal features change between people and the relevant objects, we can recognize the activity. Therefore, one promising direction of future work is to show how this method can improve activity recognition or object recognition.

References

1. Prest, A., Ferrari, V., Schmid, C.: Explicit modeling of human-object interactions in realistic videos. Technical report RT-0411, INRIA (2011)
2. Wolter, D., Wallgrün, J.O.: Qualitative spatial reasoning for applications: new challenges and the sparq toolbox. In: Qualitative Spatio-Temporal Representation and Reasoning: Trends and Future Directions. IGI Global (2010)
3. Sridhar, M., Cohn, A.G., Hogg, D.C.: Benchmarking qualitative spatial calculi for video activity analysis. In: IJCAI Workshop Benchmarks and Applications of Spatial Reasoning, pp. 15–20 (2011)
4. Sridhar, M., Cohn, A.G., Hogg, D.C.: Unsupervised learning of event classes from video. In: Association for the Advancement of Artificial Intelligence (AAAI) (2010)

5. Yao, B., Fei-Fei, L.: Modeling mutual context of object and human pose in human-object interaction activities. In: Computer Vision and Pattern Recognition (CVPR), pp. 17–24 (2010)
6. Kjellström, H., Romero, J., Kragic, D.: Visual object-action recognition: Inferring object affordances from human demonstration. Comput. Vis. Image Underst. **115**, 81–90 (2011)
7. Sokeh, H.S., Gould, S., Renz, J.: Efficient extraction and representation of spatial information from video data. In: International Joint Conferences on Artificial Intelligence (IJCAI) (2013)
8. Cohn, A.G., Renz, J.: Qualitative spatial representation and reasoning. In: van Hermelen, F., Lifschitz, V., Porter, B. (eds.) Handbook of Knowledge Representation, pp. 551–596. Elsevier, Amsterdam (2008)
9. Sridhar, M., Cohn, A.G., Hogg, D.C.: From video to RCC8: exploiting a distance based semantics to stabilise the interpretation of mereotopological relations. In: Egenhofer, M., Giudice, N., Moratz, R., Worboys, M. (eds.) COSIT 2011. LNCS, vol. 6899, pp. 110–125. Springer, Heidelberg (2011)
10. Cohn, A.G., Renz, J., Sridhar, M.: Thinking inside the box: A comprehensive spatial representation for video analysis. In: International Conference on Principles of Knowledge Representation and Reasoning (KR) (2012)
11. Hernández, D., Clementini, E., Felice, P.D.: Qualitative distances. In: Conference On Spatial Information Theory (COSIT), pp. 45–57 (1995)
12. Felzenszwalb, P.F., Girshick, R.B., McAllester, D., Ramanan, D.: Object detection with discriminatively trained part-based models. Pattern Anal. Mach. Intell. (PAMI) **32**, 1627–1645 (2010)
13. Sun, D., Roth, S., Black, M.J.: Secrets of optical flow estimation and their principles. In: CVPR, pp. 2432–2439 (2010)
14. Kalal, Z., Mikolajczyk, K., Matas, J.: Tracking-learning-detection. Pattern Anal. Mach. Intell. (PAMI) **34**, 1409–1422 (2012)
15. Dalal, N., Triggs, B.: Histograms of oriented gradients for human detection. In: Computer Vision and Pattern Recognition (CVPR), pp. 886–893 (2005)
16. Chawla, N.V., Bowyer, K.W., Hall, L.O., Kegelmeyer, W.P.: Smote: Synthetic minority over-sampling technique. J. Artif. Intell. Res. **16**, 321–357 (2002)
17. Chang, C.C., Lin, C.J.: LIBSVM: a library for support vector machines. ACM Trans. Intell. Syst. Technol. **2**, 27:1–27:27 (2011)

Enhanced Laplacian Group Sparse Learning with Lifespan Outlier Rejection for Visual Tracking

Behzad Bozorgtabar[1(✉)] and Roland Goecke[1,2]

[1] Vision and Sensing, HCC Lab, ESTeM, University of Canberra, Canberra, Australia
Behzad.Bozorgtabar@canberra.edu.au

[2] IHCC, RSCS, CECS, Australian National University, Canberra, Australia
roland.goecke@ieee.org

Abstract. Recently, sparse based learning methods have attracted much attention in robust visual tracking due to their effectiveness and promising tracking results. By representing the target object sparsely, utilising only a few adaptive dictionary templates, in this paper, we introduce a new particle filter based tracking method, in which we aim to capture the underlying structure among the particle samples using the proposed similarity graph in a Laplacian group sparse framework, such that the tracking results can be improved. Furthermore, in our tracker, particles contribute with different probabilities in the tracking result with respect to their relative positions in a given frame in regard to the current target object location. In addition, since the new target object can be well modelled by the most recent tracking results, we prefer to utilise the particle samples that are highly associated to the preceding tracking results. We demonstrate that the proposed formulation can be efficiently solved using the Accelerated Proximal method with just a small number of iterations. The proposed approach has been extensively evaluated on 12 challenging video sequences. Experimental results compared to the state-of-the-art methods demonstrate the merits of the proposed tracker.

1 Introduction

Object tracking is a well-studied problem in computer vision and has many practical applications. The problem and its difficulty depend on several factors, such as the amount of prior knowledge about the target object. Tracking of generic objects has remained challenging because an object can drastically change appearance when deforming (e.g. a pedestrian), rotating out of plane, being occluded, or when the illumination of the scene changes.

Electronic supplementary material The online version of this chapter (doi:10.1007/978-3-319-16814-2_37) contains supplementary material, which is available to authorized users. Videos can also be accessed at http://www.springerimages.com/videos/978-3-319-16813-5.

D. Cremers et al. (Eds.): ACCV 2014, Part V, LNCS 9007, pp. 564–578, 2015.
DOI: 10.1007/978-3-319-16814-2_37

Recently, sparse representation has been strongly applied to visual tracking [1,2]. In this case, the tracker represents each target candidate as a sparse linear combination of dictionary templates that can be dynamically updated to preserve an up-to-date target appearance model. However, sparse coding based trackers perform a computationally expensive l_1 minimisation at each frame. The drawback of these methods is that they ignore the underlying structure between particles and learn sparse representations of particles separately. Ignoring the relationships among particle representations tend to make the tracker more prone to drifting away from the target, especially in cases of significant appearance changes of the tracking target.

In this paper, we propose a computationally efficient Laplacian group sparse learning approach for visual tracking in a particle filter framework. Here, we consider each particle sample as a task and explore task correlation between particles. Besides, we further extend our designed objective function with the Laplacian norm to recognise the overall structure among particles with a defined similarity graph. Unlike previous methods, we also consider the consistency between tracking results in a short period of time and since the new tracking result is more likely to be similar with the most recent ones, we construct another set of dictionary items, but this time for the current candidate samples, select the most correlated ones and ignore the rest.

Finally, a new likelihood model is proposed based on two factors: **(1)** the relative location of the particles w.r.t. the current target object and **(2)** the similarity between target candidates and the dictionary templates. Consequently, once the current tracking result causes a large variance and is not occluded, we replace it with the dictionary template has less similarity with the tracking result.

2 Related Work

In general, object tracking methods can be categorised as either generative or discriminative.

2.1 Generative Trackers

Generative methods represent the target object with models that have minimum reconstruction errors, and track targets by searching for the region most similar to the models in an image frame. Examples of generative methods are eigentracker [3], mean shift tracker [4], context-aware tracker [5], fragment-based tracker (Frag) [6], incremental tracker (IVT) [7], and VTD tracker [8]. Most recent generative methods learn and maintain static or online appearance models. Black et al. [3] learn a subspace model offline to represent target objects at predefined views and build on the optical flow framework for tracking.

2.2 Discriminative Trackers

Discriminative models, which are also called tracking-by-detection methods, consider tracking as a binary classification task to separate the object from its surrounding background. The adaptive tracking-by-detection methods first train a classifier in an online manner using samples extracted from the current frame. In the next frame, a sliding window is then used to extract samples around the previous object location, before the previously trained classifier is applied to these samples. The location of the sample with the maximum classifier score is the new object location at the current frame. Examples of discriminative methods are on-line boosting (OAB) [9], ensemble tracking [10], co-training tracking [11], adaptive metric differential tracking [12] and online multiple instance learning tracking [13].

2.3 Sparse Representation for Object Tracking

The recent development of sparse representations [1,2] has attracted considerable interest in object tracking due to its robustness to occlusion and image noise. In [1], a target candidate is represented as a sparse linear combination of object templates and trivial templates. For each particle, a sparse representation is computed by solving a constrained l_1 minimisation problem with non-negativity constraints, thus, solving the inverse intensity pattern problem during tracking. Although this method yields good tracking performance, it comes at the computational expense of multiple l_1 minimisation problems that are independently solved. In Mei et al. [2], an efficient l_1 tracker with minimum error bound and occlusion detection is proposed. Zhang et al. [14] investigate convex mixed norm $l_{p,q}$ (*i.e.* $p \geq 1, q \geq 1$) to enforce joint sparsity for the particles. In [15], a particle filter based tracking formulated as a structured multi-task sparse learning problem, where particle representations, regularised by a sparsity-inducing mixed norm and a local graph term.

3 System Overview

3.1 Bayesian Inference Framework

In this paper, visual tracking is formulated within the Bayesian inference framework, in which the goal is to determine the *a posteriori* probability of the target state. In this paper, we utilise the particle filter as an effective realisation of Bayesian filtering, whereas the idea is to approximate the posterior distribution $p(s_t|z_{1:t})$ by a set of weighted particles $\left\{s_t^{(i)}, \pi_t^{(i)}\right\}_{i=1}^N$ where $z_{1:t}$ denotes the set of observations up to and including the time step t and each particle represents a possible state s_t and a weight π_t associated with it, which specifies its corresponding state's confidence. Considering Bayesian estimation scheme, the filtering distribution can be recursively updated as:

$$p(s_t|z_{1:t-1}) = \int p(s_t|s_{t-1})\, p(s_{t-1}|z_{1:t-1})\, ds_{t-1} \tag{1}$$

$$p(s_t|z_{1:t}) \propto p(z_t|s_t)\, p(s_t|z_{1:t-1}) \tag{2}$$

First, new particles are generated by sampling from a known proposal function $q\left(s_t \middle| s_{0:t-1}^{(i)}, z_{1:t}\right)$ where the simplest choice for the proposal function is the state evolution model $p(s_t | s_{t-1})$ itself for sampling. Further, the optimal state is obtained by the maximum a posteriori (MAP) estimation over a set of N samples. In our algorithm, we model the motion of a target object between two consecutive frames with an affine transformation. Let s_t be the six-dimensional parameter vector of an affine transformation. The transformation of each parameter is modelled independently by a scalar Gaussian distribution. Then, the dynamic model $p(s_t | s_{t-1})$ can be represented by a Gaussian distribution. The likelihood (observation) model $p(z_t | s_t)$ reflects the similarity measure for the tracking target. In this paper, the weights of the particles are specified by the proposed spatial score weighted by the difference in contribution of object templates and the background templates, in which a sample with a larger difference score indicates that it is more likely to be correlated with target object rather than background. The most likely sample is considered as the tracking result for that video frame.

3.2 Contribution

Inspired by the mentioned related works, we seek a particle filter based tracker using sparse representation scheme, which not only reduces the computational expense caused by regressing individual particles with respect to the defined dictionary, but also models the common structure among particle samples. Zhang et al. [15] extend the MTT framework to take into account pairwise structural correlations between particles. However, our tracker is superior and more stable. The key idea is constructing a similarity graph to better model structural information of the sampled particles. To represent the graph regularizer, the tracker in [15] only uses pairwise distance between each pair of particles by considering their spatial locations, which ignores the global structure of the whole particles and is prone to the outliers. In [16], it is extensively shown that each data point in a union of subspaces can be efficiently reconstructed by a combination of other points in the dataset. However, the spanned subspaces are usually dependent, which causes the wrong choice of inter subspaces. Based on this assumption, we consider both the mutual local and global structure of the particles. Here, we summarised our main contributions:

1. In this paper, inspired by the similar successful works in image classification e.g. [17], we formulate object tracking by proposing an enhanced Laplacian group sparse coding based scheme where the similarity among the particles specified by a graph structure, which makes the sparse codes of those particles placed close together be similar to each other (e.g. spatial smoothness). Furthermore, we investigate an enhanced similarity graph which not only considers pairwise similarity between particles, but also encode linearly representation of each particle with respect to others in a topological space. The proposed objective function for learning the sparse representation of candidate samples is rendered as a non-smooth convex (unconstrained) optimisation problem in which we implement the accelerated proximal method (APM) for solving this optimisation problem and develop efficient algorithms for computing the related proximal mapping.

2. The target object position ambiguity problem often occurs in visual tracking, which adversely influences tracking performance. The proposed tracker incorporates the particle sample importance into the observation model, which makes it able to select the most effective particles, resulting in a more stable tracker.
3. Finally, for the sake of efficient computational complexity and having a faster tracker, we introduce outlier rejection for the particle samples in the current frame where we take the advantage of this fact that the current tracking result can be well represented by the latest tracking results and pick those, which are more similar to the previous ones and more likely to be the new tracking result.

In our particle filter based tracking method, particles are randomly sampled around the current state of the tracked object according to a zero mean Gaussian distribution. In the tth frame, we consider N particle samples, whose observations (Gray scale values) are denoted in matrix form as: $Y = [y_1, \ldots, y_N] \in R^{m \times N}$[1]. We construct our dictionary $D_t = [d_1, \ldots, d_K] \in R^{m \times K}$, in which the tracked object can be represented under a variety of appearance changes by its templates $\{d_i\}_{i=1}^{K}$ (d_i is the ith dictionary item).

3.3 Joint Sparse Model

Since in particle filter based visual tracking, particle are densely sampled around the current target state, there are often underlying correlation structure between the particles. To explore these hidden structures, [14] employed multi task sparse learning to impose joint sparsity between the particles (tasks) yields a more accurate representation for the ensemble of particles where the sparse representation matrix $X = [x_1, \ldots, x_N] \in R^{K \times N}$ can be obtained by as follows:

$$\min_{X} \|Y - D_t X\|_F^2 + \lambda \|X\|_{p,q} \tag{3}$$

where $\|X\|_{p,q} = \left(\sum_{i=1}^{K} \|X_i\|_p^q\right)^{\frac{1}{q}}$, $\|X_i\|_p$ is the l_p norm of X_i, (i^{th} row of matrix X).

3.4 Laplacian Group Sparse Model

As has been discussed, in order to alleviate computationally expense caused by l_1 minimisation of each particle separately in particle filter based tracking, we seek the common structure among tasks (particle samples) in any given frame. However, considering a global structure for particles is not strong assumption. In fact, in practical application, the particles may exhibit a more sophisticated structure where the sparse representation of closely particles is more likely to be similar rather than those from different spatial locations. In this paper, we augment multi task learning framework with a graph structure to consider mutual

[1] $m = 1024 - dim$ Gray scale based features.

relation between particles. In this way, is each frame we construct the similarity graph where the particles are represented by the nodes and the edges between particles specify their correlation (feature similarity). Motivated by the success of recent work in image classification [17], we have the following representation:

$$\|Y - D_t X\|_2^2 + \frac{\lambda_1}{2} Tr\left(X \hat{L} X^T\right) + \lambda_2 \|X\|_{p,1} \tag{4}$$

where $\|X\|_{p,1} = \sum_{i=1}^{K} \|X\|_p$, λ_1 and λ_2 are the regularisation parameters. $\hat{L}$ known as the Laplacian matrix, is symmetric and positive definiteness and acts as a key factor in our proposed tracker that models the similarity graph for the particles.

3.5 Solving the Optimisation Problem

The formulated problem in Eq. 4 is a convex optimisation problem with a non-smooth objective function due to the non-negativity constraint assumption for the particles representation matrix X. In this paper, we seek to solve this optimisation problem using the accelerated proximal method (APM) [18] due to its ability of optimal convergence compared to other first-order techniques. APM iterates between two sequences of variables: **(1)** an attainable solution (updating the current representation matrix) $\left\{\hat{X}_k\right\}$ and **(2)** an aggregation matrix sequence $\left\{\nabla^k\right\}$.

Proximal mapping: At each iteration, the representation matrix X_k can be updated by the generalised proximal mapping as the following problem:

$$\min_X \frac{1}{2} \|X - H\|_2^2 + \widetilde{\lambda} \|X\|_{p,1} \tag{5}$$

where $\widetilde{\lambda} = \frac{\lambda_2}{\gamma_k}$, $H = \hat{X}_k - \frac{1}{\gamma_k} \nabla^k$ and γ_k denotes the step size.

$$\nabla^k = \hat{X}_k - \frac{1}{\gamma_k}\left(D_t^T\left(Y - D_t \hat{X}_k\right) + \lambda_1 \hat{X}_k \hat{L}\right) \tag{6}$$

Aggregation sequence: At the kth iteration of APM, the aggregation matrix is updated by linear combination of X_k and X_{k-1} from previous iterations:[2]

$$\hat{X}_{k+1} = X_{k+1} + \frac{\mu_{k+1}(1 - \mu_k)}{\mu_k}(X_{k+1} - X_k) \tag{7}$$

3.6 Enhanced Similarity Graph for the Particles

Regarding the graph structure for the particle samples in the current frame, the most existing similarity methods only consider pairwise distances of the data points. Since the pairwise distance only rely on the two connected samples

[2] μ_k is conventionally set to $\frac{2}{k+1}$.

(nodes) and ignores the global structure of the whole sample points, it is fragile to outliers. To address this problem, we propose a similarity graph, which takes advantage of a linear representation of each particle over a set of other particle samples. The proposed similarity graph not only could encode each particle feature over the other particles with less residual error, but also enforces the local representation of each particle sample using the following objective function:

$$\min_{c_i} \sum_{i=1}^{N} \rho \left\| S_i c_i \right\| + (1-\rho) \left\| y_i - A_i c_i \right\| \quad s.t. \mathbf{1}^T c_i = 1 \tag{8}$$

where we encode each particle sample by building the dictionary A_i composed of the set of remaining particles at the given frame, $A_i = [y_1, y_2, \cdots, y_{i-1}, 0, y_{i+1}, \cdots, y_N]$, S_i is a diagonal matrix whose j^{th} diagonal element is the pairwise distance from y_i to the jth particle in A_i,$(j = 1, 2, \cdots, N)$, c_i is a similarity over the corresponding dictionary, $\mathbf{1} \in \Re^N$ (N is the number of candidates) denotes the column vector whose entries are all ones and ρ is the factor controls the balance between linear representation measure and pairwise distance scheme. The similarity representation of the proposed graph can be solved as:

$$c_i = \frac{R_i^{-1} \mathbf{1}}{\mathbf{1}^T R_i^{-1} \mathbf{1}} \tag{9}$$

where $R_i = (1-\rho) \left(y_i \mathbf{1}^T - A_i \right)^T \left(y_i \mathbf{1}^T - A_i \right) + \rho S_i^T S_i$. Furthermore, in order to obtain a more discriminative correlation matrix, we keep the k strongest connections for each particle using k-nearest neighbour searching on c_i and set all other elements to zero. At the end, we use the obtained similarity matrix as our Laplacian matrix $\hat{L}$ in Eq. 4.[3]

4 Lifespan Outlier Rejection

Since the appearance of a target object is expected to be temporally correlated and does not change dramatically over a short period of time, the target object can be represented well by the more recent tracking results w.r.t. the current frame. Therefore, in each frame, we aim to select the particle samples that are highly correlated to the previous tracking results and remove the unrelated ones. In order to achieve this goal, we construct another set of dictionary templates $T = \{t_i\}_{i=1}^{n}$, in which each column represents the tracking result of the latest $n-1$ frames[4] plus the template in the first frame, which is considered as our proposal. Given the new template set, the sparse coefficient w_i for each template t^i can be computed by:

$$\min_{w_i} \left\| t^i - Y w_i \right\|_2^2 + \lambda_w \left\| w_i \right\|_1 s.t. \forall i, w_i \geq 0, i = 1, \cdots, n \tag{10}$$

[3] We denote $\widetilde{c}_i$ as a discriminative feature, then we build a similarity graph by considering each point as a vertex and assigning the connection weight between the node i and j as $|\widetilde{c}_{ij}|$.

[4] We consider every $n = 5$ frames.

where λ_w is the regularisation factor. Using l_1 minimisation of the LARS algorithm [19], we are capable of choosing the highly associated particle samples for the current frame with reduced computational complexity. The implementation also has an option to add positivity constraints on the solutions w_i, which give us a precise sparse representation. This representation reveals a small or even zero value for the jth candidate if it holds little similarity with the ith template. Therefore, we build a mask for each particle sample, in which if the sum of its sparse coefficients is zero, we set its weight ω_j to zero and ignore this particle as follows:

$$\omega_j = \begin{cases} 0 & if \sum_i^n w_{ij} = 0 \\ 1 & \text{Otherwise} \end{cases} \tag{11}$$

In this way, we build a faster tracker with the least number of particles as possible (see Fig. 1). Consequently, the selected particle samples will adaptively change according to different scenes.

5 Likelihood Model Using the Spatial Weight

We present a spatial confidence score for the particles, which can naturally integrate the particle sample importance into the tracking result. Here, we assume the tracking location at the current frame is the location of the most correct particle sample to make each particle contribute differently to the target presence probability: The closer the location is to the current tracked position, the larger probability it has and the farther it is from the tracking location, the less it contributes to the object presence probability (see Fig.2).

Up to now, the proposed tracker is entirely generative. However, in order to handle the drifting problem caused by rapid changes in appearance of the tracking object, we build up target templates with background templates randomly sampled in the first frame, which consequently should be updated in successive frames. The spatial score for the ith particle can be modelled as:

$$\psi_i = \frac{1}{C} e^{-|l_i - l^*|} \tag{12}$$

where C is the normalisation constant and $l(\cdot) \in \Re^2$ is the location function. This spatial weight is a monotone decreasing function w.r.t. the Euclidean distance between the locations of the ith particle sample and the target location l^*.

Finally, in order to obtain the overall score for the tracking result, we first divide the sparse representation matrix X into two subsets, X_{pos} and X_{neg}, each representing the candidate's similarity to the object (positive) templates $D_t^{(O)}$ and background (negative) templates $D_t^{(B)}$,respectively. Further, the weights of the particles are specified by the difference in contribution of these two parts and the tracking result z_t at time instance t is the particle y_i such that:

$$i = \arg\max y_{i=1,\dots,N} \quad \psi_i \odot \left(\|X_{pos}\|_1 - \|X_{neg}\|_1\right) \tag{13}$$

where $\odot$ is an element-wise product[5]. This likelihood function not only encourages the tracking result to be represented well by the object and *not* the background templates, it also gives more weight to the particle samples near the current tracking location (Fig. 2).

6 Dictionary Update

Updating target object templates for handling appearance change during tracking is a vital part of any visual tracking method. Neither fixed object templates nor frequently updated target templates could help the accurate representation of target appearance during tracking. Since target appearance only remains

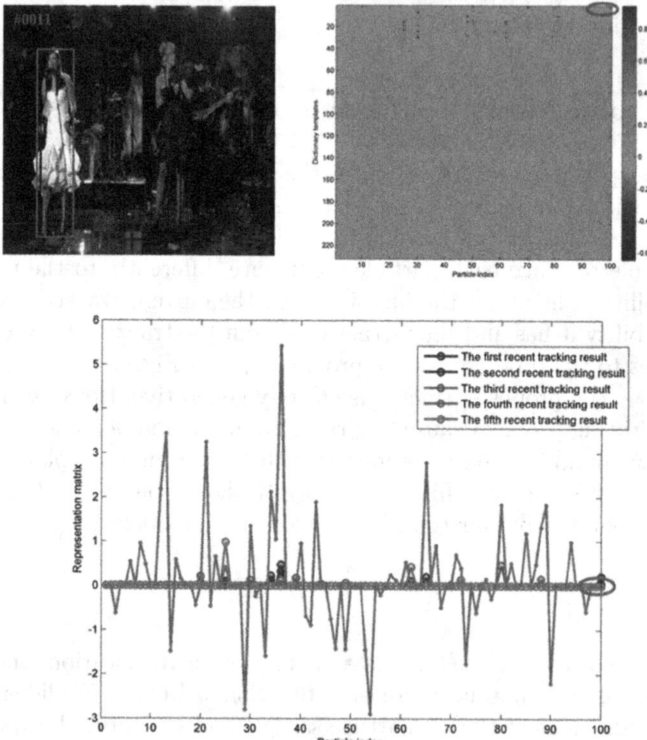

Fig. 1. Illustrating the effect of outlier rejection for the *singer 1* sequence. At the top right, the sparse representation of particles with respect to the target templates is shown, while brighter columns indicate the presence of outliers. At the bottom, sparse representations of the most recent tracking results w.r.t. the current particles are shown. As highlighted, those particles whose sum of their sparse representations is zero are removed from sampling.

[5] This is the element-wise product of two $(1 \times N)$ matrices. N is the number of sampled particles.

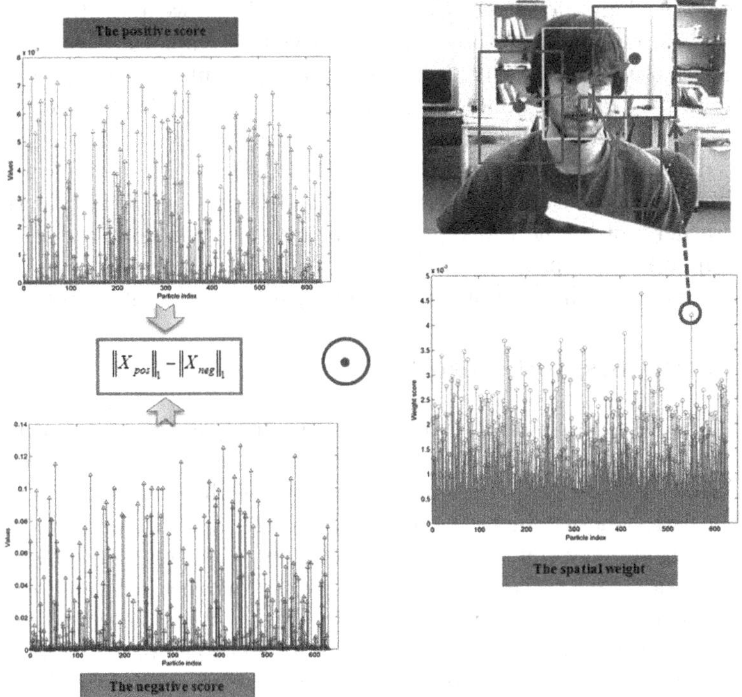

Fig. 2. This figure illustrates the principle of the proposed likelihood model. On the left side, the discriminative scores of candidates are shown. On the right side, the relative distance between particles and target object is illustrated. The yellow rectangle is the tracking result. The solid circles are the central locations of each particle and red rectangles are the particle samples. The corresponding spatial weight of the sample particle is highlighted (Colour figure online).

unchanged in just a short period of time, a stable appearance model is not reliable for long period tracking. On the other hand, if samples are updated frequently, the model will degrade. The initial dictionary comprising positive templates n_p is obtained by drawing sample images around the target location (e.g. within a radius of a few pixels) and downsampling the selected images to a normalised size (32×32 pixels in our experiments). Each downsampled image is stacked together to form the set of positive templates. Similarly, the set of n_n negative templates is composed of images further away from the labelled location (e.g. within an annular region some pixels away from the target object).

First, for the background templates $D_t^{(B)}$, since the surrounding image region of two consecutive frames are similar, we sample the negative templates from image regions away (e.g. more than 7 pixels) only from the current tracking result. Moreover, we take advantage of using our proposed target transition model to ignore those candidates as tracking result since they are involved in representing negative templates.

On the other hand, for the object template set $D_t^{(O)}$, we allocate a similarity measure μ_i that demonstrates how representative the template in tracking result is. The more a template is used to represent tracking results, the higher its weight is. Similar to [20], in each frame, we measure the similarity between the current tracking result and the object templates and if the particles are not sufficiently represented (up to a predefined threshold $\Omega = 0.4$) by the dictionary, we use the tracking result to replace the corresponding template with the new tracking result. In other words, the tracking result is added to the template set if none of the template is comparable to the tracking result. The weight of this new template is set to the median of the current normalised weight vector.

7 Experiments and Results

In this paper, we compare the performance of the proposed tracker with several state-of-the-art trackers. We use the default parameters for these trackers as they reported. These trackers can be categorized to different groups. Discriminative heuristic trackers include the STRUCK [21], the compressive tracking based CT [22] and the multiple instance learning-based tracker MIL [23]. On the opposite side, generative trackers such as the incremental subspace based IVT [7] and two channels blurring approaches DFT [24] are considered. We also utilise part-based trackers akin to the TLD [25], which estimate the new target object by combining the local motion estimates with discriminative learning of patches and Frag-Track [6], in which the target object is represented by multiple image fragments or patches. In addition, sparse representations based trackers like ASLA [26], SCM [27], MTT [14] and L1APG [28] are used. Theses trackers range from local sparse representations (ASLA tracker) to holistic sparse templates (MTT and L1APG) and both local-holistic representation method (SCM). Finally, we implement the VTD method as our last benchmark, which adapts mixture models based on sparse principal component analysis.

7.1 Parameters Setting

The parameters of the proposed tracking algorithm are fixed in all experiments. The numbers of positive templates n_p and negative templates n_n are 50 and 200, respectively. All weight parameters of Eq. 4 are set to 0.5 and the regularisation parameter λ_w in Eq. 10 is fixed to be 0.01. In Eq. (6), we set $\widetilde{\lambda}$ (by cross-validation) to 0.005 and γ_k to 1/0.01, respectively. ρ in Eq. (8) is set to 0.5. The maximum iteration of the objective function in Eq. 4 is set to 10, and 100 particles are chosen as candidate samples in each frame. An observed target image patch is partitioned into non-overlapping local fragments (image patches) of size 8×8 pixels, each of which is independently represented in gray scale values, vectorised and normalised to be a vector with unit l_2 norm. Then, we concatenate these local feature vectors so that the global structural information is maintained. The candidates and templates in this work are all represented with this locally normalized features to handle partial occlusion and to moderate appearance variation.

Table 1. Average centre location errors (in pixels). The best three results are shown in Red, Blue, and Green fonts.

Video Clip	Frag	IVT	MIL	APG	VTD	MTT	SCM	CT	TLD	ASLA	Struck	DFT	Our
Singer1	22.0	8.5	15.2	3.2	4.1	41.2	3.8	25.1	11.6	5.3	12.6	10.4	2.8
Girl	18.0	48.6	32.2	62.4	21.4	23.9	9.7	21.0	20.3	12.5	10.0	21.5	9.3
Car11	63.8	2.1	43.5	1.7	27.1	1.8	4.1	6.0	25.1	2.0	1.9	2.2	1.5
Face	48.8	69.7	134.6	57.7	140.9	127.2	125.1	144.2	67.5	95.1	25.0	26.8	15.3
David	76.7	3.6	16.1	14.3	13.6	124.2	5.1	15.3	16.3	6.0	3.1	10.2	3.4
Dudek	61.5	8.8	20.3	70.6	66.0	53.8	9.2	23.1	10.5	10.6	11.5	9.5	8.6
Woman	113.6	167.4	122.3	118.5	136.6	127.2	4.3	109.6	110.4	3.2	10.1	15.3	3.1
Bolt	240.1	170.6	163.9	225.5	22.3	106.0	73.2	115.5	34.5	56.4	98.5	102.3	16.5
Jumping	58.6	36.7	10.2	9.1	63.2	19.3	3.9	9.0	8.0	39.2	42.0	39.5	4.6
Mountain	141.6	33.2	128.3	130.2	7.5	11.3	5.9	86.7	96.5	5.1	10.5	122.4	3.3
Sylvester	98.9	70.8	31.1	112.5	49.4	14.6	9.0	21.3	17.5	9.1	20.4	34.5	8.5
Tiger1	39.5	158.7	14.2	21.5	28.9	30.9	10.5	20.0	13.9	11.4	12.2	10.0	8.9

Table 2. Average overlap rate (in pixels). The best three results are shown in Red, Blue, and Green fonts.

Video Clip	Frag	IVT	MIL	APG	VTD	MTT	SCM	CT	TLD	ASLA	Struck	DFT	Our
Singer1	0.34	0.66	0.33	0.83	0.79	0.32	0.85	0.29	0.65	0.78	0.59	0.72	0.87
Girl	0.69	0.43	0.51	0.33	0.52	0.63	0.69	0.78	0.57	0.72	0.94	0.56	0.96
Car11	0.09	0.81	0.17	0.83	0.43	0.58	0.79	0.71	0.38	0.82	0.86	0.63	0.91
Face	0.39	0.44	0.15	0.35	0.24	0.26	0.36	0.13	0.46	0.21	0.78	0.75	0.86
David	0.19	0.71	0.45	0.57	0.53	0.28	0.69	0.25	0.44	0.63	0.79	0.61	0.81
Dudek	0.46	0.81	0.64	0.61	0.46	0.36	0.76	0.51	0.71	0.73	0.75	0.68	0.83
Woman	0.20	0.18	0.16	0.06	0.15	0.17	0.77	0.16	0.07	0.81	0.86	0.74	0.85
Bolt	0.07	0.13	0.16	0.10	0.82	0.19	0.29	0.12	0.77	0.31	0.15	0.11	0.92
Jumping	0.13	0.29	0.54	0.57	0.09	0.31	0.72	0.96	0.98	0.25	0.18	0.20	0.98
Mountain	0.06	0.66	0.14	0.11	0.89	0.81	0.91	0.11	0.25	0.92	0.87	0.10	0.96
Sylvester	0.06	0.51	0.54	0.28	0.44	0.52	0.89	0.65	0.68	0.88	0.70	0.62	0.91
Tiger1	0.19	0.71	0.39	0.15	0.73	0.75	0.82	0.53	0.65	0.80	0.73	0.89	0.95

7.2 The Test Sequences

We use 12 challenging video sequences widely used in the literature and publicly available from the online object tracking benchmark[6]. Each video sequence was labelled with different attributes including five visual attributes that reflect a specific challenge in appearance humiliation: **(i)** abrupt motion, **(ii)** illumination

[6] https://sites.google.com/site/trackerbenchmark/benchmarks/v10.

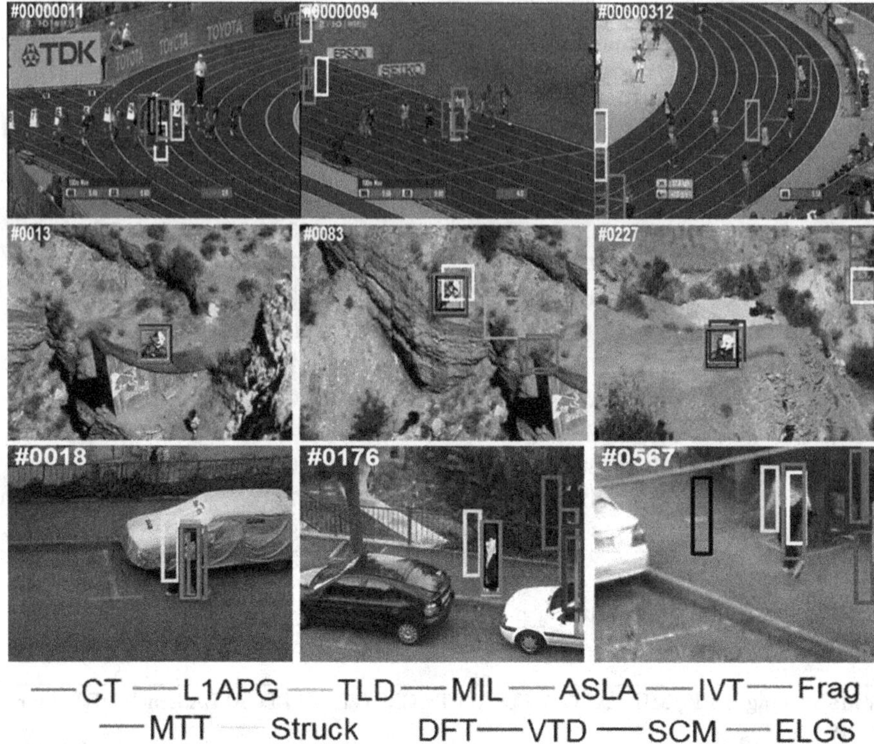

Fig. 3. Sample tracking results by our tracker (Enhanced Laplacian Group Sparse (ELGS)) compared with benchmark results in challenging sequences with rotation and non-rigid deformation (*Bolt sequence*), background clutter (*MountainBike sequence*) and heavy occlusion (*Woman sequence*).

change, **(iii)** occlusion, **(iv)** scale change and **(v)** camera motion. Their ground truths are provided. Figure 3 shows some tracking results for different video sequences.

7.3 Performance Measure

Numerous performance metrics have been proposed for visual tracking evaluation during recent years. For the purpose of measuring the performance of the proposed tracker, two criteria, the centre location error as well as the overlap ratio, are implemented here. It should be noted that a smaller average error or a bigger overlap rate means a more accurate result. The tracker's overlap rate in each frame defined as the area $\frac{area(BB_T \cap BB_G)}{area(BB_T \cup BB_G)}$, where BB_G and BB_T denote the bounding box obtained by the ground truth and a tracker, respectively. An important advantage of the overlap measure is that it accounts for both position and size of the predicted and proposal bounding boxes simultaneously and does not lead to arbitrary large errors at tracking failures. As is shown in

Tables 1 and 2, except for two sequences, the results of our tracker outperform the other trackers. Due to space limitations, we do not mention the detailed results including the average error plots and average overlap ratio plots here but do so in the supplementary material.

8 Conclusion

In this paper, we have presented an enhanced Laplacian group sparse learning method for particle filter based visual tracking. By imposing the Laplacian group sparse penalty term in our objective function, we are able to not only exploit the underlying relationship shared by different particles, but also to capture their structure ignored by previous works. Furthermore, we propose an enhanced similarity graph for the particle samples robust to outliers. In addition, since the target object can be modelled well by the more recent tracking results, in each frame, we remove the particle samples that are not correlated to the previous tracking results. Finally, a new likelihood function using the discriminative weighted particles is proposed where the particle importance is considered. In comparison with 12 state-of-the-art trackers, our tracker shows superior performance in both accuracy measures used.

References

1. Mei, X., Ling, H.: Robust visual tracking and vehicle classification via sparse representation. IEEE Trans. Pattern Anal. Mach. Intell. **33**, 2259–2272 (2011)
2. Mei, X., Ling, H., Wu, Y., Blasch, E., Bai, L.: Minimum error bounded efficient ? 1 tracker with occlusion detection. In: 2011 IEEE Conference on Computer Vision and Pattern Recognition (CVPR), pp. 1257–1264. IEEE (2011)
3. Black, M.J., Jepson, A.D.: Eigentracking: robust matching and tracking of articulated objects using a view-based representation. In: Buxton, B., Cipolla, R. (eds.) ECCV 1996. LNCS, vol. 1064, pp. 329–342. Springer, Heidelberg (1996)
4. Comaniciu, D., Ramesh, V., Meer, P.: Kernel-based object tracking. IEEE Trans. Pattern Anal. Mach. Intell. **25**, 564–577 (2003)
5. Yang, M., Wu, Y., Hua, G.: Context-aware visual tracking. IEEE Trans. Pattern Anal. Mach. Intell. **31**, 1195–1209 (2009)
6. Adam, A., Rivlin, E.: Robust fragments-based tracking using the integral histogram. In: Computer Vision and Pattern Recognition (CVPR), pp. 798–805 (2006)
7. Ross, D., Lim, J., Lin, R.S., Yang, M.H.: Incremental learning for robust visual tracking. Int. J. Comput. Vis. **77**, 125–141 (2008)
8. Kwon, J., Lee, K.M.: Visual tracking decomposition. In: 2010 IEEE Conference on Computer Vision and Pattern Recognition (CVPR), pp. 1269–1276. IEEE (2010)
9. Grabner, H., Grabner, M., Bischof, H.: Real-time tracking via online boosting. In: British Machine Vision Conference (BMVC), pp. 47–56 (2006)
10. Avidan, S.: Ensemble tracking. IEEE Trans. Pattern Anal. Mach. Intell. **29**, 261–271 (2007)
11. Liu, R., Cheng, J., Lu, H.: A robust boosting tracker with minimum error bound in a co-training framework. In: 2009 IEEE 12th International Conference on Computer Vision, pp. 1459–1466. IEEE (2009)

12. Jiang, N., Liu, W., Wu, Y.: Adaptive and discriminative metric differential tracking. In: 2011 IEEE Conference on Computer Vision and Pattern Recognition (CVPR), pp. 1161–1168. IEEE (2011)
13. Babenko, B., Yang, M., Belongie, S.: Visual tracking with online multiple instance learning. In: Computer Vision and Pattern Recognition (CVPR) (2009)
14. Zhang, T., Ghanem, B., Liu, S., Ahuja, N.: Robust visual tracking via multi-task sparse learning. In: 2012 IEEE Conference on Computer Vision and Pattern Recognition (CVPR), pp. 2042–2049. IEEE (2012)
15. Zhang, T., Ghanem, B., Liu, S., Ahuja, N.: Robust visual tracking via structured multi-task sparse learning. Int. J. Comput. Vis. **101**, 367–383 (2013)
16. Elhamifar, E., Vidal, R.: Sparse subspace clustering: algorithm, theory, and applications. IEEE Trans. Pattern Anal. Mach. Intell. **35**, 2765–2781 (2013)
17. Gao, S., Tsang, I.H., Chia, L.T.: Laplacian sparse coding, hypergraph laplacian sparse coding, and applications. IEEE Trans. Pattern Anal. Mach. Intell. **35**, 92–104 (2013)
18. Beck, A., Teboulle, M.: A fast iterative shrinkage-thresholding algorithm for linear inverse problems. SIAM J. Imaging Sci. **2**, 183–202 (2009)
19. Efron, B., Hastie, T., Johnstone, I., Tibshirani, R., et al.: Least angle regression. Ann. Stat. **32**, 407–499 (2004)
20. Zhang, T., Ghanem, B., Liu, S., Ahuja, N.: Low-rank sparse learning for robust visual tracking. In: Fitzgibbon, A., Lazebnik, S., Perona, P., Sato, Y., Schmid, C. (eds.) ECCV 2012, Part VI. LNCS, vol. 7577, pp. 470–484. Springer, Heidelberg (2012)
21. Hare, S., Saffari, A., Torr, P.H.: Struck: structured output tracking with kernels. In: 2011 IEEE International Conference on Computer Vision (ICCV), pp. 263–270. IEEE (2011)
22. Zhang, K., Zhang, L., Yang, M.-H.: Real-time compressive tracking. In: Fitzgibbon, A., Lazebnik, S., Perona, P., Sato, Y., Schmid, C. (eds.) ECCV 2012, Part III. LNCS, vol. 7574, pp. 864–877. Springer, Heidelberg (2012)
23. Babenko, B., Yang, M.H., Belongie, S.: Robust object tracking with online multiple instance learning. IEEE Trans. Pattern Anal. Mach. Intell. **33**, 1619–1632 (2011)
24. Sevilla-Lara, L., Learned-Miller, E.: Distribution fields for tracking. In: 2012 IEEE Conference on Computer Vision and Pattern Recognition (CVPR), pp. 1910–1917. IEEE (2012)
25. Kalal, Z., Matas, J., Mikolajczyk, K.: Pn learning: bootstrapping binary classifiers by structural constraints. In: 2010 IEEE Conference on Computer Vision and Pattern Recognition (CVPR), pp. 49–56. IEEE (2010)
26. Jia, X., Lu, H., Yang, M.H.: Visual tracking via adaptive structural local sparse appearance model. In: 2012 IEEE Conference on Computer Vision and Pattern Recognition (CVPR), pp. 1822–1829. IEEE (2012)
27. Zhong, W., Lu, H., Yang, M.H.: Robust object tracking via sparsity-based collaborative model. In: 2012 IEEE Conference on Computer Vision and Pattern Recognition (CVPR), pp. 1838–1845. IEEE (2012)
28. Bao, C., Wu, Y., Ling, H., Ji, H.: Real time robust l1 tracker using accelerated proximal gradient approach. In: 2012 IEEE Conference on Computer Vision and Pattern Recognition (CVPR), pp. 1830–1837. IEEE (2012)

Cross-view Action Recognition via Dual-Codebook and Hierarchical Transfer Framework

Chengkun Zhang, Huicheng Zheng(✉), and Jianhuang Lai

School of Information Science and Technology, Sun Yat-sen University, Guangzhou 510006, China
zhangchk@mail2.sysu.edu.cn
{zhenghch,stsljh}@mail.sysu.edu.cn

Abstract. In this paper, we focus on the challenging cross-view action recognition problem. The key to this problem is to find the correspondence between source and target views, which is realized in two stages in this paper. Firstly, we construct a Dual-Codebook for the two views, which is composed of two codebooks corresponding to source and target views, respectively. Each codeword in one codebook has a corresponding codeword in the other codebook, which is different from traditional methods that implement independent codebooks in the two views. We propose an effective co-clustering algorithm based on semi-nonnegative matrix factorization to derive the Dual-Codebook. With the Dual-Codebook, an action can be represented based on Bag-of-Dual-Codes (BoDC) no matter it is in the source view or in the target view. Therefore, the Dual-Codebook establishes a sort of codebook-to-codebook correspondence, which is the foundation for the second stage. In the second stage, we observe that, although the appearance of action samples will change significantly with viewpoints, the temporal relationship between atom actions within an action should be stable across views. Therefore, we further propose a hierarchical transfer framework to obtain the feature-to-feature correspondence at atom-level between source and target views. The framework is based on a temporal structure that can effectively capture the temporal relationship between atom actions within an action. It performs transfer at atom levels of multiple timescales, while most existing methods only perform video-level transfer. We carry out a series of experiments on the IXMAS dataset. The results demonstrate that our method obtained superior performance compared to state-of-the-art approaches.

1 Introduction

Recently, action recognition has gained much attention in computer vision due to its extensive applications in video surveillance [26], human-machine interaction,

Electronic supplementary material The online version of this chapter (doi:10.1007/978-3-319-16814-2_38) contains supplementary material, which is available to authorized users.

D. Cremers et al. (Eds.): ACCV 2014, Part V, LNCS 9007, pp. 579–592, 2015.
DOI: 10.1007/978-3-319-16814-2_38

medical assistance for elders [1,25], etc. Previous work has proposed some popular features for recognizing actions, such as space-time point features [5,14,19], shape features [3,17,18,32], optical-flow features [6,17]. These features have led to remarkable action recognition performance for typical scenarios where there are only limited viewpoint variations. However, when the view point changes significantly, traditional approaches for action recognition would suffer from serious drop of performance [10,11].

Several approaches have been proposed to address action recognition across views. One category of approaches rely on 3D reconstruction [9,21,27,30]. Some other approaches directly use 2D image or geometric constraints across different views [8,16,22,23,31]. Besides, temporal self-similarities have also been exploited for view-invariant feature extraction [12,13].

Recently, some works seek to transfer action model from the source view to the target view, and have received satisfactory results. Farhadi et al. [7] proposed to use Maximum Margin Clustering to build split-based features for frames. Then, they transfer them among corresponding frames across different views. Liu et al. [20] constructed "bilingual words" by using the co-occurrence of visual words from source and target views. By representing the videos as a bag of bilingual words (BoBW), they can transfer the action model at the video-level across different views. Zheng et al. [34] proposed to build a transferable dictionary pair by forcing the videos of the same action to have the same sparse coefficients across views. These approaches are attractive, for they have little dependence on the 3D model reconstruction of actions, reliable body joints detection and tracking, and the geometric information across different views.

However, existing approaches generally implement codebooks separately trained in the source and target views, which cannot guarantee reliable correspondence between visual words. This will degrade the performance of these approaches on transferring action models from the source view to the target view. In this paper, we propose to construct a Dual-Codebook for the source and target views. Unlike traditional codebook learning approaches, we model the construction of Dual-Codebook as a co-clustering problem and propose an effective algorithm to solve it. Our Dual-Codebook consists of two codebooks, one for each of the two views. Since it is obtained by co-clustering, not isolated clustering in source and target views, each codeword in one codebook has a corresponding codeword in the other codebook. This means that our Dual-Codebook contains basic view-correspondence, i.e., a codebook-to-codebook correspondence across two views. To our knowledge, this has never been explored before.

Furthermore, existing approaches usually transfer action models at the video-level, ignoring the sequential composition of atom actions during the execution of the full action. Such a strategy will not be discriminative enough when multiple actions contain similar atom actions following different occurrence orders, such as sit down and get up. To resolve this problem, we propose a novel hierarchical framework for transferring action models across different views. Specifically, we divide action videos into several segments along the time dimension at each level of this framework. Each segment contains an atom action within a short time interval. Then, we enforce similar sparse representations for each pair of corresponding segments from the source and target views by learning a transferable pairwise dictionary. The inputs of the learning procedure are the Bag-of-Dual-Codes (BoDC) of these segments. This is different from implementations of existing dictionary learning strategies, which are usually based on separately generated codebooks. The representation generated in this way is more robust to view changes, as demonstrated experimentally.

This paper presents the following contributions.

1. A Dual-Codebook is constructed for source and target views. We propose an effective co-clustering algorithm to learn the Dual-Codebook. The Dual-Codebook achieves the codebook-to-codebook correspondence across different views.
2. We propose a hierarchical transfer framework based on Dual-Codebook. The framework transfers the action model at the atom-level on different timescales and achieves the feature-to-feature correspondence across different views.
3. We evaluate our method on the IXMAS dataset, and demonstrate the superiority of our method compared to state-of-the-art methods.

2 Dual-Codebook Construction

In this section, we firstly model the process of learning Dual-Codebook as a co-clustering problem. Then, we propose an iterative algorithm to solve this problem effectively, which is based on semi-nonnegative matrix factorization.

We consider two kinds of actions: shared actions and orphan actions as in [7]. *Shared actions* are observed in both source and target views, and *orphan actions* are only observed in the source view during training. We only use shared actions to construct Dual-Codebook in the training phase, and use the samples of orphan action in the target view as test samples in the classification phase. This setting means that we do not use the correspondence across pairwise views for the orphan action.

2.1 Problem Formulation

The classical k-means algorithm aims to minimize the representation error of the given set of data points, and can be modeled as follows. Let $Y \in R^{d\times N}$ be the set of N d-dimensional data points. Then, the codebook of K-cluster centroids $C \in R^{d\times K}$ can be obtained by solving the following optimization problem

$$\{C^*, X^*\} = \arg\min_{C,X} \|Y - CX\|_F^2 \tag{1}$$

where $X \in R^{K\times N}$ is the cluster indicators of the N data points. Here, $\|.\|_F$ is the Frobenius norm of a matrix. Since C contains both positive and negative entries, and the entries in X should be nonnegative, if we allow the entries in X to range over $(0, 1)$, the k-means clustering can be seen as semi-nonnegative matrix factorization [4].

Existing methods for cross-view action recognition usually implement codebooks obtained by k-means clustering separately in source and target views. As a result, these codebooks cannot guarantee correspondence with each other. We propose to construct a Dual-Codebook across two different views, which is composed of two codebooks, one in each view. Each pair of codewords that hold the same column number in these two codebooks is a pair of corresponding codewords across source and target views. The codewords in the Dual-Codebook are generated while maintaining pairwise associations across two views, which is very different from traditional codebook learning approaches.

To establish the association, we reduce the distance between the histograms of each pair of corresponding frames in the source and target views. We argue that, if two codewords from these two views correspond to each other, their frequency in the corresponding action videos should be close. Hence, by reducing the distance between the corresponding histograms from the source and target views, we can obtain corresponding codewords across the two views.

Suppose there are N_s, N_t feature points extracted from the videos of shared actions in source and target views, respectively. Let $Y_s \in R^{d\times N_s}, Y_t \in R^{d\times N_t}$ denote the sets of these feature points in source and target views. The Dual-Codebook $\{C_s, C_t\}$, where $C_s, C_t \in R^{d\times K}$ correspond to source and target views, respectively, can be learned by minimizing the following objective function

$$f(C_s, C_t, X_s, X_t) = \alpha \|X_s A_s - X_t A_t\|_F^2 + \|Y_s - C_s X_s\|_F^2 + \|Y_t - C_t X_t\|_F^2 \quad s.t.\ X_s \geq 0_{K\times N_s}, X_t \geq 0_{K\times N_t} \tag{2}$$

where $X_s \in R^{K\times N_s}$, $X_t \in R^{K\times N_t}$ denote the cluster indicators of the feature points in source and target views, respectively. α is a positive constant. Besides, $A_s \in \{0,1\}^{N_s\times T}$, T is the total number of frames in source and target views. $A_s(i,j) = 1$ indicates that the i-th feature point is located in the j-th frame in the source view. The matrix $A_t \in \{0,1\}^{N_t\times T}$ is defined similarly in the target view. Thus, $X_s A_s$, $X_t A_t$ denote the histograms of all frames in source and target views, respectively.

The first term of Eq. (2) reflects the difference of the histograms of all corresponding frames in source and target views. The second and third terms of Eq. (2) are the representation errors of Y_s and Y_t, respectively.

It should be noted that Eq. (2) can be seen as a co-clustering problem, because codebooks C_s, C_t are generated simultaneously and the clustering on one of them induces that of the other, maintaining pairwise associations across source and target views. Specifically, for $i = 1, 2, \ldots, K$, the i-th columns of C_s and C_t are two codewords that correspond to each other.

2.2 Optimization

Since C_s, C_t contain both positive and negative entries, and the entries in X_s, X_t are nonnegative, Eq. (2) can be seen as a constrained joint semi-nonnegative matrix factorization. Inspired by [4], we propose an iterative algorithm to solve the problem as follows. Let $X_s = [x_{s1}, x_{s2}, \ldots, x_{sN_s}] \in R^{K\times N_s}$, $X_t = [x_{t1}, x_{t2}, \ldots, x_{tN_t}] \in R^{K\times N_t}$.

Step 1: Initialize X_s, X_t.

We first apply k-means clustering separately in the source and target views to obtain visual words in the two views. Then, we use these visual words as vertexes to build a bipartite graph for matching the visual words preliminarily across the two views. Afterwards, we can initialize X_s, X_t according to the matching result of visual words.

Step 2: Update C_s, C_t while fixing X_s, X_t as follows

$$C_s = Y_s X_s^T (X_s X_s^T)^{-1} \tag{3}$$

$$C_t = Y_t X_t^T (X_t X_t^T)^{-1} \tag{4}$$

Eqs. (3) and (4) are obtained by letting the partial derivatives of Eq. (2) with respect to C_s, C_t be zero, respectively.

Step 3: Update X_s column by column using Eq. (5) while fixing X_t, for $m = 1, 2, \ldots, K$,

$$x_{si(m)}^{(t+1)} = x_{si(m)}^{(t)} \sqrt{\frac{\alpha \left[X_t^{(t)}(A_t A_s^{\mathrm{T}})_{\bullet i}\right]_{(m)} + \left[(C_s^{\mathrm{T}} C_s)^{-} x_{si}^{(t)}\right]_{(m)} + \left[(C_s^{\mathrm{T}} Y_s)_{\bullet i}^{+}\right]_{(m)}}{\alpha \left[X_s^{*}(A_s A_s^{\mathrm{T}})_{\bullet i}\right]_{(m)} + \left[(C_s^{\mathrm{T}} C_s)^{+} x_{si}^{(t)}\right]_{(m)} + \left[(C_s^{\mathrm{T}} Y_s)_{\bullet i}^{-}\right]_{(m)}}} \tag{5}$$

To obtain Eq. (5), we use the auxiliary function approach as in [15] to find the auxiliary function of Eq. (2), which is the upper bound of Eq. (2) and is a convex function in X_s. Then, to find the minima of this auxiliary function, we set its partial derivative with respect to X_s to be zero. In Eq. (5), $x_{si(m)}^{(t+1)}$ is the updated value of the m-th entry in the i-th column of X_s at iteration $t+1$. $(\cdot)_{\bullet i}$ denotes the i-th column of the matrix in the parentheses. $[\cdot]_{(m)}$ is the m-th entry of the vector in the brackets. The matrix X_s^* is the result of X_s where the first $i-1$ columns have been updated in the iteration $t+1$. So we can see that, the updated result of the i-th column of X_s is related to the updated results of the first $i-1$ columns of X_s.

Besides, in Eq. (5),

$$(C_s^T C_s)^{+} = \frac{1}{2}[|(C_s^T C_s)| + (C_s^T C_s)] \tag{6}$$

$$(C_s^T C_s)^{-} = \frac{1}{2}[|(C_s^T C_s)| - (C_s^T C_s)] \tag{7}$$

where $(C_s^T C_s)^{+}$ and $(C_s^T C_s)^{-}$ are the positive and negative parts of matrix $C_s^T C_s$, respectively. All superscripts "+" and "−" in Eq. (5) are defined similarly.

Note that $X_s^*(A_s A_s^T)_{\bullet i}$ in Eq. (5) corresponds to the histogram of the frame that contains the i-th feature point in the source view. And $X_t^{(t)}(A_t A_s^T)_{\bullet i}$ in Eq. (5) represents the histogram of a frame in the target view while the corresponding frame in the source view contains the i-th feature point. Consequently, the iterative process of updating each column of X_s (i.e., the cluster indicator of each feature point in the source view) is constrained by the interaction between the histograms of corresponding frames in source and target views. This means that Eq. (5) maintains the pairwise associations across source and target views.

Step 4: Update X_t column by column using Eq. (8) while fixing X_s, for $m = 1, 2, \dots, K$,

$$x_{ti(m)}^{(t+1)} = x_{ti(m)}^{(t)} \sqrt{\frac{\alpha \left[X_s^{(t+1)}(A_s A_t^{\mathrm{T}})_{\bullet i}\right]_{(m)} + \left[(C_t^{\mathrm{T}} C_t)^{-} x_{ti}^{(t)}\right]_{(m)} + \left[(C_t^{\mathrm{T}} Y_t)_{\bullet i}^{+}\right]_{(m)}}{\alpha \left[X_t^{*}(A_t A_t^{\mathrm{T}})_{\bullet i}\right]_{(m)} + \left[(C_t^{\mathrm{T}} C_t)^{+} x_{ti}^{(t)}\right]_{(m)} + \left[(C_t^{\mathrm{T}} Y_t)_{\bullet i}^{-}\right]_{(m)}}} \tag{8}$$

Eq. (8) is obtained in a similar way as Eq. (5).

We iteratively perform Step 1 to 4 until Eq. (2) converges. The convergence proof of the above algorithm can be found in the supplementary material. After the Dual-Codebook is obtained, we can replace traditional Bag-of-Visual-Words (BoVW) with Bag-of-Dual-Codes (BoDC), which contains the codebook-to-codebook correspondence across views.

3 Hierarchical Temporal-Structure Transfer

In this section, we firstly propose the action temporal-structure model that can effectively capture the information about atom actions within a full action. Then, based on this model, we propose the hierarchical temporal-structure transfer framework.

3.1 Action Temporal-Structure Modeling

The execution of an action is typically considered to be composed of several atom actions. Each of these atom actions corresponds to a short time interval and their sequential order forms the temporal pattern of an action. Thus, the categories and sequential composition of the atom actions can reflect the nature of an action [1]. More specifically, both the categories and sequential order of the atom actions will not change with viewpoints. For instance, the action "sit down" can be seen as an atom-action sequence "stand-stoop-sit" in whatever viewpoint it is observed. Consequently, we consider that these significant invariabilities should be fully utilized for solving the cross-view action recognition problem. Before doing this, it is necessary to construct a model that can effectively capture the atom actions and the temporal relationship among them within an action.

To exploit the temporal information, we divide actions into several segments along the time dimension. Each segment can be assumed to contain an atom action, which can be described by a BoDC. For example, when three segments are implemented, the action "sit down" can be divided into "stand", "stoop", and "sit". While for the action "stand up", the atom-action-sequence "sit", "stoop", and "stand" will be obtained instead. In this way, the sequential orders of the segment-BoDCs can be used to distinguish these two actions effectively.

Modeling Details: Based on the above analysis, we consider multiple timescales to construct the action temporal-structure model. For action videos that are approximately aligned in time dimension, at the l-th scale, $l = 1, 2, \ldots, L$, we divide an action into 2^{l-1} segments of equal duration along the time dimension. As a result, an action can be modeled as a sequence of increasingly finer segments at levels $1, 2, \ldots, L$. Based on this action temporal-structure model, we propose a novel hierarchical transfer framework in Sect. 3.2.

3.2 Hierarchical Transfer Framework

In this section, we propose a hierarchical transfer framework that exploits the previous temporal-structure model. In each level of proposed transfer framework, only the shared actions are used to construct the transferable relationship across different views, while orphan actions are utilized to test the effectiveness of this relationship.

In the training stage, we divide two action videos of the same class from source and target views into several segments as in Sect. 3.1. Then we construct the common representation of corresponding segments within these two videos. The basic idea is "pairwise dictionary learning". It has also been explored in cross-domain face recognition [32], and in cross-view action recognition for video-level correspondence [34].

Incorporating this basic idea into the temporal-structure model, we propose a novel hierarchical transfer framework. As illustrated in Fig. 1, both action videos are assumed to have a 2-level temporal structure. For each level of the models in two views, we aim to learn a transferable pairwise dictionary based on the Dual-Codebook. In other words, what we utilize to learn the transferable pairwise dictionary are the BoDCs of all pairs of corresponding segments from shared actions in the source and target views. This is different from existing implementations of dictionary learning strategies that are based on separately generated codebooks. In this hierarchical framework, each level has its own pairwise dictionary, i.e., $\{D_{si}, D_{ti}\}$ shown in Fig. 1, such that all pairs of corresponding segments across source and target views are converted to similar sparse representations, such as $x_{11}, x_{11}^{'}$ in Fig. 1. Thus, these sparse representations are view-invariant, and only depend on atom actions within the segments. This means that, the hierarchical framework is capable to transfer at the atom-level effectively. At last, for each action video in the source and target views, we obtain its full view-invariant sparse representation by concatenating the sparse representations of all segments at all levels of the temporal-structure model, i.e., $[x_{11}, x_{21}, x_{22}]$ and $\left[x_{11}^{'}, x_{21}^{'}, x_{22}^{'}\right]$ shown in Fig. 1.

In the following, we explain the procedure of learning a transferable pairwise dictionary at each level. Let $B_s, B_t \in R^{K \times N}$ denote the K-dimensional BoDCs of N segments of shared actions in the source and target views, respectively. The transferable pairwise dictionary $\{D_s, D_t\}$ is learned by solving the following optimization problem

$$\arg\min_{D_s, D_t, S} \{\|B_s - D_s S\|_2^2 + \|B_t - D_t S\|_2^2\}, \quad s.t. \ \forall i, \|s_i\|_0 \leq T_0 \qquad (9)$$

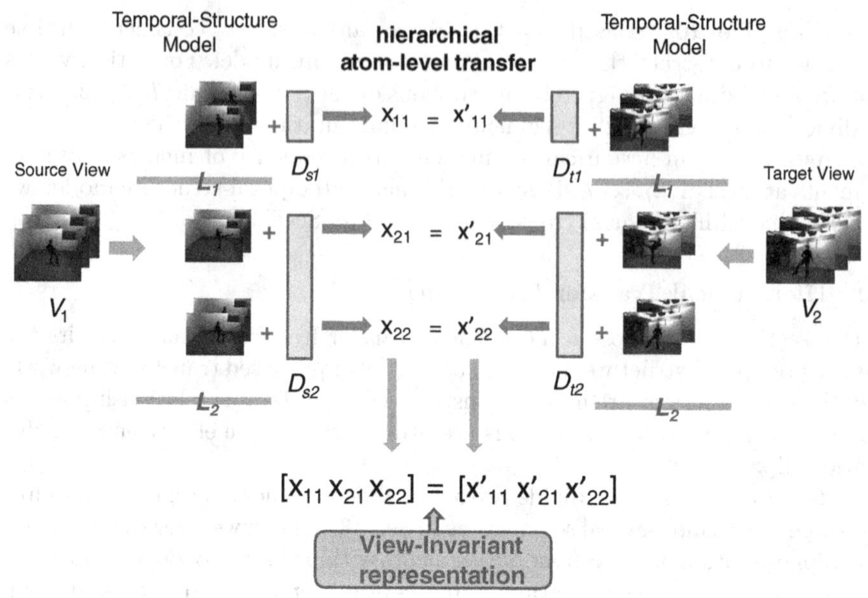

Fig. 1. The proposed hierarchical transfer framework, where we perform transfer at atom-level, converting the corresponding segments to similar sparse representations.

where $D_s, D_t \in R^{K \times J}$ denote, respectively, the dictionaries with J items in the source and target views. The matrix $S = [s_1, s_2, \ldots, s_N] \in R^{J \times N}$ denotes the common sparse representations of B_s and B_t, which satisfies the sparsity constraint $\|s_i\|_0 \leq T_0$. The terms $\|B_s - D_s S\|_2^2$ and $\|B_t - D_t S\|_2^2$ are the reconstruction errors of source and target views, respectively.

Furthermore, by constructing $B = \left[B_s^T \ B_t^T\right]^T$, $D = \left[D_s^T \ D_t^T\right]^T$, we formulate Eq. (9) equivalently as

$$\arg\min_{D,S} \{\|B - DS\|_2^2\}, \quad s.t. \ \forall i, \|s_i\|_0 \leq T_0 \tag{10}$$

The K-SVD algorithm can be used to solve Eq. (10) [2].

When the transferable pairwise dictionary $\{D_s, D_t\}$ is obtained, we calculate the sparse representations of all segments (from either shared actions or orphan actions) in source and target views by solving Eqs. (11) and (12), respectively,

$$S_s = \arg\min_{S_s} \{\|B_s^* - D_s S_s\|_2^2\}, \quad s.t. \ \forall i, \|s_{si}\|_0 \leq T_0 \tag{11}$$

$$S_t = \arg\min_{S_t} \{\|B_t^* - D_t S_t\|_2^2\}, \quad s.t. \ \forall i, \|s_{ti}\|_0 \leq T_0 \tag{12}$$

where M denotes the number of all segments both in the source and target views, $S_s = [s_{s1}, s_{s2}, \ldots, s_{sM}] \in R^{J \times M}$ and $S_t = [s_{t1}, s_{t2}, \ldots, s_{tM}] \in R^{J \times M}$ refer to the sparse representations of all the M segments in source and target views, respectively. The matrices $B_s^*, B_t^* \in R^{K \times M}$ denote the K-dimension BoDCs of all the

M segments in source and target views, respectively. Both Eqs. (11) and (12) can be efficiently solved by orthogonal matching pursuit (OMP) algorithm [24].

In our hierarchical transfer framework, what we obtain ultimately are the sparse representations at the atom-level of the action videos, which guarantees that the information of all the segments as well as the temporal relationship therein can be preserved. As a result, the invariance across different views are fully utilized during the transfer procedure, which contributes to the feature-to-feature correspondence at atom-level through our framework.

4 Experiments

4.1 Dataset and Experimental Setup

We use the multi-view dataset IXMAS [25] in our experiment. This dataset contains eleven action categories, each of which is observed by five different cameras, and is performed by twelve people for three times. We denote the five different camera views of this dataset as $C1, C2, \ldots, C5$ respectively.

We extract spatial-temporal interest-point-based features [5] to describe actions in each viewpoint. The protocol for calculating these features is the same as in [34] and [20]. Specifically, while constructing the codebook, the size of our Dual-Codebook is chosen from 50, 100, 250, and 500.

In our experiments, we observed that the 3-level temporal-structure model obtained relatively better results than other choices. Hence, we set our action temporal-structure model to 3-levels, and the action videos at these three levels have one, two, and four segments respectively.

The selection strategies of the parameters in our method are as follows. At each level of the hierarchical transfer framework, the number of dictionary atoms is set to be the same as that of training samples. The sparsity constraint T_0 is set to 36, since each action class has 36 samples in the IXMAS dataset, and we assume that each sample can be well represented by other samples of the same class. Moreover, α is empirically fixed to be 1 according to the experiments.

In order to have a fair comparison to [34] and [20], we follow their leave-one-action-class-out scheme, where each time we only consider one action category for testing (i.e., as an orphan action). Accordingly, we utilize all other action categories to learn the Dual-Codebook and the transferable pairwise dictionary at each level of our transfer framework.

In the classification phase, we take all action videos in the source view as training samples, and use the nearest-neighbor classifier to recognize the target-view video of the orphan action.

4.2 Experimental Results

Firstly, we conduct two controlled experiments to verify the effectiveness of the proposed framework. In the first experiment, we implement codebooks separately trained with k-means in the two views instead of Dual-Codebook, followed by the

Table 1. The results of controlled experiments. Column A, B and "Ours" are the results of "k-means codebooks + hierarchical transfer framework", "Dual-Codebook + video-level transfer", and our method, respectively.

%	target view														
	C1			C2			C3			C4			C5		
	A	B	Ours	A	B	Ours	A	B	Ours	A	B	Ours	A	B	Ours
C1				89.9	74.0	**99.0**	92.2	77.3	**99.2**	86.1	69.7	**98.2**	91.2	76.0	**98.7**
C2	89.6	67.4	**99.2**				92.7	66.4	**98.7**	87.6	68.4	**98.7**	91.2	77.0	**99.7**
C3	91.2	78.5	**98.7**	88.6	73.7	**97.7**				92.7	74.7	**98.7**	93.4	82.6	**99.0**
C4	86.6	76.0	**99.0**	87.4	70.5	**96.7**	92.4	80.1	**99.2**				91.2	74.0	**99.2**
C5	88.4	79.8	**99.5**	88.6	78.0	**98.5**	94.7	87.9	**99.0**	88.9	77.8	**98.0**			
Ave.	89.0	75.4	**99.1**	88.6	74.1	**98.0**	93.0	77.9	**99.0**	88.8	72.7	**98.4**	91.8	77.4	**99.2**

proposed hierarchical transfer framework, to verify the effectiveness of the proposed Dual-Codebook. In the second experiment, the Dual-Codebook is implemented, but action videos are not segmented, i.e., only video-level transfer is performed. The results are listed in Table 1.

Comparing Column A to "Ours", we can see that our method performs better in all twenty pairwise view combinations. The average accuracy of our method is about 8.5 % higher than that using separate k-means codebooks instead. This indicates that our Dual-Codebook is a better foundation than separate k-means codebooks for transferring actions models across pairwise views. Moreover, comparing Column B to "Ours", we can also see that our method performs better in all twenty pairwise view combinations. The average accuracy of our method is about 23.2 % higher than that not splitting the action videos at all. This indicates that the atom-level transfer in our hierarchical framework is more discriminative than the usual video-level transfer in most existing work.

Additionally, in Table 2, we compare our method to three state-of-the-art approaches for all twenty pairwise view combinations on the IXMAS dataset. The size of Dual-Codebook is set to 500. As can be observed, our method has obtained recognition rates of higher than 98 % in eighteen pairwise view combinations. Compared to the results of [20] and [34], our method performs better in all twenty pairwise view combinations. Compared to [33], the proposed method obtained higher recognition rates in fifteen pairwise view combinations. The reason is that, the proposed Dual-Codebook contains codebook-to-codebook correspondence across two views, while codebooks separately trained in each view cannot guarantee the same level of correspondence. Moreover, the atom-level transfer strategy in the hierarchical framework is more discriminative than the video-level transfer in [33].

In Table 2, the recognition rates of [20] and [34] dropped dramatically when camera 5 was the source or target view. The reason might be that camera 5 is set above the actors. The action observations obtained in this camera is dramatically different from those in other cameras, which is very challenging. It is interesting

Table 2. Performance comparison between our method and state-of-the-art approaches.

%	target view																			
	C1				C2				C3				C4				C5			
	[33]	[20]	[34]	Ours	[33]	[20]	[34]	Ours	[33]	[20]	[34]	Ours	[33]	[20]	[34]	Ours	[33]	[20]	[34]	Ours
C1					**99.1**	79.9	96.7	99.0	90.9	76.8	97.9	**99.2**	88.7	76.8	97.6	**98.2**	95.5	74.8	84.9	**98.7**
C2	97.8	81.2	97.3	**99.2**					91.2	75.8	96.4	**98.7**	78.4	78.0	89.7	**98.7**	88.4	70.4	81.2	**99.7**
C3	**99.4**	79.6	92.1	98.7	97.6	76.6	89.7	**97.7**					91.2	79.8	94.9	**98.7**	**100.0**	72.8	89.1	99.0
C4	87.6	73.0	97.0	**99.0**	**98.2**	74.1	94.2	96.7	**99.4**	74.4	96.7	99.2					95.4	66.9	83.9	**99.2**
C5	87.3	82.0	83.0	**99.5**	87.8	68.3	70.6	**98.5**	92.1	74.0	89.7	**99.0**	90.0	71.1	83.7	**98.0**				
Ave.	93.0	79.0	92.4	**99.1**	95.6	74.7	87.8	**98.0**	93.4	75.2	95.1	**99.0**	87.1	76.4	91.2	**98.4**	95.1	71.2	84.8	**99.2**

to note that the proposed method obtained high accuracies under camera 5. We consider the reason is that, the key of our method is fully utilizing the information of the categories and sequential composition of the atom actions within an action during transfer, and this information is invariant to the viewpoint.

The average recognition accuracies of each action category for different target views are demonstrated in Fig. 2 (the size of Dual-Codebook is 500). We can see that the action "get-up" gains 100 % recognition accuracies in all five target views. Besides, the action "kick" and "punch" achieve 100 % recognition accuracies in four target views, although they tend to be mistaken for each other in some viewpoints. The recognition accuracies of the action "pick up" are relatively low compared to other actions, but still higher than 85 %. We find that it is often mistaken for the action "sit-down". The possible reason is that, the observations of these two actions are extremely similar while seen in most of the viewpoints, since they contain the similar atom-action sequences "stand-stoop-squat" and "stand-stoop-sit". And our hierarchical transfer framework relies on

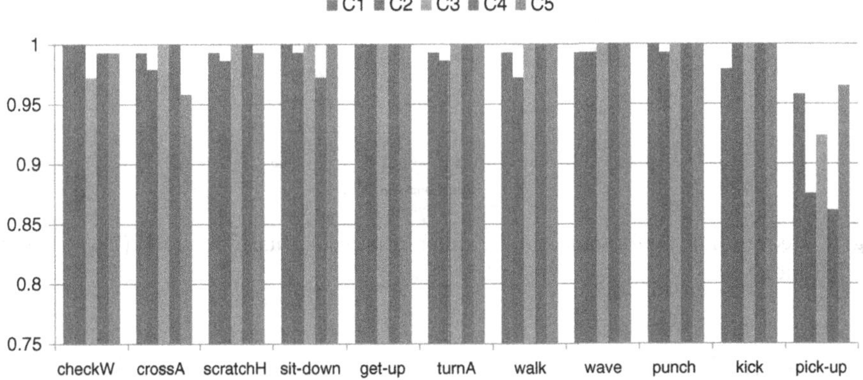

Fig. 2. The recognition accuracy of each action category in different target views (best viewed in PDF file).

the categories and sequential composition of atom actions, so it confuses "pick up" with "sit-down" in some cases.

We also conduct experiments studying recognition performance under Dual-Codebooks of different sizes. As shown in Fig. 3, in all source views, the recognition rates of our method increase quickly with the size of Dual-Codebook when the size is under 250. When the codebook size is greater than 250, the recognition rate curves tend to be flat. This indicates that, a larger Dual-Codebook generally contains more accurate codebook-to-codebook correspondence across two views and more discriminative information.

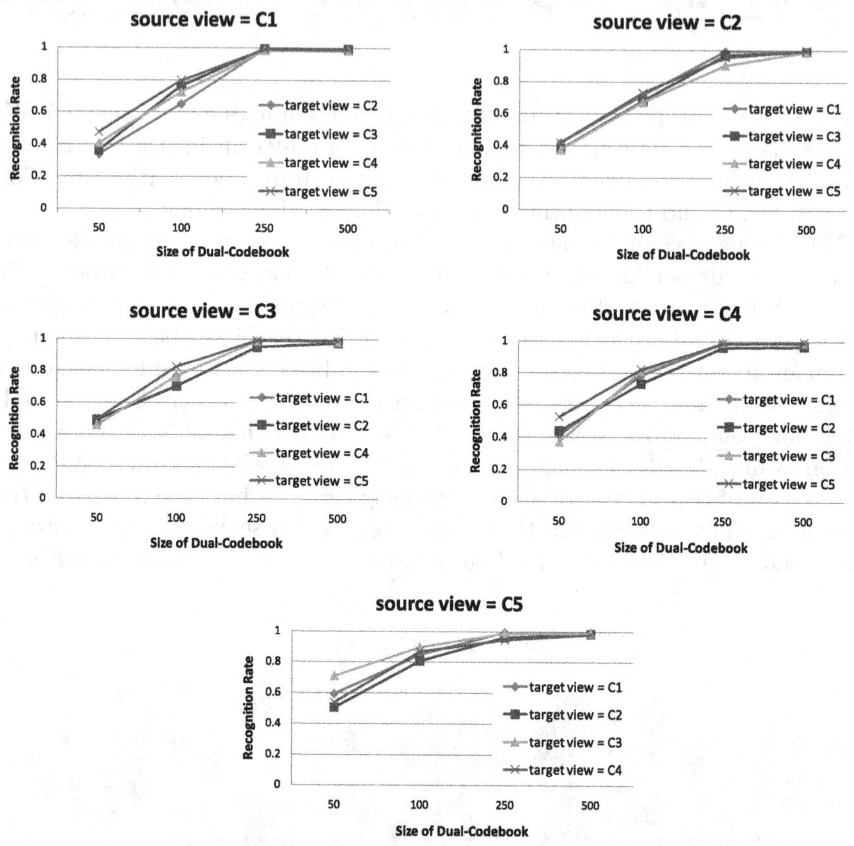

Fig. 3. Recognition performance under different size of Dual-Codebook (best viewed in PDF file).

5 Conclusion

In this paper, we explore the challenging cross-view action recognition problem. For this purpose, we firstly propose a Dual-Codebook that achieves codebook-to-codebook correspondence across different views. With the Dual-Codebook, each action can be represented based on Bag-of-Dual-Codes (BoDC). We further introduce a hierarchical transfer framework, which performs atom-level transfer on multiple timescales. This framework guarantees that each pair of corresponding video segments from pairwise views obtain similar sparse representations, and achieves feature-to-feature correspondence at atom-level. This contributes to a more accurate transfer relationship than the simple video-level transfer. At last, we conduct a series of experiments on the IXMAS dataset. The experimental results demonstrate that our method can achieve superior performance over state-of-the-art approaches.

Acknowledgement. This work is supported by National Natural Science Foundation of China (No. 61172141), Key Projects in the National Science & Technology Pillar Program during the 12th Five-Year Plan Period (No. 2012BAK16B06), and Science and Technology Program of Guangzhou, China (2014J4100092).

References

1. Aggarwal, J., Ryoo, M.: Human activity analysis: a review. ACM Comput. Surv. **43**, 1–43 (2011)
2. Aharon, M., Elad, M., Bruckstein, A.: K-SVD: an algorithm for designing overcomplete dictionaries for sparse representation. TSP **54**, 4311–4322 (2006)
3. Cheung, G., Baker, S., Kanade, T.: Shape-from-silhouette of articulated objects and its use for human body kinematics estimation and motion capture. In: CVPR (2003)
4. Ding, C., Li, T.: Convex and semi-nonnegative matrix factorizations. PAMI **32**, 45–55 (2010)
5. Dollar, P., Rabaud, V., Cottrell, G., Belongie, S.: Behavior recognition via sparse spatio-temporal features. In: VS-PETS (2005)
6. Efros, A., Berg, A., Mori, G., Malik, J.: Recognizing action at a distance. In: ICCV (2003)
7. Farhadi, A., Tabrizi, M.K.: Learning to recognize activities from the wrong view point. In: Forsyth, D., Torr, P., Zisserman, A. (eds.) ECCV 2008, Part I. LNCS, vol. 5302, pp. 154–166. Springer, Heidelberg (2008)
8. Farhadi, A., Tabrizi, M., Endres, I., Forsyth, D.: A latent model of discriminative aspect. In: ICCV (2009)
9. Gavrila, D., Davis, L.S.: 3D model-based tracking of humans in action: a multi-view approach. In: CVPR (1996)
10. Holte, M.B., Moeslund, T.B., Tran, C., Trivedi, M.: Human action recognition using multiple views: a comparative perspective on recent developments. In: HGBU (2011)
11. Ji, X., Liu, H.: Advances in view-invariant human motion analysis: a review. TCSVT **40**, 13–24 (2010)
12. Junejo, I., Dexter, E., Laptev, I., Patrick, P.: View-independent action recognition from temporal self-similarities. PAMI **33**, 172–185 (2011)
13. Junejo, I.N., Dexter, E., Laptev, I., Pérez, P.: Cross-view action recognition from temporal self-similarities. In: Forsyth, D., Torr, P., Zisserman, A. (eds.) ECCV 2008, Part II. LNCS, vol. 5303, pp. 293–306. Springer, Heidelberg (2008)
14. Laptev, I., Lindeberg, T.: Space-time interest points. In: ICCV (2003)

15. Lee, D., Seung, H.: Algorithms for non-negative matrix factorization. In: Advances in Neural Information Processing Systems, vol. 13. MIT Press, Cambridge (2001)
16. Li, R., Zickler, T.: Discriminative virtual views for cross-view action recognition. In: CVPR (2012)
17. Lin, Z., Jiang, Z., Davis, L.: Recognizing actions by shape-motion prototype trees. In: ICCV (2009)
18. Liu, J., Ali, S., Shah, M.: Recognizing human actions using multiple features. In: CVPR (2008)
19. Liu, J., Shah, M.: Learning human actions via information maximization. In: CVPR (2008)
20. Liu, J., Shah, M., Kuipers, B., Savarese, S.: Cross-view action recognition via view knowledge transfer. In: CVPR (2011)
21. Lv, F., Nevatia, R.: Single view human action recognition using key pose matching and viterbi path searching. In: CVPR (2007)
22. Paramesmaran, V., Chellappa, R.: View invariance for human action recognition. IJCV **66**, 83–101 (2006)
23. Rao, C., Yilmaz, A., Shah, M.: View-invariant representation and recognition of actions. IJCV **50**, 203–226 (2002)
24. Tropp, J., Gilbert, A.: Signal recovery from random measurements via orthogonal matching pursuit. TIT **53**, 4655–4666 (2007)
25. Turaga, P., Chellappa, R., Subrahmanian, V., Udrea, O.: Machine recognition of human activities: a survey. TCSVT **18**, 1473–1488 (2008)
26. Valera, M., Velastin, S.: Intelligent distributed surveillance systems: a review. VISP **152**, 192–204 (2005)
27. Weinland, D., Boyer, E., Ronfard, R.: Action recognition from arbitrary views using 3D examplars. In: ICCV (2007)
28. Weinland, D., Ozuysal, M., Fua, P.: Making action recognition robust to occlusions and viewpoint changes. In: ECCV (2010)
29. Wright, J., Yang, A., Ganesh, A., Sastry, S., Ma, Y.: Robust face recognition via sparse representation. PAMI **31**, 210–227 (2009)
30. Yan, P., Khan, S.M., Shah, M.: Learning 4D action feature models for arbitrary view action recognition. In: CVPR (2008)
31. Yilmaz, A., Shah, M.: Actions sketch: a novel action representation. In: CVPR (2005)
32. Zhang, Z., Wang, Y., Zhang, Z.: Face synthesis from near-infrared to visual light via sparse representation. In: IJCB (2011)
33. Zheng, J., Jiang, Z.: Learning view-invariant sparse representations for cross-view action recognition. In: ICCV (2013)
34. Zheng, J., Jiang, Z., Phillips, P., Chellappa, R.: Cross-view action recognition via a transferable dictionary pair. In: BMVC (2012)

Stereo, Physics, Video and Events

Stereo Ground Truth with Error Bars

Daniel Kondermann[1], Rahul Nair[1(✉)], Stephan Meister[1], Wolfgang Mischler[1], Burkhard Güssefeld[1], Katrin Honauer[1], Sabine Hofmann[2], Claus Brenner[2], and Bernd Jähne[1]

[1] Heidelberg Collaboratory for Image Processing at IWR, Ruprecht-Karls-Universität Heidelberg, Heidelberg, Germany
{daniel.kondermann,rahul.nair,stephan.meister,wolfgang.mischler, burkhard.gussefeld,katrin.honauer,bernd.jahne}@iwr.uni-heidelberg.de

[2] Institute of Cartography and Geoinformatics, Leibniz Universität Hannover, Hanover, Germany
{sabine.hofmann,claus.brenner}@ikg.uni-hannover.de

Abstract. Creating stereo ground truth based on real images is a measurement task. Measurements are never perfectly accurate: the depth at each pixel follows an error distribution. A common way to estimate the quality of measurements are error bars. In this paper we describe a methodology to add error bars to images of previously scanned static scenes. The main challenge for stereo ground truth error estimates based on such data is the nonlinear matching of 2D images to 3D points. Our method uses 2D feature quality, 3D point and calibration accuracy as well as covariance matrices of bundle adjustments. We sample the *reference data error* which is the 3D depth distribution of each point projected into 3D image space. The *disparity distribution* at each pixel location is then estimated by projecting samples of the reference data error on the 2D image plane. An analytical Gaussian error propagation is used to validate the results. As proof of concept, we created ground truth of an image sequence with 100 frames. Results show that disparity accuracies well below one pixel can be achieved, albeit with much large errors at depth discontinuities mainly caused by uncertain estimates of the camera location.

1 Introduction

Reference data is needed when quantitative performance evaluations are a requirement; this is for example the case for safety-relevant applications such as driver assistance systems. Whenever real data needs to be augmented with ground truth, measurement devices such as 3D scanners are used. These devices come with their own limits of accuracy. 3D scanners are for example limited in accuracy at objects with low reflectance, glossy surfaces or high geometric detail. Therefore, ground truth is never perfect - we need to understand the limits of the measurement devices in order to judge the quality of a ground truth dataset.

Electronic supplementary material The online version of this chapter (doi:10. 1007/978-3-319-16814-2_39) contains supplementary material, which is available to authorized users.

D. Cremers et al. (Eds.): ACCV 2014, Part V, LNCS 9007, pp. 595–610, 2015.
DOI: 10.1007/978-3-319-16814-2_39

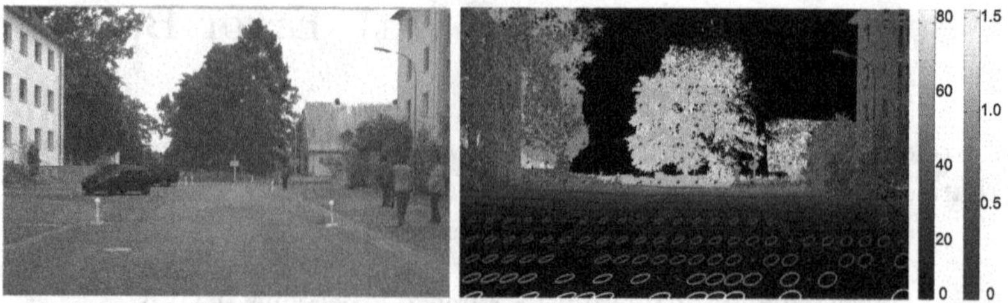

Fig. 1. Ground truth needs error bars. Left: left stereo image with overlay of dynamic objects. Right: ground truth disparities with sparse overlay of 3σ uncertainty ellipses. The disparity error is encoded in the color of the ellipse. Since the measured reference data is always subject to measurement errors the resulting ground truth dataset can contain uncertainties (Color figure online).

As a rule of thumb, a measurement device should be one order of magnitude more accurate than the required accuracy for the system to be evaluated. Many current stereo benchmarks analyze the number of pixels with a disparity error of one or more pixels [1]. Hence, to create stereo ground truth, the disparity map coming with the camera images should be around a tenth of a pixel accurate. The 3D data acquired by a scanner needs to be analyzed in pixel disparity space, resulting in mainly two errors: first, a depth-dependent error is introduced by the 3D-to-2D projection. This error becomes smaller with distance in case the scanner has a constant accuracy with respect to spatial coordinates. Second, a matching-dependent error occurs caused by bad alignment of the 2D image with the 3D scene. This results in very large, mostly bimodal error distribution near depth discontinuities. Both error sources cause highly different errors at individual pixel locations, rendering a general approximate error estimate for the full dataset relatively meaningless.

For this paper, we set up a high-end camera stereo system and reconstructed a large outdoor set using the best LIDAR system available for this task. Our aim is to focus on accuracy: how accurate can our real-world ground truth become at individual pixels when all involved systems are state of the art? To this end, we devised a method to estimate the accuracy of our ground truth at the pixel level. This paper does not propose a new dataset. Instead, we propose *a method* to create arbitrary stereo ground truth datasets with reliable per-pixel error bars (cf. Fig. 1). Although our approach generalizes to arbitrary 3D scanners and camera setups in static scenes, we focus on large-scale outdoor scenes (>30.000 m^2) which can to date only be acquired by LIDAR systems.

Our approach is illustrated in Fig. 2 and is divided into the following steps: The static scene is scanned first and then a calibrated stereo sequence is recorded within this scene. The camera location for each frame is locally estimated based on manually selected 2D-3D-correspondences. All cameras and correspondences are inserted into a bundle adjustment model considering all error sources appropriately based on Gaussian errors in 2D feature localization, LIDAR accuracy and camera calibration parameters. Finally, the covariance of the functional

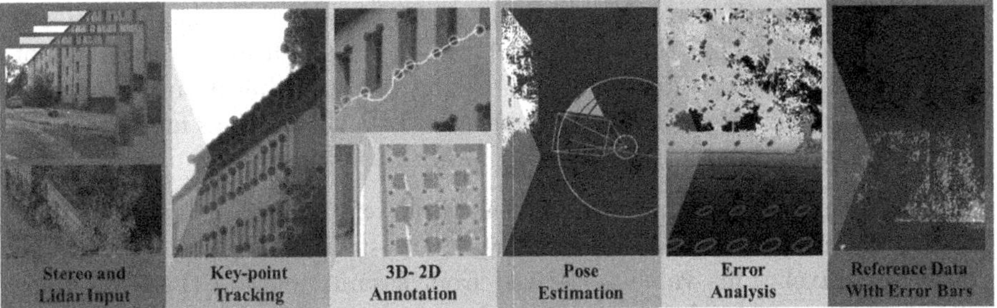

Fig. 2. Workflow stages: Starting with a LIDAR scan and an image sequence we compute 2D feature tracks. These are matched manually with landmark 3D points using manual annotations (Sect. 3.1). Using these annotations and the other 2D feature tracks we estimate the pose of each frame (Sect. 3.1). By means of covariance analysis and uncertainty propagation we then obtain uncertainties in the localization of reprojected 3D point cloud (Sect. 4). We then combine these localization uncertainties with the reprojections to finally output reference disparity maps and per pixel disparity distributions (Sect. 5).

is evaluated at the solution to assess the uncertainty in the derived camera extrinsics. The resulting error distributions of the inputs (LIDAR, image data, intrinsics) and derived inputs (extrinsics) are mapped into image space and, subsequently, into disparity space using both analytic error propagation and Monte Carlo sampling. As a result, our method comprises a full error propagation, starting with Gaussian error assumptions of the involved measurement devices and ending at per-pixel non-parametric disparity distributions.

2 Related Work

Generation Techniques: Ground truth generation implies two parts: an evaluation dataset and a reference dataset with superior accuracy. Different techniques differ in the way these datasets are obtained [2].

Synthetic imagery [3–5] allows for generation of reference data with little uncertainty and makes white box testing of algorithms feasible by varying parameters such as geometry, light and materials. Yet, it remains to be shown whether content and renderer model reality well enough [6,7].

Another option is to record real data and use *manual annotations*. While relatively new to low-level vision, efforts have been undertaken with some success [8]. With the advent of crowd-sourcing platforms [9], generation of such data has also become scalable. While the accuracy is reported to be good in general, possible biases introduced by humans are yet to be investigated.

Finally, reference data can also be obtained by *measurement* e.g. by using more than two cameras [10], additional devices such as the Kinect [11] a LIDAR scanner [12] or by using multiple exposures and UV-paint as in [1]. The approach of using more data sources is not as costly and sometimes scales very well because existing vision algorithms only need to be slightly modified. It should be noted however that in any case the reference data is itself obtained by measurement and therefore subject to uncertainty. Assessing this uncertainty in our opinion is of utmost importance as statements such as "LIDAR is always more accurate than stereo" do not hold in general [13].

Stereo Datasets[1]**:** General-purpose real-world reference data has been published in the Middlebury database [1] with an estimated accuracy of around 1/60th of a pixel. This value is derived from assumptions on the used block matching scheme and a down-sampling of originally larger images.

The EISATS database comprises a variety of sequences both real and synthetic [10,14]. Using a third camera in the real dataset for additional redundancy proved to be beneficial for achieving an improved quality, but the accuracy of this data has not been thoroughly evaluated.

The closest approach to ours in terms of experimental setup is the KITTI dataset [12]: here, a stereo setup was combined with a car-mounted laser scanner. Mounting a LIDAR on the car has two main advantages. The scene can be recorded both in 2D and 3D at the same time and the density of 3D measurements is maximized as the LIDAR is very close to the optical axis of the stereo cameras. A disadvantage is that the system is moving while scanning, introducing a possibly low point density at high speed as well as motion artifacts. Although the accuracy was not explicitly evaluated in the original publication, it is reported by the authors to be less than three disparities for most of the pixels.

In our approach, the scene is scanned first and recorded later. Hence, motion artifacts cannot occur and the sampling is spatially roughly uniform. In both KITTI and our setup LIDAR was chosen as the most accurate and viable option to obtain depth in large scenes. Note, however, that our approach can be applied to any measurement technique with known uncertainty. Also all the main focus of all these databases is the creation of the ground truth database and the evaluation of algorithms. We focus on neither of both: Our aim is to exemplify error bar computation for real-world stereo ground truth using an appropriate statistical model.

Finally, the work most similar to ours in terms of scope is [13]. Here uncertainties in camera intrinsics/extrinsics, LIDAR measurements and image key-point estimation are propagated to obtain reconstruction uncertainties for multiple view stereo. While the authors make extensive use of sampling to estimate uncertainty we provide an analytical solution for both camera pose estimation and the uncertainty of the disparity maps. This makes handling large numbers of frames (more than 1000 vs 25 in [13]) tractable in the first place. While comparing a re-implemented version of their method with the proposed method we not only see a considerable speed up, even for small problems - we also observe tighter bounds on the camera pose uncertainty (cf. Sect. 3.2).

[1] Although most of the following works comprise additional datasets next to stereo data, we only focus on the latter.

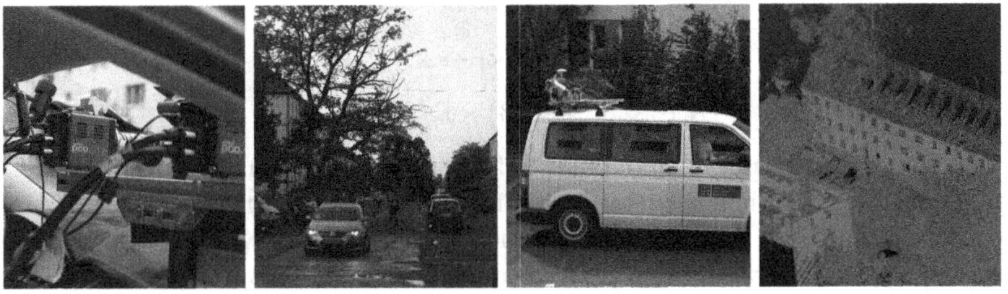

Fig. 3. From left to right: stereo rig, set photo, LIDAR mounted on car and resulting data.

Uncertainty Estimation for Bundle Adjustment: A rich body of work exists on the theory of uncertainty estimation in the related field of bundle adjustment [15–18]. Most techniques use local features of the bundle adjustment energy in the optimum e.g. covariance analysis. A lot of effort is then put into tackling the inherent gauge ambiguity issue of the structure from motion problem. While we do use a bundle adjustment variant for estimating the camera parameters we circumvent the gauge ambiguity issue by fixing the gauge to the LIDAR reference frame. Also, it should be noted that our final goal is not the reconstruction of the camera parameters but rather stereo disparity maps with a per pixel uncertainty. To assess the quality of our camera reconstructions we build on work in [19].

3 Ground Truth Acquisition

The acquisition modalities are depicted in Fig. 3. A reference 3D point cloud of a street of houses was collected using a RIEGL VMX-250-CS6. The stereo system consists of two cameras with a 30 cm baseline with 12 mm lenses With a sensor size of 16.64 mm × 14.04 mm, this corresponds to a field of view of 69.5°. The image sequences were acquired at 200 Hz with a resolution of 2560 × 1080 pixels. Preprocessing steps of the stereo data involved a lossless compression [20] of the 16 bit pixel data to 8 bits as well as camera calibration using [21]. Further details of the acquisition system can be found in the supplemental material.

3.1 2D-3D Alignment

All measurement based reference data acquisition systems rely on a 2D-3D alignment step at some point of the processing pipeline. To build on this step for both explaining our alignment process as well as on how we derive error bars, we will now review the basic pose estimation and calibration process.

With K we refer to the set of possible internal camera parameters and with $\mathbf{so}(3)$ the group of rotations. For a distortion free perspective camera with 4 parameters[2] $K = \mathbb{R}^4$. Let

$$\pi : (\mathbf{X}, \mathbf{t}, \kappa) \rightarrow \mathbf{x}, \tag{1}$$

$$\mathbf{X} \in \mathbb{R}^3, \mathbf{t} \in \mathbf{so}(3) \times \mathbb{R}^3, \kappa \in K, \tag{2}$$

be the projective mapping of point $\mathbf{X}$ from the world to image coordinate system using the extrinsic parameters $\mathbf{t}$ and intrinsics κ. Furthermore, let $\{(\mathbf{X_i}, \mathbf{x_i^j})\}$ be a set of 3D-2D correspondences of p measured 3D points $\mathbf{X_i}$ and their projections $\mathbf{x_i^j}$ in the jth frame of an image sequence containing n images. Then, the optimal intrinsic parameter κ^* and set of extrinsics $T^* = \{\mathbf{t^j}^*\}$ for each of the n frames is given by

$$(T^*, \kappa^*) = \underset{T,\kappa}{\operatorname{argmin}} \sum_{j=0}^{n} \sum_{i \in V(j)} \left\| \pi\left(\mathbf{X_i}, \mathbf{t^j}, \kappa\right) - \mathbf{x_i^j} \right\|^2, \tag{3}$$

where $V(j) \subset [0...p]$ is the subset of 3D points that are visible in the jth frame. For a fixed camera - LIDAR setup such as KITTI this is done once in a calibration step with calibration targets before acquisition. Both geometry and projection of salient points are known here such that P can be obtained automatically. In our case the LIDAR and the camera rig measure independently. This has the advantage of having LIDAR data at a much higher point density and allows for capturing image sequences from other camera modalities (e.g. Time-of-Flight, Plenoptic cameras) without requiring all cameras to be mounted on the same rig. In this setup, however, 2D-3D correspondences cannot be automatically aligned anymore. Picking individual points out of eight million options is an extremely tedious and error-prone task. We propose an annotation and processing pipeline minimizing the risk of false correspondences (cf. Fig. 2).

2D-3D Correspondence Estimation/Annotation: 2D feature tracks ($\mathbf{x_i^j}$) were automatically obtained with Voodoo Tracker[3] using the Harris Corner detector and a cross correlation based feature tracking.[4] A subset of the tracks was matched manually with 3D points. This is difficult since each point in the 2D projection of the cloud corresponds to many 3D points at different depths. One solution would be to automatically mesh the point clouds, but it turns out that current approaches do not work well enough on our kind of data and also modify the location of the points in a non-linear way introducing unknown biases to the measurements. To ease point picking, we reduced the 3D point cloud to a 2D representation in two steps:

Map Annotation: We manually select landmark 3D points which were also always found by the 2D feature tracker. These points are visualized in a "fold-out" map of the measurement perimeter. Correspondences are established by connecting map landmarks with 2D features in the images.

[2] Horizontal vertical focal lengths (f_x, f_y), principle point (c_x, c_y).
[3] http://www.digilab.uni-hannover.de/docs/manual.html.
[4] Cross correlation window: 21×21. Search neighborhood 21×21.

Range Annotation: Using an initial pose estimate computed from these correspondences, a range image with LIDAR reflectance information was created, containing at most one point per pixel from which additional correspondences can be chosen[5].

Camera Estimation with Known Variances: Neither the feature tracks nor the 3D points or internal camera parameters are perfect. Also the intrinsic calibration routine usually delivers a good initial guess $\hat{\kappa}$ for the intrinsics. We assume Gaussian errors in each of these values:

$$\mathbf{X}_\mathrm{i} = \mathbf{Z}_\mathrm{i} + \epsilon_{\mathbf{X}_\mathrm{i}}, \epsilon_{\mathbf{X}_\mathrm{i}} \sim \mathcal{N}_3(0, \Sigma_{\mathbf{X}_\mathrm{i}}) \tag{4}$$

$$\hat{\kappa} = \kappa + \epsilon_\kappa, \epsilon_\kappa \sim \mathcal{N}_4(0, \Sigma_\kappa) \tag{5}$$

$$\mathbf{x}_\mathrm{i}^\mathrm{j} = \mathbf{z}_\mathrm{i}^\mathrm{j} + \epsilon_{\mathbf{z}_\mathrm{i}^\mathrm{j}}, \epsilon_{\mathbf{x}_\mathrm{i}^\mathrm{j}} \sim \mathcal{N}_2(0, \Sigma_{\mathbf{x}_\mathrm{i}^\mathrm{j}}) \tag{6}$$

To accommodate for these errors we modify Eq. 3:

$$(\{\mathbf{Z}_\mathrm{i}\}^*, T^*, \kappa^*) = \underset{(\{\mathbf{Z}_\mathrm{i}\}, T, \kappa)}{\operatorname{argmin}} \; \Phi(\{\mathbf{Z}_\mathrm{i}\}, T, \kappa), \tag{7}$$

with

$$\Phi(\{\mathbf{Z}_\mathrm{i}\}, T, \kappa) = \sum_{j=0}^{n} \sum_{i \in V(j)} \Bigg(\left\| \pi\left(\mathbf{Z}_\mathrm{i}, \mathbf{t}^\mathrm{j}, \kappa\right) - \mathbf{x}_\mathrm{i}^\mathrm{j} \right\|_{\Sigma_{\mathbf{x}_\mathrm{i}^\mathrm{j}}}^2 + \left\| \mathbf{X}_\mathrm{i} - \mathbf{Z}_\mathrm{i} \right\|_{\Sigma_{\mathbf{X}_\mathrm{i}}}^2 + \left\| \hat{\kappa} - \kappa \right\|_{\Sigma_\kappa}^2 \Bigg). \tag{8}$$

$\|.\|_\Sigma^2$ denotes the squared Mahalanobis distance. Note the quadratic penalty terms in Eq. 8 and explicit usage of latent variables $\mathbf{Z}_\mathrm{i}$ and κ. These are required as the first residual term is not linear in $\mathbf{X}_\mathrm{i}$ and $\hat{\kappa}$ whereas it is in $\mathbf{x}_\mathrm{i}^\mathrm{j}$. This splitting of variables is often used to be able to better treat nonlinearities in Gaussian energy functionals [22,23]. Also, note that the first term corresponds to a bundle adjustment problem and the last two terms to priors on $\mathbf{X}_\mathrm{i}$ and $\mathbf{x}_\mathrm{i}^\mathrm{j}$. In the optimization, it is therefore possible to include 2D feature tracks without 3D correspondences. Parameter estimation was done using the open source Ceres Solver [24] library.

3.2 Consistency and Precision of the Pose Estimation with Synthetic Data

To assess the precision and consistency of our pose estimation system we borrow ideas from [19]. Here, a method is proposed to compute consistency and precision of a dataset with respect to a reference dataset with lower but nonzero uncertainty. As the output of our system has the highest available precision we have to resort to synthetic data and make some changes to the formulas in [19] to cater to the zero uncertainty of our reference.

[5] Screenshots and usage videos of the tools can be found in the supplemental material.

Consistency is a measure for the likelihood that both reference and synthetic datasets have the same parameters. As in [19] we report the Mahalanobis distance between the synthetic reference and the methods using the estimated pose covariance.

Precision refers to the certainty of the method of the correctness of its parameter estimate. Given two parameter estimates with a similar consistency with regard to the reference, the estimate with the smaller uncertainty should be favoured. Here, we report the trace of the estimated covariances.

Table 1 summarizes the results. The reference data was generated by randomly picking p key points in the first frame, randomly choosing a depth for each key point between 5 and 70 m and finally, by rejecting 3D points not visible in the $n-1$ other camera frames. The evaluation dataset was obtained by adding Gaussian noise according to the *noise* column on key point position and 3D point. We compare our method to a sampling based strategy similar to [13] where the 2D and 3D points are perturbed around the estimated solution (s times), the best new parameter set obtained by minimizing the bundle adjustment functional (keeping 2D and 3D measurements fixed) and estimating the sample mean and covariance. In the result columns, we report mean consistency, precision and run times in seconds after 30 runs. The standard deviation for consistency was always around 1, for precision and run time an order of magnitude smaller than the reported values. While we observe mostly similar consistency values between both methods - with the sampling consistency deteriorating with higher noise levels and larger datasets - our method produces a tighter precision bound on the parameter estimate with much faster run times. Further parameter sweeps can be found in the supplementary material.

4 Reference Data with Error Bars

Once the pose estimation in Eq. 8 has been solved we can proceed in creating reference data by computing a range image based on κ, T and the LIDAR point cloud by means of Eq. 1. This reference data contains holes with no information whenever no LIDAR measurements map to the corresponding pixel location. In the following we consider the extended reference data mapping

$$\tilde{\pi}_b : (\mathbf{X}, \mathbf{t}, \kappa) \rightarrow (\mathbf{x}, d) \tag{9}$$

Table 1. Pose estimation results on synthetic data. The tuples reported in the right 3 columns correspond to consistency, precision and run time. Lower values are better.

Noise [cm, px]	Number of points p	Number of frames n	Sampling s = 100	Sampling s = 1000	Ours
(5, 0.1)	100	5	(5.1, 3.9e-4, 0.4)	(5.1, 4.0e-4, 4.7)	(5.3, 1.1e-4, 0.1)
(5, 0.5)	100	10	(7.7, 1.7e-2, 0.8)	(7.6, 1.7e-2, 8.2)	(7.6, 5.5e-3, 0.2)
(1, 0.1)	1000	10	(8.1, 7.8e-5, 9.5)	(7.9, 7.9e-5, 96)	(8.5, 2.2e-5, 2.4)
(5, 0.5)	1000	10	(8.2, 1.8e-3, 9.5)	(8.0, 1.8e-3, 97)	(7.2, 5.2e-4, 2.1)

which not only computes the projected image location of a 3D point but also the disparity of this point given stereo baseline b. With $\mathbf{d} = (\mathbf{x}, d)$ we will denote the vector containing image coordinates and disparity. We omit the subscript b in the further discussion as it remains constant for each sequence.

The inputs in $\tilde{\pi}(\mathbf{X_i}, \mathbf{t^j}, \kappa)$ are either measurements or values derived from measurements. As measurements always contain errors the reference point $\tilde{\pi}(...)$ will also have an error. To assess theses errors quantitatively we need to first obtain error estimates for $\mathbf{X_i}, \mathbf{t^j}$ and κ.

1. For the **3D point position** $\mathbf{X_i}$ we assume that the components are independently distributed such that $\Sigma_{\mathbf{X_i}} = \sigma^2_{\mathbf{X_i}} I$. In our case this is the measurement error of the LIDAR scanner. For point clouds consisting of multiple LIDAR scans that were merged [12] via iterative closest points (ICP) or similar methods the error should be the error propagated from the ICP fit.
2. For the **camera pose** $\mathbf{t^j}^*$ we assume that $\mathbf{t^j} \sim \mathcal{N}_6(\mathbf{t^j}^*, \Sigma_{\mathbf{t^j}})$. As $\mathbf{t^j}$ is a value derived from a least squares fit, $\Sigma_{\mathbf{t^j}}$ can be obtained by evaluating the covariance matrix of Φ at the solution $s^* = \{\mathbf{t^j}, ..., \}$ with
$$COV_{\Phi}(s^*) = (J_{\Phi(s*)} J^T_{\Phi(s*)})^{-1}. \tag{10}$$
Here, $J_{\Phi(s*)}$ is the Jacobian of the residual vector of Φ evaluated at solution s^*. $\Sigma_{\mathbf{t^j}}$ is the diagonal block of $COV_{\Phi}(s^*)$ corresponding to the parameter block belonging to $\mathbf{t^j}$. Note that a regular bundle adjustment scenario has an inherent scale ambiguity which leads to $J_{\Phi(s*)}$ being rank deficient. In contrast, our functional has full rank as the scale is given by the 2D-3D correspondences. Also note that by supplying the correct error estimates during the alignment fit COV is properly scaled.
3. For the **camera intrinsics** κ we either use the same approach as chosen for $\mathbf{t^j}$ or use variances estimated by external calibration tools. Again the distribution is assumed to be Gaussian with $\kappa \sim \mathcal{N}_4(\kappa, \Sigma_\kappa)$.

The error distribution in $\tilde{\pi}$ of the reference point and the error in the disparity measure can be obtained via error propagation. This is achieved either via sampling input realizations from the above distributions or by analytical linear error propagation. For the latter, the full covariance matrix of the inputs evaluates to:

$$COV_{IN} = \begin{pmatrix} \Sigma_{\mathbf{X_i}} & & \\ & \Sigma_{\mathbf{t^j}} & \\ & & \Sigma_\kappa \end{pmatrix} \tag{11}$$

The error in $\tilde{\pi}$ is then obtained by linearizing $\tilde{\pi}$ at the reference point. Under assumption of a Gaussian distribution of the input variables the output is again Gaussian with covariance given by

$$COV_{\mathbf{d}} = J_{\tilde{\pi}(\mathbf{x},d))} COV_{IN} J^T_{\tilde{\pi}(\mathbf{x},d)}. \tag{12}$$

The choice between sampling and linear propagation depends on the available computational resources as sampling will deliver more accurate output error distributions given enough samples while linear error propagation is analytical and thus fast.

4.1 Reference Data Sensitivity

In the following we will give an analysis of our reference data using the tools provided above. We will first discuss the error values used for the inputs. The **LIDAR accuracy** is obtained from the data sheet as $\sigma_{\mathbf{X}_i} = 1\,\text{cm}$. We use this accuracy measure for the error propagation step. For the contribution of the 3D points towards pose uncertainty (cf. Eq. 10) we have to assume a larger error due to the point spacing. Therefore, the localization of a manually picked point (e.g. a window corner) is only accurate up to the mean distance between points. This was determined to be $\sigma'_{\mathbf{X}_i} = 3.5\,\text{cm}$ by estimating the point density on building facades where the landmark points were chosen from. The **feature track accuracy** was empirically estimated to be $\sigma_{xij} = 0.5\,\text{px}$, while errors in**focal length and principal point** were obtained from our calibration routine as $\sigma_{\mathcal{K}(f_x,f_y)} = 1.97\,\text{px}$ for the focal length and $\sigma_{\mathcal{K}(c_x,c_y)} = 1.46\,\text{px}$ for the principal point. For the **pose estimation accuracy**, we report the square root of the diagonal entries of $\Sigma_{\mathbf{t}j}$ obtained from covariance analysis to be $(r_x, r_y, r_z) = (3, 3, 2)\times 10^{-4}$ for the rotation and $(t_x, t_y, t_z) = (1.23, 2.53, 2.17)\,\text{cm}$ for the translation over 100 frames. The rotation is parametrized using a three dimensional angle-axis representation. The error has an upper bound[6] of 0.026°. For a LIDAR point at 50 m distance this corresponds to a localization error of around 2 cm. The error in the translation also amounts to 2 cm. Using the errors obtained from the input we can compute the uncertainty in the reference data by means of error propagation. For each reference point the full covariance in $\mathbf{d}$ (i.e. pixel localization and disparity error) was computed using both linear error propagation and sampling. In Fig. 4 the square roots of the diagonal entries are reported for an example scene. The first two rows correspond to the localization error and the third row is the disparity error in logarithmic scale. For both linear propagation and sampling we see the expected inverse distance reduction of all errors. While the disparity error for most parts is under a pixel the localization error exceeds five pixels for points closer than a few meters. Also noticeable is the rise in x localization error towards the image edges observable in all our sequences. We believe that this is related to a rotational error of the camera localization. Finally, we can see by comparing sampling and linear propagation that the sampling propagation in general gives a tighter bound on the reference data error while preserving the general shape. As both propagation methods yield similar results we conclude that linear error propagation can be used to obtain a quick though looser bound on the reference data error.

5 Disparity Maps with Error Bars

So far we discussed the reference data quality in terms of the localization and disparity error of each reference point. For evaluating a stereo algorithm we are faced with a slightly different question as we are concerned with the question

[6] Based on the maximum deviation of the angle-axis vector.

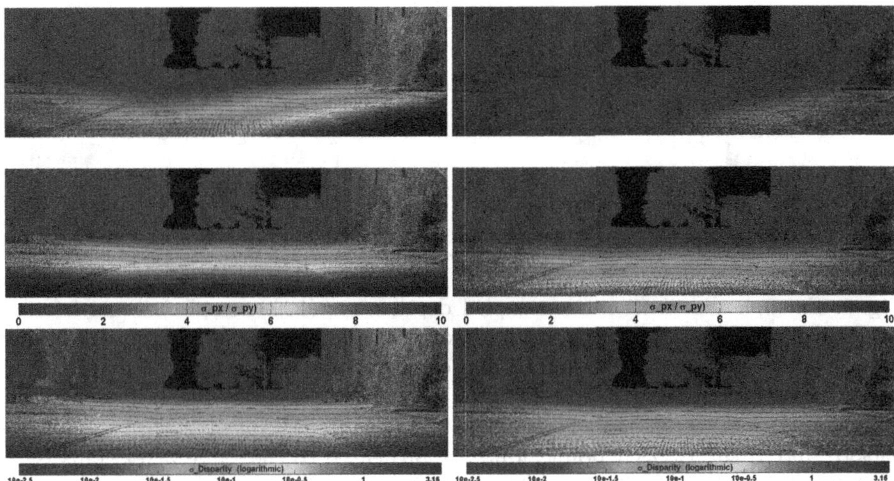

Fig. 4. Diagonal entries of uncertainty $\Sigma_{\mathbf{d}}$ obtained by **linear error propagation (left)** and **sampling (right)**. From top to bottom: localization error in x and y as well as disparity error of reference data points. Note that the bottom row is scaled logarithmically. While the general form of the error distribution is the same for both analytic and sampling based propagation, we obtain tighter bounds on all errors using sampling.

how good a given disparity map is. We hence need a distribution of possible disparity values in each pixel. Given a set of reference data points with uncertainty $R = \{(\mu_{\mathbf{r}}, \Sigma_r)\}$ computed as described in Sect. 4, we define the probability of a disparity map $\mathbf{D}$ to be

$$p(\mathbf{D}|R) = \prod_{\mathbf{x_i} \in \mathbf{D}} \frac{1}{N} \sum_{(\mu_{\mathbf{r}}, \Sigma_r) \in R} \exp\left((\mathbf{x_i} - \mu_{\mathbf{r}})^T \Sigma_r^{-1} (\mathbf{x_i} - \mu_{\mathbf{r}})\right) \tag{13}$$

with $\mathbf{x_i} = (\mathbf{p_i}, d)$ the disparity d at pixel position $\mathbf{p_i}$ and normalization N. The Gaussian distribution in Eq. 13 is multivariate (in pixel position and disparity). This distribution can alternatively be computed by either sampling from the reference data distribution or analytically from the input data distribution directly using Gaussian error propagation. The main drawback of a linear error propagation is that the projection of Gaussian disparity distribution into image space yields multi-modal per-pixel distributions which cannot be accounted for using linear propagation. Figure 5 shows such distributions at example pixel locations. We can distinguish three error cases: first, due to extrinsic camera parameter uncertainty the locations of depth edges are projected to different pixel locations. This causes bimodal disparity distributions since either the background or the foreground is sampled. The result is a very high variance, i.e. a large, though correct error bar on the ground truth.

Second, multi-modal distributions can occur caused by back surfaces: multiple surfaces such as the front and back of a house as well as the houses in the

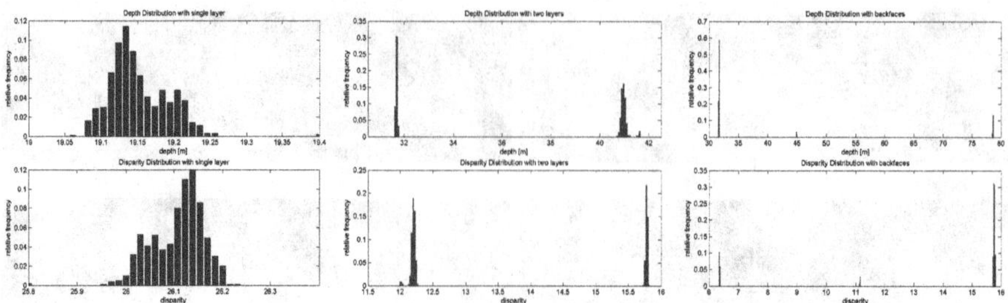

Fig. 5. Example distributions on sampled depth maps (1000 samples). From left to right: pixel with single depth layer, edge pixel with two depth layers, pixel with unresolved back faces. Top row: depth distribution. Bottom row: disparity distribution.

background of the LIDAR point cloud are projected to the same pixel. This is a fundamental limitation of point clouds - yet established meshing tools can not deal with our data as was explained in Sect. 3.1. In these situations, the ground truth is not wrong per se - but more reasoning is required to decide whether the multi-modality of the distribution is caused either by a depth edge or back surfaces.

Third, in case the scanner did not measure a foreground object, for example due to limited resolution (landlines, small twigs on trees), the disparity distribution becomes unimodal but still displays the wrong depth of the object behind the small foreground object. This case can only be dealt with by more accurate measurement devices which not yet exist at least for our application. The problem can only be alleviated by manual segmentation of foreground objects which are visible in the image, but not in the 3D scan.

Once the per-pixel distributions in disparity space are sampled, we can reduce their information to per-pixel scalar values. Figure 6 displays two such options: the top image contains the median of the disparity distribution. Assuming that the number of foreground samples outweighs the number of back-surfaces by a factor of at least two, this is a robust ground truth depth. Note however, that this approach fails at depth boundaries when foreground and background can easily become equally likely. Therefore, the lower image displays the standard deviation of the disparity distributions. We can for example use it to define a ground truth mask as is common for stereo benchmarks such as Middlebury or KITTI: we choose a threshold defining when we cannot trust the ground truth any longer. To obtain meaningful ground truth for a pixel-accurate algorithm, one would typically choose a maximum standard deviation of 1 pixels.

It is important to mention that this type of masking is not necessarily the best option for performance evaluation. A simple performance metric based on the full distribution could be $m(\mathbf{D}|R) = -\log(p(\mathbf{D}|R))$. For reference data with localization error much smaller than the pixel size the sum in Eq. 13 can be replaced with a single normal distribution belonging to the reference point in the respective pixel. The negative logarithm of the term then yields a per-pixel weighted sum of a squared distance metric. A more appropriate evaluation would

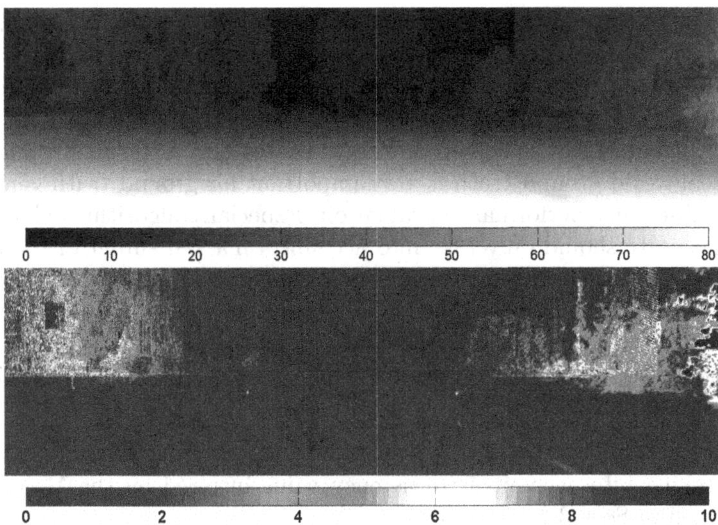

Fig. 6. Top: median of disparity distribution. Bottom: standard deviation of disparity distribution. High variances show regions with unreliable ground truth mainly caused by vegetation and camera misalignments. Regions looking like artifacts are caused by backsurfaces as explained in the text. In all other regions, the standard deviation is below two disparities.

require the stereo algorithm to propose a disparity distribution as well; then, the performance metric would compare ground truth and computed disparity distribution e.g. by a Kolmogorov-Smirnov test.

6 Conclusion and Outlook

We have presented a methodology to add error bars to image sequences with disparity ground truth. It is based on previously measured point clouds and arbitrary calibrated cameras and therefore highly versatile for all kinds of indoor as well as outdoor applications. However, due to the chosen 3D scanning device our approach is limited to static scenes.

Based on intuitive inputs such as calibration, 2D feature and 3D LIDAR accuracy we estimated the covariance matrix of our model at the solution to derive per-pixel depth-distributions. The results were used to define error bars, e.g. by computing the depth variance at each pixel.

Results with a recently recorded scene showed that the localization error caused by suboptimal camera estimates significantly deteriorates quality by introducing multi-modal depth distributions at depth edges, especially at objects close to the camera. Even with arguably the best hardware available today and highly tuned manual alignment tools, the disparity standard deviation exceeds several pixels at nearby objects. Objects with high geometric detail cannot be measured with LIDAR reliably, causing additional artifacts in the ground truth. In this paper we used the accuracy claimed in the LIDAR manufacturer's data sheet which should be a very good approximation. More detailed studies such as [25] will be incorporated in future work. Only in the background accuracies well below one pixel can be achieved. This indicates that a per-pixel quality estimate of real-world ground truth is very important for ground truth generation and any subsequent performance evaluation. Especially algorithms claiming to be pixel-accurate should only take into account a masked subset of the ground truth with standard deviations of less than 1 pixels. It should be noted however that thresholding the reference data is only one simple way of harnessing known error distributions of reference data for purposes of performance analysis. By analyzing not only the absolute difference between stereo output $\mathbf{D}_s$ with reference depth image $\mathbf{D}_r$

$$\mathbf{R} = |\mathbf{D_R} - \mathbf{D_S}|, \tag{14}$$

but also taking into account a consistency value inspired by the Mahalanobis distance used in Sect. 3.2

$$\mathbf{C} = |\mathbf{D_R} - \mathbf{D_S}|/\mathbf{S_R}, \tag{15}$$

where $\mathbf{S_R}$ is the interquartile range of the reference data distribution, it is possible to gain more insights into the performance characteristics of a stereo algorithm; especially, it is possible to identify situations where the algorithm is achieving the same accuracy as the reference data measurements yet other areas where no statements can be made about the algorithm performance. We give a more detailed discussion of the metrics as an outlook in the supplementary material, as the results presented there are only intended as a proof of concept and require further investigation to be conclusive.

In terms of our experimental setup, the accuracy could be improved in smaller scenes by using our approach with a micrometer-accurate structured light scanner delivering object meshes rather than point clouds. Then, the limiting factor becomes camera pose estimation, which is a matter of future studies. We will further add ground truth with error bars for optical flow and look at improved methods for backface analysis of large point clouds such as manual meshing, usage of camera motion and point normal analysis. The results and presented here as well as a supplementary video are available on the dataset homepage[7].

Acknowledgments. We thank Wolfgang Niehsen and his Team at Robert Bosch GmbH, Computer Vision Research Lab, Hildesheim, for supplying the test car, camera mount and tons of input regarding meaningful content of the scenes we recorded. We further thank Jens Taupadel, Jakob Knauer and Moritz Wandsleb at Universität Hannover for acquiring and processing the scans. Finally, we thank our lab members Karsten Krispin, Alexandro Sanchez-Bach, Ekaterina Melnik for their assistance in data processing, Florian Becker and Frank Lenzen for helpful discussions as well as AEON Verlag&Studio GmbH for the organization of all helpers and facilities.

[7] http://hci.iwr.uni-heidelberg.de/Benchmarks/document/StereoErrorBars/.

References

1. Baker, S., Scharstein, D., Lewis, J.P., Roth, S., Black, M.J., Szeliski, R.: A database and evaluation methodology for optical flow. Int. J. Comput. Vis. **92**, 1–31 (2011)
2. Kondermann, D.: Ground truth design principles: an overview. In: Proceedings of the International Workshop on Video and Image Ground Truth in Computer Vision Applications, p. 5. ACM (2013)
3. Onkarappa, N., Sappa, A.D.: Synthetic sequences and ground-truth flow field generation for algorithm validation. Multimedia Tools Appl. **4**, 1–15 (2013)
4. Haltakov, V., Unger, C., Ilic, S.: Framework for generation of synthetic ground truth data for driver assistance applications. In: Weickert, J., Hein, M., Schiele, B. (eds.) GCPR 2013. LNCS, vol. 8142, pp. 323–332. Springer, Heidelberg (2013)
5. Butler, D.J., Wulff, J., Stanley, G.B., Black, M.J.: A naturalistic open source movie for optical flow evaluation. In: Fitzgibbon, A., Lazebnik, S., Perona, P., Sato, Y., Schmid, C. (eds.) ECCV 2012, Part VI. LNCS, vol. 7577, pp. 611–625. Springer, Heidelberg (2012)
6. Meister, S., Kondermann, D.: Real versus realistically rendered scenes for optical flow evaluation. In: Proceedings of 14th ITG Conference on Electronic Media Technology, Informatik Centrum Dortmund e.V. (2011)
7. Güssefeld, B., Kondermann, D., Schwartz, C., Klein, R.: Are reflectance field renderings appropriate for optical flow evaluation? In: IEEE International Conference on Image Processing 2014 (ICIP 2014), Paris, France (2014)
8. Liu, C., Freeman, W.T., Adelson, E.H., Weiss, Y.: Human-assisted motion annotation. In: IEEE Computer Society Conference on Computer Vision and Pattern-Recognition, CVPR 2008, pp. 1–8 (2008)
9. Donath, A., Kondermann, D.: Is crowdsourcing for optical flow ground truth generation feasible? In: Chen, M., Leibe, B., Neumann, B. (eds.) ICVS 2013. LNCS, vol. 7963, pp. 193–202. Springer, Heidelberg (2013)
10. Morales, S., Klette, R.: A third eye for performance evaluation in stereo sequence analysis. In: Jiang, X., Petkov, N. (eds.) CAIP 2009. LNCS, vol. 5702, pp. 1078–1086. Springer, Heidelberg (2009)
11. Meister, S., Izadi, S., Kohli, P., Hämmerle, M., Rother, C., Kondermann, D.: When can we use kinectfusion for ground truth acquisition? In: Proceedings Workshop on Color-Depth Camera Fusion in Robotics (2012)
12. Geiger, A., Lenz, P., Urtasun, R.: Are we ready for autonomous driving? The kitti vision benchmark suite. In: Computer Vision and Pattern Recognition (CVPR), Providence, USA (2012)
13. Strecha, C., von Hansen, W., Van Gool, L., Fua, P., Thoennessen, U.: On benchmarking camera calibration and multi-view stereo for high resolution imagery. In: IEEE Conference on Computer Vision and Pattern Recognition, CVPR 2008, pp. 1–8. IEEE (2008)
14. Vaudrey, T., Rabe, C., Klette, R., Milburn, J.: Differences between stereo and motion behaviour on synthetic and real-world stereo sequences. In: Proceedings of 23rd International on Conference Image and Vision Computing New Zealand (IVCNZ 2008), pp.1–6 (2008)
15. Kanatani, K.: Statistical optimization for geometric fitting: theoretical accuracy bound and high order error analysis. Int. J. Comput. Vis. **80**, 167–188 (2008)
16. Kanatani, K.: Uncertainty modeling and model selection for geometric inference. IEEE Trans. Pattern Anal. Mach. Intell. **26**, 1307–1319 (2004)

17. Triggs, B., McLauchlan, P.F., Hartley, R.I., Fitzgibbon, A.W.: Bundle adjustment – a modern synthesis. In: Triggs, B., Zisserman, A., Szeliski, R. (eds.) ICCV-WS 1999. LNCS, vol. 1883, pp. 298–372. Springer, Heidelberg (2000)
18. Förstner, W.: Reliability analysis of parameter estimation in linear models with applications to mensuration problems in computer vision. Comp. Vis. Graph. Image Proc. **40**, 273–310 (1987)
19. Dickscheid, T., Läbe, T., Förstner, W.: Benchmarking automatic bundle adjustment results. In: 21st Congress of the International Society for Photogrammetry and Remote Sensing (ISPRS), Part B3a, pp. 7–12 (2008)
20. Jähne, B.: Digitale Bildverarbeitung, 7th edn. Springer, Heidelberg (2012)
21. Abraham, S., Hau, T.: Towards autonomous high-precision calibration of digital cameras. In: Videometrics, V. (ed.) Proceedings of SPIE Annual Meeting, vol. 3174, pp. 82–93. Citeseer (1997)
22. Afonso, M.V., Bioucas-Dias, J.M., Figueiredo, M.A.: Fast image recovery using variable splitting and constrained optimization. IEEE Trans. Image Process. **19**, 2345–2356 (2010)
23. Zach, C., Pock, T., Bischof, H.: A duality based approach for realtime TV-L^1 optical flow. In: Hamprecht, F.A., Schnörr, C., Jähne, B. (eds.) DAGM 2007. LNCS, vol. 4713, pp. 214–223. Springer, Heidelberg (2007)
24. Agarwal, S., Mierle, K., Others: ceres solver. (http://ceres-solver.org)
25. Boehler, W., Bordas Vicent, M., Marbs, A.: Investigating laser scanner accuracy. Int. Arch. Photogrammetry Remote Sens. Spat. Inf. Sci. **34**, 696–701 (2003)

Separation of Reflection Components by Sparse Non-negative Matrix Factorization

Yasuhiro Akashi(✉) and Takayuki Okatani

Tohoku University, Miyagi, Japan
akashi@vision.is.tohoku.ac.jp

Abstract. This paper presents a novel method for separating reflection components in a single image based on the dichromatic reflection model. Our method is based on a modified version of sparse non-negative matrix factorization (NMF). It simultaneously performs the estimation of body colors and the separation of reflection components through optimization. Our method does not use a spatial prior such as smoothness of colors on the object surface, which is in contrast with recent methods attempting to use such priors to improve separation accuracy. Experimental results show that as compared with these recent methods that use priors, our method is more accurate and robust. For example, it can better deal with difficult cases such as the case where a body color is close to the illumination color.

1 Introduction

This paper considers the problem of separating reflection components (i.e., specular and diffuse reflections) in a single image. It is useful for several purposes. One is the use with photometric methods, such as shape-from-shading [1,2] and photometric stereo [3]. As these methods often assume the surfaces of objects to be perfectly diffuse, it is necessary to eliminate specular component before applying them to real objects having specular reflectance. The separation of reflection components are also useful for the visual recognition of materials of objects; the highlights extracted from images are used as features for the recognition.

A large number of studies have been conducted to develop a method for accurately and robustly separating reflection components in a single image [4–13]. Most of them assume the dichromatic reflection model, which states that the light reflected on an object surface is given by a linear sum of a specular component and a diffuse component [4]. Specifically, the 3-vector $\mathbf{i}_p$ containing the RGB values of a pixel p is given by

$$\mathbf{i}_p = \alpha_p \mathbf{i}_s + \beta_p \mathbf{i}_d, \tag{1}$$

where $\mathbf{i}_s$ is the color of the only illumination existing in the scene and $\mathbf{i}_d$ is the body color (i.e., the color caused by diffuse reflection) of the object surface.

If multiple pixels p share the same illumination color $\mathbf{i}_s$ and the same body color $\mathbf{i}_d$, then Eq. (1) gives constraints on the variables on the right hand side. This is the principle on which color-based methods for separating components

D. Cremers et al. (Eds.): ACCV 2014, Part V, LNCS 9007, pp. 611–625, 2015.
DOI: 10.1007/978-3-319-16814-2_40

in a single image rely. More specifically, they commonly consider the following setting:

- The object surface consists of multiple regions with different body colors, each of which consists of a number of pixels with a single color $\mathbf{i}_d$.
- The illumination color $\mathbf{i}_s$ is known. The body color $\mathbf{i}_d$ of each region and also which region each pixel belongs to are unknown. The coefficients α_p and β_p are different for each pixel p, both of which are also unknown.

Early studies [7,8,14] attempt to solve the problem within this setting. More recent studies [9–13,15] attempt to utilize spatial information to improve separation accuracy. To do so, they incorporate spatial priors such as the smoothness of the body colors and/or the specular reflections on the object surface.

Our method separates reflection components based on sparse non-negative matrix factorization. It simultaneously performs the estimation of body colors and the separation of reflection components through optimization. It is notable that our method does not use an additional prior or assumption as those used in the recent studies. In this respect, our study runs counter to the recent trend of research, which is also the argument we make in this paper. That is, the above setting with the dichromatic model (1) alone might be more sufficient than expected for accurate separation of reflection components. In fact, as shown in the experimental results, our method is more accurate and robust than the state-of-the-art that uses additional priors. As an additional prior is not necessary, our method is free from tuning a number of hyper parameters.

2 Related Work

The early approach to the problem is to determine body colors by analyzing the color space. A number of studies [7,8,14] are fallen in this category, and they solve the problem in two steps: (i) they determine the body colors first by analyzing the color space onto which all the image pixels are projected, and (ii) then determine the other unknowns using the results. The method of Klinker et al. [7] performs clustering of all the pixels in the RGB color space to determine body colors. Bajscy et al. [8] used the Hue-Saturation-Lightness color space instead of the RGB space. The method of Tan and Ikeuchi [14] projects pixel colors along the direction of the illumination color to a point of the lowest observed intensity to determine the body color. However, all these methods tend to be vulnerable to the clutters in the color space, such as image noises and color blending along the border of body colors.

To cope with this difficulty, more recent methods attempt to utilize spatial information in the image [9–13,15]. Instead of determining body colors first, most of these methods search for all the parameter values simultaneously through optimization. Some of them use a specular-free image (or its extension), an image free from specular components but with distorted diffuse components. It is created from the input image usually by a simple, pixel-wise operation.

Tan and Ikeuchi [9] first proposed a method of this category. They showed a method of creating the specular-free image by setting the maximum chromaticity of each pixel to an arbitrary value. Based on this, they presented a method that iteratively separates the reflection components by using a relation of two neighboring pixels. In their method, body colors are estimated gradually in such a way that information propagates from outside highlight regions to inside them. This propagation often fails on the boundary of body colors. It also cannot correctly deal with body colors having the same hue but different saturation. To solve these problems, Tan et al. [10] proposed a method for recovering diffuse components by using the texture information around highlights, but it requires the positions of highlights to be known.

Yang et al. [12] extends the method of Tan and Ikeuchi by incorporating a more explicit prior that the body colors should be smooth on the object surface. Their method separates reflection components by applying a bilateral filter to the image of chromaticity. The bilateral filter, whose range filter is determined according to chromaticity information, smoothes out specular reflections while maintaining the edges in the chromaticity image.

There are more studies that follow a similar approach. Shen et al. [11] proposed another specular-free image that is obtained by subtracting the minimum of the RGB values from them for each pixel. They proposed a simple separation method based on it and also on an incorporated prior that the body color changes smoothly around highlights. Although it is simple and fast, their method is less accurate than the above methods, as it simplifies the problem too much, resulting in that Eq. (1) will no longer be satisfied. Kim et al.'s [13] have recently proposed an optimization-based approach that uses three different priors (i.e., the spatial smoothness of specular reflections and body colors, and the number of body colors being as small as possible). They also propose to apply the dark channel prior [16] to obtain another specular-free image, although it is exactly the same as the one of Shen et al. [11]. Their method alternately performs the following steps in an iterative manner: (i) cluster image pixels based on the latest estimate of their chromaticity and (ii) apply an edge-preserving filter to the result, followed by reassignment of labels. However, it remains unclear how accurate their method is, since their experiments compare mostly with the method of Tan and Ikeuchi [9] alone and not with that of Yang et al. [12], which is more close to their method in that the smoothness of body colors is assumed and an edge-preserving filter is used. Moreover, their method requires a number of hyperparameters (and it is unclear how to choose them) and also the assumed three priors are too much and could narrow the range of applicability.

3 Non-negative Matrix Factorization (NMF)

Our method is based on sparse non-negative matrix factorization (sparse NMF). Before describing our method, this section briefly summarizes sparse NMF and its numerical algorithm.

3.1 Basic NMF

NMF is a general-purpose method for multi-variate analysis. For data consisting of non-negative values such as images and speech signals, it factorizes the data into additive components. To be specific, a $M \times N$ matrix $\mathbf{V}$ containing only non-negative elements is factored into a product of a $M \times R$ matrix $\mathbf{W}$ and a $R \times N$ matrix $\mathbf{H}$, both of which similarly contain only non-negative elements:

$$\mathbf{V} \simeq \mathbf{WH}, \tag{2}$$

or the j-th column vector $\mathbf{v}_j$ of $\mathbf{V}$ is represented by a linear combination of the column vectors $\mathbf{w}_k$'s of $\mathbf{W}$ weighted by the (k, j) element $H_{k,j}$ of $\mathbf{H}$ as

$$\mathbf{v}_j \simeq \sum_{k=1}^{R} \mathbf{w}_k H_{k,j}. \tag{3}$$

The factorization is obtained by minimizing some cost $D(\mathbf{W}, \mathbf{H})$ measuring the difference between $\mathbf{V}$ and its reproduction $\mathbf{WH}$. For $D(\mathbf{W}, \mathbf{H})$, L_2 norm

$$D(\mathbf{W}, \mathbf{H}) = \|\mathbf{V} - \mathbf{WH}\|_2^2 \tag{4}$$

is widely used for general purposes, so is in our method. The generalized KL divergence [17] and Itakura-Saito divergence [18] are sometimes used depending on problems.

Since an efficient iterative algorithm was developed by Lee et al. [17], NMF has been applied to all sorts of problems, and various extensions have been made to the cost function depending on problems [18–24].

3.2 Sparse NMF

An important extension is the sparse NMF that incorporates the sparse regularization into the minimization [19]. It minimizes the following cost for the purpose of obtaining $\mathbf{H}$ having as small a number of non-negative elements as possible.

$$F(\mathbf{W}, \mathbf{H}) = \frac{1}{2}\|\mathbf{V} - \mathbf{WH}\|_2^2 + \lambda \sum_{i,j} H_{i,j}. \tag{5}$$

The second term on the right hand side follows the same relaxation as sparse coding [25] that L_0 norm is replaced by L_1 norm. The minimization of this cost results in that each data vector $\mathbf{v}_j$ is represented by a linear combination of as small a number of bases (i.e., the column vector of $\mathbf{W}$) as possible, as in sparse coding. Its difference from sparse coding is that the resulting quantities are all non-negative.

A numerical algorithm for this sparse NMF, i.e., minimizing this cost under the constraints that $\mathbf{W}$ and $\mathbf{H}$ both have only non-negative entries is as follows. Starting from initial values $\mathbf{W}$ and $\mathbf{H}$ that are usually initialized in a random manner, it alternately iterates the following two updating rules until convergence:

$$\mathbf{H} \leftarrow \mathbf{H} \odot \frac{\bar{\mathbf{W}}^\top \mathbf{V}}{\bar{\mathbf{W}}^\top \bar{\mathbf{W}}\mathbf{H} + \lambda}, \tag{6a}$$

$$\mathbf{W} \leftarrow \mathbf{W} \odot \frac{\mathbf{V}\mathbf{H}^\top + \bar{\mathbf{W}} \odot \mathbf{A}\bar{\mathbf{W}}\mathbf{H}\mathbf{H}^\top}{\bar{\mathbf{W}}\mathbf{H}\mathbf{H}^\top + \bar{\mathbf{W}} \odot \mathbf{A}\mathbf{V}\mathbf{H}^\top}, \tag{6b}$$

where $\bar{\mathbf{W}}$ represents a matrix obtained by normalizing each column vector of $\mathbf{W}$; $\mathbf{A}$ is the $M \times M$ matrix whose entries are all 1; $\odot$ indicates the Hadamard product (entry-wise product) and the division is similarly performed in the entry-wise manner. It is shown [19] that this iteration always reaches a local minimum in a finite counts of iterations.

4 Separation of Specular Components by Sparse NMF

4.1 Problem Formulation

In this section, we present our formulation of the problem of separating reflection components in a given image. Letting $R-1$ be the number of body colors in the image (or equivalently, R be the body colors plus one illumination color), we denote the body colors by $\mathbf{i}_k$ for $k = 1, \ldots, R-1$. We assume that there is only a single illumination color and denote it by a normalized vector $\mathbf{i}_s$ (i.e., $\|\mathbf{i}_s\|_2 = 1$). Following the dichromatic model (1), the color $\mathbf{i}_p$ of a pixel p can be represented as

$$\mathbf{i}_p = \alpha_p \mathbf{i}_s + \sum_{k=1}^{R-1} \beta_{k,p} \mathbf{i}_k, \tag{7}$$

where $\beta_{k,p}$ has a nonzero value only for a unique k in $[1, \ldots, R-1]$ and is zero for all other k's, as the pixel color should be a linear sum of one body color and the illumination color. Using L_0 (counting) norm, this can be represented as

$$\sum_{k=1}^{R-1} \|\beta_{k,p}\|_0 = 1, \tag{8}$$

for any p. Note that the entries of $\mathbf{i}_p$, $\mathbf{i}_s$, and $\mathbf{i}_k$ as well as α_p and $\beta_{k,p}$ have non-negative values.

For the moment, we assume that the number of body colors to be known, or equivalently, that R is known. Then, the separation problem is to estimate all the variables but $\mathbf{i}_s$ on the right hand side of Eq. (7), under the constraint of Eq. (8) along with the non-negativeness of these variables, given $\mathbf{i}_p$ for a number of pixels $p = 1, \ldots$.

This problem can be expressed compactly in a matrix form as the following constrained non-negative matrix factorization:

$$\mathbf{V} = \mathbf{W}\mathbf{H}, \tag{9a}$$

$$\text{s.t.} \sum_{i=2}^{R} \|H_{i,j}\|_0 = 1 \; (j = 1, \ldots, N), \tag{9b}$$

where $\mathbf{V}$ a $3 \times N$ matrix (N is the number of image pixels) whose columns store the pixel colors $\mathbf{i}_p$'s for $p = 1, \dots, N$; $\mathbf{W}$ is a $3 \times R$ matrix defined to be

$$\mathbf{W} = [\mathbf{i}_s, \mathbf{i}_1, ..., \mathbf{i}_{R-1}]; \tag{10}$$

$\mathbf{H}$ is a $R \times N$ matrix storing α_p and $\beta_{k,p}$'s in its columns as

$$\mathbf{H} = \begin{bmatrix} \alpha_1 & \alpha_2 & \cdots & \alpha_N \\ \beta_{1,1} & \beta_{1,2} & \cdots & \beta_{1,N} \\ \vdots & \vdots & \ddots & \vdots \\ \beta_{R-1,1} & \beta_{R-1,2} & \cdots & \beta_{R-1,N} \end{bmatrix}, \tag{11}$$

where the order of the columns (i.e., the pixels) is the same as $\mathbf{V}$; $H_{i,j}$ is the (i, j) entry of $\mathbf{H}$. Note that the second equation is merely a rewritten version of Eq. (8). Note also that the constraints of non-negative values are naturally implemented in the inherent requirement of NMF. However, there is also a difference from usual NMF, which is that not all the entries of $\mathbf{W}$ are unknown; when separating $\mathbf{W}$ into the body and illumination colors and denoting it by

$$\mathbf{W} = [\mathbf{i}_s, \mathbf{W}_d], \tag{12}$$

we are to determine only the submatrix $\mathbf{W}_d$.

In the presence of noises, it is natural to minimize

$$F(\mathbf{W}_d, \mathbf{H}) \equiv \|\mathbf{V} - \mathbf{W}\mathbf{H}\|_2^2 \tag{13}$$

under the constraint of (9b). The choice of L_2 norm is rationalized if we assume i.i.d. additive Gaussian noises with zero mean for each RGB value of each pixel. Then, the problem turns to finding a solution to this constrained NMF.

4.2 Relaxation of the Problem

The presence of the constraint with L_0 norm makes it hard to directly solve the constrained minimization. Instead, we consider

$$F(\mathbf{W}_d, \mathbf{H}) = \frac{1}{2}\|\mathbf{V} - \mathbf{W}\mathbf{H}\|_2^2 + \lambda \sum_{j=1}^{N} \sum_{i=2}^{R} \|H_{i,j}\|_0. \tag{14}$$

If there were no noise, the minimizer to this clearly gives the correct solution (i.e., the minimizer $(\mathbf{W}, \mathbf{H})$ yields the exact $\mathbf{V}(= \mathbf{W}\mathbf{H})$ and $\mathbf{H}$ satisfies the constraint (9b)), as long as we choose a small λ. (We exclude here the case where there are two or more possible factorizations for the given $\mathbf{V}$.) The same argument basically remains true in the presence of noises unless they are very large. However, one problem emerges in that case, which originates from the fact that the illumination color can be used 'for free.' For example, the illumination color could be wrongly used to explain noises. Even worse, it could also be used to explain pure diffuse colors, particularly for pixels having dark colors. If a pixel's color is dark (i.e., it is close to the origin in the RGB space), then which color to choose tends not to change the L_2 error much.

This necessitates imposing a certain penalty on choosing the illumination color. For this purpose, we employ the same regularization for the illumination color and rewrite the cost into

$$F(\mathbf{W_d}, \mathbf{H}) = \frac{1}{2}\|\mathbf{V} - \mathbf{W}\mathbf{H}\|_2^2 + \lambda_s \sum_{j=1}^{N} \|H_{1,j}\|_0 + \lambda_d \sum_{j=1}^{N}\sum_{i=2}^{R} \|H_{i,j}\|_0. \tag{15}$$

The newly added term requires as small a number of pixels as possible to have specular components. Although the regularization parameters λ_s and λ_d can be arbitrarily chosen, they have the same nature that they should be determined based on the comparison against the strength of the noises. Thus, we set

$$\lambda = \lambda_s = \lambda_d. \tag{16}$$

Equation (15) is still difficult to directly minimize, because of the existence of L_0 norm. Following the popular relaxation strategy of replacing L_0 norm with L_1 norm, we consider the minimization of

$$F(\mathbf{W}_d, \mathbf{H}) = \frac{1}{2}\|\mathbf{V} - \mathbf{W}\mathbf{H}\|_2^2 + \lambda \sum_{j=1}^{N}\sum_{i=1}^{R} \|H_{i,j}\|_1. \tag{17}$$

Then, this is mostly the same as the cost for sparse NMF (Eq. (5)), although there is a difference that not all entries of $\mathbf{W}$ are unknown in the above cost.

4.3 Modifying Sparse NMF Algorithm for Separating Reflection Components

To deal with the difference of our problem from sparse NMF, we modify the algorithm so that only the unknown submatrix $\mathbf{W}_d$ in $\mathbf{W}$ will be updated. To be specific, we revise Eq. (6b) as

$$\mathbf{W}_d \leftarrow \mathbf{W}_d \odot \frac{\mathbf{V}'\mathbf{H}_d^\top + \bar{\mathbf{W}}_d \odot \mathbf{A}\bar{\mathbf{W}}_d\mathbf{H}_d\mathbf{H}_d^\top}{\bar{\mathbf{W}}_d\mathbf{H}_d\mathbf{H}_d^\top + \bar{\mathbf{W}}_d \odot \mathbf{A}\mathbf{V}'\mathbf{H}_d^\top}, \tag{18}$$

where

$$\mathbf{V}' = \mathbf{V} - \mathbf{i}_s\mathbf{h}_s, \tag{19a}$$

$$\mathbf{h}_s = \begin{bmatrix}\alpha_1 \cdots \alpha_N\end{bmatrix}, \tag{19b}$$

and

$$\mathbf{H_d} = \begin{bmatrix} \beta_{1,1} & \cdots & \beta_{1,N} \\ \vdots & \ddots & \vdots \\ \beta_{R-1,1} & \cdots & \beta_{R-1,N} \end{bmatrix}. \tag{20}$$

Here, $\mathbf{A}$ is the $M \times M$ matrix of all 1's. This revised updating rule does not change $\mathbf{i}_s$, for which we set the known illumination color.

4.4 Determining R

We have assumed R (i.e., the number of body colors plus one) to be known so far. It is unknown in reality, and thus needs to be determined.

Our problem is originally to factorize a matrix containing the image into a product of non-negative matrices under the constraint (8); the constraint is such that a pixel color should be given by a linear combination of the illumination color and a single body color chosen from multiple candidates. This is relaxed to the minimization of (17), which we expect to give a good solution. If it indeed gives a good solution, the solution will satisfy the constraint (8) at least approximately.

Thus, we incorporate a measure of how well a solution satisfies this constraint and search for R in an exhaustive manner using the measure. Specifically, computing a number of solutions for multiple different R's, we choose the solution with the highest measure. For this measure, we define

$$\text{score}(\mathbf{H}) = \frac{1}{N}\sum_{j=1}^{N} \frac{\max_{i\in[2,R]} H_{i,j}}{\sum_{i=2}^{R} H_{i,j}}. \tag{21}$$

This score is in the range [0,1] and returns 1 if the above constraint is fully satisfied. For a dark pixel without specular component, however, its diffuse component could be zero, making the score of the pixel also zero. Therefore, we choose the solution returning the highest score.

It seems difficult to determine the number of body colors for real images, because a certain amount of ambiguity has to be involved in the determination. Fortunately, our method tends not to be sensitive to the choice of R. As shown in Fig. 1, it yields almost the same separation result for a certain range of R.

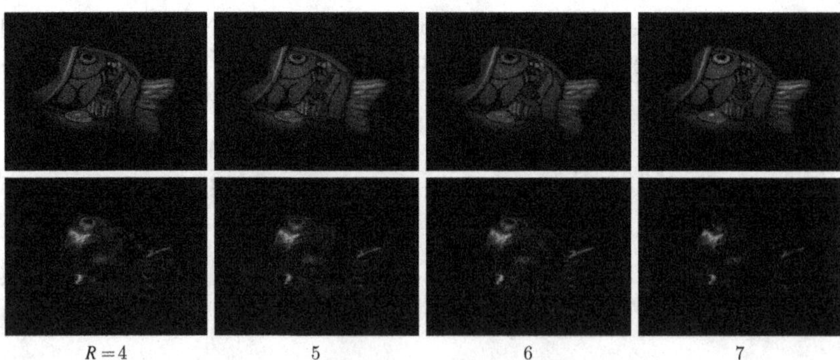

Fig. 1. The separation results obtained by our method for different R's. Upper row: Diffuse components. Lower row: Specular components. The original image is shown in the top-left corner of Fig. 6.

5 Experimental Results

We conducted several experiments to examine the effectiveness of the proposed method and compare its performance with existing methods. For them, we choose Tan-Ikeuchi [9] and Yang et al. [12]; we used the authors' code[1,2] in the experiments. We exclude Kim et al. [13], since its repeatability is limited due to lack of information. The method has a lot of tunable parameters, and the paper does not show how to choose them. (For example, the threshold of chromaticity distance between regions to be merged, after k-means clustering, in Sect. 6.1 of [13]; it is unclear what edge-preserving filter is used for computing λ in Sect. 6.2; the convergence threshold κ is not shown, and so on.) Note also that no authors' implementation is available.

5.1 Parameters and Initial Values

We set the weight of the sparse regularization $\lambda = 3$ throughout the experiments. For each image, we iterated the modified sparse NMF until it converges. The convergence is judged by

$$|F_t - F_{t-1}| < \epsilon |F_t|, \tag{22}$$

where F_t and F_{t-1} are the values of the cost (17) at iteration count t and $t-1$, respectively; we set ϵ to be $\exp(-18)$.

The initial values of $\mathbf{H}$ and $\mathbf{W}_d$ are generated by uniform random numbers over $[1, 255]$, and each column vector of $\mathbf{W}_d$ is normalized to have length 1. We set the illumination color $\mathbf{i}_s$ to be $\frac{1}{\sqrt{3}}[1,1,1]^\top$ in all the experiments. As is described in Sect. 4.4, we choose the solution yielding the best score (21) among those obtained for different R in the range [3,12]. The (modified) sparse NMF is not guaranteed to find the global optimum. In fact, we confirmed in our experiments that it was occasionally trapped in apparent local minima. Thus, we run it three times with different initial values for each value of R, and choose the solution yielding the best score among all the solutions thus obtained.

From $\mathbf{W}_d$ and $\mathbf{H}$ of the best solution, the specular and diffuse components are reconstructed by

$$\mathbf{I}_s = \mathbf{i}_s \mathbf{h}_s, \tag{23}$$

and

$$\mathbf{I}_d = \mathbf{W}_\mathbf{d} \mathbf{H}_\mathbf{d}, \tag{24}$$

respectively.

5.2 Synthetic Images

We first applied the three methods to a synthetic image shown in Fig. 2 and its results also are shown in there. The parenthesis below each image show the error

[1] http://www.staff.science.uu.nl/~tan00109/code.html.

[2] http://www.cs.cityu.edu.hk/~qiyang/publications.html.

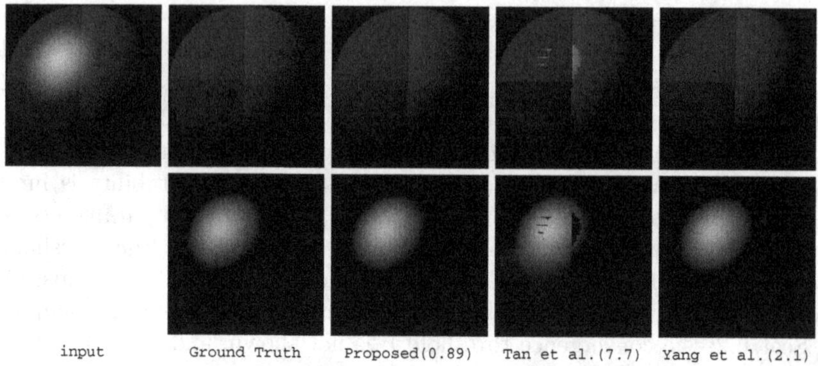

Fig. 2. Input image, ground truth, and separation results by the three methods. The numbers in the parentheses indicate the errors of the separated specular components.

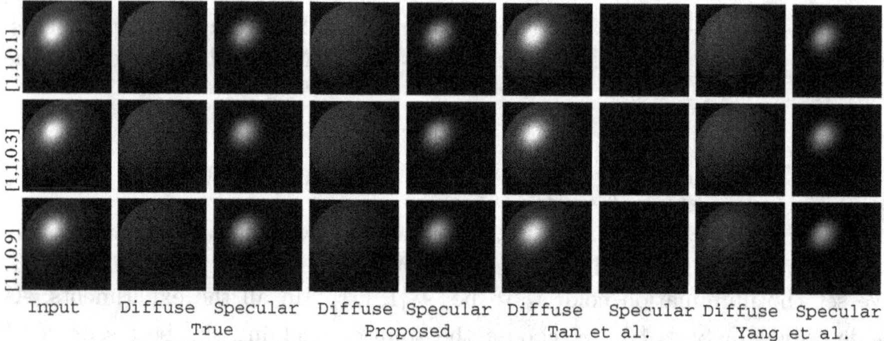

Fig. 3. The results when the body color is close to the illumination color. From top row to bottom, $[R, G, B] = [1, 1, 0.1]$, [1, 1, 0.3], and [1, 1, 0.9].

(RMSE) of the separated specular components. From the separation results, our method is the best in terms of accuracy; Tan-Ikeuchi is clearly erroneous, and Yang et al. is better than Tan-Ikeuchi but has an erroneous horizontal line between the two regions on the left. These are also confirmed by the error values in the parentheses.

When a body color is close to the illumination color, the separation will be difficult. We compare the behaviors of the three methods in such situations. We created the images of a sphere with a single body color $[R, G, B] = [1, 1, x]$ by varying $x = 0.1$, 0.3, and 0.9. As the illumination color is $[1, 1, 1]$, the separation is more difficult as x goes to 1. Figure 3 shows the results for these images. Tan-Ikeuchi could not separate the components at all, as they assume $R \neq G \neq B$ for every pixel. The results of Yang et al. tend to be worse with increasing x; the separated specular components appear to be smaller than their true values. Our method yields clearly better separation results.

5.3 Real Images

We then show results for real images. We first show the results for the dataset of [9] that is available from the author's site[3] and is widely used in previous studies.

We first tested robustness to image noises. We added zero-mean Gaussian noise with $\sigma = 0.1$, 1.0, and 5.0 to each pixel (ranging in [0, 255]) of each channel of an input image. Figure 4 shows the results for different levels of the noise. It is seen that the three methods are almost equally robust to noises, although Tan et al. is slightly less robust than the other two.

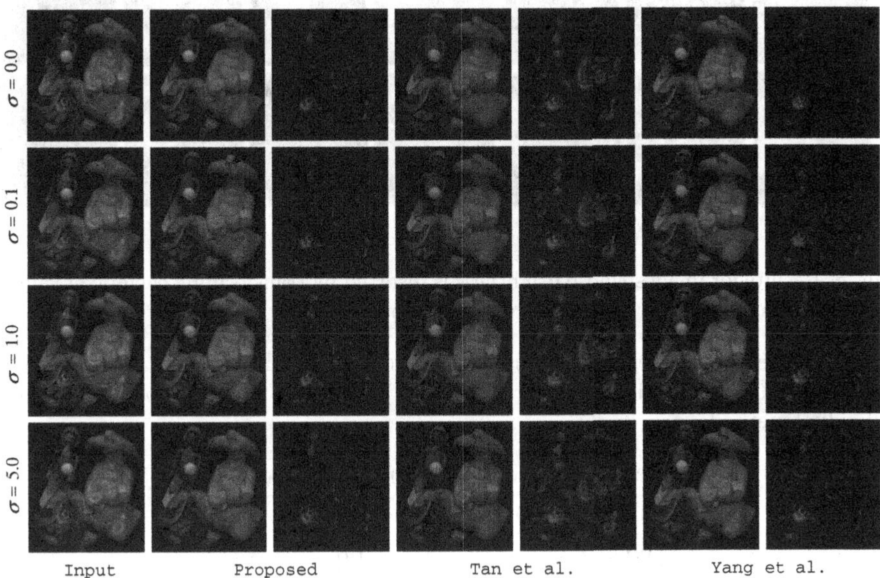

Fig. 4. Results for noisy input images. Zero-mean Gaussian noises with $\sigma = 0.1$, 1.0, and 5.0 are added to each pixel of each channel of the original image of the top row.

Many existing methods assume a linear mapping between the image irradiance and the corresponding pixel value. Calibrating the response function of the camera will make the assumption true, but the calibration will include a certain amount of errors. We may simulate such errors by transforming each pixel value x into $x^{1/\gamma}$. To examine the performance of the methods in the presence of such calibration errors, we generated a number of images in this way and applied the three methods to the images. The results are shown in Fig. 5.

We may consider a separation result for each γ value to be more accurate if it is closer to that for $\gamma = 1.0$ (the original image). Table 1 shows the errors in this accuracy measure. It is seen that our method is significantly better than Tan-Ikeuchi and is slightly better than Yang et al.

[3] http://www.staff.science.uu.nl/~tan00109/code.html.

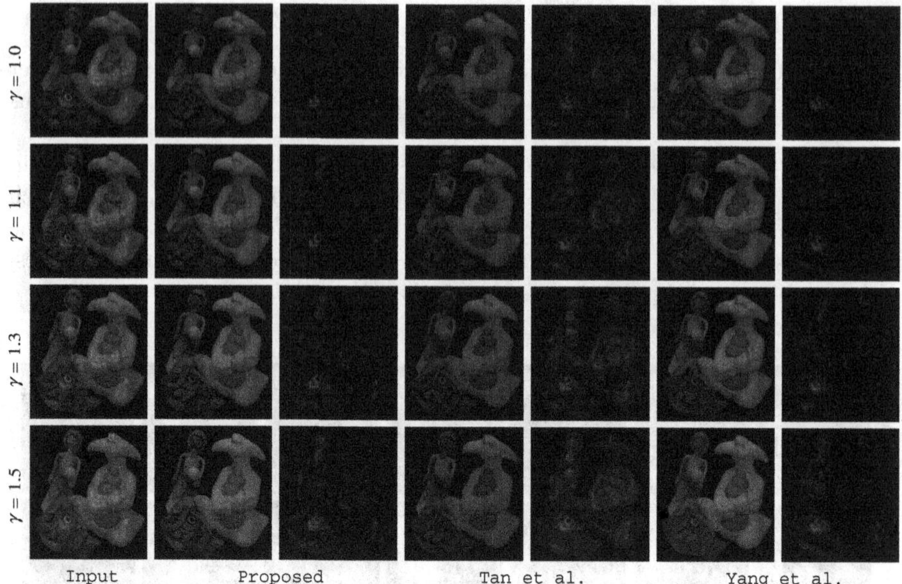

Fig. 5. Results for images whose brightness is disorted by transforming each pixel value x to $x^{1/\gamma}$. See Table 1 for quantitative comparisons.

Table 1. The errors of separation results for each γ. Each number shows the difference of the separation result (i.e., specular component) from that for $\gamma = 1$ obtained by the individual method.

γ	Proposed	Tan-Ikeuchi [9]	Yang et al. [12]
1.0	0.0	0.0	0.0
1.1	0.77	5.3	1.8
1.3	1.9	9.5	4.0
1.5	3.3	14.7	5.7

Unlike other methods, our method does not assume a prior on spatial information such as the smoothness of body colors. To show the difference of our method from others, we intentionally destroyed the spatial relationship of pixels and applied the three methods to the resulting images. To be specific, we transform an image by dividing it into patches of $w \times w$ pixels in a grid manner and then randomly shuffle these patches to generate an image. Figure 6 shows the results. Note that the displayed images have been transformed back by the inverse of the above transformation (except for the input images). The three rows correspond to $w = \infty$(no shuffle), 5×5, and 1×1(pixelwise), respectively. Tan-Ikeuchi is somewhat robust to this geometric transformation, as it uses only the relationship between the neighboring pixels, whereas Yang et al. is less robust; it completely fails separation at $w = 1$.

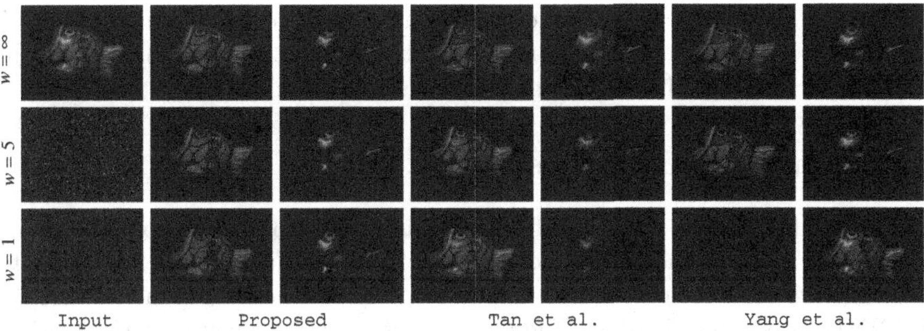

Fig. 6. The results for images undergoing patch-wise geometric shuffling. The image at the top-left corner is divided into $w \times w$ patches and randomly shuffled (the leftmost column). The separation results are transformed back by the inverse of the shuffling.

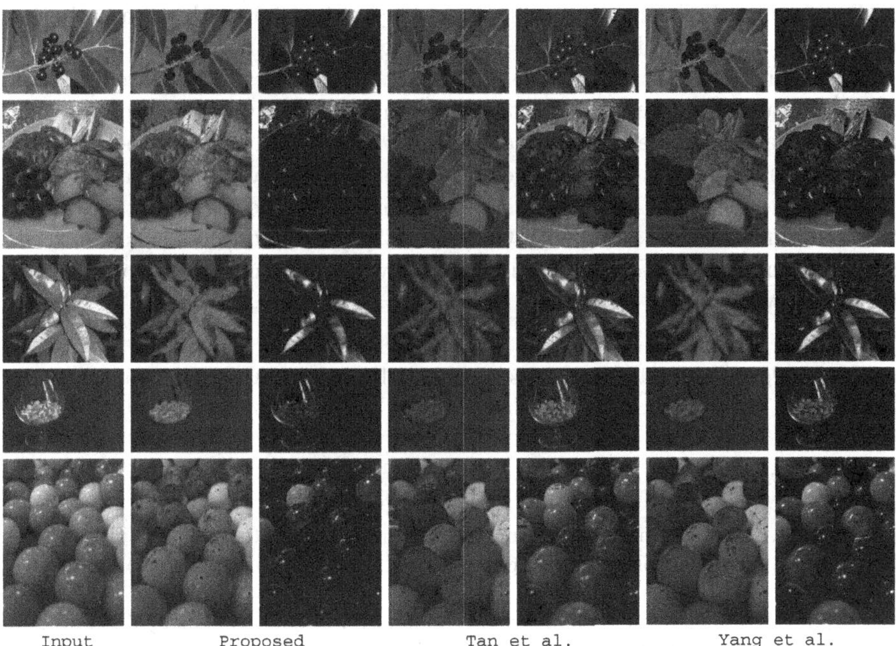

Fig. 7. The results for other real images.

Finally, we show the results for other real images in Fig. 7. Although there is no ground truth and thus it is difficult to evaluate separation accuracy, it is observed that Tan-Ikeuchi clearly yields excessive amount of specular components; the results of Yang et al. are slightly better, but its tendency is the same; our method provides much better results than the others. It should be noted that in the results from third to fifth rows, some of the pixels have zero diffuse components, which are caused by saturation of the brightness. It violates the assumed model, and it is no wonder that the correct results are not obtained. We nevertheless show the result to demonstrate how the methods can handle the real-world images having saturated pixels.

6 Summary and Discussions

This paper has shown a method for separating reflection components based on sparse NMF. The method is characterized by that it simultaneously performs the estimation of body colors and the separation of reflection components through the NMF-based optimization. The experimental results show that the method yields more accurate separation results than the state-of-the-art that incorporates spatial priors such as the smoothness of body colors. This shows that the basic problem setting with the dichromatic model alone might be more sufficient than expected for accurate separation of reflection components. Our sparse NMF-based method can successfully find an accurate solution through optimization, owing to the good numerical property of NMF.

The main contribution of this study is not necessarily the proposed method itself but rather the finding that the problem can be solved more simply than thought. Earlier studies use spatial priors, whereas our method does not use spatial information at all, and nevertheless yields reasonably better results. We suspect that our NMF formulation can better utilize the constraints given by the dichromatic model along with the implicit surface color model (i.e., surfaces consist of multiple uni-colored regions). This will be further investigated in our future study.

Acknowledgement. This work was supported by JSPS KAKENHI Grant Number 25135701.

References

1. Horn, B.K.P.: Obtaining shape from shading information. In: Winston, H.P., Horn, B. (eds.) The Psychology of Computer Vision, pp. 115–155. MIT Press, Cambridge (1975)
2. Prados, E., Faugeras, O.: Shape from shading. In: Paragios, N., Chen, Y., Faugeras, O. (eds.) Handbook of Mathematical Models in Computer Vision, pp. 1–17. Springer, US (2006)
3. Woodham, R.: Photometric method for determining surface orientation from multiple images. Opt. Eng. **19**, 139–144 (1980)
4. Shafer, S.: Using color to separate reflection components. Color Res. Appl. **10**, 43–51 (1985)
5. Swaminathan, R., Kang, S.B., Szeliski, R., Criminisi, A., Nayar, S.K.: On the motion and appearance of specularities in image sequences. In: Heyden, A., Sparr, G., Nielsen, M., Johansen, P. (eds.) ECCV 2002, Part I. LNCS, vol. 2350, pp. 508–523. Springer, Heidelberg (2002)
6. Feris, R., Raskar, R., Turk, M.: Specular reflection reduction with multi-flash imaging. In: 17th Brazilian Symposium on Computer Graphics and Image Processing. IEEE Computer Society (2004)

7. Klinker, G., Shafer, S., Kanade, T.: The measurement of highlights in color images. IJCV **2**, 7–32 (1988)
8. Bajcsy, B., Lee, S., Leonardis, A.: Detection of diffuse and specular interface reflections and inter-reflections by color image segmentation. IJCV **17**, 241–272 (1996)
9. Tan, R.T., Ikeuchi, K.: Separating reflection components of textured surfaces using a single image. PAMI **27**, 178–193 (2005)
10. Tan, P., Lin, S., Quan, L.: Separation of highlight reflections on textured surfaces. In: CVPR (2006)
11. Shen, H.L., Cai, Q.Y.: Simple and efficient method for specularity removal in an image. Appl. Opt. **48**, 2711–2719 (2009)
12. Yang, Q., Wang, S., Ahuja, N.: Real-time specular highlight removal using bilateral filtering. In: Daniilidis, K., Maragos, P., Paragios, N. (eds.) ECCV 2010, Part IV. LNCS, vol. 6314, pp. 87–100. Springer, Heidelberg (2010)
13. Kim, H., Jin, H., Hadap, s., Kweon, I.: Specular reflection separation using dark channel prior. In: CVPR (2013)
14. Tan, R.T., Katsushi, I.: Reflection components decomposition of textured surfaces using linear basis functions. In: CVPR (2005)
15. Mallick, S.P., Zickler, T.E., Belhumeur, P.N., Kriegman, D.J.: Specularity removal in images and videos: a PDE approach. In: Leonardis, A., Bischof, H., Pinz, A. (eds.) ECCV 2006, Part I. LNCS, vol. 3951, pp. 550–563. Springer, Heidelberg (2006)
16. He, K., Sun, J., Tang, X.: Single image haze removal using dark channel prior. In: CVPR (2009)
17. Lee, D.D., Seung, H.S.: Learning the parts of objects by non-negative matrix factorization. Nature **401**, 788–791 (1999)
18. Févotte, C., Bertin, N., Durrieu, J.: Nonnegative matrix factorization with the itakura-saito divergence: with application to music analysis. Neural Comput. **21**, 793–830 (2009)
19. Eggert, J., Korner, E.: Sparse coding and NMF. Neural Netw. **2**, 2529–2533 (2004)
20. Hoyer, P.: Non-negative matrix factorization with sparseness constraints. Mach. Learn. Res. **5**, 1457–1469 (2004)
21. Virtanen, T.: Monaural sound source separation by nonnegative matrix factorization with temporal continuity and sparseness criteria. Audio Speech Lang. Process. **15**, 1066–1074 (2007)
22. Schmidt, M.: Speech separation using non-negative features and sparse non-negative matrix factorization. In: Computer Speech and Language (2008)
23. Choi, S.: Algorithms for orthogonal nonnegative matrix factorization. In: International Joint Conference on Neural Networks, pp. 1828–1832 (2008)
24. Bertin, N., Badeau, R., Vincent, E.: Enforcing Harmonicity and Smoothness in Bayesian Non-Negative Matrix Factorization Applied to Polyphonic Music Transcription. Audio Speech Lang. Process. **18**, 538–549 (2010)
25. Olshausen, B., Field, D.J.: Sparse coding of sensory inputs. Curr. Opin. Neurobiol. **14**, 481–487 (2004)

Spatiotemporal Derivative Pattern: A Dynamic Texture Descriptor for Video Matching

Farshid Hajati[1(✉)], Mohammad Tavakolian[1], Soheila Gheisari[1,2], and Ajmal Saeed Mian[3]

[1] Electrical Engineering Department, Tafresh University, Tafresh, Iran
{hajati,m_tavakolian}@tafreshu.ac.ir
[2] Electrical Engineering Department, Central Tehran Branch, Islamic Azad University, Tehran, Iran
s.gheisari@iauctb.ac.ir
[3] Computer Science and Software Engineering, The University of Western Australia, Crawley, WA 6009, Australia
ajmal.mian@uwa.edu.au

Abstract. We present Spatiotemporal Derivative Pattern (SDP), a descriptor for dynamic textures. Using local continuous circular and spiral neighborhoods within video segments, SDP encodes the derivatives of the directional spatiotemporal patterns into a binary code. The main strength of SDP is that it uses fewer frames per segment to extract more distinctive features for efficient representation and accurate classification of the dynamic textures. The proposed SDP is tested on the Honda/UCSD and the YouTube face databases for video based face recognition and on the Dynamic Texture database for dynamic texture classification. Comparisons with existing state-of-the-art methods show that the proposed SDP achieves the overall best performance on all three databases. To the best of our knowledge, our algorithm achieves the highest results reported to date on the challenging YouTube face database.

1 Introduction

Automatic visual motion analysis has attracted the interest of many researchers [1,2]. In nature, visual motions are classified into three categories [3]: motions, activities, and dynamic textures. Motions are one-time occurring phenomena, such as a door closing, that are not repetitive in either spatial or temporal domains. Activities are events, such as running, that are temporally periodic while spatially restricted. Dynamic textures present a statistical regularity having indeterminate spatial and temporal extent [4]. In other words, image sequences of moving scenes that exhibit certain stationary time properties are defined as dynamic texture [5]. Dynamic textures such as smoke, fire, sea-waves, blowing flags, and waterfalls are periodic in the temporal domain and repetitive in the spatial domain. In some cases, dynamic textures such as smoke can be partially transparent and the object's spatiotemporal appearance may change over time. In other cases, the shape and appearance of an object may be fixed but

D. Cremers et al. (Eds.): ACCV 2014, Part V, LNCS 9007, pp. 626–641, 2015.
DOI: 10.1007/978-3-319-16814-2_41

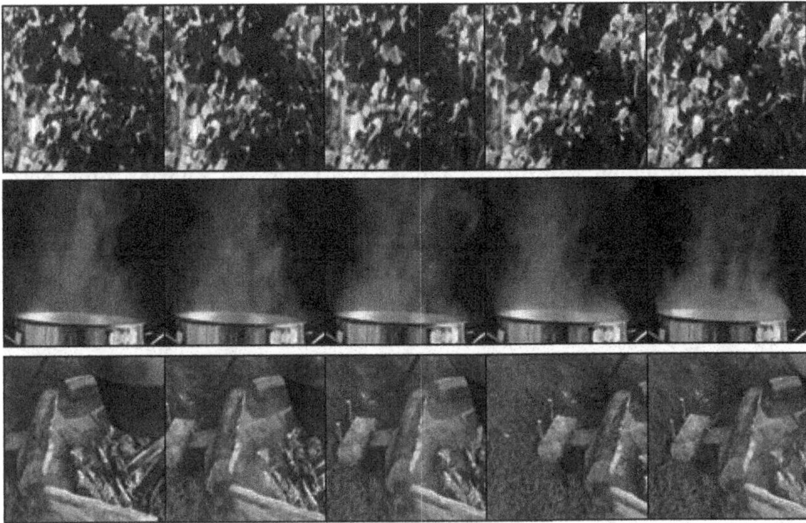

Fig. 1. Examples of the dynamic texture from the DynTex database [6]. **Top:** shaking leaves as dynamic texture with fixed shape. **Middle:** rising steam as a translucent dynamic texture. **Bottom:** the camera's panning.

the camera may exhibit motions such as zooming, rotation, or panning. Figure 1 illustrates three examples of dynamic textures; shaking leaves, rising steam, and moving camera.

Representation of dynamic textures has attracted the attention of computer vision community because of its applications in surveillance systems, video retrieval, space-time texture synthesis, and image registration. Dynamic textures are able to abstract a wide range of complicated appearances and motions into a spatiotemporal model. Research has shown that the redundancy contained in dynamic textures can improve an algorithm's performance [7]. Considering the above mentioned intrinsic properties of dynamic textures, more effective representations can be obtained from image sequences. However, due to its unknown and stochastic spatial and temporal properties, dynamic texture representation is more challenging compared to static textures.

2 Related Work

Earlier dynamic texture approaches were based on still images. Their goal was to select representative frames from a given sequence and applying traditional still-image based algorithms on the selected frames. Principle Component Analysis (PCA) [8], Linear Discriminant Analysis (LDA) [9], Local Binary Pattern (LBP) [10], Locality Preserving Projections (LPP) [11], and Local Directional Number pattern (LDN) [12] are examples of the still-image based methods that have been used in dynamic texture recognition. The major drawback of these methods is that they are not able to capture the temporal periodic properties of the image sequences. Moreover, when there are only a few frames per video in the training set, the performance of the still-image based methods decreases dramatically and popular still image methods such as LBP cannot extract discriminative features for matching.

Existing methods in dynamic texture representation can be divided into two categories: those which completely ignore the temporal relationships between the frames and those which assume that adjacent frames are temporally contiguous. The first category mainly consists of image set classification approaches [13,14] that only consider the spatial cues and treat the images as points on a high dimensional manifold. In image set classification, each class is represented by multiple images and the algorithm assigns a label to the query image set by measuring the minimum distance to the gallery sets. Hu et al. [15] proposed the Sparse Approximate Nearest Point (SANP) for image set classification. SANPs are the nearest points of two image sets that can be sparsely approximated by a subset of the corresponding image set. Wang et al. [16] proposed Covariance Discriminative Learning (CDL) to represent image sets as a covariance matrix. They treat the image set classification problem as the problem of point classification on a Riemannian manifold spanned by symmetric positive-definite matrices. Wang et al. [17] represented an image set by a nonlinear manifold and proposed Manifold to Manifold Distance (MMD) to measure the similarity between manifolds. A manifold learning technique which represented a manifold by a set of locally linear subspaces was proposed to compute the MMD. They used MMD to integrate the distances between each pair of subspaces. Coviello et al. [18] introduced Bag-of-Systems (BoS) representation for motion description in the dynamic texture. In their framework, the dynamic texture codewords represents the typical motion patterns in spatiotemporal patches extracted from the video. They proposed the BoS Tree which constructs a bottom-up hierarchy of codewords that enables mapping of videos to the BoS codebook.

The methods in the second category attempt to represent the dynamic textures by capturing both spatial and temporal cues of the image sequence. We can further divide these approaches into holistic and local methods. Liu et al. [19] used an adaptive Hidden Markov Model (HMM) [20] to learn the statistics and the temporal dynamics of the training video. Global temporal features of the query video were represented over time and the recognition task is performed by the likelihood score computed using the HMMs' comparison. Rahman et al. [1] proposed a motion-based temporal texture characterization technique using first-order global motion co-occurrence features. Doretto et al. [21] extended the Active Appearance Model (AAM) [22] to represent dynamic shapes, motions, and appearances globally by conditionally linear models using the joint variations of shape and appearance of portions in the image sequence. Derpanis et al. [23] investigated the impact of multi-scale orientation measurements on scene classification. These measurements in visual space, $x - y$, and spacetime, $x - y - t$, were recovered by a bank of spatiotemporal oriented energy filters.

Compared to global representations, local spatiotemporal representations can capture temporal relationships more effectively [2]. Xu et al. [24] assumed dynamic textures as the product of nonlinear stochastic dynamic systems. Based on the assumption, they proposed a dynamic texture descriptor using an extension of dynamic fractal analysis called Dynamic Fractal Spectrum (DFS). DFS captures the stochastic self-similarities in the local structure of the dynamic textures for classification. Zhao et al. [2] proposed two variants of the LBP features namely Volume Local Binary Pattern (VLBP) and Local Binary Pattern from Three Orthogonal Planes (LBP-TOP). VLBP is an extension of the LBP to dynamic textures by combining the appearance and the motion. VLBP is extracted by considering a local volumetric neighborhood around each pixel. Comparing the gray-level of the center pixel and the neighbors, VLBP generates a binary representative code. Local Binary Pattern from Three Orthogonal Planes (LBP-TOP) models the textures by concatenating the extracted LBPs on the three orthogonal planes ($x - y$ plane, $x - t$ plane, and $y - t$ plane) and considering the co-occurrence statistics on the three planes. The main drawback of VLBP and LBP-TOP is that they only represent the first-order derivative pattern of an image sequence and cannot extract detailed information of the image sequence. Moreover, they sample the image for coding on a discrete rectangular grid which can have aliasing effects. However, high-order derivatives, such as second order derivatives, capture more detailed spatial and temporal discriminant information contained in the image sequence. Similarly, extracting derivative patterns based on continuous circular neighborhoods are likely to generate more robust features.

We present a novel dynamic texture descriptor called Spatiotemporal Derivative Pattern (SDP) that overcomes the above two limitations. SDP describes dynamic textures by characterizing image sequences by a feature vector computed from the high-order spatiotemporal derivative patterns within local neighborhoods. Neighborhoods are defined using continuous circular and spiral regions to avoid the aliasing effects. Using the high-order spatiotemporal derivatives, SDP captures more detailed information about the given image sequence. Comprehensive experiments are conducted on the Honda/UCSD [25], the YouTube [26], and the DynTex [6] datasets. Comparisons with existing state-of-the-art techniques show the effectiveness of the proposed method for dynamic texture analysis. To the best of our knowledge, our proposed technique achieves the highest recognition rate reported on the challenging YouTube database [26]. Our experiments demonstrate that the SDP needs fewer numbers of frames for dynamic texture recognition compared to existing methods.

3 Spatiotemporal Derivative Pattern (SDP)

Video-based dynamic texture recognition is a sequential process where every incoming frame adds to the information provided by the previous frames [27]. However, the limitation of system memory is an important issue in dynamic texture recognition. Therefore, representing the dynamic texture with the least number of frames is desirable but challenging at the same time. This can be done by considering only the M number of contiguous frames that optimally

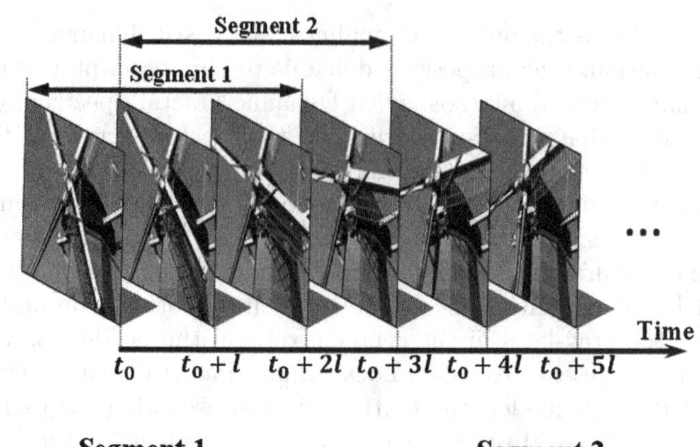

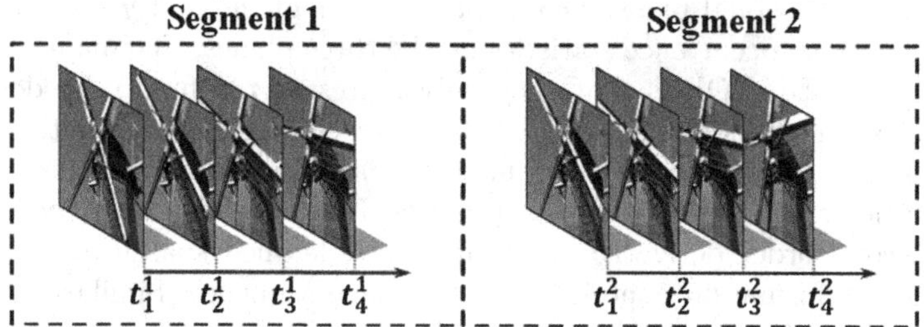

Fig. 2. Definition of segments in an image sequence from the DynTex database [6].

represent the scene. SDP characterizes the image segments by encoding them into binary patterns based on the spatiotemporal directional variations within segments. A segment is a subset of the image sequence with a determined number of frames. Figure 2 illustrates the definition of two 4-frame segments in a given image sequence.

We partition the given image sequence into M-frame overlapping segments (see Fig. 2). Let $f(x, y, t)$ be a texture point in the given image sequence, where x and y are the spatial coordinates of the texture point, and t denotes the time of the frame in which the texture point is located. The k-th frame of the s-th segment, $f_{s,k}(x, y, t_k^s)$, is defined as

$$f_{s,k}(x, y, t_k^s) = f(x, y, t_0 + (s + k - 2)l) \\ s = 1, 2, \cdots, (L - M + 1) \;\; \& \;\; k = 1, \cdots, M \quad (1)$$

where L is the length of the image sequence and l is the time interval between two successive frames. M and s denote the total number of frames in the segment and the segment's index number, respectively. t_k^s denotes the time of the k-th frame in the s-th segment.

We define the first frame of each segment as the reference frame of the segment. The SDP algorithm considers the texture points of the s-th segment's reference frame, $f_{s,1}(x, y, t_1^s)$, as the reference point of a spatiotemporal 'Spiral Route' with radius r. The spiral route starts from the reference point and passes through all the segment's frames, making a spiral path. A spiral route

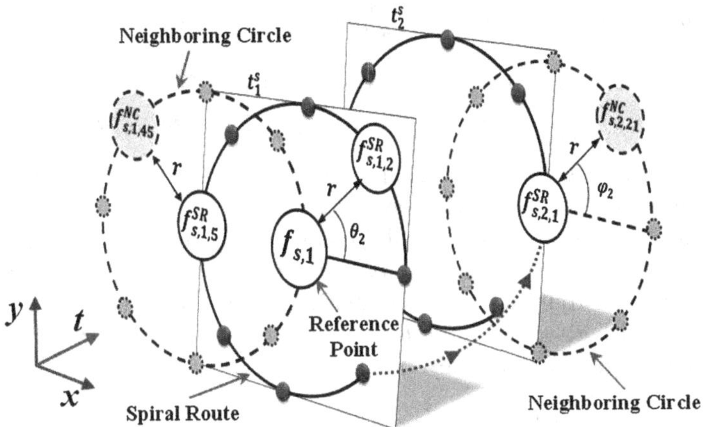

Fig. 3. Defining the spiral route and the neighboring circle in a two-frame segment. A neighboring (planar) circle is defined for every point in the spiral route.

with radius r has $8r$ points in each frame; the total number of spiral route's points in a M-frame segment is $8r \times M$. Figure 3 illustrates the spiral route's points (solid points) and the reference point in a two-frame segment. The spiral route specifies a local spatiotemporal neighborhood for the reference point. To compute the local spatiotemporal derivatives within segments, we consider another circular neighborhood for each point of the spiral route with a similar radius r. We call this circular neighborhood as the 'Neighboring Circle'. We consider $8r$ neighboring points on a neighboring circle with radius r. Examples of the neighboring circle are also illustrated in Fig. 3. Since the effectiveness of the circular neighborhood has been proven in 2D image description [28], we use circular schemes in both the space and the time domains to represent dynamic textures.

We move the neighboring circle on the spiral route and compute the derivatives using the points along its circumference. Using the k-th frame of s-th segment, $f_{s,k}(x, y, t^s_k)$, the i-th texture point in the k-th frame of the spiral route, $f^{SR}_{s,k,i}(x_i, y_i, t^s_k)$, is defined as

$$f^{SR}_{s,k,i}(x_i, y_i, t^s_k) = f_{s,k}(x + r\cos(\theta_i), y + r\sin(\theta_i), t^s_k)$$
$$i = 1, \cdots, 8r \;\&\; k = 1, \cdots, M \quad (2)$$

where t^s_k, is the time of the k-th frame in the s-th segment. r is the radius of the spiral route and $\theta_i = 2\pi(i-1)/8r$ is the angle of the i-th spiral route's point with respect to the x axis. x_i and y_i are the coordinates of the i-th texture point of the spiral route.

As already mentioned, each texture point of the spiral route is surrounded by $8r$ neighbors on the neighboring circle. Denoting the k-th frame of the s-th segment as $f_{s,k}(x, y, t^s_k)$, the j-th neighboring texture points of the i-th spiral route's point in the s-th segment, $f^{NC}_{s,k,ji}(x_j, y_j, t^s_k)$, is defined as

$$f^{NC}_{s,k,ji}(x_j, y_j, t^s_k) = f_{s,k}(x_i + r\cos(\varphi_{ji}), y_i + r\sin(\varphi_{ji}), t^s_k)$$
$$i = 1, \cdots, 8r \;\&\; j = 1, \cdots, 8r \;\&\; k = 1, \cdots, M \quad (3)$$

where $\varphi_{ji} = 2\pi(j-1)/8r$ is the angle of the j-th neighboring texture point of the i-th spiral route's point with respect to the x axis.

SDP considers the spatiotemporal directional texture transitions within segments for description. Here, we have two directions: θ and φ. Using the texture points of the spiral route and the neighboring circles, the first-order spatiotemporal directional derivatives along θ direction, $\partial f_{s,1,a}(x, y, t^s_1)/\partial\theta$, and along φ direction, $\partial f_{s,k,bc}(x, y, t^s_k)/\partial\varphi$, are defined as

$$\partial f_{s,1,a}(x, y, t^s_1)/\partial\theta = f_{s,1}(x, y, t^s_1) - f^{SR}_{s,1,a}(x_a, y_a, t^s_1)$$
$$a = 1, \cdots, 4r \quad (4)$$

$$\partial f_{s,k,bc}(x, y, t^s_k)/\partial\varphi = f^{NC}_{s,k,bc}(x_b, y_b, t^s_k) - f^{SR}_{s,k,c}(x_c, y_c, t^s_k)$$
$$c = 1, \cdots, 8r \;\&\; b = 1, \cdots, 4r \quad (5)$$

where $f_{s,1}(x, y, t^s_1)$ denotes the texture point of the s-th segment's reference point and $f^{SR}_{s,1,a}(x_a, y_a, t^s_1)$ is the a-th spiral route's texture point in the reference frame. In order to compute the directional derivatives, we only consider the first $4r$ points ($a = 1, \cdots, 4r$) on the spiral route in the reference frame and the first $4r$ points ($b = 1, \cdots, 4r$) on each neighboring circle. The remaining neighboring points are considered in the derivative calculation by changing the spatial coordinates of the reference point.

We compute the second-order spatiotemporal directional derivatives from the first-order derivatives. The second-order spatiotemporal directional derivatives along θ direction, $\partial^2 f_{s,1,a}(x, y, t^s_1)/\partial\theta^2$, and along φ direction, $\partial^2 f_{s,k,bc}(x, y, t^s_k)/\partial\varphi^2$, are computed as

$$\partial^2 f_{s,1,a}(x, y, t^s_1)/\partial\theta^2 = \partial f_{s,1}(x, y, t^s_1)/\partial\theta - \partial f^{SR}_{s,1,a}(x_a, y_a, t^s_1)/\partial\theta$$
$$a = 1, \cdots, 4r \quad (6)$$

$$\partial^2 f_{s,k,bc}(x, y, t^s_k)/\partial\varphi^2 = \partial f^{NC}_{s,k,bc}(x_b, y_b, t^s_k)/\partial\varphi - \partial f^{SR}_{s,k,c}(x_c, y_c, t^s_k)/\partial\varphi$$
$$c = 1, \cdots, 8r \;\&\; b = 1, \cdots, 4r \quad (7)$$

where $\partial f_{s,1}(x, y, t^s_1)/\partial\theta$, $\partial f^{SR}_{s,1,a}(x_a, y_a, t^s_1)/\partial\theta$, and $\partial f^{NC}_{s,k,bc}(x_b, y_b, t^s_k)/\partial\varphi$ are the first-order directional derivative along θ direction in the reference point, the first-order directional derivative of the a-th spiral route's texture point along θ direction in the reference frame, and the first-order directional derivative of the b-th neighbor of the c-th spiral route's texture points along φ direction, respectively, computed as

$$\partial f_{s,1}(x, y, t^s_1)/\partial\theta = f_{s,1}(x, y, t^s_1) - f_{s,1}(x + r\cos(\theta), y + r\sin(\theta), t^s_1) \quad (8)$$

$$\partial f_{s,k,a}^{SR}(x_a, y_a, t_k^s)/\partial\theta = f_{s,k,a}^{SR}(x_a, y_a, t_k^s) - f_{s,k}(x_a + r\cos(\theta), y_a + r\sin(\theta), t_k^s) \quad (9)$$

$$\partial f_{s,k,bc}^{NC}(x_b, y_b, t_k^s)/\partial\varphi = f_{s,k,bc}^{NC}(x_b, y_b, t_k^s) - f_{s,k}(x_b + r\cos(\varphi), y_b + r\sin(\varphi), t_k^s) \quad (10)$$

Generally, the nth-order spatiotemporal directional derivatives are computed from the $(n-1)^{th}$-order spatiotemporal directional derivatives along θ and φ direction using the following recursive equations:

$$\partial^n f_{s,1,a}(x, y, t_1^s)/\partial\theta^n = \partial^{n-1} f_{s,1}(x, y, t_1^s)/\partial\theta^{n-1} - \partial^{n-1} f_{s,1,a}^{SR}(x_a, y_a, t_1^s)/\partial\theta^{n-1} \quad a = 1, \cdots, 4r \quad (11)$$

$$\partial^n f_{s,k,bc}(x, y, t_k^s)/\partial\varphi^n = \partial^{n-1} f_{s,k,bc}^{NC}(x_b, y_b, t_k^s)/\partial\varphi^{n-1} - \partial^{n-1} f_{s,k,c}^{SR}(x_c, y_c, t_k^s)/\partial\varphi^{n-1} \quad c = 1, \cdots, 8r \;\&\; b = 1, \cdots, 4r \quad (12)$$

where $\partial^{n-1} f_{s,1}(x, y, t_1^s)/\partial\theta^{n-1}$ and $\partial^{n-1} f_{s,1,a}^{SR}(x_a, y_a, t_1^s)/\partial\theta^{n-1}$ are the $(n-1)^{th}$-order directional derivative along θ direction in the reference point and the $(n-1)^{th}$-order directional derivative of the a-th spiral route's texture point along θ direction in the reference frame, respectively. $\partial^{n-1} f_{s,k,bc}^{NC}(x_b, y_b, t_k^s)/\partial\varphi^{n-1}$ denotes the $(n-1)^{th}$-order spatiotemporal directional derivative of the b-th neighbor of the c-th spiral route's texture points along φ direction.

We encode the computed derivatives into binary bits using the unit step function, thereby forming a binary bit pattern analogous to LBP features. Essentially, we are only encoding the direction of derivative which is more robust to changes compared to the derivative value itself. By concatenating the coded spatiotemporal directional derivatives, we define the nth-order Derivative Pattern (DP) along $\alpha_b = 2\pi(b-1)/8r$ direction for the s-th segment of the given image sequence, $DP_{s,\alpha_b}^{(n)}(f(x, y, t))$, as

$$DP_{s,\alpha_b}^{(n)}(f(x, y, t)) = \{u(\frac{\partial^n f_{s,1,b}(x, y, t_1^s)}{\partial\alpha_b^n} \times \frac{\partial^n f_{s,k,bc}(x, y, t_k^s)}{\partial\alpha_b^n}) \;|c = 1, \cdots, 8r\,;\, k = 1, \cdots, M\} \quad b = 1, \cdots, 4r \quad (13)$$

where $u(\cdot)$ is the unit step function which encodes the transitions' direction.

Using the nth-order derivative pattern along α_b direction, we compute the nth-order Spatiotemporal Derivative Pattern (SDP) within the s-th segment along α_b direction as

$$SDP_{s,\alpha_b}^{(n)}(f(x, y, t)) = \frac{1}{2^{8r\times M}} \sum_{q=1}^{8r\times M} 2^{(8r\times M)-q} \times DP_{s,\alpha_b,q}^{(n)}(f(x, y, t)) \quad b = 1, \cdots, 4r \quad (14)$$

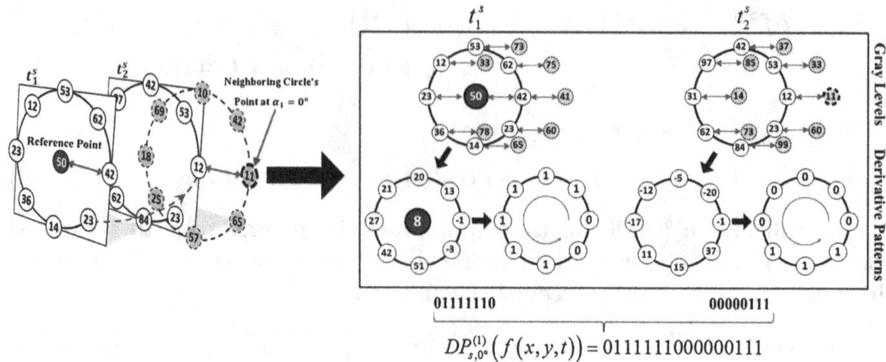

Fig. 4. Example of obtaining the first-order SDP along 0° direction in a two-frame segment. **Left:** the texture points on the spiral route and a sample neighboring circle. **Right:** derivative pattern calculation in 2D plane.

where $DP^{(n)}_{s,\alpha_b,q}(f(x,y,t))$ is the q-th component of the nth-order derivative pattern along α_b direction computed using Eq. (13).

An example of computing the first-order SDP along $\alpha_1 = 0°$ direction in a two-frame segment is illustrated in Fig. 4. For better illustration, the neighboring circles are omitted in the right and just the points on each neighboring circle along the 0° direction are shown. The shaded circles denote the gray level of the points on the neighboring circle along the 0° direction. The first-order spatiotemporal directional derivatives are calculated using Eqs. (4) and (5). Then, a 16-bit binary code $DP^{(1)}_{s,0°}(f(x,y,t)) = 0111111000000111$ is generated by concatenating the two 8-bit derivative patterns from the two frames in the segment. Using Eq. (14), the first-order SDP along 0° direction, $SDP^{(1)}_{s,0°}(f(x,y,t))$, is determined as 0.4923.

According to the described algorithm, SDP generates a feature vector for each segment of the image sequence along α_b ($b = 1, \cdots, 4r$) directions. Figure 5 illustrates the extracted SDPs along 0° direction for a 10-frame segment from the Honda/UCSD face database [25]. As can be seen, more details are extracted from the image sequence as the order of the derivatives increases. By increasing the radius r, the number of texture points on the spiral route and the neighboring circle increases and the derivatives are taken in a larger local area. Hence, the accuracy of the descriptor decreases and less detailed information is extracted from the given image sequence.

SDP extracts high-order local features for each segment's texture points. We model the distribution of the SDP by the spatial histogram [29] because of its robustness against variations [28]. For this purpose, the SDP along α_b ($b = 1, \cdots, 4r$) directions is partitioned into P non-overlapping equal-sized square regions represented by $R_1, \cdots, R_P$ and the spatial histograms of the regions are concatenated using Eq. (15).

$$HSDP_{s,\alpha_b} = \{H_{SDP_{s,\alpha_b}}(R_p) | p = 1, \cdots, P\} \qquad b = 1, \cdots, 4r \tag{15}$$

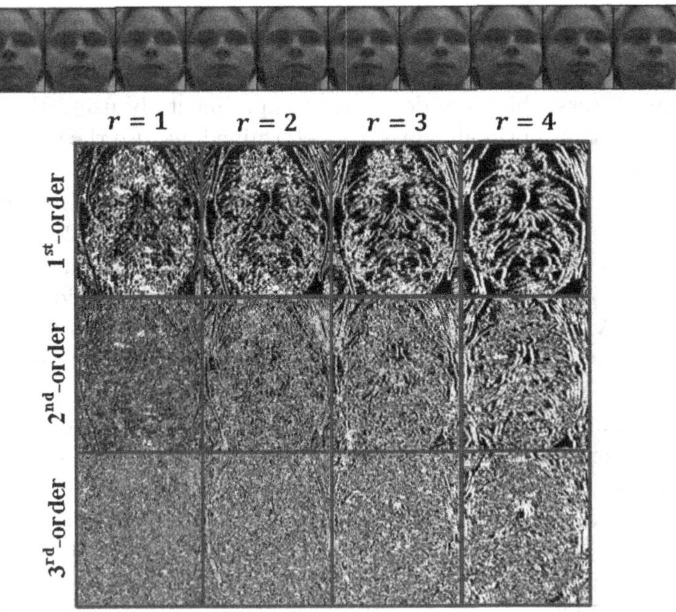

Fig. 5. Visualization of SDPs along 0° direction for a 10-frame segment from Honda/UCSD face database. **Top:** the given segment. **Bottom:** SDPs with different orders and radii.

where $HSDP_{s,\alpha_b}$ denotes the spatial histogram of the SDP of the s-th segment along α_b direction, and $H_{SDP_{s,\alpha_b}}(R_p)$ is the spatial histogram of the p-th region in the SDP of the s-th segment along α_b direction. After calculating the spatial histograms along all directions, we concatenate the computed histograms to extract a histogram vector for the whole segment as

$$HSDP_s(f(x,y,t)) = \{HSDP_{s,\alpha_b}|b = 1, \cdots, 4r\} \tag{16}$$

where $HSDP_s(f(x,y,t))$ denotes the histogram vector of the s-th segment in the given image sequence.

We partition a given image sequence into M-frame query segments using Eq. (1). For each query segment, the matching is performed by considering the minimum Euclidean distance between the histogram of the segment computed using Eq. (16) and the histogram of M-frame model segments in the gallery. The model in the gallery with the minimum distance is considered as the correct match.

4 Experimental Results

We evaluate the performance of the proposed method using the Honda/UCSD [25], the YouTube [26], and the DynTex [6] databases. The Honda/UCSD and the YouTube databases are designed for video-based face recognition while the DynTex dataset is used for dynamic texture recognition task.

4.1 Parameters Determination

The spiral route and the neighboring circles' radius, r, and the SDP's order are two free parameters which are determined experimentally using Honda/UCSD database. Once their optimal values are determined, we use the same values for all experiments.

The Honda/UCSD video database is widely used for evaluating face tracking and recognition algorithms. It contains 59 video sequences of 20 different subjects. The video sequences are recorded in an indoor environment for at least 15 seconds at 15 frames per second. The resolution of each video sequence is 640×480 in AVI format. All the video sequences contain both in-plane and in-depth head rotations. In this paper, we use the standard training/test configuration provided in [25]; 20 sequences (one per subject) are used as the gallery and the remaining 39 sequences are used as the probes. All gallery and probe sequences are partitioned into M-frame overlapping segments using Eq. (1). To have a better comparison with the benchmarks, all the faces in the video segments are detected, cropped, and resized to 40×40 frames using the algorithm proposed in [15].

The average rank-1 recognition rate of the proposed algorithm is computed using SDPs with different radius of the spiral route and the neighboring circles, r, versus the SDP's order (see Fig. 6). In this experiment, we computed the average rank-1 recognition rate of SDP for different segment's length (i.e. 5, 10, 50, and 100 frames and full length of image sequence). As can be seen, the recognition rate is significantly improved when the order of local pattern is increased from the first-order SDP to the second-order SDP for all radii. Then, the performance drops when the SDP's order increases. On the other hand, as the radius of the spiral route and the neighboring circles increase the accuracy of the SDP drops. This means that SDP captures more detailed information in small local regions. The results prove the effectiveness of the second-order SDP in extracting more distinctive features from the given video segment. Moreover, the best value of the radius of the spiral route and the neighboring circles' radius is $r = 1$. Therefore, we used the second-order SDP with radius $r = 1$ in all the remaining experiments.

4.2 Results on the Honda/UCSD Database

The rank-1 recognition rate of SDP using query segments with different length on the Honda/UCSD face databases is compared to the state-of-the-art approaches in Table 1. As can be seen, SDP achieves 21.7 %, 10.9 %, 4.0 %, and 3.1 % improvement over Volume Local Binary Pattern (VLBP) [2], VLBP + AdaBoost [30], Extended Volume Local Binary Pattern (EVLBP + AdaBoost) [30], and Manifold-Manifold Distance (MMD) [17], respectively. Notice that Sparse Approximated Nearest Point (SANP) [15] and Kernel Approximated Nearest Point (KSANP) [15] achieved 100 % recognition rate but using the full length image sequences (varying between 275 and 1168 for each sequence). On the other hand, SDP achieved 100 % recognition rate using only 70 frames per each query segment.

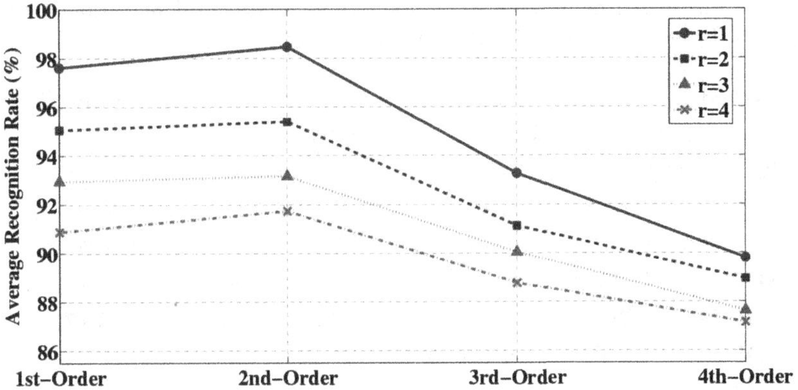

Fig. 6. Average rank-1 recognition rate versus SDP's order and the radius.

Table 1. Comparison of rank-1 recognition rates (%) on the Honda/UCSD dataset [25].

Method	Number of frames per segment	Recognition rate (%)
[a]VLBP [2]	N/A	78.30
[a]VLBP+AdaBoost [30]	N/A	89.10
[a]EVLBP+AdaBoost [30]	N/A	96.00
MMD [17]	300 – 400	96.90
SANP [15]	Full Length (275 – 1168)	100
KSANP [15]	Full Length (275 – 1168)	100
SDP	**10**	**95.32**
SDP	**50**	**97.51**
SDP	**70**	**100**

[a]The results are from [30].

4.3 YouTube Database

The YouTube database [26] contains 3,425 videos of 1,595 individuals. All the videos are from the YouTube website containing the subjects of the Labeled Faces in the Wild LFW database [31]. The videos have a frame rate of 24 frames/second, and an average of 2.15 videos are available for each subject. The shortest video duration is 48 frames, while the longest one is 6,070 frames, and the average length of a video sequence is 181.3 frames. The faces are detected, cropped, and resized using the procedure in [26].

In order to make a direct comparison with the results reported in [26], the same experimental strategy used in [26] is adopted in our experiments. We conduct ten-fold experiments by splitting the data randomly similar to [26]. The average rank-1 recognition rate, the standard deviation, and the Equal Error Rate (EER) of the SDP and the benchmark approaches on YouTube database are summarized in Table 2. The results demonstrate that the proposed method

Table 2. Comparison of average recognition rates ± standard deviations (%) and Equal Error Rates (%) on the YouTube database [26].

Method	Number of frames per segment	Average recognition rate ± deviation (%)	EER (%)
[a]CSLBP [32]	N/A	63.10 ± 1.1	37.40
[a]FPLBP [33]	N/A	65.60 ± 1.8	35.60
[a]LBP [18]	N/A	65.70 ± 1.7	35.20
SDP	**10**	**90.00 ± 1.5**	**12.24**
SDP	**20**	**90.24 ± 1.5**	**12.17**
SDP	**Full length (48–6070)**	**91.42 ± 1.2**	**10.31**

[a]The results are from [26].

consistently achieves the highest recognition rate and the smallest EER compared to the benchmarks. SDP improves the average recognition accuracy by 28.32 %, 25.82 %, and 25.72 % over Center-Symmetric Local Binary Pattern (CSLBP) [32], Four-Path Local Binary Pattern (FPLBP) [33], and Local Binary Pattern (LBP) [18]. It also improves the EER by 24.89 % compared to the smallest EER of the benchmarks. To the best of our knowledge, these are the highest recognition rates achieved on the challenging YouTube database.

4.4 DynTex Database

DynTex (Dynamic Texture) [6] is a standard database for dynamic texture research containing high-quality dynamic texture videos. It contains over 650 dynamic texture shots in different conditions. Dynamic texture sequences were recorded in PAL format at 25 frames per second with a frame resolution of 720×576. DynTex's standard video length is 250 frames.

Table 3 compares the rank-1 recognition rate of the SDP for different query segment's lengths with the dynamic texture benchmark approaches. SDP achieves

Table 3. Comparison of rank-1 recognition rates (%) on the dynamic texture database [6].

Method	Number of frames per segment	Recognition rate (%)
VLBP [2]	N/A	95.71
LBP-TOP [2]	N/A	97.14
DFS [24]	N/A	97.63
BoS Tree [18]	N/A	98.86
SDP	**10**	**97.94**
SDP	**100**	**98.23**
SDP	**Full length (250)**	**99.10**

0.9 % error rate which is equivalent to 21.05 % reduction in error rate compared to the nearest competitor BoS Tree [18] (1.14 %).

5 Conclusion

In this paper, we proposed a novel dynamic texture descriptor namely Spatiotemporal Derivative Pattern (SDP). SDP captures the spatiotemporal variations of a video segment using the spatiotemporal directional high-order derivatives. The SDP algorithm encodes the video segments into directional patterns based on the spatiotemporal directional derivatives computed within segments. The spatiotemporal directional derivatives are computed using continuous circular and spiral paths to avoid the aliasing effects. A binary code is obtained by comparing the gray-level transitions of the segment's points. The most important characteristic of the SDP is using fewer training sample frames compared to the benchmark methods.

The proposed SDP was tested on three standard datasets: the Honda/UCSD and the YouTube databases for video-based face recognition and the DynTex database for dynamic texture classification. In all experiments, the algorithm was compared with state-of-the-art benchmarks. It is a very encouraging finding that the SDP performs consistently superior to all benchmarks under the video-based face recognition and the dynamic texture classification tasks. Especially, our results demonstrate that the proposed method consistently achieves the best performances for the challenging YouTube database. This research reveals that the Spatiotemporal Derivative Pattern provides a new solution for the dynamic texture description.

References

1. Rahman, A., Murshed, M.: A temporal texture characterization technique using block-based approximated motion measure. IEEE Trans. Circ. Syst. Video Technol. **17**, 1370–1382 (2007)
2. Zhao, G., Pietikainen, M.: Dynamic texture recognition using local binary patterns with an application to facial expressions. IEEE Trans. PAMI **29**, 915–928 (2007)
3. Polana, R., Nelson, R.: Temporal texture and activity recognition. Motion-Based Recognition, Computational Imaging and Vision, vol. 9, pp. 87–124. Springer, Heidelberg (1997)
4. Chetverikov, D., Peteri, R.: A brief survey of dynamic texture description and recognition. In: Proceedings of International Conference on Computer Recognition Systems, pp. 17–26 (2005)
5. Doretto, G., Chiuso, A., Wu, Y.N., Soatto, S.: Dynamic textures. IJCV **51**, 91–109 (2003)
6. Peteri, R., Fazekas, S., Huiskes, M.J.: Dyntex: A comprehensive database of dynamic textures. Pattern Recogn. Lett. **31**, 1627–1632 (2010)
7. O'Toole, A.J., Roark, D.A., Abdi, H.: Recognizing moving faces: A psychological and neural synthesis. Trends Cognitive Sci. **6**, 261–266 (2002)
8. Turk, M., Pentland, A.: Eigenfaces for recognition. J. Cognitive Neurosci. **3**, 71–86 (1991)

9. Etemad, K., Chellappa, R.: Discriminant analysis for recognition of human face images. J. Optical Soc. Am. A **14**, 1724–1733 (1997)
10. Ojala, T., Pietikainen, M., Maenpaa, T.: Multiresolution gray-scale and rotation invariant texture classification with local binary patterns. IEEE Trans. PAMI **24**, 971–987 (2002)
11. He, X., Yan, S., Hu, Y., Niyogi, P., Zhang, H.J.: Face recognition using laplacianfaces. IEEE Trans. PAMI **27**, 328–340 (2005)
12. Rivera, A.R., Castillo, R., Chae, O.: Local directional number pattern for face analysis: Face and expression recognition. IEEE Trans. Image Process. **22**, 1740–1752 (2013)
13. Cevikalp, H., Triggs, B.: Face recognition based on image sets. In: IEEE CVPR, pp. 2567–2573 (2010)
14. Kim, T.K., Kittler, J., Cipolla, R.: Discriminative learning and recognition of image set classes using canonical correlations. IEEE Trans. PAMI **29**, 1005–1018 (2007)
15. Hu, Y., Mian, A.S., Owens, R.: Face recognition using sparse approximated nearest points between image sets. IEEE Trans. PAMI **34**, 1992–2004 (2012)
16. Wang, R., Guo, H., Davis, L.S., Dai, Q.: Covariance discriminative learning: A natural and efficient Approach to image set classification. In: IEEE CVPR, pp. 2496–2503 (2012)
17. Wang, R., Shan, S., Chen, X., Gao, W.: Manifold-manifold distance with application to face recognition based on image set. In: IEEE CVPR, pp. 1–8 (2008)
18. Coviello, E., Mumtaz, A., Chan, A., Lanckriet, G.: Growing a bag of systems tree for fast and accurate classification. In: IEEE CVPR, pp. 1979–1986 (2012)
19. Liu, X., Chen, T.: Video-based face recognition using adaptive hidden markov models. In: Proceedings of IEEE CVPR, pp. 340–345 (2003)
20. Rabiner, L.R.: A tutorial on hidden markov models and selected applications in speech recognition. Proc. IEEE **77**, 257–286 (1989)
21. Doretto, G., Soatto, S.: Dynamic shape and appearance models. IEEE Trans. PAMI **28**, 2006–2019 (2006)
22. Cootes, T.F., Edwards, G.J., Taylor, C.J.: Active appearance models. IEEE Trans. PAMI **23**, 681–685 (2001)
23. Derpanis, K., Lecce, M., Daniilidis, K., Wildes, R.: Dynamic scene understanding: The role of orientation features in space and time in scene classification. In: IEEE CVPR, pp. 1306–1313 (2012)
24. Xu, Y., Quan, Y., Ling, H., Ji, H.: Dynamic texture classification using dynamic fractal analysis. In: IEEE ICCV, pp. 1219–1226 (2011)
25. Lee, K.C., Ho, J., Yang, M.H., Kriegman, D.: Video-based face recognition using probabilistic appearance manifolds. In: Proceedings of IEEE CVPR, pp. 313–320 (2003)
26. Wolf, L., Hassner, T., Maoz, I.: Face recognition in unconstrained videos with matched background similarity. In: IEEE CVPR, pp. 529–534 (2011)
27. Mian, A.S.: Online learning from local features for video-based face recognition. Pattern Recogn. **44**, 1068–1075 (2011)
28. Ahonen, T., Hadid, A., Pietikainen, M.: Face description with local binary patterns: Application to face recognition. IEEE Trans. PAMI **28**, 2037–2041 (2006)
29. Zhang, H., Gao, W., Chen, X., Zhao, D.: Object detection using spatial histogram features. Image Vis. Comput. **24**, 327–341 (2006)
30. Hadid, A., Pietikainen, M.: Combining appearance and motion for face and gender recognition from videos. Pattern Recogn. **42**, 2818–2827 (2009)

31. Huang, G.B., Ramesh, M., Berg, T., Miller, E.L.: Labeled faces in the wild: A database for studying face recognition in unconstrained environments. Technical report, University of Massachusetts, Amherst (2007)
32. Heikkilä, M., Pietikäinen, M., Schmid, C.: Description of interest regions with center-symmetric local binary patterns. In: Kalra, P.K., Peleg, S. (eds.) ICVGIP 2006. LNCS, vol. 4338, pp. 58–69. Springer, Heidelberg (2006)
33. Wolf, L., Hassner, T., Taigman, Y.: Descriptor based methods in the wild. In: Real-Life Images Workshop in ECCV (2008)

Weakly Supervised Action Recognition and Localization Using Web Images

Cuiwei Liu(✉), Xinxiao Wu, and Yunde Jia

Beijing Laboratory of Intelligent Information Technology,
School of Computer Science, Beijing Institute of Technology,
Beijing 100081, People's Republic of China
{liucuiwei,wuxinxiao,jiayunde}@bit.edu.cn

Abstract. This paper addresses the problem of joint recognition and localization of actions in videos. We develop a novel Transfer Latent Support Vector Machine (TLSVM) by using Web images and weakly annotated training videos. In order to alleviate the laborious and time-consuming manual annotations of action locations, the model takes training videos which are only annotated with action labels as input. Due to the non-available ground-truth of action locations in videos, the locations are treated as latent variables in our method and are inferred during both training and testing phrases. For the purpose of improving the localization accuracy with some prior information of action locations, we collect a number of Web images which are annotated with both action labels and action locations to learn a discriminative model by enforcing the local similarities between videos and Web images. A structural transformation based on randomized clustering forest is used to map Web images to videos for handling the heterogeneous features of Web images and videos. Experiments on two publicly available action datasets demonstrate that the proposed model is effective for both action localization and action recognition.

1 Introduction

Action recognition is an active research topic in computer vision and plays an important role in wide applications such as intelligent video surveillance, content-based video retrieval and human computer interaction. Most of the existing action recognition methods [1–4] focus on recognizing which action exists in a video, regardless of where the action really takes place. In recent years, action recognition and localization have attracted extensive research interests, and some literatures [5–8] engage in jointly predicting which action is performed (recognition) and where the action occurs (localization) in videos. However, most of the action recognition and localization methods require both the annotations of action classes and action locations in each frame for training.

In this work, we aim to build an action recognition and localization system which takes training videos only annotated with action labels as input for alleviating the arduous and time-consuming manual annotations of action locations.

D. Cremers et al. (Eds.): ACCV 2014, Part V, LNCS 9007, pp. 642–657, 2015.
DOI: 10.1007/978-3-319-16814-2_42

Some recent literatures [9,10] also consider to localize and recognize actions using weakly annotated training videos. These methods generate candidate spatiotemporal regions without supervision and take one or more spatiotemporal regions discriminative for action recognition as the results of action localization. These methods assume that the most discriminative parts of videos are actually the spatiotemporal regions of the actions. However, for many actions such as diving and bowling, instances usually share similar scenarios. Consequently, regions of background are more discriminative than regions of motions for action recognition, which would lead to incorrect localizations.

To address this problem, we propose a novel Transfer Latent Support Vector Machine (TLSVM) for jointly recognizing and localizing actions in videos by using training videos only annotated with action labels and Web images annotated with both action labels and action locations. The model takes the spatiotemporal regions of actions as latent variables and selects the best one from a set of region candidates in both training and test videos. During the training stage, the local similarities between spatiotemporal regions of interest from training videos and the annotated regions of interest from Web images are enforced to boost both action recognition and localization. At test time, the proposed model is able to automatically predict both the action label and location in an input video. In this paper, bag-of-words representations based on randomized clustering forest are adopted to characterize videos and Web images. Since videos and Web images are represented by heterogeneous features generated from different code books, we introduce a structural transformation based on randomized clustering forest to transform the image feature space to the video feature space. An overview of our approach is illustrated in Fig. 1.

The remainder of this paper is organized as follows. Section 2 reviews the related work. In Sect. 3, we describe the representation of videos and Web images, including the bag-of-words framework based on randomized clustering forest and the structural transformation from images to videos. The detailed implementation of the proposed TLSVM model is introduced in Sect. 4. In Sect. 5, we evaluate the proposed method on the UCF sports dataset and the Olympic sports dataset. Finally, Sect. 6 gives the conclusions drawn from the experimental results.

2 Related Work

Some recent literatures [5–8] focus on simultaneously predicting the action label and localizing the action within a video. Yao et al. [5] presented an approach to classify and localize actions using a Hough transform voting framework. They annotated each frame of training examples with a bounding box, in order to obtain normalized action tracks to build a hough forest. An implicit representation of the spatiotemporal shape of an activity is proposed in [6] for localizing and recognizing human actions in unsegmented image sequences, in which the upper and lower bounds of the subjects are manually annotated at each frame. Lan et al. [7] proposed a discriminative model coupling action recognition with

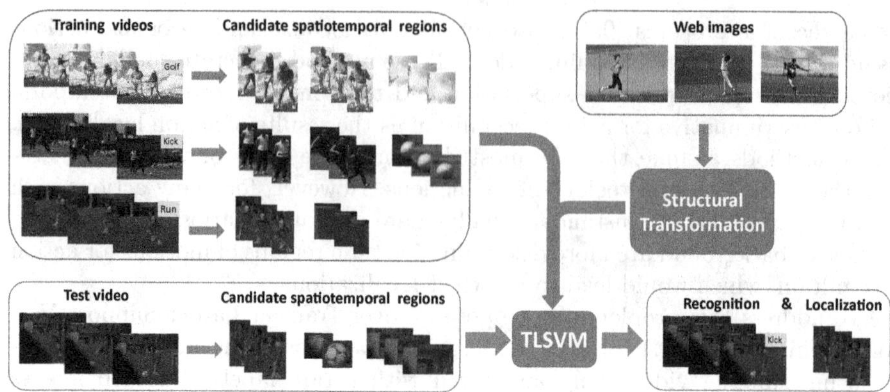

Fig. 1. Overview of the proposed method.

person localization. Although this method utilizes a latent region of interest to indicate the action location, it still requires the supervision of latent region in each frame of training videos. Raptis et al. [8] focused on discovering discriminative action parts from clusters of local trajectories that are densely sampled from the videos for action recognition and localization. In their work, strongly supervised bounding boxes of all training frames are extracted to restrict the selection of action parts. All of the aforementioned approaches require the manual annotation of action location for each frame as well as the action label for the whole video.

Shapovalova et al. [9] proposed a SCLSVM model for weakly supervised action recognition and localization. This model aims to advance the recognition performance by enforcing the consistency of local regions among training data, and uses the regions that are most discriminative for recognition as localization results. Ma et al. [10] presented to generate Hierarchical Space-Time Segments in an unsupervised manner, and these segments are utilized as the action representation for classification. In their work, localization of the action is achieved by outputting space-time segments that have positive contributions to the classification. However, in many cases, a region from the background may be chosen as the action localization result due to the similar scenarios shared among training videos with the same action label. Our approach conquers this problem by introducing Web images which are annotated with both action labels and action locations. Local similarities between spatiotemporal regions of interest from training videos and annotated regions of interest from Web images are enforced to boost both action recognition and localization.

There has been recent interests in transferring visual knowledge from images to videos. Duan et al. [11] developed a multiple source domain adaptation method for event recognition in consumer videos by leveraging a large number of Web images from different sources. Chen et al. [12] proposed an event recognition model for consumer videos, using a large number of loosely labeled Web videos and Web images. Both of these methods focus on event recognition without considering the localization task, while the proposed approach can simultaneously recognize and localize the action in a video. Ikizler-Cinbis and Sclaroff [13] employed action pose classifiers trained with a large image dataset to detect actions in each frame of an input video. A key difference between our approach and [13] is that [13] focuses on transferring knowledge from images to images, while our model is able to transfer knowledge from Web images to videos for recognizing and localizing actions in videos.

3 Representation of Videos and Images

In this section, we first describe how to represent videos and Web images in a bag-of-words framework based on randomized clustering forest [14], and then we present a structural transformation to map images to videos.

3.1 Bag-of-words Representation Based on Randomized Clustering Forest

Bag-of-words model [2] is a popular and powerful method for classification and recognition, which quantizes the low-level local descriptors as a histogram of visual words to get a discriminative mid-level representation. In our work, we use the randomized clustering forest [14] to quantize low-level descriptors effectively.

Web images are characterized by a set of densely sampled low-level HOG descriptors [15] $\{z_l^{HOG}\}_{l=1:N_I}$, and videos are described by dense trajectories [16] $\{z_k^{traj}\}_{k=1:N_V}$. For trajectory k, a descriptor z_k^{traj} is extracted within a space-time volume around the trajectory, and a HOG descriptor z_k^{HOG} is extracted to characterize the spatial patch. The trajectory descriptors $\{z_k^{traj}\}_{k=1:N_V}$ are utilized to construct the randomized clustering forest for videos, while two sets of HOG descriptors $\{z_k^{HOG}\}_{k=1:N_V}$ and $\{z_l^{HOG}\}_{l=1:N_I}$ are integrated to build the randomized clustering forest for images. Moreover, the correspondence between z_k^{traj} and z_k^{HOG} are exploited to learn a transformation from images to videos, which will be described in detail in Sect. 3.2.

Randomized clustering forest is an ensemble of decision trees, and the tree hierarchies provide a means of clustering low-level local descriptors. Nodes of each tree constitute the hierarchical clusters, namely, the visual words in bag-of-words model. Histograms of visual words in videos are generated from clustering forests built upon trajectory descriptors, while histograms of visual words in images are created from forests built upon HOG descriptors.

Construction of trees. Each tree in a clustering forest is independently grown from a random subset D' of the labeled training low-level descriptors D in a top-down manner. We assume that low-level descriptors share the same label with the video or image they are sampled from. All the training data in D' are dropped down from the root of a tree. In order to split a node n, we randomly generate a set of N_H hypotheses $\{(c_k^n, t_k^n)_{k=1:N_H}\}$, where c_k^n denotes one feature candidate and t_k^n is the corresponding threshold for splitting. Each hypothesis divides the training data arriving at the node n into two subsets, and the one

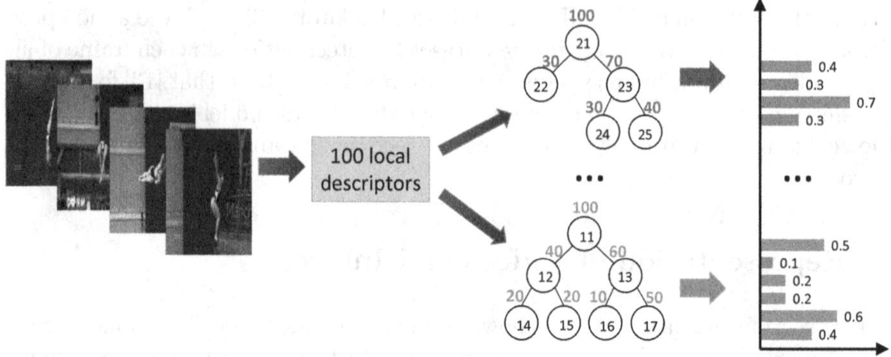

Fig. 2. Generating the mid-level representation for a video.

maximizing the expected information gain is chosen for node split. Growth of a tree is controlled by a maximum tree depth and a minimum amount of samples, so a node stops splitting in the following three cases: (1) The limited tree depth is reached; (2) There are not enough data for splitting; (3) All the data belong to the same class. If one of the above three conditions is satisfied, the node will be treated as a leaf.

Data coding. We take all the nodes (except the root) of each tree, including split nodes and leaf nodes as hierarchical visual words in our framework. Randomized forests for videos and images are built separately by their corresponding training low-level descriptors, we quantize the visual words for videos and images in the same way. Taking a video for example, all the extracted local trajectory descriptors are dropped down from the root of each tree, and the occurrences of nodes across all trees are concatenated to create a normalized histogram H, as shown in Fig. 2. Suppose $\mathbf{H}(n)$ to be the occurrence of split node n, then $\mathbf{H}(n)$ can be calculated as

$$\mathbf{H}(n) = \mathbf{H}(n_L) + \mathbf{H}(n_R), \tag{1}$$

where n_L and n_R denote the left and right children nodes of node n, respectively. The hierarchical histogram encodes the structure of each tree, and the relationship among father node and children nodes (defined in Eq. 1) is employed to learn a linear transformation in the next section.

3.2 Structural Transformation

In order to cope with the heterogeneous features of images and videos, a class specific structural transformation is introduced to map the image feature space to the video feature space.

Assume that $RF^V = \{T_r^V\}_{r=1:N_T}$ and $RF^I = \{T_r^I\}_{r=1:N_T}$ are randomized clustering forests for videos and images, respectively, where T_r denotes the r th tree in a forest and N_T is the number of trees. Training trajectory descriptors of videos $\{z_k^{traj}\}_{k=1:N_V}$ are passed through T_r^V from the root, and the corresponding HOG descriptors $\{z_k^{HOG}\}_{k=1:N_V}$ are dropped down to T_r^I simultaneously.

We first learn a set of class specific mapping matrices $\{\mathbf{L}_r^y\}_{y \in Y} \in R^{Nl_r^V \times Nl_r^I}$ among the leaf nodes of T_r^I and T_r^V by using the correspondence between low-level descriptors, where Nl_r^V is the number of leaf nodes in tree T_r^V, and Nl_r^I is the number of leaf nodes in tree T_r^I. Each element $\mathbf{L}_r^y(p,q)$ in matrix $\mathbf{L}_r^y$ is obtained by calculating the amount of samples k of action y, that z_k^{traj} reaches leaf node p of tree T_r^V and z_k^{HOG} goes to leaf node q of tree T_r^I. Normalization is performed on each column of $\mathbf{L}_r^y$ afterwards.

Suppose $\mathbf{H}_r^I$ to be the histogram of an image with action label y, generated by tree T_r^I, and $\mathbf{Hl}_r^I \in R^{Nl_r^I \times 1}$ to be a sub-histogram of $\mathbf{H}_r^I$ corresponding to leaf nodes, we can get a transformed sub-histogram $\mathbf{Hl}_r^V \in R^{Nl_r^V \times 1}$ by defining each element in $\mathbf{Hl}_r^V$ as

$$\mathbf{Hl}_r^V(p) = \sum_{q=1:Nl}^{I_r} \mathbf{L}_r^y(p,q) \cdot \mathbf{Hl}_r^I(q). \tag{2}$$

With the transformed sub-histogram $\mathbf{Hl}_r^V$ of leaf nodes, we can create the transformed histogram $\mathbf{H}_r^V$ of all nodes according to Eq. 1.

Since both of the transformations defined by Eqs. 1 and 2 are linear, the whole transformation from $\mathbf{H}_r^I$ to $\mathbf{H}_r^V$ is also a linear transformation. Transformed histograms of all trees $\{\mathbf{H}_r^V\}_{r=1:N_T}$ are concatenated to form the transformed mid-level representation of the Web image. In the following, we use a matrix $\mathbf{A}$ to represent the linear transformation from the feature space of images to that of videos, for convenience.

4 Transfer Latent SVM Model

The Transfer Latent SVM (TLSVM) Model is able to predict both which action happens and where this action locates in an action video. A few Web images annotated with both the action labels and action locations are employed to learn a discriminative model. Since the annotations of action locations are not available for training videos, the model takes the action location as a latent variable and could automatically select a region of interest from a set of spatiotemporal region candidates. In the rest of this section, we first describe the generation of candidate spatiotemporal regions of interest, and then we present the model formulation, the learning procedure and the inference.

4.1 Candidate Spatiotemporal Regions of Interest

Our goal is to generate a reduced set of candidate spatiotemporal regions of interest for a given video. One intuitive strategy is to extract global 3-dimensional bounding boxes covering the whole action. However, this constrained structure is only applicable for actions with stable locations in a video (i.e., boxing and handshake), and does not work well on drastic actions such as running and walking. In this paper, we independently detect bounding boxes from each frame by using both the static appearance information and the motion information, and then a two-stage cluster algorithm is introduced to group the bounding boxes into different spatiotemporal regions of interest.

Given an input video, an "objectness" detector [17] is utilized to extract bounding boxes that are likely to contain an object of interest from each frame of the video. Appearance information characterizes the static pattern of an image, while motion information captures the focus of action and allows to discard some irrelevant parts from the background. In order to take advantage of both the static appearance information and the motion information, we compute the boundary map [18] for each frame by merging six appearance channels (i.e., color and soft-segmentation [18]) and two optical flow [19] channels, then the "objectness" detector operates on the boundary maps and returns the potential bounding boxes.

With the detected bounding boxes from each frame, we utilized a two-stage cluster algorithm based on Affinity Propagation [20] to group the bounding boxes into different spatiotemporal regions of interest. Affinity Propagation is an exemplar based cluster algorithm, taking a similarity matrix between samples as input.

In the first stage, Affinity Propagation cluster algorithm is employed to group the bounding boxes into hundreds of clusters based on their appearance similarities and spatiotemporal distances. Intuitively, bounding boxes that are both similar in appearance and adjacent in space and time fall in the same cluster. Given two bounding boxes $B_i = (\mathbf{h}_i, \mathbf{a}_i, \mathbf{c}_i, \mathbf{t}_i)$ and $B_j = (\mathbf{h}_j, \mathbf{a}_j, \mathbf{c}_j, \mathbf{t}_j)$, where $\mathbf{h}_i$ is the color histogram, $\mathbf{a}_i$ denotes the area, $\mathbf{c}_i$ denotes the spatial coordinates for the center point, and $\mathbf{t}_i$ represents the temporal coordinate. The similarity between B_i and B_j is defined as

$$S_B(B_i, B_j) = -\mathcal{D}_h(\mathbf{h}_i, \mathbf{h}_j) - \mathcal{D}_a(\mathbf{a}_i, \mathbf{a}_j) - \mathcal{D}_s(\mathbf{c}_i, \mathbf{c}_j) - \mathcal{D}_t(\mathbf{t}_i, \mathbf{t}_j), \quad (3)$$

where $\mathcal{D}_h$, $\mathcal{D}_a$, $\mathcal{D}_s$ and $\mathcal{D}_t$ denote the χ^2 distance between two color histograms, the difference between the area, the spatial Euclidean distance between two center points and the temporal distance between two bounding boxes, respectively. Due to the temporal distance $\mathcal{D}_t$, bounding boxes extracted from temporally distant frames will fall into different clusters, and each cluster is composed of similar bounding boxes from adjacent frames.

In the second stage, Affinity Propagation cluster algorithm is performed on the first-stage clusters, according to the similarities between bounding boxes in different first-stage clusters. This results in tens of second-stage clusters, and bounding boxes appear in the same second-stage cluster form a spatiotemporal region of interest. The similarity between two first-stage clusters C_k^1 and C_l^1 is defined as

$$S_C(C_k^1, C_l^1) = \max_{i,j:B_i \in C_k^1, B_j \in C_l^1} -\mathcal{D}_h(\mathbf{h}_i, \mathbf{h}_j) - \mathcal{D}_a(\mathbf{a}_i, \mathbf{a}_j) - \mathcal{D}_s(\mathbf{c}_i, \mathbf{c}_j). \quad (4)$$

Different from Eq. 3, the similarity measure in Eq. 4 does not take the temporal distance $\mathcal{D}_t$ of bounding boxes into consideration. Accordingly, similar bounding boxes from adjacent frames are grouped into clusters in the first stage, and then distant first-stage clusters with similar appearances are allowed to be clustered together in the second stage.

4.2 Model Formulation

Let $\mathcal{D}^V = \{(x_i, y_i)_{i=1:N}\}$ be the training videos, where $y_i \in Y$ is the action label of video x_i, and the unobserved action locations $\{h_i\}_{i=1:N}$ of videos are treated as latent variables in our model. The latent variable h_i specifies a local spatiotemporal region in video x_i. Our method aims to learn a discriminative compatibility function $F(x, y)$ which measures how compatible the action label y is suited to an input video x:

$$F(x, y) = \max_{h} f_\omega(x, y, h),$$

$$f_\omega(x, y, h) = \omega^T \Phi(x, y, h),$$

where ω is the learned parameter of the model, and $\Phi(x, y, h)$ is a joint feature vector which describes the relationship between the action video x, the action label y, and the latent action location h.

The model parameter includes two parts $\omega = \{\alpha; \beta\}$. The relationship between an action video x, an action label y and the latent region h is formulated as

$$\begin{aligned} \omega^T \Phi(x, y, h) &= \alpha^T \varphi_1(x, y) + \beta^T \varphi_2(x, h, y), \\ \alpha^T \varphi_1(x, y) &= \sum_{t=1}^{N_y} \alpha_t^T \cdot \phi(x) \cdot \mathbf{I}(y = t), \\ \beta^T \varphi_2(x, h, y) &= \sum_{t=1}^{N_y} \beta_t^T \cdot \psi(x, h) \cdot \mathbf{I}(y = t), \end{aligned} \tag{5}$$

where $\mathbf{I}(y = t)$ is an indicator function, with $\mathbf{I}(y = t) = 1$ if $y = t$ and 0 otherwise. The potential function $\alpha^T \varphi_1(x, y)$ captures the global relationship between an action video x and the action label y, where $\phi(x)$ denotes a mid-level representation obtained by the random clustering forest using low-level trajectory descriptors extracted from the whole video. The potential function $\beta^T \varphi_2(x, h, y)$ measures the compatibility between a local region h and the action label y, where $\psi(x, h)$ is also a mid-level feature vector, but only using low-level trajectory descriptors extracted from a local region of x specified by the latent variable h.

4.3 Learning

Given a set of weakly labeled training videos $\mathcal{D}^V = \{(x_i, y_i)_{i=1:N}\}$ and a few Web images $\mathcal{D}^I = \{(x_j^I, y_j^I, h_j^I)_{j=1:M}\}$, where $y_j^I \in Y$ is the action label of image x_j^I and h_j^I indicates the spatial location of the person, our goal is to learn the model parameter ω. Since the unobserved action locations of training videos

$\{h_i\}_{i=1:N}$ are treated as latent variables, the model is formulated in a latent structural SVM framework for learning:

$$\min_{\omega,\xi_i,\xi_j^I,\xi_i^s} \frac{1}{2}\|\omega\|^2 + C_1\sum_{i=1}^{N}\xi_i + C_2\sum_{j=1}^{M}\xi_j^I + C_3\sum_{i=1}^{N}\xi_i^S, \tag{6}$$

$$\text{s.t.} \quad f_\omega(x_i, y_i, h_i) - f_\omega(x_i, y', h') \geq \Delta(y_i, y') - \xi_i; \forall y', \forall h', \forall i; \tag{7}$$

$$g_\omega(x_j^I, y_j, h_j) - g_\omega(x_j^I, y', h_j) \geq \Delta(y_j, y') - \xi_j^I; \forall y', \forall j; \tag{8}$$

$$\min_{j:y_i=y_j} \frac{1}{Z_{x_i}} \cdot \Theta((x_i, h_i), (x_j^I, h_j)) \leq \xi_i^S \tag{9}$$

where ξ_i and ξ_i^S are slack variables for training video x_i, and ξ_j^I is the slack variable for Web image x_j^I. The normalization factor Z_{x_i} for video x_i is defined by

$$Z_{x_i} = \max_h \min_{j:y_i=y_j} \Theta((x_i, h), (x_j^I, h_j)). \tag{10}$$

Equation 7 represents the usual latent SVM max margin constraints which optimize ω by classifying training videos correctly. The loss function $\Delta(y, y')$ measures the cost of predicting the truth label y as action label y'. We define $\Delta(y, y')$ as a simple Hamming loss: $\Delta(y, y')$ is 1 if $y \neq y'$ and 0 otherwise.

Equation 8 denotes the max margin constraints for the transferred Web images. The constraints defined in Eqs. 7 and 8 compel the model to classify both the Web images and the training videos. Different from the training videos, the Web images are annotated with the regions of actions, therefore Eq. 8 does not include any latent variables. $g_\omega(x^I, y, h)$ is the score function for Web images, defined by

$$g_\omega(x^I, y, h) = \sum_{t=1}^{N_y} \alpha_t^T \cdot \mathbf{A} \cdot \phi(x^I) + \sum_{t=1}^{N_y} \beta_t^T \cdot \mathbf{A} \cdot \psi(x^I, h).$$

where $\mathbf{A}$ is a learned mapping matrix transforming the image feature space to the video feature space, as Web images and videos are represented by heterogeneous features with different dimensions.

Equation 9 enforces the local similarities between training videos and Web images, which means that the latent regions of training videos should resemble the regions of actions annotated in Web images. According to this constraint, TLSVM model is inclined to choose latent regions with more similarity or less distance to the annotated local regions of images, which benefits both classification and localization. Here we define the loss function $\Theta((x_i, h_i), (x_j^I, h_j^I))$ as a pair-wise distance to estimate the similarity between a local region of image and a latent region of video, which can be directly calculated using mapping matrix $\mathbf{A}$ as

$$\Theta((x_i, h_i), (x_j^I, h_j^I)) = d(\psi(x_i, h_i), \mathbf{A} \cdot \psi(x_j^I, h_j^I)),$$

A variety of distance functions can be employed to measure the similarity between a video and an image, and we adopt the χ^2 distance which is suitable for histogram similarity estimation.

The optimization problem in Eq. 6 is non-convex since the latent variables $\{h_i\}_{i=1:N}$ are not observed during learning. Therefore we employ the non-convex bundle optimization algorithm [21]. This algorithm iteratively builds a gradually accurate piecewise quadratic approximation, and converges to an optimal solution of parameter ω. At each iteration, calculation of the subgradient is required to add a new linear cutting plane to the piecewise quadratic approximation.

The objective function in Eq. 6 can be rewritten in an unconstrained form:

$$O(\omega) = \min_{\omega} \frac{1}{2}\|\omega\|^2 + \sum_{i=1}^{N}(L_i - R_i) + \sum_{j=1}^{M} P_j^I, \tag{11}$$

where L_i, R_i and P_j^I are defined by

$$L_i = C_1 \max_{y',h'}[f_\omega(x_i, y', h') + \Delta(y', y_i)],$$
$$R_i = \max_{h_i}[C_1 f_\omega(x_i, y_i, h_i) - \frac{C_3}{Z_{x_i}} \min_{j} \Theta((x_i, h_i), (x_j^I, h_j))],$$
$$P_j^I = C_2\{\max_{y'}[g_\omega(x_j^I, y', h_j^I) + \Delta(y', y_j)] - g_\omega(x_j^I, y_j, h_j^I)\}.$$

Assume that (y_i^*, h_i^*), h_i and y_j^* are solutions to L_i, R_i, and P_j^I, respectively, the subgradient of $O(\omega)$ in Eq. 11 can be calculated by

$$\begin{aligned}\partial_\omega(O(\omega)) =& C_1 \sum_{i=1}^{N}(\Phi(x_i, y_i^*, h_i^*) - \Phi(x_i, y_i, h_i)) \\ &+ C_2 \sum_{j=1}^{M}(\Phi(x_j^I, y_j^*, h_j^I) - \Phi(x_j^I, y_j, h_j^I)).\end{aligned}$$

We enumerate y', h' and h_i to find the optimal (y_i^*, h_i^*), h_i and y_j^*.

4.4 Inference

With the learned parameter ω, the inference problem is to simultaneously find the best action label y^* and the best latent region h^* given an input video x. The inference is equal to the following optimization problem:

$$(y^*, h^*) = \arg\max_{y,h} \omega^T \Phi(x, y, h). \tag{12}$$

We can solve Eq. 12 by enumerating all the possible action labels y and latent regions h for a test video x, as the set of possible values for y and h is limited.

5 Experiments

5.1 Dataset and Settings

We evaluate our method on the UCF sports dataset [22] and the Olympic sports dataset [23]. The UCF sports dataset contains 150 sports videos of 10 different

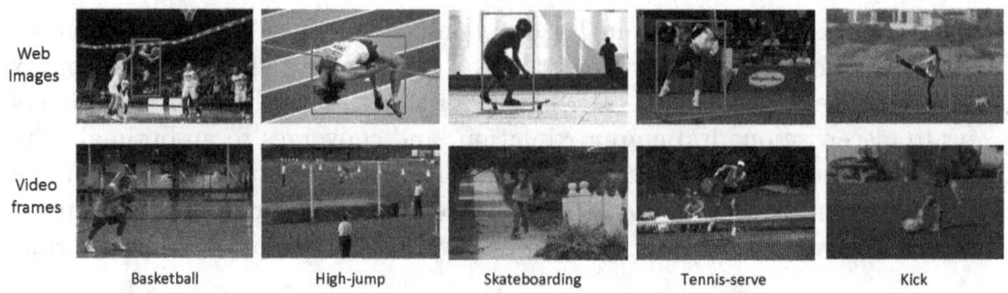

Fig. 3. Examples of the web images and the video frames.

human actions. Videos in this dataset are extracted from sports broadcasts, and bounding boxes of the person performing the action are provided for each frame. The test strategy proposed in [7] is adopted, in which one third of the videos are selected for testing, leaving the rest for training. The Olympic sports dataset consists of 783 sports videos of 16 action classes. Complex sports actions, drastic camera motions, poor light and large variations of human appearance augment the difficulty of both action recognition and localization. The whole dataset is split into 649 videos for training and 134 videos for testing. We annotate the Olympic sports dataset with bounding boxes in order to quantify our localization performance. We use Image Search Engine to download images from the Web taking the action class labels as query keywords, and annotate a bounding box around the person of interest for each Web image. Examples of the Web images are shown in Fig. 3.

In our implementation, HOG and MBH descriptors of dense trajectory [16] are extracted from videos, and HOG descriptors are densely sampled from the Web images. We randomly select 100,000 training descriptors to build the clustering forests for videos and images. The clustering forest of Web images consists of five trees, and the depth of each tree is limited to 12. The clustering forest of videos consists of five trees, and the depth of each tree is limited to sixteen and eleven for the UCF sports dataset and the Olympic sports dataset, respectively.

We compare the proposed approach with three baseline methods:

Global linear SVM model without images. It only considers the first potential function $\alpha^T \varphi_1(x, y)$ in Eq. 5, which captures the global relationship between a video x and the action label y. A linear SVM classifier is trained on the global representations of training videos. Note that this method can only assign an action label to a test video, without predicting the location of person.

Latent SVM model without images. It is similar to our method, except that no Web images are employed. Regions of interest are also treated as latent variables, but the local similarities between training videos and Web images are not enforced in this model. Particularly, only the parameter ω under the constraint in Eq. 7 is optimized, and the constraints in Eqs. 8 and 9 are neglected.

TLSVM model using frames from the training videos. Instead of using Web images, this baseline method employs frames randomly selected from the

Table 1. Action recognition accuracy comparison with three baselines.

Method	UCF	Olympic
Linear SVM	0.711	0.643
Latent SVM	0.794	0.695
TLSVM (Video frames)	0.844	0.715
TLSVM (Web images)	0.869	0.727

Table 2. Mean action recognition accuracy of each class for different methods on the UCF sports dataset.

Method	Accuracy
Lan et al. [7]	0.731
Shapovalova et al. [9]	0.753
Raptis et al. [8]	0.794
Ma et al. [10]	0.817
Our method	0.869

training videos to learn the model. With this baseline method, we aim to assess the benefit of introducing Web images for training.

5.2 Experimental Results

Action Recognition. The proposed approach is compared with the three baseline methods, and the results are summarized in Table 1. It is observable that the proposed approach significantly improves the recognition accuracy compared with the first two baseline methods, which demonstrates the effectiveness of leveraging annotated images for training the model. Meanwhile, our method performs slightly better than the third baseline method, in which the Web images are replaced by images selected from the training videos. A major cause of the performance improvement is that our method avoids the problem of overfitting. Furthermore, the Latent SVM method achieves better performance than the Linear SVM method, which leads a conclusion that incorporating local spatiotemporal information benefits the recognition of action videos.

Table 2 compares the proposed approach with state-of-the-art methods [7–10] on the UCF sports dataset. As is shown in Table 2, our approach achieves the best result among all the listed methods. We also compare our method with other methods on the Olympic sports dataset. We evaluate the mean average precision for all categories and show the results of different methods in Table 3. It is observable that the proposed method achieves better performance than the methods listed in Table 3.

Action Localization. We adopt the evaluation criterion in [7] and compute the ROC curves of each action class. Given a video, the IOU (intersection-over-union) score is computed for each frame, and the average IOU score over all test

Table 3. Mean Average Precision (MAP) of each class for different methods on the Olympic Sports dataset.

Method	MAP
Niebles et al. [23]	0.625
Tang et al. [24]	0.668
Liu et al. [25]	0.743
Li et al. [26]	0.765
Our method	0.771

frames is compared to a predefined threshold ν to decide whether this video is successfully localized. A test video is considered to be correctly predicted if it is correctly classified and the average IOU score is larger than ν. The action localization results on the UCF sports dataset and the Olympic sports dataset are shown in Fig. 4 and Fig. 5, respectively. Figures 4(a) and 5(a) depict the average ROC curves for all action classes with $\nu = 0.2$. The Area Under ROC curve (AUC) is evaluated with ν varying from 0.1 to 0.5, and the curves are shown in Figs. 4(b) and 5(b).

From Figs. 4 and 5, we can see that our method outperforms the last two baseline methods, which demonstrates the effectiveness of introducing the Web images for learning. Our method is also compared with the method of [7] on the UCF sports dataset. As is shown in Fig. 4, although [7] is trained on videos annotated with bounding boxes for each frame, our method could outperform [7] by using a few annotated images. Moreover, in many cases, the proposed approach using Web images performs better than the third baseline method which employs images from training data, especially for $\nu = 0.2$. These results demonstrate the positive effect of introducing Web images into training for action localization.

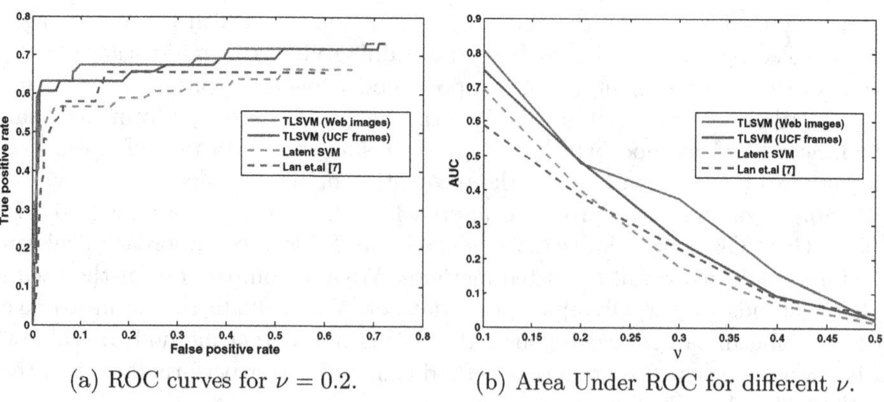

(a) ROC curves for $\nu = 0.2$. (b) Area Under ROC for different ν.

Fig. 4. Comparison of action localization performance on the UCF sports dataset.

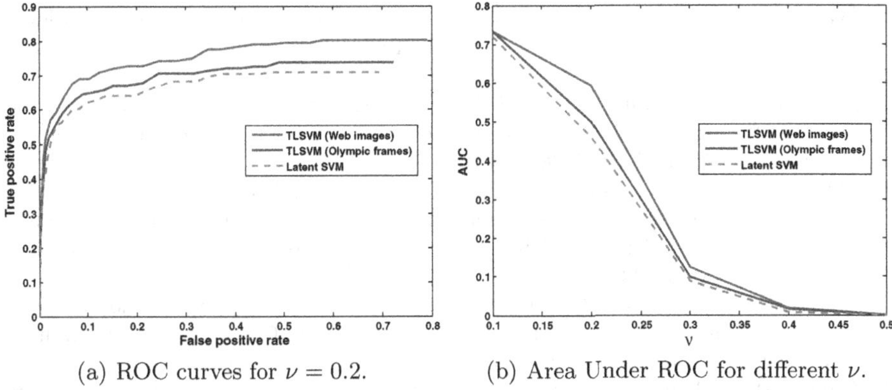

(a) ROC curves for $\nu = 0.2$. (b) Area Under ROC for different ν.

Fig. 5. Comparison of action localization performance on the Olympic sports dataset.

6 Conclusions

We have presented a discriminative Transfer Latent Support Vector Machine (TLSVM) for jointly recognizing and localizing actions in videos. The model is trained on videos only annotated with action labels, and a few Web images annotated with both action labels and action locations are introduced into the learning framework. The spatiotemporal region capturing the action being performed is treated as a latent variable in the proposed model. Since images and videos are represented by different types of features, we introduce a structural transformation that maps images to videos. Experimental results on the UCF sports dataset and the Olympic sports dataset demonstrate that our model can effectively recognize and localize actions in videos.

Acknowledgement. The research was supported in part by the Natural Science Foundation of China (NSFC) under Grant 61203274, the Specialized Research Fund for the Doctoral Program of Higher Education of China (20121101120029), the Specialized Fund for Joint Building Program of Beijing Municipal Education Commission and the Excellent Young Scholars Research Fund of Beijing Institute of Technology.

References

1. Efros, A.A., Berg, A.C., Mori, G., Malik, J.: Recognizing action at a distance. In: IEEE International Conference on Computer Vision, pp. 726–733 (2003)
2. Niebles, J.C., Fei-Fei, L.: A hierarchical model of shape and appearance for human action classification. In: IEEE Conference on Computer Vision and Pattern Recognition (CVPR), pp. 1–8 (2007)
3. Laptev, I., Marszalek, M., Schmid, C., Rozenfeld, B.: Learning realistic human actions from movies. In: IEEE Conference on Computer Vision and Pattern Recognition (CVPR), pp. 1–8 (2008)

4. Wu, X., Xu, D., Duan, L., Luo, J., Jia, Y.: Action recognition using multilevel features and latent structural svm. IEEE Trans. Circ. Syst. Video Technol. **23**, 1422–1431 (2013)
5. Yao, A., Gall, J., Van Gool, L.: A hough transform-based voting framework for action recognition. In: IEEE Conference on Computer Vision and Pattern Recognition (CVPR), pp. 2061–2068 (2010)
6. Oikonomopoulos, A., Patras, I., Pantic, M.: An implicit spatiotemporal shape model for human activity localization and recognition. In: IEEE Computer Society Conference on Computer Vision and Pattern Recognition Workshops (CVPR Workshops), pp. 27–33 (2009)
7. Lan, T., Wang, Y., Mori, G.: Discriminative figure-centric models for joint action localization and recognition. In: IEEE International Conference on Computer Vision (ICCV), pp. 2003–2010 (2011)
8. Raptis, M., Kokkinos, I., Soatto, S.: Discovering discriminative action parts from mid-level video representations. In: IEEE Conference on Computer Vision and Pattern Recognition (CVPR), pp. 1242–1249 (2012)
9. Shapovalova, N., Vahdat, A., Cannons, K., Lan, T., Mori, G.: Similarity constrained latent support vector machine: an application to weakly supervised action classification. In: Fitzgibbon, A., Lazebnik, S., Perona, P., Sato, Y., Schmid, C. (eds.) ECCV 2012, Part VII. LNCS, vol. 7578, pp. 55–68. Springer, Heidelberg (2012)
10. Ma, S., Zhang, J., Ikizler-Cinbis, N., Sclaroff, S.: Action recognition and localization by hierarchical space-time segments. In: IEEE International Conference on Computer Vision (2013)
11. Duan, L., Xu, D., Chang, S.F.: Exploiting web images for event recognition in consumer videos: a multiple source domain adaptation approach. In: IEEE Conference on Computer Vision and Pattern Recognition (CVPR), pp. 1338–1345 (2012)
12. Chen, L., Duan, L., Xu, D.: Event recognition in videos by learning from heterogeneous web sources. In: IEEE Conference on Computer Vision and Pattern Recognition (CVPR), pp. 2666–2673 (2013)
13. Ikizler-Cinbis, N., Sclaroff, S.: Web-based classifiers for human action recognition. IEEE Trans. Multimed. **14**, 1031–1045 (2012)
14. Moosmann, F., Nowak, E., Jurie, F.: Randomized clustering forests for image classification. IEEE Trans. Pattern Anal. Mach. Intell. **30**, 1632–1646 (2008)
15. Dalal, N., Triggs, B.: Histograms of oriented gradients for human detection. In: IEEE Conference on Computer Vision and Pattern Recognition (CVPR), pp. 886–893 (2005)
16. Wang, H., Klaser, A., Schmid, C., Liu, C.L.: Action recognition by dense trajectories. In: IEEE Conference on Computer Vision and Pattern Recognition (CVPR), pp. 3169–3176 (2011)
17. Alexe, B., Deselaers, T., Ferrari, V.: Measuring the objectness of image windows. IEEE Trans. Pattern Anal. Mach. Intell. **34**, 2189–2202 (2012)
18. Leordeanu, M., Sukthankar, R., Sminchisescu, C.: Efficient closed-form solution to generalized boundary detection. In: Fitzgibbon, A., Lazebnik, S., Perona, P., Sato, Y., Schmid, C. (eds.) ECCV 2012, Part IV. LNCS, vol. 7575, pp. 516–529. Springer, Heidelberg (2012)
19. Liu, C.: Beyond pixels: exploring new representations and applications for motion analysis. Ph.D. thesis, Massachusetts Institute of Technology (2009)
20. Frey, B.J., Dueck, D.: Clustering by passing messages between data points. Sci. Am. Assoc. Adv. sci. **315**, 972–976 (2007). American Association for the Advancement of Science

21. Do, T.M.T., Artières, T.: Large margin training for hidden markov models with partially observed states. In: Proceedings of the 26th Annual International Conference on Machine Learning, pp. 265–272 (2009)
22. Rodriguez, M., Ahmed, J., Shah, M.: Action mach: a spatio-temporal maximum average correlation height filter for action recognition. In: IEEE Conference on Computer vision and pattern recognition (CVPR), pp. 1–8 (2008)
23. Niebles, J.C., Chen, C.-W., Fei-Fei, L.: Modeling temporal structure of decomposable motion segments for activity classification. In: Daniilidis, K., Maragos, P., Paragios, N. (eds.) ECCV 2010, Part II. LNCS, vol. 6312, pp. 392–405. Springer, Heidelberg (2010)
24. Tang, K., Fei-Fei, L., Koller, D.: Learning latent temporal structure for complex event detection. In: IEEE Conference on Computer Vision and Pattern Recognition (CVPR), pp. 1250–1257 (2012)
25. Liu, J., Kuipers, B., Savarese, S.: Recognizing human actions by attributes. In: IEEE Conference on Computer Vision and Pattern Recognition (CVPR), pp. 3337–3344 (2011)
26. Li, W., Vasconcelos, N.: Recognizing activities by attribute dynamics. In: NIPS, pp. 1115–1123 (2012)

A Game-Theoretic Probabilistic Approach for Detecting Conversational Groups

Sebastiano Vascon[1(✉)], Eyasu Zemene Mequanint[2], Marco Cristani[1,3], Hayley Hung[4], Marcello Pelillo[2], and Vittorio Murino[1,3]

[1] Department of Pattern Analysis and Computer Vision (PAVIS), Istituto Italiano di Tecnologia, Genova, Italy
sebastiano.vascon@iit.it

[2] Department of Environmental Sciences, Informatics and Statistics, University Ca' Foscari of Venice, Venezia, Italy

[3] Department of Computer Science, University of Verona, Verona, Italy

[4] Faculty of Electrical Engineering, Mathematics and Computer Science, Technical University of Delft, Delft, The Netherlands

Abstract. A standing conversational group (also known as F-formation) occurs when two or more people sustain a social interaction, such as chatting at a cocktail party. Detecting such interactions in images or videos is of fundamental importance in many contexts, like surveillance, social signal processing, social robotics or activity classification. This paper presents an approach to this problem by modeling the socio-psychological concept of an F-formation and the biological constraints of social attention. Essentially, an F-formation defines some constraints on how subjects have to be mutually located and oriented while the biological constraints defines the plausible zone in which persons can interact. We develop a game-theoretic framework embedding these constraints, which is supported by a statistical modeling of the uncertainty associated with the position and orientation of people. First, we use a novel representation of the affinity between pairs of people expressed as a distance between distributions over the most plausible oriented region of attention.Additionally, we integrate temporal information over multiple frames to smooth noisy head orientation and pose estimates, solve ambiguous situations and establish a more precise social context. We do this in a principled way by using recent notions from multi-payoff evolutionary game theory. Experiments on several benchmark datasets consistently show the superiority of the proposed approach over state of the art and its robustness under severe noise conditions.

Electronic supplementary material The online version of this chapter (doi:10.1007/978-3-319-16814-2_43) contains supplementary material, which is available to authorized users. Videos can also be accessed at http://www.springerimages.com/videos/978-3-319-16813-5.

H. Hung—Author has been partially supported by the European Commission under contract number FP7-ICT-600877 (SPENCER) and is affiliated with the Delft Data Science consortium.

D. Cremers et al. (Eds.): ACCV 2014, Part V, LNCS 9007, pp. 658–675, 2015.
DOI: 10.1007/978-3-319-16814-2_43

1 Introduction

After decades of research on the automated modeling of individuals, the computer vision community has recently started focusing on the new problem of analyzing groups [1–10]. In this paper, we focus on standing conversational groups, also known as *F-formations* [11], that is, groups of people who spontaneously decide to be in each other's immediate presence to converse with each and every member of that group. Standing conversational groups are of primary importance in many contexts, from video surveillance [7] to social signal processing [1,2,4,6], from multimedia [3] to social robotics [12] and activity recognition, as we will discuss extensively in Sect. 2. Many studies have been carried out by social psychologists to understand how people behave in public. By exploiting the theory behind these findings, we propose novel and more socio-psychologically principled ways of designing methods for automatically analyzing human behavior. For example, Hall [13] proposed that relationships and levels of interactions could be inferred by considering different social distances. Goffman [14] observed that group interactions can be categorized into those that are 'focused' and those that are 'unfocused'. Focused interactions concern the gathering of people to participate in an activity where there is a common focus, such as playing and watching a football match, conversing, or marching in a band. Unfocused encounters involves light interactions such as avoiding people on a street, briefly greeting a colleague while passing them in the corridor, or indicating to let someone pass when boarding a train.

Within the class of focused encounters, the F-formation is a specific type of group interaction which requires more attention from our senses. Specifically, an F-formation arises "whenever two or more individuals in close proximity orient their bodies in such a way that each of them has an easy, direct and equal access to every other participant's transactional segment, and when they maintain such an arrangement" [15, p. 243]. Some example of F-formations from real-world images are illustrated in Fig. 1a. There can be different F-formations as shown in Fig. 2a–e. In the case of two participants, typical F-formation arrangements are vis-a-vis, L-shape, and side-by-side. From an F-formation, three social spaces emerge: the o-space, the p-space and the r-space. The most important part is the o-space

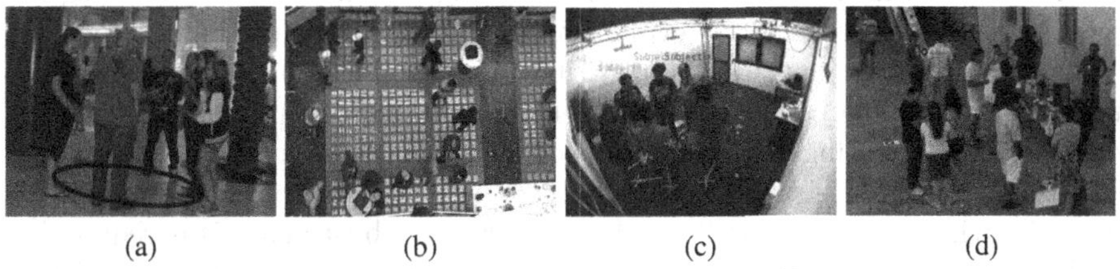

(a) (b) (c) (d)

Fig. 1. Standing conversational groups: (a) in black, graphical depiction of overlapping space within an F-formation: the o-space; (b) a poster session in a conference, where different groupings are visible; (c) circular F-formation; (d) a typical surveillance setting where camera is located at 2.5–3 m from the floor, for which detecting groups is challenging.

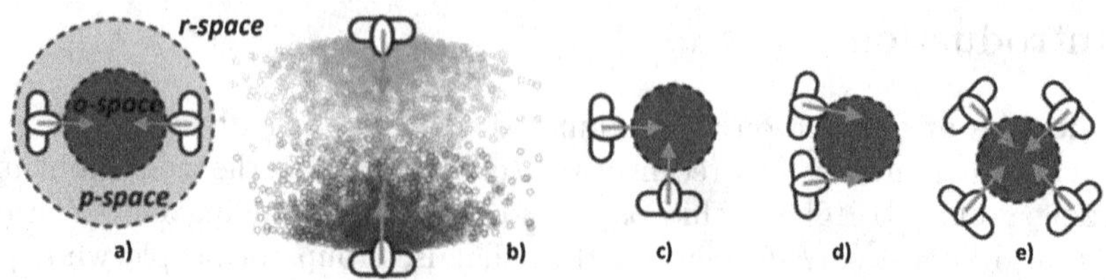

Fig. 2. F-formations; (a) components of an F-formation: o-space, p-space, r-space; in this case, a face-to-face F-formation is sketched; (b) modeling the frustum of attention by particles: in the intersection stays the o-space; (c) L-shape F-formation; (d) side-by-side F-formation; (e) circular F-formation.

(see Fig. 2), a convex empty space surrounded by the people involved in a social interaction, in which every participant looks inward, and no external people are allowed. The p-space is a narrow strip that surrounds the o-space, and that contains the bodies of the conversing people, while the r-space is the area beyond the p-space.

Our goal in this paper is to develop a robust approach to automatically detect F-formations from images and videos employing a single monocular camera. As input, the approach requires the position of the persons in the scene on the ground plane as well as their body orientation, although in most cases, head orientation is more readily captured, even under heavy occlusion. These cues are easily obtainable nowadays, even if they are not estimated very accurately, and many approaches are devoted to these goals [4,16,17]. A recent experimental work of Setti et al. [18] shows that substantial improvement in the performance of F-formation detection algorithms can be achieved by combining a probabilistic approach such as the one developed in [7] and graph-based clustering methods [6]. Motivated by these findings, we develop a new, robust, psychologically-principled approach which combines in a natural way the modeling of the uncertainty in the position and orientation of a subject and a game-theoretic clustering approach which allows one to extract coherent groups in edge-weighted graphs, digraphs and hypergraphs [19,20]. The game-theoretic setting provides a conceptual framework which allows also us to integrate temporal information in a principled way, in an attempt to reliably extract groups in video sequences under severe tracking noise. This is done by using a recent approach to integrate multiple payoff functions in an evolutionary game-theoretic setting [21].

Our approach is a substantial contribution for the computer vision community: so far, grouping behaviors have been analyzed mainly in dynamic situation via tracking, exploiting the oriented velocity as a primary cue, for example by associating individuals' tracklets [22–30]. In our case, F-formation are manifested primarily when people are still, so that a finer yet robust analysis is required.

To test the effectiveness of the proposed approach, we performed extensive experiments over five different datasets, each of which represents a particular scenario. In particular, we used a synthetic dataset [7], the Coffee Break dataset [7], the GDet dataset [7], the Idiap Poster data dataset [6], and the Cocktail Party [5] dataset. We also carried out systematic noise resistance experiments to fully investigate the stability of our method. The results consistently show the superiority of the proposed approach over the state of the art.

The rest of the paper is organized as follows. A detailed review of the literature on group detection approaches is presented in Sect. 2. Our approach is detailed in Sect. 3. In Sect. 4 we describe the game-theoretic clustering approach we use to extract F-formations and its extension to multiple affinity matrices. Finally, Sect. 5 presents the experimental results and Sect. 6 concludes the paper.

2 Literature Review

2.1 Groups

During multi-party activities, we expect that there is a different underlying structure that governs the behavior of groups compared to individuals acting independently. For example, there has been considerable prior work on estimating group activities by modeling behavior at the individual as well as group level [8–10]. However, unlike works that treat all group structures equivalently, our premise is that there are fundamental semantic differences in what this prior work has considered to be a 'group' and what we refer (from the social psychological literature) as an 'F-formation' [11]. These prior definitions of a group of people assume that they are necessarily close together because they are for example, forming a queue, watching a football match, crossing the road together, or asked to mingle in a specific location. Some of these principles informed early socially-motivated methods of people tracking [31] by the social force model [32], that originated from pedestrian simulation research.

In more semantically meaningful social cases, one can attribute meaning to groupings based on some form of acquaintanceship, such as for detecting when people are traveling together [24] or when people are conversing in a lecture hall [2]. However in free standing scenarios, when people come together physically in order to make conversation, a specific, unspoken, and mutual agreement is made between all those involved that they wish to converse for some extended but finite period of time. Such an interaction requires a focusing of the senses, compared to the other group behaviors which can rely more on peripheral and unfocused sensing.

Importantly, the region in front of the body in which limbs can reach easily, and hearing and sight is most effective was defined as the *transactional segment*. A necessary condition of the F-formation was that the transactional segments of all members of an F-formation should overlap. Such a region can be considered an individual's frustum of social attention.

2.2 Exploiting Visual Attention

Considering this idea of frustum of attention, computer vision researchers have considered how the head pose can be used as a proxy for visual attention [33]. For visually led tasks such as looking at adverts [33], considering the visual attentional mechanisms is useful. However, when considering social contexts, the concept of social attention is a relatively new domain in the social sciences [34]. More specifically, head pose is actually equally if not more perceptually salient as a cue for gaze direction in humans [34, Ch. 6]. Moreover Kendon studied the role of gaze direction during conversational interactions suggesting that it functions as a cue for turn-taking, holding, or yielding [35]. Jovanovic and Op den Akker also found that addressees could be identified using gazing cues [36], while Duncan found that speakers attracted the gaze of listeners [37] during conversations. Ba and Odobez [38] exploited findings in primate social behavior by modeling plausible eye-in-head positions for gaze estimation to estimate the visual focus of attention of participants during meetings using only head pose while Subramanian et al. [39] used both gaze and head pose to estimate social attention in meetings.

2.3 Conversational Groups Detection

For the specific task of detecting F-formations, different approaches have been proposed. Groh et al. [1] proposed to use the relative shoulder orientations and distances (using markers attached to the shoulders) between each pair of people as a feature vector for training a binary classification task. Cristani et al. [7] proposed to solve the task using a Hough voting strategy which accumulated a density estimating the location of the o-space. Concurrently, Hung and Kröse [6] proposed to consider an F-formation as a dominant-set cluster [40] of an edge-weighted graph where each node in the graph was a person, and the edges between them measures the affinity between pairs.

Later these two approaches were compared by Setti et al. [18] to investigate the strengths and weaknesses of both approaches for the F-formation task. They found that while the method of Cristani et al. [7] was more stable using head orientation information in the presence of noise, the method of Hung and Kröse [6] performed better when only position (and not orientation) information was available. Setti et al. [41] also proposed to handle the physical effect that different cardinalities of the F-formations sizes would have on the most plausible physical spatial layout of each member of the group. By taking this into account using separate accumulation spaces for each size, they were able to improve over the original Hough voting strategy proposed in [7]. A similar density-based approach has also been proposed by Gan et al. [3] where the final purpose of the task was to dynamically select camera angles for automated event recording. Tran et al. have subsequently analyzed temporal patterns of activities [10].

3 Our Approach

Given a dataset of frames with positions of the persons and head/body orientations, the pipeline of the algorithm can be summarized in the following steps:

1. For each person $p_i \in P$ in a frame/scene, generate a frustum f_i based on his position and orientation as modeled by a 2-dimensional histogram (see Sect. 3.1).

2. Compute a pairwise affinity matrix for each $p_i \in P$ (see Sect. 3.2).
3. Extract F-formation (clusters) using evolutionary stable strategy-clusters (see Sect. 4).

3.1 Frustum of Attention Modeling

Our frustum of social attention is inspired by Kendon's definition of a transactional segment. This takes into account both the field of view of the person and also the locus of attention of all other senses for a given body orientation. Since it is typically easier to obtain head pose rather than body or gaze orientation in crowded environments (due to occlusions), the head pose provides an approximation of the direction of the social attention frustum. It is characterized by a direction θ (which is the person's head orientation), an aperture α (we used $\alpha = 160°$ which was reported by Ba and Odobez [38], who used the same measure for approximating the range of possible eye gaze directions given a specific head pose) and a length l. These three elements determine the socio-attentional frustum of a person. Given the parameters (θ, α and l) the frustum is modeled as a 2-dimensional (x and y position in the ground plane) Gaussian distribution in which each of the dimensions are generated independently. The parameter l corresponds to the variance of the Gaussian distribution centered around the location of a person. Therefore, a denser sampling is possible at locations closer to the person and decrease in density further away (after $3 * \sigma$ the number of sample are close to zero). The frustum is generated by drawing samples from the above Gaussian kernel and by keeping only those that fall within the cone (see Fig. 3). Given a person located at $p(x, y)$, with head orientation θ, a sample $s(x, y)$ is inside the frustum if

$$acos\left(\frac{s \cdot f_L}{||s|| * l}\right) \leq \frac{\alpha}{2} \tag{1}$$

where $f_L = \{\cos(\theta) * l, \sin(\theta) * l\}$ is the line of symmetry of the frustrum, a vector of length l and angle θ. This sampling process is iterated until the

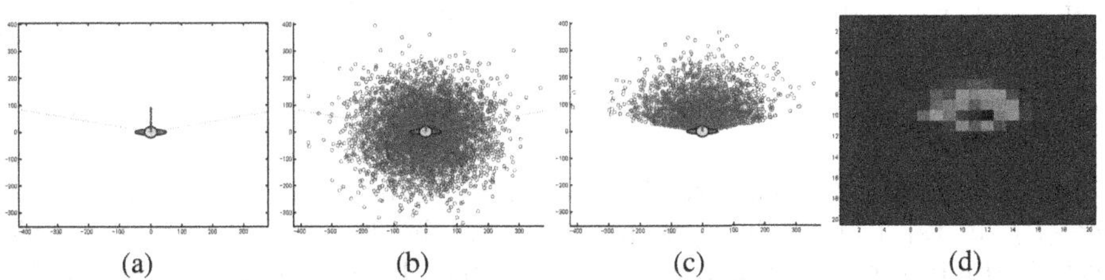

(a) (b) (c) (d)

Fig. 3. In figure is shown the process of generating the frustum: (a) given the i-th person position and orientation a cone of aperture $\alpha = 160°$ is over imposed (b) the 2D Gaussian set of samples are generated (c) only the biologically feasible samples are kept (d) binning of the space on a 20×20 grid to get the final histogram representation h_i.

desired number of samples that falls in the cone is reached. The region that these samples represent intuitively models the transactional segment of a person. Each person in a scene is thus modeled using his frustum represented as 2-dimensional histogram h_i of size $N_c \times N_r$ normalized by the number of samples (s), where N_c and N_r span over the area of the scene captured by the camera. Experimentally, changing the value of the granularity such that $N_c \times N_r = 400, 2500, 10000$ did not change the overall performance (on the benchmarks we tried). Therefore, we keep the granularity fixed at 400 bins.

3.2 Quantifying Pairwise Interactions

Two persons are more likely to be interacting if their social attention frustums overlap. By quantifying the pairwise interaction as a distance between distributions, we are able to encode the uncertainty about the true transactional segment of the person given their head pose. Since we are dealing with histograms that represent discrete probability distributions, it is natural to consider information-theoretic measures to model the distance between them.

Given a pair of discrete probability distributions $P = \{p_1, \dots, p_n\}$ and $Q = \{q_1, \dots, q_n\}$, the first natural choice to measure their distance is given by the well-known Kullback-Leibler (KL) divergence, which is defined as:

$$D(P||Q) = \sum_{i=1}^{n} \log p_i \frac{p_i}{q_i} \tag{2}$$

The KL-divergence is known to be asymmetric. A symmetric version of the KL-divergence measure is the Jensen-Shannon (JS) divergence, which is defined as:

$$J(P, Q) = \frac{D(P||M) + D(Q||M)}{2} \tag{3}$$

where $M = \frac{1}{2}(P + Q)$ is the mid-point between P and Q. Hence, given two persons i and j in a scene and their vectorized histograms h_i and h_j, the distance between i and j can be calculated either as $D(h_i||h_j)$ or as $JS(h_i, h_j)$.

To obtain a measure of affinity, rather than distance, between each pair of histograms we used the classical Gaussian kernel:

$$\gamma(i, j) = \exp\left\{-\frac{d(h_i, h_j)}{\sigma}\right\} \tag{4}$$

where the funtion "*d*" refers to either the KL- or the JS-divergence. The parameter σ in Eq. 4 allows intrinsic properties of the scene (e.g., how far people usually stand from each other when they are in an F-formation) to be taken into account. Once we calculate this measure, it becomes possible to find groups of persons that are interacting by exploiting a grouping game, as described in the next section.

4 Grouping as a Non-cooperative Game

In this work we cast the approach proposed in [19,20] in the problem of detecting F-formations in terms of a non-cooperative *clustering game*. We choose this clustering algorithm for a series of nice properties:

- The distance function is not required to be symmetric, e.g. the Kullback-Leibler divergence.
- An a-priori number of clusters, like k-means, is not needed to be set since the algorithm let the cluster to emerge by data similarities. This represents a necessary condition since the number of groups in a scene is unknown.
- It search for maximal clique in a weighted graph which is an accepted definition of F-formation in the computer science community [6].
- Game-theory domain provides us the theoretical foundation to integrates multiple payoff matrices, thing of valuable importance when dealing with different temporal instants (see Sect. 4.1).

Given a set of elements $O = \{1 \dots n\}$ and an $n \times n$ (possibly asymmetric) affinity matrix $A = (a_{ij})$ which quantifies the pairwise similarities between the objects in O, we envisage a situation whereby two players play a game which consists of simultaneously selecting an element from O. After showing their choice the players get a reward which is proportional to the similarity of the chosen elements. In game-theoretic jargon the elements of set O are the "pure strategies" available to both players and the affinity matrix A represents the "payoff" function (specifically, a_{ij} represents the payoff received by an individual playing strategy i against an opponent playing strategy j). In our application, the objects to to be grouped (namely, the pure strategies of this grouping game) correspond to the persons detected in a scene, the payoff function being the similarity measure between subjects as described in the previous sections.

A central notion in game theory is that of a *mixed strategy*, which is simply a probability distribution $\boldsymbol{x} = (x_1, \dots, x_n)^T$ over the set of pure strategies O. Mixed strategies clearly belong to the $(n-1)$-dimensional standard simplex:

$$\Delta = \left\{ \boldsymbol{x} \in \mathbb{R}^n : \sum_{i=1}^{n} x_i = 1 \text{ and } x_i \geq 0,\ i = 1, \dots, n \right\}. \tag{5}$$

Given a mixed strategy $\boldsymbol{x} \in \Delta$, we define its *support* as $\sigma(\boldsymbol{x}) = \{i \in O : x_i > 0\}$.

The expected payoff received by an individual playing mixed strategy $\boldsymbol{y}$ against an opponent playing mixed strategy $\boldsymbol{x}$ is given by $\boldsymbol{y}^T A \boldsymbol{x}$. The set of *best replies* against a mixed strategy $\boldsymbol{x}$ is defined as $\beta(\boldsymbol{x}) = \{\boldsymbol{y} \in \Delta : \boldsymbol{y}^T A \boldsymbol{x} = \max_{\boldsymbol{z}} \boldsymbol{z}^T A \boldsymbol{x}\}$. Finally, a mixed strategy $\boldsymbol{x} \in \Delta$ is said to be a *Nash equilibrium* if it is a best reply to itself, namely if $\boldsymbol{x} \in \beta(\boldsymbol{x})$ or, in other words, if

$$\boldsymbol{x}^T A \boldsymbol{x} \geq \boldsymbol{y}^T A \boldsymbol{x} \tag{6}$$

for all $\boldsymbol{y} \in \Delta$. If inequality holds strictly, then $\boldsymbol{x}$ is said to be *strict* Nash equilibrium. Intuitively, at a Nash equilibrium no player has an incentive to unilaterally deviate from it. The clustering game is supposed to be played within an evolutionary setting wherein the two players, each of which is assumed to play a pre-assigned strategy, are repeatedly drawn at random from a large population. Here, given a mixed strategy $\boldsymbol{x} \in \Delta$, x_j ($j \in O$) is assumed to represent the proportion of players that is programmed to select pure strategy j. A dynamic evolutionary selection process will then make the population state $\boldsymbol{x}$ evolve according to a survival-of-the-fittest principle in such a way that, eventually, the better-than-average (pure) strategies will survive while the others will get extinct. Within this context, a mixed strategy $\boldsymbol{x} \in \Delta$ is said to be an *evolutionary stable strategy* (ESS) if it is a Nash equilibrium and if, for each best reply $\boldsymbol{y}$ to $\boldsymbol{x}$, we have $\boldsymbol{x}^T A\boldsymbol{y} > \boldsymbol{y}^T A\boldsymbol{y}$. Intuitively, ESS's are strategies such that any small deviation from them will lead to an inferior payoff (see [42] for an excellent introduction to evolutionary game theory).

In [19,20] a combinatorial characterization of ESS's is given which make them plausible candidates for the notion of a cluster (which they call ESS-cluster). The motivation behind this claim resides in the property that ESS-clusters do incorporate the two basic features which characterize a cluster, i.e.,

- *internal coherency*: elements belonging to the cluster should have high mutual similarities;
- *external incoherency*: the overall cluster internal coherency decreases by introducing external elements.

We refer to [19,20] for details. One of the distinguishing features of this approach is its generality as it allows one to deal in a unified framework with a variety of scenarios, including cases with asymmetric, negative, or high-order affinities. Note that, when the affinity matrix A is symmetric (that is, $A = A^T$) the notion of an ESS-cluster coincides with that of a dominant set [40], which amounts to finding a (local) maximizer of $\boldsymbol{x}^T A\boldsymbol{x}$ over the standard simplex Δ.

Algorithmically, to find an ESS-cluster one can use the classical *replicator dynamics* [42], a class of dynamical systems which mimic a Darwinian selection process over the set of pure strategies. The discrete-time version of these dynamics is given by the following update rule:

$$x_i(t+1) = x_i(t)\frac{(A\boldsymbol{x}(t))_i}{\boldsymbol{x}(t)^T A\boldsymbol{x}(t)} \tag{7}$$

for all $i \in O$. The process starts from a point $\boldsymbol{x}(0)$ usually close to the barycenter of the simplex Δ, and it is iterated until convergence (typically when distance between two successive states is smaller than a given threshold). It is clear that the whole dynamical process is driven by the payoff function which, in our case, is defined precisely to favor the evolution of highly coherent objects. Accordingly, the support $\sigma(\boldsymbol{x})$ of the converged population state $\boldsymbol{x}$ does represent a cluster, the non-null components of which providing a measure of the degree of membership of its elements.

The support of an ESS corresponds to the indices of the elements in the same group. To extract all the ESS-clusters we implemented a simple peel-off strategy:

when an ESS-cluster is computed the corresponding elements are removed from the original and the replicator dynamics is executed again on the remaining elements.

4.1 Integrating Multiple Frames in Video Sequences

When dealing with videos, the inter-frame smoothness between consecutive frames can be exploited to face cases of noisy data, such as wrong positions or head orientations. The idea is simply to consider a buffer of K frames: at time t, we will have knowledge of the frames at time $t-K+1,\ldots,t$, which can be used jointly for a more robust group estimation. This keeps the process of group modeling on-line (it can lie on top of the tracking algorithm), while permitting to prune out noise in an effective way. Assuming that the movement of the same person between frames is smooth, given a set of K consecutive frames, the problem is then to somehow integrate the corresponding affinity matrices to perform the grouping process.

From our game-theoretic perspective this problem can be seen in the context of multiple-payoff (or multi-criteria) games, a topic which has been the subject of intensive studies by game theorists since the late 1950's [43–46]. Under this setting, payoffs are no longer scalar quantities but take the form of vectors whose components represent different commodities. Clearly, the main difficulty which arises here is that the players' payoff spaces now can be given only a partial ordering. Although in "classical" game theory several solution concepts have been proposed during the years, the game theory community has typically given little attention to the evolutionary setting. Recently, a solution to this problem has been put forward by Somasundaram and Baras [21] who extended the notion of replicator dynamics and that of an ESS using the concept of Pareto-Nash equilibrium. Another recent attempt towards this direction, though more theoretical in nature, can be found in [47].

In the work reported in this paper, we follow the idea proposed in [21] which provides a principled solution to the problem of integrating multiple payoff functions. Using concepts from multi-criteria linear programming (MCLP) [48] they proposed a notion of Pareto reply and of Pareto-Nash equilibrium and showed the equivalence with "weighted sum scalarization", a classical technique from multi-objective optimization (see, e.g., [48]). Basically, this means that a Pareto-Nash equilibrium can be achieved by integrating the K affinity matrices as follows:

$$\hat{A} = \sum_{i=1}^{K} w_i A_i \tag{8}$$

where the w_i's ($i = 1\ldots K$) represent appropriate non-negative trade-off weights associated to the different matrices, subject to the constraint $\sum_i w_i = 1$. Formulated in this way, the problem of determining a Pareto-Nash equilibrium in a multi-payoff scenario is now reduced to the problem of determining the correct trade-off weights, and this in turn can be done by solving a multi-objective linear programming problem (MOLP). To this end, following [21], in our experiments we used the multi-objective simplex method (we refer the reader to Chap. 7 of [48] and to the original paper [21] for details).

5 Experiments and Results

We carried out experiments considering both the *single* (Sect. 5.3) and *multiple*-frame methods (Sect. 5.4) under ideal and noisy situation. In the former, F-formations are estimated on each single frame independently, while in the latter we perform integration over consecutive frames in order to smoothing noisy detection. Moreover we test the resilience of the method injecting increasing level of noise (Fig. 5). Source code available at http://www.iit.it/en/datasets-and-code/code/gtcg.html.

5.1 Datasets

The five datasets used (see Table 1) are the currently publicly available benchmarks for detecting F-formations, where for each individual in a scene his x, y position and the head orientation are provided. Consecutive frames are available for two of them with a low frame rate. In three cases the annotation has been done via automatic tracking while other two were manually annotated by the respective authors as stated in Table 1.

PosterData [6]: It consists of 3 h of aerial video of over 50 people during a scientific meeting involving poster presentations and a coffee break. 82 distinct image frames were selected based on maximizing differences between images, ambiguity in group membership and varying levels of crowdedness. 21 trained annotators were split into 8 trios who annotated 10–11 images for F-formations, leading to a subjective representation of the ground truth.

CocktailParty [5]: The CocktailParty dataset contains 16 min of video recordings of a cocktail party in a 30 m^2 lab environment involving 7 subjects. The party was recorded using four synchronized angled-view cameras (15 Hz, $1024 \times 768px$, jpeg) installed in the corners of the room. The dataset is challenging for video analysis due to frequent and persistent occlusions, in a highly cluttered scene. Subject's positions and horizontal head orientations were logged using a particle filter-based body tracker with head pose estimation. Groups in one frame every 3 s were annotated manually by an trained expert, resulting in a total of 320 distinct frames for evaluation.

Table 1. Datasets: multiple #Frame indicate diverse sequences, in these cases the final results are averaged over the sequences and normalized by the number of frames.

Dataset	#Sequences	#Frames × seq	Consecutive Frames	Automated Tracking
CoffeeBreak	2	45,74	Y	Y
CocktailParty	1	320	Y	Y
GDet	5	132,115,79,17,60	N	Y
PosterData	82	1	N	N
Synth	10	10	N	N

CoffeeBreak [7]: The dataset focuses on a coffee-break scenario of a social event, with max 14 individuals organized in groups of 2–3 people. People's positions were estimated by exploiting multi-object tracking on the heads, and head detection has been performed afterward, considering solely 4 possible orientations (Front, Back, Left, Right). The tracked positions were projected onto the ground plane. A trained expert annotated the videos indicating the groups present in the scenes (in combination with questionnaires that the subjects filled in about the number of people they spoke with)on two different coffee breaks, for a total of 45 frames for *Seq1* and 75 frames for *Seq2*, acquired in a period of 3 s.

Synth [7]: A trained expert synthesised 10 different *situations*, with F-formation and singletons Each situation is repeated 10 times, with slightly varying position and orientation of the subjects. Here, noise in the position and orientations are absent.

GDet [7]: these videos consider a vending machines area where people take coffee and other drinks, and chat. In this case the head orientation considers solely 4 possible alternatives. Here the frame rate is very low, so that the multiple frame approach cannot be applied.

As comparative approaches, we consider the Hough-based approach of [7] in its renewed version of [18] (HFF), the hierarchical extension of the Hough-based approach of [41] (MULTI), and the dominant-set-based technique of [6](DS). Comparison with other baselines are not reported in Table 2 since are already carried out and overcomed in [7,18].

5.2 Evaluation Metrics and Parameter Exploration

In terms of evaluation, as in [18], we consider a group as correctly estimated if at least $\lceil (T \cdot |G|) \rceil$ of their members are found by the grouping method were correctly detected by the algorithm, and if no more than $1 - \lceil (T \cdot |G|) \rceil$ false subjects are identified, where $|G|$ is the cardinality of the labeled group G, and $T = 2/3$. Based on this metrics, we produce *precision*, *recall* and *F measure* per frame; averaging these values over the frames gives the final scores.

Different combination of parameters are explored and validated on each dataset. In particular we examine the response of our approach when using the similarity functions (Eqs. 2 and 3), by changing the value of $\sigma = \{0.1, 0.2, 0.3, 0.4, 0.5, 0.7, 0.9\}$ and the length of the frustum $l = \{20, 25, 30, 40, 50, 60, 80, 150\}$.

5.3 Single Frame Experiment

Table 2 shows the parameters used and the quantitative results obtained in the single-frame modality while in Fig. 4 qualitative results of our group detector is shown compared with other method. As done in the comparative approaches, we show here the performances obtained with the best parameter settings, using both the Kullback-Leibler divergence (KL) and the Jensen-Shannon (JS) and averaged over 5 runs to evaluate the stability. As shown, the only case where

Table 2. Results on single frame: only the best results are shown while the parameters are discussed in the paper (σ in Eq. 4 and l in Eq. 1). The comparative methods are: HFF [7], DS [18], MULTISCALE [41], JS or KL is our method using respectively the Jensen-Shannon (Eq. 4) and the Kullback-Leibler (Eq. 3) divergence. Maximum value for standard deviation for precision is 0.74 % and for recall is 0.75 %.

Method	CoffeeBreak (S1+S2)			PosterData			Gdet		
	Prec	Rec	F1	Prec	Rec	F1	Prec	Rec	F1
HFF [18]	0,82	0,83	0,82	**0,93**	**0,96**	**0,94**	0,67	0,57	0,62
DS ([6,18][a])	0,68	0,65	0,66	**0,93**	0,92	0,92	-	-	-
MULTISCALE [41]	0,82	0,77	0,80	-	-	-	-	-	-
Our KL	0,80	0,84	0,82	0,90	0,94	0,92	**0,76**	**0,75**	**0,75**
	$\sigma = 0.2$, $l = 40$			$\sigma = 0.2$ $l = 30$			$\sigma = 0.5$ $l = 80$		
Our JS	**0,83**	**0,89**	**0,86**	0,92	**0,96**	**0,94**	**0,76**	**0,76**	**0,76**
	$\sigma = 0.2$, $l = 50$			$\sigma = 0.3$, $l = 25$			$\sigma = 0.5$ $l = 80$		
	Cocktail Party			**Synth**					
Method	Prec	Rec	F1	Prec	Rec	F1			
HFF ([7,41])	0,59	0,74	0,66	0,73	0,83	0,78			
MULTISCALE [41]	0,69	0,74	0,71	0,86	0,94	0,90			
Our KL	**0,85**	**0,81**	**0,83**	**1,00**	**1,00**	**1,00**			
Our JS	**0,86**	**0,82**	**0,84**	**1,00**	**1,00**	**1,00**			
	$\sigma = 0.5$, $l = 60$			$\sigma = 0.1$, $l = 30$					

[a]Note that in [18] the parameters for the DS method were not fully optimised.

we do not outperform the state of the art is on the Poster Data, with a difference of 1 % in the precision with respect to HHF [18] and DS [6], a difference which is close to the maximum estimated variance of our approach. In the other cases, the results are definitely superior, saturating for example the synthetic benchmark, and outperforming by over 10 % the *F-measure* on the GDet and the CocktailParty. It is worth noting that the performances across the different runs of the algorithm have been quite stable, with a mean standard deviation of $\simeq$0.74 % for both the precision and recall values.

5.4 Multiple Frame Experiment

The results are reported in Fig. 5. Compared with the single-frame approach, in a noiseless tracking situation (blue curve), this version gives comparable results. As shown, the temporal integration varies almost uniformly except a slight increase in the CoffeeBreak Seq.1. In the case of noise (green,red and cyan curves) the single frame (first point on the curves) provides a low F score and is completely dominated by the multi-frame version, irrespective of the number of frames considered in the buffer. To emphasize this fact a noise analysis on the CoffeeBreak and Cocktailparty datasets has been done. In these sequences, to

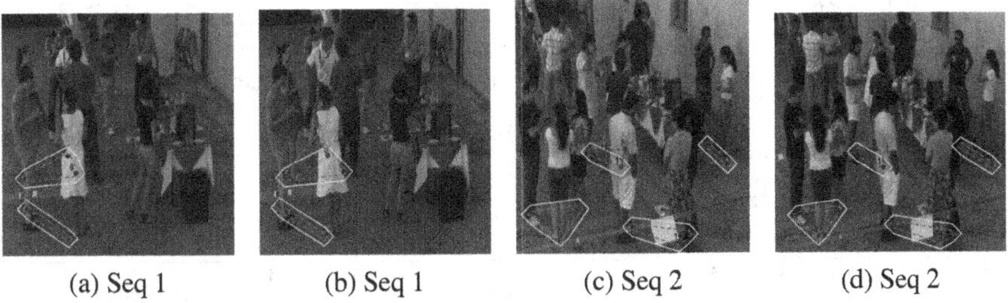

(a) Seq 1 (b) Seq 1 (c) Seq 2 (d) Seq 2

Fig. 4. Qualitative results on the CoffeeBreak dataset compared with the state of the art HFF [7]. In yellow the groundtruth, in green our method and in red HFF. As evident from (a, b, c, d) HFF often fails in detecting groups of more than two persons while our approach is more stable (Colour figure online).

simulate cluttered situations or noisy detector, we injected noise in the orientation of persons by randomly selecting the frames to corrupt and the number of people to consider. In particular, the added orientation noise (γ) was 0-mean Gaussian, with a standard deviation varing in $\{\frac{\pi}{8}, \frac{\pi}{4}, \frac{\pi}{2}, \frac{2}{3}\pi\}$. The amount of frames and persons affected by noise was set by selecting from these percentages: $F = \{0\,\%, 25\,\%, 50\,\%, 75\,\%\}$, where the percentages indicate both the number of frames to be corrupted (whose time indexes have been sampled uniformly without replacement from the entire sequence) and the number of people affected by the noise. For example, in a sequence with 100 frames and 8 persons, setting a noise of 25 % means to have 25 random frames where 2 random individual per frame are affected by noise. Considering the following size of the window $K = \{1, 2, 3, 4, 5\}$ of frames, we explore our approach applying the temporal integration. The Jensen-Shannon divergence has been used to generate the similarity matrices because it produces the better results in the single-frame experiments, outperforming the KL divergence in both the datasets. To combine the different similarity matrices in a buffer of K-frames, we used the average of the possible weights produced by the algorithm (Sect. 4.1) normalized by their sum.

5.5 Discussion

Having these experimental evidences we can provide an overall final analysis. The proposed approach is to be preferred over the others under a wide variety of different scenarios. The performance are incredibly stable under both noisy (real) and ideal (synthetic) set. For example we have highest performance in the CoffeeBreak even if it is a very noisy dataset in terms of head orientation since only 4 orientations are possible while the Synthetic is an ideal case in which we reach 100 % in precision and recall. From the single frame experiments it is clear that the Jensen-Shanon measure produces the highest and more stable performance. This seems to suggest that, while modeling a pairwise social interaction, it is reasonable to assume that both the individuals want to maintain a connection with the same strength, implying a symmetric affinity.

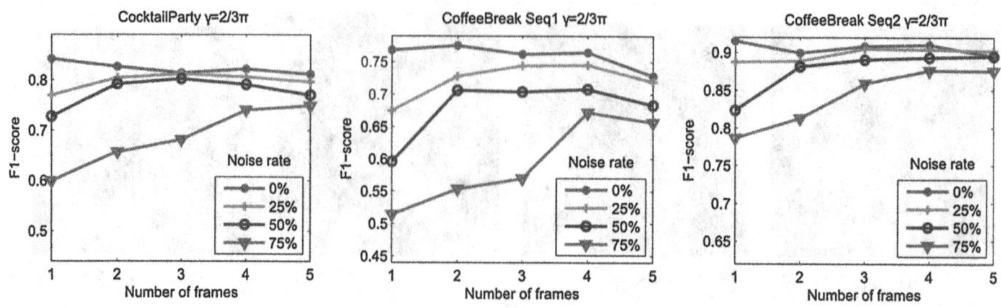

Fig. 5. Multiple-frame results: lines report the multiple-frame approach, with different level of noise: 0 %, 25 %, 50 % and 75 %. In this plot we show the worst case in which noise variance $\gamma = \frac{2}{3}\pi$. As visible, when noise is injected, the multiple-frame consistently outperforms the single-frame approach (first point of each curve). Mean value of the standard deviation for the precision is 1.61 % and for recall is 1.73 %.

Moreover the comparison between the multi frame and the single frame with noise reveals the meaningfulness of considering consecutive instants of the same scene to strengthen noisy detections. Concluding the blocks that absolutely contributed the most in this work and that represents the main novelty, has been the biologically inspired model of the frustum, which capture far better the sociological interaction between individual with respect to the previous approaches, and the game-theoretic temporal integration which provides a principled way to efficiently prune noise by smoothing data across multiple frame.

6 Conclusions

In this paper we have proposed a new method for detecting conversational groups (F-Formations) that can be included in a typical surveillance pipeline or on top of a persons detector. The method has been designed to cope with very diverse realistic scenarios, dealing with both single/multi frame sequences, noisy tracking, missing detections, inaccurate face orientations and groups of any cardinality. This impacts several domains, like surveillance&security, behavior analysis, group detection, scene understanding and social signal processing. The approach improves upon existing methods by building a stochastic model of social attention from which the probability of an o-space existing between candidate pairs can be quantified using entropic measures. The resulting affinity matrix turns out to be more accurate than the ones used in the literature outperforming the actual state of the art. F-formations are extracted using a game-theoretic clustering approach which is able to efficiently find coherent groups in edge-weighted graphs. This game-theoretic perspective allowed us to integrate in a principle way the information coming from multiple consecutive frames, in an attempt to deal with noisy situations, like in a crowded scenario or due to inaccuracy of the detection algorithms. Our extensive experiments on single-frame showed improvements over other methods on five different datasets, while the integration with multiple frames allowed to augment the overall group detection accuracy, especially in the case of strong noise. Moreover encoding the frustum using an histogram makes the approach non-parametric and thus able to accommodate newer frustum models without changing the rest of the method. In the future, we plan to address the problem of modeling F-formations more deeply by considering points of instability when people leave or join groups and to integrate multiple cues (like gaze or body orientation) during the grouping process.

References

1. Groh, G., Lehmann, A., Reimers, J., Frieß, M.R., Schwarz, L.: Detecting social situations from interaction geometry. In: 2010 IEEE Second International Conference on Social Computing (SocialCom), pp. 1–8. IEEE (2010)
2. Li, R., Porfilio, P., Zickler, T.: Finding group interactions in social clutter. In: IEEE Conference on Computer Vision and Pattern Recognition (CVPR) (2013)
3. Gan, T., Wong, Y., Zhang, D., Kankanhalli, M.S.: Temporal encoded F-formation system for social interaction detection. In: Proceedings of the 21st ACM International Conference on Multimedia, MM 2013, pp. 937–946. ACM, New York, NY, USA (2013)
4. Marin-Jimenez, M., Zisserman, A., Ferrari, V.: Here's looking at you, kid. Detecting people looking at each other in videos. In: British Machine Vision Conference (2011)
5. Zen, G., Lepri, B., Ricci, E., Lanz, O.: Space speaks: towards socially and personality aware visual surveillance. In: 1st ACM International Workshop on Multimodal Pervasive Video Analysis, pp. 37–42 (2010)
6. Hung, H., Kröse, B.: Detecting F-formations as dominant sets. In: ICMI (2011)
7. Cristani, M., Bazzani, L., Paggetti, G., Fossati, A., Tosato, D., Del Bue, A., Menegaz, G., Murino, V.: Social interaction discovery by statistical analysis of F-formations. In: Proceedings of the BMVC, pp. 23.1–23.12. BMVA Press (2011)
8. Lan, T., Wang, Y., Yang, W., Robinovitch, S.N., Mori, G.: Discriminative latent models for recognizing contextual group activities. IEEE Trans. Pattern Anal. Mach. Intell. **34**, 1549–1562 (2012)
9. Yu, T., Lim, S., Patwardhan, K.A., Krahnstoever, N.: Monitoring, recognizing and discovering social networks. In: CVPR (2009)
10. Tran, K., Gala, A., Kakadiaris, I., Shah, S.: Activity analysis in crowded environments using social cues for group discovery and human interaction modeling. Pattern Recogn. Lett. **44**, 49–57 (2013)
11. Kendon, A.: Conducting Interaction: Patterns of Behavior in Focused Encounters (Studies in Interactional Sociolinguistics). Cambridge University Press, Cambridge (1990)
12. Hüttenrauch, H., Eklundh, K.S., Green, A., Topp, E.A.: Investigating spatial relationships in human-robot interaction. In: 2006 IEEE/RSJ International Conference on Intelligent Robots and Systems, pp. 5052–5059. IEEE (2006)
13. Hall, E.T.: The Hidden Dimension. Anchor, New York (1990)
14. Goffman, E.: Behavior in Public Places: Notes on the Social Organization of Gatherings. Free Press, New York (1966)
15. Ciolek, T.M., Kendon, A.: Environment and the spatial arrangement of conversational encounters. Sociol. Inq. **50**, 237–271 (1980)
16. Chen, C., Odobez, J.: We are not contortionists: coupled adaptive learning for head and body orientation estimation in surveillance video. In: 2012 IEEE Conference on Computer Vision and Pattern Recognition (CVPR), pp. 1544–1551. IEEE (2012)

17. Jain, V., Crowley, J.L.: Head pose estimation using multi-scale gaussian derivatives. In: Kämäräinen, J.-K., Koskela, M. (eds.) SCIA 2013. LNCS, vol. 7944, pp. 319–328. Springer, Heidelberg (2013)
18. Setti, F., Hung, H., Cristani, M.: Group detection in still images by F-formation modeling: a comparative study. In: WIAMIS (2013)
19. Torsello, A., Rota Bulò, S., Pelillo, M.: Grouping with asymmetric affinities: a game-theoretic perspective. In: IEEE Computer Society Conference on Computer Vision and Pattern Recognition (CVPR), vol. 1, pp. 292–299 (2006)
20. Rota Buló, S., Pelillo, M.: A game-theoretic approach to hypergraph clustering. IEEE Trans. Pattern Anal. Mach. Intell. **35**, 1312–1327 (2013)
21. Somasundaram, K., Baras, J.S.: Achieving symmetric Pareto Nash equilibria using biased replicator dynamics. In: 48th IEEE Conference Decision Control, pp. 7000–7005 (2009)
22. Pellegrini, S., Ess, A., Van Gool, L.: Improving data association by joint modeling of pedestrian trajectories and groupings. In: Daniilidis, K., Maragos, P., Paragios, N. (eds.) ECCV 2010, Part I. LNCS, vol. 6311, pp. 452–465. Springer, Heidelberg (2010)
23. Yamaguchi, K., Berg, A., Ortiz, L., Berg, T.: Who are you with and where are you going? In: IEEE Conference on Computer Vision and Patter Recognition (CVPR) (2011)
24. Ge, W., Collins, R.T., Ruback, R.B.: Vision-based analysis of small groups in pedestrian crowds. IEEE Trans. Pattern Anal. Mach. Intell. **34**, 1003–1016 (2012)
25. Qin, Z., Shelton, C.R.: Improving multi-target tracking via social grouping. In: IEEE Conference on Computer Vision and Pattern Recognition (CVPR) (2012)
26. Chang, M., Krahnstoever, N., Ge, W.: Probabilistic group-level motion analysis and scenario recognition. In: IEEE ICCV (2011)
27. Leal-Taixé, L., Pons-Moll, G., Rosenhahn, B.: Everybody needs somebody: modeling social and grouping behavior on a linear programming multiple people tracker. In: IEEE International Conference on Computer Vision Workshops (ICCVW). 1st Workshop on Modeling, Simulation and Visual Analysis of Large Crowds (2011)
28. Mckenna, S.J., Jabri, S., Duric, Z., Wechsler, H., Rosenfeld, A.: Tracking groups of people. Comput. Vis. Image Underst. **80**, 42–56 (2000)
29. Cupillard, F., Bremond, F., Thonnat, M.: Tracking groups of people for video surveillance. In: Remagnino, P., Jones, G.A., Paragios, N., Regazzoni, C.S. (eds.) Video-Based Surveillance Systems, pp. 89–100. Springer, Heidelberg (2002)
30. Marques, J.S., Jorge, P.M., Abrantes, A.J., Lemos, J.M.: Tracking groups of pedestrians in video sequences. In: IEEE Conference on Computer Vision and Patter Recognition Workshops (CVPR Workshops), vol. 9, pp. 101–101 (2003)
31. Pellegrini, S., Ess, A., Schindler, K., Gool, L.J.V.: You'll never walk alone: modeling social behavior for multi-target tracking. In: ICCV 2009, pp. 261–268 (2009)
32. Helbing, D., Molnar, P.: Social force model for pedestrian dynamics. Phys. Rev. E **51**, 4282 (1995)
33. Smith, K., Ba, S.O., Odobez, J.M., Gatica-Perez, D.: Tracking the visual focus of attention for a varying number of wandering people. IEEE Trans. Pattern Anal. Mach. Intell. **30**, 1212–1229 (2008)
34. Adams, R.B.: The Science of Social Vision, vol. 7. Oxford University Press, New York (2011)
35. Kendon, A.: Some functions of gaze-direction in social interaction. Acta Psychol (Amst) **26**, 22–63 (1967)

36. Jovanovic, N., op den Akker, R.: Towards automatic addressee identification in multi-party dialogues. In: Proceedings of the 5th SIGdial Workshop on Discourse and Dialogue, pp. 89–92, Pennsylvania, USA. Association for Computational Linguistics (2004). Imported from HMI
37. Duncan, S.: Some signals and rules for taking speaking turns in conversations. J. Pers. Soc. Psychol. **23**, 283–292 (1972)
38. Ba, S.O., Odobez, J.: Multiperson visual focus of attention from head pose and meeting contextual cues. IEEE Trans. Pattern Anal. Mach. Intell. **33**, 101–116 (2011)
39. Subramanian, R., Staiano, J., Kalimeri, K., Sebe, N., Pianesi, F.: Putting the pieces together: multimodal analysis of social attention in meetings. In: Proceedings of the International Conference on Multimedia, MM 2010, pp. 659–662. ACM, New York, NY, USA (2010)
40. Pavan, M., Pelillo, M.: Dominant sets and pairwise clustering. IEEE Trans. Pattern Anal. Mach. Intell. **29**, 167–172 (2007)
41. Setti, F., Lanz, O., Ferrario, R., Murino, V., Cristani, M.: Multi-scale F-formation discovery for group detection. In: International Conference on Image Processing (ICIP) (2013)
42. Weibull, J.W.: Evolutionary Game Theory. MIT Press, Cambridge (2005)
43. Blackwell, D.: An analog of the minimax theorem for vector payoffs. Pacific J. Math. **6**, 1–8 (1956)
44. Shapley, L.S.: Equilibrium points in games with vector payoffs. Naval Res. Logist. Q. **6**, 57–61 (1959)
45. Contini, B.M.: A decision model under uncertainty with multiple objectives. In: Mensch, A. (ed.) Theory of Games: Techniques and Applications. American Elsevier, New York (1966)
46. Zeleny, M.: Games with multiple payoffs. Int. J. Game Theory **4**, 179–191 (1975)
47. Kawamura, T., Kanazawa, T., Ushio, T.: Evolutionarily and neutrally stable strategies in multicriteria games. IEICE Trans. Fundam. Electr. Commun. Comp. Sci. **E96–A**, 814–820 (2013)
48. Ehrgott, M.: Multicriteria Optimization, 2nd edn. Springer, Berlin (2005)

Author Index